Fifth Edition

The Development of Language

Jean Berko Gleason
Boston University

Allyn and Bacon

Boston • London • Toronto • Sydney • Tokyo • Singapore

Executive Editor: Stephen D. Dragin
Editorial Assistant: Barbara Strickland
Senior Editiorial-Production Administrator: Joe Sweeney
Editorial-Production Service: Walsh & Associates, Inc.
Composition Buyer: Linda Cox
Manufacturing Buyer: Chris Marson
Cover Administrator: Brian Gogolin
Electronic Composition: Omegatype Typography, Inc.

Copyright © 2001, 1997, 1993, 1989 by Allyn & Bacon
A Pearson Education Company
160 Gould Street
Needham Heights, MA 02494
www.abacon.com

Library of Congress Cataloging-in-Publication Data
Gleason, Jean Berko.
   The development of language / Jean Berko Gleason. — 5th ed.
     p. cm.
   Includes bibliographical references and indexes.
   ISBN 0-205-31636-0
   1. Language acquisition.   2. Psycholinguistics.   3. Sociolinguistics.   I. Title.

P118.D44   2000
401'.93—dc21   00-035562

Printed in the United States of America
10 9 8 7 6 5   04 03

Contents

**4   *Semantic Development:
Learning the Meanings of Words*   125**

Barbara Alexander Pan, Harvard Graduate School of Education
Jean Berko Gleason, Boston University

**5   *Putting Words Together: Morphology
and Syntax in the Preschool Years*   162**

Helen Tager-Flusberg, University of Massachusetts at Boston
and Eunice Kennedy Shriver Center

**6   *Language in Social Contexts: Communicative
Competence in the Preschool Years*   213**

Judith Becker Bryant, University of South Florida

7   *Theoretical Approaches to Language Acquisition*   254

John N. Bohannon III, Butler University
John D. Bonvillian, University of Virginia

8   *Individual Differences: Implications for the Study of Language Acquisition*   315

Beverly A. Goldfield, Rhode Island College
Catherine E. Snow, Harvard Graduate School of Education

9   *Atypical Language Development*   347

Nan Bernstein Ratner, University of Maryland

Preface

This is the fifth edition of *The Development of Language,* which is intended for anyone with an interest in how children acquire language and in how language develops over the life span. Readers will learn about what the fetus hears prenatally, what happens to language in the aging brain, and everything in between. Our emphasis on change over the life span is even more important now than it was when we first began to write this book, since developments in cognitive neuroscience have made it evident that language, once acquired, is not static, but rather, undergoes constant neural reorganization.

Every chapter has been written by an expert in that area of research, but in a way that is accessible to educated nonexperts. The book has been designed as a text for upper-level undergraduate or graduate courses in language development, or as readings for courses in psycholinguistics, cognitive development, developmental psychology, speech pathology, and related subjects. The book also serves as a resource for professionals in all of the fields just noted.

This edition has been revised extensively to contain state-of-the-art knowledge on all the topics that are covered. The fifth edition also contains material that we have added in response to suggestions from students, colleagues, and reviewers; this will enhance its value as a text and resource. In addition to all the features that characterized the fourth edition, this edition has an expanded new chapter on language in society. As our understanding of developmental pragmatics and developmental sociolinguistics has grown, we have been able to provide much new information on research in these areas. This edition also contains contemporary information on language questions that are being asked in the society at large—for instance, the newly written chapter on language in society discusses African American Vernacular English and provides the reader with information from the Linguistic Society of America that puts questions about AAVE into pedagogical perspective. We also have new and exhaustive references that will make this book a valuable addition to our readers' libraries.

In order to benefit from the book, previous study of linguistics on the part of the reader is not assumed, and each chapter presents its material along with whatever linguistic background information is necessary for understanding. On the other hand, we assume that readers will be familiar with basic concepts in psychology (e.g., *object permanence*) and with the work of major figures such as Jean Piaget and B. F. Skinner. Many books on language development are concerned only with language acquisition by children and have tended to assume that development is complete when the most complex syntactic structures have been attained. But linguistic development, like psychological development, is a lifelong process, and so we have set out to illuminate the nature of language development over the life span.

It would be hard for a single author to write this book. The study of language development has grown so rapidly in recent years that there are now many topics that are highly specialized, and it is rare for one person to be an expert in all areas of this expanding field. For instance, there are few investigators who are authorities on the language of both infants and elderly people. Yet, both topics are covered here. Fortunately, a number of researchers specializing in major subfields have agreed to contribute to the book; the chapters, therefore, are written by authors who not only know their topic well, but are known for their research in it. They present what they consider to be the salient ideas and the most recent and relevant studies in their own areas.

Since development is always the result of an interaction between innate capacities and environmental forces, we take an interactive perspective, one that takes into account both the biological endowment that makes language possible and the environmental factors that foster development. Our theoretical perspective has remained the same—both interactive and eclectic—but we have tried to add new material that represents the field, even if it does not necessarily represent our own views. Theory remains a controversial area in psycholinguistics; the most important theoretical positions are presented here, along with their strengths and weaknesses, in what we hope is an even-handed but thought-provoking approach. We count proponents of each of the divergent theories among our personal friends and value their continued friendship.

We have had to be selective in our choice of major topics, and some of our favorite subjects have, of necessity, been omitted. There are so many different topics that are now recognized in the study of language development that it is impossible to include them all in one cohesive book. And we have not attempted to include cross-cultural and bilingual studies that rely on knowledge of languages other than English.

Instructors will be happy to learn that we also have a newly revised instructor's manual prepared by Pam Gleason, available to those who adopt the book as a text. The manual provides exam questions, helpful outlines of the chapters, emphasis on key points, and suggestions for classroom activities. A number of the authors here can be seen in the Public Broadcasting Service NOVA production on language development called "Babytalk," which is still available in some areas; more recently, PBS has made available a videotaped college course called "Discovering Psychology," with a half-hour program (#6) devoted to early language development. Students and instructors will want to visit the web sites related to language, particularly the Child Language Data Exchange System (CHILDES), which can be found easily by entering its name into any search engine.

It is impossible to edit a book without becoming indebted to many people. I am grateful, first of all, to the authors who agreed to revise their earlier contributions to this volume, and I welcome Judith Becker Bryant, who is a new contributor. Thanks also to Steve Dragin, our editor at Allyn and Bacon, and to Mary Perry at Boston University, who, as ever, has been immensely helpful in every way.

My family is due thanks as well: my husband, Andrew Gleason, for his patience, and my daughters Katherine, Pam, and Cynthia, now grown, whose developing language was a source of inspiration and joy.

I know the other authors will join me as well in thanking Roger Brown, who, though gone, remains in our hearts.

Chapter 1

The Development of Language: An Overview and a Preview

Jean Berko Gleason
Boston University

Why do we study language development? This phenomenal yet basically universal human achievement poses some of the most challenging theoretical and practical questions of our times: How and why do young children acquire complex grammar? What if no one spoke to them—would children invent language by themselves? Are humans unique, or can language be taught to higher primates? Are there theories or models that can adequately account for language development? Is language a separate capacity, or is it simply one facet of our general cognitive ability? What is it that individuals actually must know in order to have full adult competence in language, and to what extent is the development of those skills representative of universal processes? What about individual differences? What happens when language develops atypically, and is there anything we can do about it? What happens to language skills as one grows older—what is acquired, and what is lost? These are some of the questions that intrigue language-development researchers, and they have led to the plan of this book.

By the time they are three or four years old, children in every part of the world acquire the major components of their native languages, regardless of how complex their grammar and sound systems may be. By the time they are of school age and begin the formal study of grammar, they already can vary their speech to suit the social and communicative nature of a situation; they know the meaning and pronunciation of literally thousands of words, and they use quite correctly the grammatical forms—subjects, objects, verbs, plurals, and tenses—whose names they learn only in the late elementary years. Language development, however, does not cease when the individual reaches school age or, for that matter, adolescence or maturity—the developmental process continues throughout the life cycle. The reorganization and reintegration of mental processes that are typical of other intellectual functions can also be seen in language, as the changing conditions that accompany maturity lead to modification of linguistic capacity. This book, therefore, is written from a developmental perspective that encompasses the life span. Since most studies of language development have centered on children, this preponderance is reflected in the research reported here. The major questions addressed, however, are not limited to what can be learned from the study of children and, in fact, require the study of mature individuals as well.

This chapter is divided into four major sections: The first section provides a brief overview of *the course of language development* from early infancy to old age. It serves as a preview of the chapters that follow (the major topics included are treated at length in later chapters of the book).

The second section notes some of the unique *biological foundations* for language that make its development possible in humans. Our biological endowment is necessary, but not sufficient to ensure language development, which does not occur without social interaction. The third section describes the major *linguistic systems* that individuals must acquire. No particular linguistic theory is advocated here; instead, descriptive information is presented that has provided the framework for much basic research in language acquisition, and more technical linguistic material is presented in the appropriate substantive chapter. If there is a unifying perspective that the authors of this book share, it is the view that individuals acquire during their lives an **internalized representation** of language that is systematic in nature and amenable to study. This does not imply that inner representation could be established in the absence of social contact, or without several different types of learning (as Chapter 7 on theoretical perspectives makes clear).

The fourth and final section of this chapter focuses on the background and methods of the *study of language development.*

An Overview of the Course of Language Development

Communication Development in Infancy

During their first months, infants begin to acquire the communicative skills that underlie language, long before they say their first words. Babies are intensely social beings; they gaze into the eyes of their caregivers and are sensitive to the emotional tone of the voices around them. They pay attention to the language spoken to them; they take their turn in conversation, even if that turn is only a burble (Masataka, 1993; Snow, 1977). If they want something, they learn to make their intentions known. In addition to possessing the social motivations that are evidenced so early in life, data now show that infants are also physiologically equipped to process incoming speech signals; they are even capable of making fine distinctions among speech sounds that are both rare in the world's languages and previously unknown to them (Eimas, 1975; Werker & Tees, 1984). By the age of six months, babies have already begun to categorize the sounds of their own language, much as adult speakers do (Kuhl, Williams, Lacerda, Stevens, & Lindblom, 1992). By the age of about eleven months, many babies understand fifty or more common words, and point happily at the right person when someone asks "Where's daddy?" (Fenson, Dale, Reznick, Bates, Thal, & Pethick, 1994).

Midway through their first year, infants begin to babble, playing with sound much as they play with their fingers and toes. At approximately the same age that they take their first steps, many infants produce their first words. Like walking, early language appears at around the same age and in much the same way all over the world, regardless of the degree of sophistication of the society. The relative ease of pronunciation of a language and its degree of grammatical complexity do not appear to affect the age at which children begin to speak (Lenneberg, 1967). The early precursors of language that develop during the first year of life are discussed in Chapter 2.

Phonological Development: Learning Sounds and Sound Patterns

Early in their second year, the babbling of the prelinguistic infant gives way to words, for most children. There has been considerable controversy over the relation between babbling and talking (Blake & Boysson-Bardies, 1992; de Boysson-Bardies & Vihman, 1991; Jakobson, 1968); however, most researchers now agree that babbling blends into early speech and may continue even after the appearance of recognizable words (Stoel-Gammon, 1998). Once infants have begun to speak, the course of language development appears to have some universal characteristics (Brown, 1973). Typically, toddlers' early utterances are only one word long, and the words are simple in pronunciation and concrete in meaning (Stoel-Gammon & Cooper, 1984). They refer to the objects, events, and people in the child's immediate surroundings—words like *hi, doggie, mommy,* and *juice* (Bloom, 1970; Clark, 1993; Nelson & Lucariello, 1985). Here, as in other areas of linguistic research, it is important to recognize that different constraints act upon the child's **comprehension** and **production** of a particular form. Some sounds are more difficult to pronounce than others, and combinations of consonants may prove particularly problematic. Within a given language, children solve the phonological problems they encounter in varying ways. A framework for the study of children's growing ability to both recognize and produce the sounds of their language is provided in Chapter 3.

Semantic Development: Learning the Meanings of Words

The ways in which speakers relate words to their referents and their meanings are the subject matter of **semantic development.** Just as there are constraints on the phonological shapes of children's early words, there appear to be limits on the kinds of meanings that those early words embody—for instance, very young children's vocabularies are more likely to contain words that refer to objects that move (*bus*) than objects that are immobile (*bench*). Their vocabularies reflect their daily lives and are unlikely to refer to events that are distant in time or space or to anything of an abstract nature. As they enter the school years, children's words become increasingly complex and interconnected, and children also gain a new kind of knowledge: **metalinguistic awareness.** This new ability makes it possible for them to think about their language, understand what words are, and even define them (Papandropoulou & Sinclair, 1974; Snow, 1990). Investigations of children's first words and their meanings, as well as the ways in which early meaning systems become elaborated into complex semantic networks, are discussed in Chapter 4.

Putting Words Together: Morphology and Syntax in the Preschool Years

Sometime during their second year, after they know about fifty words, most children progress to a stage of two-word combinations (Brown, 1973). Words that they said in the one-word stage are now combined into these **telegraphic** utterances, without articles, prepositions, inflections, or any of the other grammatical modifications that adult language requires. The child can now say such things as "That doggie," meaning "That is a doggie," and "Mommy juice," meaning "Mommy's juice" or "Mommy, give me my juice" or "Mommy is drinking her juice."

An examination of children's two-word utterances in many different language communities (Brown, 1973; Slobin, 1979) has shown that everywhere in the world children at this age are expressing the same kinds of thoughts and intentions in the same kinds of utterances. They ask for more of something; they say no to something; they notice something, or they notice that it has disappeared. This leads them to produce utterances like "More milk!" "No bed!" "Hi, kitty!" and "All-gone cookie!"

A little later in the two-word stage, another dozen or so kinds of meanings appear. For instance, children may name an actor and a verb: "Daddy eat." They modify a noun: "Bad doggie." They specify a location: "Kitty table." They name a verb and an object, leaving out the subject: "Eat lunch." At this stage, children are expressing these basic meanings but they cannot use the language forms that indicate number, gender, and tense. Even in a highly inflected language (such as Hebrew) in which it would be impossible to speak the root word without some of these markers, children settle on one form, which they use indiscriminately: Girls, for example, frequently use the feminine form of words, regardless of the grammatical requirements (Dromi & Berman, 1982). Toddler language is in the here and now; there is no tomorrow and no yesterday in language at the two-word stage. What children can say is closely related to their level of cognitive and social development, and a child who cannot conceive of the past is unlikely to speak of it. As the child's utterances grow longer, grammatical forms begin to appear. In English, articles, prepositions, and inflections representing number, person, and tense begin to be heard. Although the two-word stage has some universal characteristics across all languages, what is acquired next depends on the features of the language being learned. English-speaking children learn the articles *a* and *the,* but in a language such as Russian there are no articles. Russian grammar, on the other hand, has features that English grammar does not. One remarkable finding has been that children acquiring a given language do so in essentially the same order. In English, for instance, children learn *in* and *on* before other prepositions such as *under.* After they learn regular plurals and pasts, like *nooses* and *heated,* they create some **overregularized** forms of their own, like *gooses* and *eated.*

Researchers account for children's early utterances in varying ways, however. The work of the 1960s, inspired by grammatical theory (Chomsky, 1957, 1965), interpreted early word combinations as evidence that the child was a young cryptographer, endowed with a cognitive impetus to develop syntax and a grammatical system. More recently, the child's intentions and need to communicate them to others have been looked to for explanations of grammatical development. But children's unique ability to acquire complex grammar, regardless of the motivation behind it, remains at the heart of linguistic inquiry. The learning of morphological systems, such as the plural or past tense (Berko, 1958), remains some of the strongest evidence we have that children are not simply learning bits and pieces of the adult linguistic system but are constructing generative systems of their own. Early sentences and the acquisition of morphology are examined in Chapter 5.

Language in Social Contexts: Communicative Competence in the Preschool Years

Language development includes acquiring the ability to use language appropriately in a multiplicity of social situations. The system of rules that dictates the way language is used to accomplish social ends is often called **pragmatics.** An individual who acquires the phonology, morphology, syntax, and semantics of a language has acquired **linguistic competence.** A sentence such as "Excuse me, but might I borrow your pencil for a moment?" certainly shows that the speaker has linguistic competence, since it is obviously perfectly grammatical. If, however, this sentence is addressed to a two-year-old, it is just as certainly inappropriate; more appropriate would be something like "Give me the pencil—that's right, give it to me." Linguistic competence is not sufficient; speakers must also acquire **communicative competence** (Hymes, 1972), or the ability to vary their language appropriately in a variety of situations; in other words, it requires knowledge of the social rules for language use, or pragmatics. During the preschool years, young children learn to express a variety of **speech acts,** such as polite requests, or clarification of their own utterances. Their parents are particularly eager that they learn to be polite (Snow, Perlmann, Berko Gleason, & Hooshyar, 1990). Speakers ultimately learn important variations in language that serve to mark their gender, regional origin, social class, and occupation. Other necessary variations are associated with such things as the social setting, topic of discourse, and characteristics of the person being addressed. The use of language in social contexts is discussed in Chapter 6.

Theoretical Approaches to Language Acquisition

In general, explaining what it is that children acquire during the course of language development is easier than explaining how they do it. Do parents shape their children's early babbling into speech through reinforcement and teaching strategies? Or is language, perhaps, an independent and **innate** faculty, built into the human biobehavioral system? Learning theorists and linguistic theorists do not agree on these basic principles. Between the theoretical poles represented by learning theorists on the one hand and linguistic theorists on the other lie three different interactionist perspectives: (1) *Cognitive developmentalists* believe that language is just one facet of human cognition, and that children in acquiring language are basically learning to put words to concepts they have already acquired. (2) *Information theorists* who study language are also interested in human cognition, but from the perspective of the neural architecture that supports it. They see children as processors of information, and they use the computer to model the ways neural connections supporting language are strengthened through exposure to adult speech. (3) *Social interactionists* emphasize the child's motivation to communicate with others. They emphasize the role that the special features of **child-directed speech** (CDS) may play in facilitating children's language acquisition. A discussion and an evaluation of the theories that have been put forth to explain language development are included in Chapter 7.

Individual Differences: Implications for the Study of Language Acquisition

Even though this brief overview has emphasized the regularities and continuities that have been observed in the development of language, it is important to know that individual differences have been found in almost every aspect, even during the earliest period of development. In the acquisition of phonology, for instance, some children are quite conservative and avoid words they have difficulty pronouncing; others are willing to take a chance. Early words and early word combinations reveal different strategies in acquiring language. Although much of linguistic inquiry has been directed at finding commonalities across children in language acquisition, it is important to remember that there is also variation in the onset of speech, the rate at which language develops, and the style of language used by the child. This should not surprise us, since we know that babies differ in temperament, cognitive style, and in many other ways; variation is a very healthy part of our genetic heritage. In addition, children's early language may reflect the preferences of adults in a society—for instance, American parents stress the names of things, but nouns might not be so important in all societies. Individual differences must be accounted for by any comprehensive theory of language development, and they must be taken into account by those who work with children. Individual differences are the topic of Chapter 8.

Atypical Language Development

Language has been a human endowment for so many millennia that it is exceptionally robust; as we shall see, it is under most circumstances almost impossible to suppress. There are conditions, however, that may lead to atypical language development—for instance, sensory problems such as deafness. In this case the capacity for language is intact, but lack of accessible auditory input makes the acquisition of oral language difficult; children with hearing impairments who learn a manual language such as **American Sign Language** (ASL), however, are able to communicate in a complete and sophisticated language.

Children who are diagnosed as mentally retarded, such as most children with **Down syndrome,** may show rather typical patterns of language development, but at a slower rate than normally developing children. Children with **autism** frequently exhibit patterns of language development that are atypical in multiple ways; they may have particular problems, for instance, using language that deals with the emotional states of others (Tager-Flusberg, 1999). Occasionally children suffer from **specific language impairment,** problems in language development accompanied by no other obvious physical, sensory, or emotional difficulties. Still other children have particular problems producing speech, even though their internal representation of language is intact: They may stutter or have motor impairments. Atypical language development, and its relation to the processes described in earlier chapters, is the subject of Chapter 9.

Language and Literacy in the School Years

By the time they get to kindergarten, children have amassed a vocabulary of about 8,000 words and almost all of the basic grammatical forms of their language. They can handle questions, negative statements, dependent clauses, compound sentences, and a great variety of other constructions. They have also learned much more than vocabulary and grammar—they have learned to use language in many different social situations. They can, for instance, talk baby talk to babies, be rude to their friends, and act somewhat polite with their grandparents. Their communicative competence is growing.

During the school years, children are increasingly called upon to interact with peers; peer speech is quite different from speech to parents, and it is often both humorous and aggressive. Jokes, riddles, and play with language constitute a substantial portion of their spontaneous speech. Faced with many new models, school-aged children also learn from television and films, and their speech may be marked by expressions from their favorite entertainments.

New cognitive attainments in the school years make it possible for children to talk in ways that they could not as preschoolers, and to think about language itself—they may even have favorite words (like *barracuda*) that are not necessarily their favorite things. They become increasingly adept at producing connected, multi-utterance speech and can produce interesting narratives that describe their past experience. In order to succeed in school, children must also learn to use **decontextualized language**—language that is not tied to the here and now. In addition to their narrative skills, they now develop the ability to provide explanations and descriptions using decontextualized language (Snow, 1983).

The attainment of literacy marks a major milestone in children's development, and it calls upon both their metalinguistic abilities (for instance, they must understand what a word is), and their new abilities to use decontextualized language. Study of the cognitive processes involved in reading and the development of adequate models that represent the acquisition of this skill are two topics that actively involve researchers in developmental psycholinguistics.

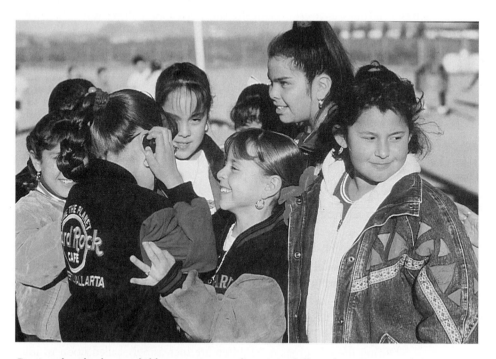

During the school years children acquire new linguistic skills as they interact with peers. Explaining how to take the bus or telling a joke requires connected discourse and decontextualized language.

Children who come from literate households know a great deal about reading and writing before formal instruction begins, and thus are at an advantage in school. Once children have acquired the ability to read and write, these new skills, in turn, have profound effects upon their spoken language. Learning to read is not an easy task for all children; this extremely complex activity requires intricate coordination of a number of separate abilities. Humans have been speaking since the earliest days of our prehistory, but reading has been a common requirement only in very modern times; we should not be surprised, therefore, that reading skills vary greatly in the population. Reading problems as exemplified in the **dyslexias** pose serious theoretical and practical problems for the psycholinguistic researcher. The acquisition of language and the development of literacy skills during the school years and through adolescence are discussed in Chapter 10.

Development and Loss: Changes in the Adult Years

In the normal course of events, language development, like cognitive development, moral development, or psychological development, continues beyond the point where the individual has assumed the outward appearance of an adult. During the teen years, young people acquire their own special style, and part of being a successful teenager rests in knowing how to talk like one. Now, in adulthood, there are new linguistic attainments.

Language is involved in psychological development; psychiatrist Erik Erikson (1959) pointed out that one of the major life tasks facing young people is the formation of an identity, a sense of who they are. A distinct personal linguistic style is part of one's special identity. Further psychological goals of early adulthood that call for expanded linguistic skills include beginning an occupation and establishing intimate relations with others.

Language development during the adult years varies greatly among individuals, depending on such things as level of education and social and occupational roles. Actors, for instance, must learn not only to be heard by large audiences but to speak the words of others using varying voices and regional dialects. Working people learn the special tones of voice and terminology associated with their own occupational register or code.

With advancing age, numerous linguistic changes take place. For instance, some word-finding difficulty is inevitable—the inability to produce a name that is "on the tip of the tongue" is a phenomenon that becomes increasingly familiar as one approaches retirement age. Hearing loss and impairments of memory can affect an older person's ability to communicate. But not all changes are for the worse—vocabulary increases, as does narrative skill. In preliterate societies, for instance, the official storytellers are typically older members of the community. Although most individuals remain linguistically vigorous in their later years, language deterioration becomes severe for some, and they may lose both comprehension and voluntary speech. The aphasias and dementias exact their linguistic toll on affected individuals, whose speech may become as limited as that of young children. Language development in adulthood and the later years is described in Chapter 11.

The Biological Bases of Language

Animal Communication Systems

Human language has special properties that have led many researchers to conclude that such language is both **species specific** and **species uniform;** that is, it is unique to humans and essentially similar in all humans (Lenneberg, 1967; Marler, 1990). The characteristics that distinguish human language are illuminated when they are compared with those of animal communication systems. Animals are clearly able to communicate at some level with one another as well as with humans. Cats and dogs meow and bark for attention and are able to convey a variety of messages by methods such as scratching at the door or looking expectantly at their dishes. Scratching, meowing, and gazing hopefully are clearly not language, however; the messages are very limited in scope and can be interpreted only in the context of the immediate situation.

Bee Communication

Insects such as bees have been shown to have an elaborate communication system. Ethologist Karl von Frisch (1950) began to study bees in the 1920s and won a Nobel Prize in 1973 for his studies of communication among these highly social insects. Unlike the expressive meowing of a hungry cat, in many senses the communication system of the bee is referential—it tells other bees about something in the outside world. A bee returning to the hive after finding nectar-filled flowers collects an audience and then performs a dance that indicates the direction and the approximate distance of the nectar from the hive. Other bees watch, join the dance, and then head for the flowers. The bee's dance is actually a miniature form of the trip to the flowers, rather than a symbolic statement. There is nothing symbolic or arbitrary about dancing toward the north to indicate that other bees should fly in that direction. Moreover, although the movements of the dance have structure and meaning, there is only one possible conversational topic— where to find nectar. Even this repertoire is seriously limited; bees cannot, for instance, tell one another that the flowers are pretty or that they just hate gathering nectar.

Sea Mammals and Birds

Many animals have ways of communicating with other members of their species. Whales and dolphins employ elaborate systems of whistles and grunts that are clearly meaningful to other whales and dolphins (Herman, 1981; Savage-Rumbaugh, 1993).

Some birds have been shown to have a variety of meaningful calls. Jackdaws, for instance, were studied by Konrad Lorenz (1971), who shared von Frisch's Nobel Prize. Lorenz showed that these relatives of the crow have courting calls, a call for flying away, and one for flying home. They also have a warning rattle that they sound before attacking any other creature carrying a dangling black object. (He discovered this while carrying [dangling] his black swimsuit!)

All of these communication systems have clear utility for the animals that use them, and each one resembles human language in some respect, but they are all tied to the stimulus situation, limited to the here and now and to a restricted set of messages. Human language has characteristics not found in their entirety in these other systems.

Researchers concerned with criteria for what constitutes *language* have produced lists of characteristics that vary somewhat in both length and scope. Most would agree, however, on at least these three cited by Roger Brown (1973):

1. True language is marked by *productivity* in the sense that speakers can make many new utterances and can recombine the forms they already know to say things they have never before heard.
2. It also has *semanticity;* that is, it can represent ideas, events, and objects symbolically.
3. It offers the possibility of *displacement*—messages need not be tied to the immediate context.

Human language enables its users to comment on any aspect of their experience and to consider the past and the future, as well as referents that may be continents away or only in the imagination. The natural communication systems of bees and lower animals do not meet these criteria of language.

Recent attempts to teach language to talking birds, however, have produced some extremely provocative results. For instance, an African grey parrot named Alex has been trained to recognize objects, colors, and shapes and to answer questions about them in English. Faced with an array of things, he is asked, "What object is green?" Alex says, correctly, "wood." He is right about 80 percent of the time (Pepperberg, 1991). Experiments with young grey parrots have shown that they can learn to label common objects if they have human tutors who provide interactive lessons; they do not learn from passive listening to lessons on audiotape or from watching videotapes, but do best when the words are presented in context by a friendly and informative person (Pepperberg, 1994). Do African grey parrots have the same sort of linguistic skill human children do? One view is that they do not, and that the birds are responding to complex learned cues. Another interpretation of the evidence is that language is a continuum on which grey parrots have clearly alighted. These parrots are all relatively young (Alex's twenty-fifth birthday is in 2001), and they have a life span of as much as eighty years, so we can afford to reserve judgment on these remarkable birds.

Primate Language

During the past half-century, a great deal of curiosity has focused on the possibility that the higher primates might be capable of learning human language. Chimpanzees are intelligent, social, and communicative animals (Maple & Cone, 1981; Miles, 1983). They use a variety of vocal cries in their life in the wild, including a food bark and a danger cry. Chimpanzees possess genetic structures very similar to our own and are our closest relatives in the animal world (Diamond, 1992). There have been numerous attempts to teach language to chimpanzees and at least one major gorilla language project that is still ongoing (Bonvillian & Patterson, 1997; Patterson & Cohn, 1990). The ape studies have provided us with much useful and controversial data on the ability of nonhumans to acquire our language forms. Some of these studies have taught chimpanzees to use colored plastic shapes in order to communicate with humans, or to use a computer console to send messages (Premack, 1976; Rumbaugh, 1977). We will concentrate here on some studies that have set out to teach natural language to chimpanzees.

Gua and Viki

In 1931, Professor and Mrs. W. N. Kellogg became the first American family to raise a chimpanzee and a child together (Kellogg, 1980). The Kelloggs brought into their home Gua, a seven-month-old chimpanzee, who stayed with them and their infant son Donald for nine months. No special effort was made to teach Gua to talk; like their human baby, she was simply exposed to a speaking household. During this period, Gua came to use some of her natural chimpanzee cries rather consistently; for instance, she used her food bark not just for food but for anything at all that she wanted. Although Gua was rather better than Donald in most physical accomplishments, unlike Donald she did not babble and did not learn to say any English words.

In the 1940s, psychologists Catherine and Keith Hayes (Hayes, 1951) set out to improve upon the Kelloggs' experiment by raising a chimpanzee named Viki as if she were their own child. This included outfitting her in little dresses and introducing her to strangers as their daughter. She lived with them for a number of years, beginning at the age of six weeks. The Hayeses made explicit efforts to teach Viki to talk; they had assumed that chimpanzees were rather like institutionalized retarded children, and that love and patient instruction would afford Viki the opportunity for optimal language development. After six years of training, Viki appeared to understand a great deal, but she was able to produce, with great difficulty, only four words: *mama, papa, cup,* and *up.* She was never able to say more, and in order to pronounce a /p/, she had to hold her lips together with her fingers. Since speech is an **overlaid function**, that is, the organs involved in its production (such as the tongue and lungs) all have primary functions other than language, it requires an extraordinary degree of physiological coordination to articulate while continuing with functions such as breathing and swallowing. From the Hayeses' research it became clear that chimpanzees do not have the specialized articulatory and physiological abilities that make spoken language possible.

In more recent times, other researchers have concluded that the inability to speak may not preclude the possibility of having language. The deaf community in the United States, for instance, uses a gestural rather than a spoken language, American Sign Language (ASL). ASL is a complete language, with its own elaborated grammar and a rich vocabulary, all of which can be conveyed by the shape and movement of the hands in front of the body; it is the equal of vocal language in its capacity to communicate complex human thought (Fischer, 1993; Klima & Bellugi, 1979). A new appreciation of the richness of ASL led to innovative experiments with chimpanzees.

Washoe

The first attempt to capitalize on the ability to comprehend language and the natural gestural ability of a chimpanzee by teaching her signed human language (ASL) was made by Drs. Beatrice and Allen Gardner at the University of Nevada in 1966 (Gardner & Gardner, 1969). The Gardners moved a young chimpanzee named Washoe into a trailer behind their house and began to teach her ASL. Washoe was ten months old at the time and had been captured in the wild in Africa. During the time she was involved in this project, she learned over 130 ASL signs, as well as how to combine them into utterances of several signs (Gardner & Gardner, 1980; see also 1984a, 1984b). On seeing her trainer, she was able to sign, "Please tickle hug hurry," "Gimme food drink," and similar requests.

Washoe was able to sign many of the same things that are said by children in the very early stages of language acquisition, before they learn the grammatical refinements of their own language (Brown, 1970; Van Cantfort & Rimpau, 1982). She appeared to use her signs in a creative way: On seeing a duck for the first time, she signed "water bird." Since her utterances were typically answers to questions posed to her (e.g., "What is that?"), it is not clear whether she was attempting to make a new word, or simply saying that it was water *and* a bird. Unlike English-speaking children, she did not pay attention to word order, and at the time her training ceased in the fifty-first month, it was not clear if her sign language was actually grammatically structured in the sense that even a young child's is (Brown, 1970; Klima & Bellugi, 1972). However, through vocabulary tests of Washoe, as well as of subsequent chimpanzee subjects, the Gardners were able to demonstrate that children's and chimpanzees' first fifty words are very similar.

Moreover, the chimpanzees extended or generalized their words in much the same way that humans do—for instance, once they knew the ASL sign, calling a hat they had never seen before *hat* (Gardner & Gardner, 1984a; 1984b). The question of whether a chimpanzee was capable of syntax remained open. This is an important theoretical question, because syntax makes *productivity,* one of the hallmarks of human language, possible. On the practical side, the remarkable successes attained with chimps have led to innovative programs that teach sign language to communicatively handicapped children.

Nim Chimpsky

An attempt to answer the question of whether chimpanzees can make grammatical sentences was made by Columbia University professor Herbert S. Terrace (1980). Terrace adopted a young male chimp, whom he named Nim Chimpsky (no doubt with apologies to the famous linguist Noam Chomsky.) The plan was to raise Nim in a rich human environment, teach him ASL, and then analyze the chimp's emerging ability to combine signs into utterances, paying special attention to any evidence that he could indeed produce grammatical signed sentences. Nim began to sign early: He produced his first sign, "drink," when he was only four months old. But his later utterances never progressed much beyond the two- or three-sign stage. He signed, "Eat Nim," and, "Banana me eat," but when he made four-sign utterances, he added no new information and, unlike even young children, he used no particular word order. He signed, "Banana me eat banana," in which the additional word is merely repetitive. Analyzing the extensive data collected in this project, Terrace concluded that there was no evidence that the chimp could produce anything that might be called a sentence.

An even more serious question regarding the chimpanzee's linguistic capability was raised after Terrace and his associates studied the videotaped interactions of young Nim and his many teachers. They found that Nim understood little about conversational turn-taking, often interrupting his teachers, and that very little of what Nim signed actually originated with the chimp. Most of what he signed was prompted by the teacher and contained major constituents of the teacher's signed utterance to him.

Terrace carried his study further by analyzing films made available to him by other ape-language projects and arrived at the same conclusion: Much of what the chimps signed had just been signed to them. The signing chimps appeared to be responding at least in part to subtle cues from their trainers. Armed with this information, some critics went so far as to suggest that the chimps were modern equivalents of Clever Hans. Clever Hans was a horse who became famous for his mental powers in turn of the century Germany, until it was discovered that, rather than doing arithmetic, he was sensitive to minute physical cues in the people around him who knew the answers to the questions he was being asked (Brown, 1958). The question of the apes' potential was not completely settled by this study, since, as other researchers pointed out, children also interrupt and repeat parts of what adults say, and as Terrace himself was aware, the project had various shortcomings; for instance, Nim may have had too many trainers, and not all of them were equally proficient in ASL. In March, 2000, Nim Chimpsky died at the Black Beauty Reserve in Tyler, Texas. He was 26 years old.

Kanzi

Although it may be true that apes are not capable of adult language as we know it, the chimpanzee studies have indicated that there are substantial similarities between very young children's and chimpanzees' abilities to engage in symbolic communication (Greenfield & Savage-Rumbaugh, 1991).

Current research by D. M. Rumbaugh and E. S. Savage-Rumbaugh with a pygmy chimp named Kanzi at the Yerkes Center in Atlanta (Savage-Rumbaugh, 1990; Savage-Rumbaugh, Shanker, & Taylor, 1998) has given rise to new hope and speculation about primate linguistic ability. Prior chimpanzee studies used the common chimp (*pan troglodytes*). The pygmy chimpanzee or bonobo (*p. paniscus*) was virtually unheard of until the mid-1970s.

Pygmy chimpanzees are found only in the remote rain forests of the Democratic Republic of Congo (formerly known as Zaire). They are smaller, less aggressive, more social, more intelligent, and more communicative than the common chimp. Kanzi surprised his trainers when he acquired some manual signs merely by observing his mother's lessons. He is currently the subject of an intensive longitudinal study.

Kanzi has a large, free area in which to roam, and many opportunities to learn both spoken and signed language, as well as how to make tools and carry out everyday activities like cooking dinner. He is nineteen years old (in 2000) and weighs around 130 pounds. Although he is sexually mature, the Rumbaughs believe they will be able to

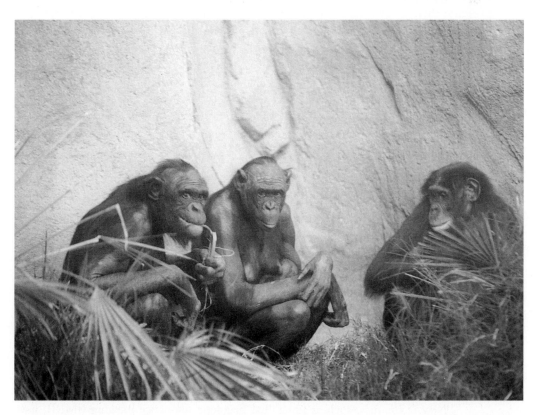

The bonobo, or pygmy chimpanzee, possesses a genetic stucture much like our own. Bonobos are sociable, interactive, and have shown remarkable abilities to communicate. Photo courtesy Roberta Gallagher ©.

continue working with him. Studies of his understanding of spoken English show that he comprehends many unusual utterances and can carry out the acts described in them with remarkable accuracy. For instance, if asked to "put the mushroom in the potty," Kanzi obligingly does so, proving that he is attending to language and not simply carrying out activities that are evident from the nonverbal situation. Current work with Kanzi has led his trainers to be very optimistic about the chimp's progress. Whether the pygmy chimpanzee is the hope of the future in animal language studies remains to be seen.

The Biological Base: Humans

Language in humans is clearly dependent on their having a society in which to learn it, other humans to speak to, and the emotional motivation and intelligence to make it possible; humans have also evolved with specialized capacities for speech and neural mechanisms that subserve language. Human beings who are physiologically and psychologically intact will acquire the language of those around them if they grow up among people who speak to them (Locke, 1990). This human interaction seems necessary; there is no evidence that infants can acquire language from watching television, for instance. There are some strong arguments for the case that human language is biologically determined—that it owes its existence to specialized structures in the brain and in the neurological systems of humans. Some of these biological specifications underlie the social and affective characteristics of infants that tie them to the adults around them and serve as precursors to language development. For instance, infants are intensely interested in human faces, and there is now evidence that the infant brain contains neurons that are specialized for the identification of human faces and for the recognition of affect in faces (Locke, 1993).

Language Areas in the Brain

Unlike our relatives the apes, humans have areas in the cerebral cortex that are known to be associated with language. The two hemispheres of the brain are not symmetrical (Geschwind, 1982). Most individuals, about 85 percent of the population, are right-handed, and almost all right-handers have their language functions represented in their left hemisphere. Of the left-handed population, perhaps half also have their language areas in the left hemisphere; therefore, the vast majority of the populace is **lateralized** for language in the left hemisphere. The right hemisphere, however, also participates in some aspects of language processing. For instance, recognition of the emotional tone of speech appears to be a right hemisphere function; moreover, when populations other than literate white males are studied, the cerebral asymmetry for language is less pronounced (Caplan, Lecours, & Smith, 1984).

New techniques, such as functional magnetic resonance imaging (fMRI), have made it possible to study the normal brain in action. Shaywitz and colleagues (1995) reported finding sex differences in the neural organization of the brain for language. Females activate areas in both hemispheres during phonological processing, whereas males use a comparatively restricted area of the left hemisphere. Until recently, however, most of our information about specialized areas came from the study of what happens when the brain is injured, either through a traumatic accident or from a stroke, aneurysm, or other cerebrovascular event. Damage to the language areas of the brain results in **aphasia,** a generalized communication disorder with varying characteristics depending on the site of the lesion (Berko Gleason & Goodglass, 1984; Goodglass, 1993). There are at least three well-established major language areas in the left hemisphere (see Figure 1.1).

- **Broca's area** in the left frontal region is very near to that part of the motor strip that controls the tongue and lips, and damage to Broca's area results in a typical aphasic syndrome, called Broca's aphasia, in which the patient has good comprehension but much difficulty with pronunciation and producing the little words of the language, such as articles and prepositions. Speech

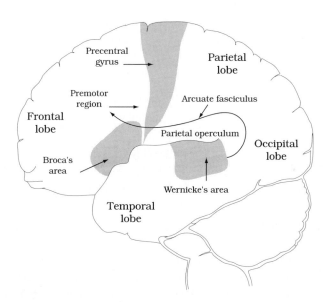

Figure 1.1

Language areas in the left hemisphere. *Broca's area, at the foot of the motor strip, is involved in the programming of speech for production. Wernicke's area, adjacent to the auditory cortex, is involved in the comprehension of language we hear. The arcuate fasciculus is a bundle of subcortical fibers that connects Broca's and Wernicke's areas. In order to repeat a word we hear (e.g., "cat"), we process it first in Wernicke's area, and then send a representation of it via the arcuate fasciculus to Broca's area, where its spoken form is organized. Damage to the arcuate fasciculus results in conduction aphasia, characterized by an inability to repeat words.*

tends to be *telegraphic*—it contains only the most important words. For instance, when one patient seen in Boston was asked how he planned to spend the weekend at home, he replied, with labored articulation, "Boston College. Football. Saturday."

- **Wernicke's area** is located in the posterior left temporal lobe, near the auditory association areas of the brain. Damage to Wernicke's area produces an aphasia that is characterized by fluent speech with many **neologisms** (nonsense words) and poor comprehension. One Wernicke's aphasic, when asked to name an ashtray, said, "That's a fremser." When he was later asked to point to the fremser, however, he had no idea what the examiner meant.

- The **arcuate fasciculus** is a band of subcortical fibers that connects Wernicke's area with Broca's area (see Figure 1.1). If you ask someone to repeat what you say, the incoming message is processed in Wernicke's area and then sent out over the arcuate fasciculus to Broca's area, where it is programmed for production. Patients with lesions in the arcuate fasciculus are unable to repeat; their disorder is called **conduction aphasia.** There are also areas of the brain known to be associated with written language: Damage to the angular gyrus, for instance, impairs the ability to read.

A child of five or six who suffers left-brain damage will in all likelihood recover complete language. However, adults who become aphasic are liable to remain so if they do not recover in the first half-year after their injury.

Specialized language areas of the brain are found in adults, but there is evidence that in young children either the areas are not yet so firmly specialized or the nonlanguage hemisphere can take over in case of damage to the dominant hemisphere. The brains of infants are not fully formed and organized at birth. The brains of newborns have many fewer synapses (connections) than those of adults. By the age of about two, the number of synapses reaches adult levels, and then increases rapidly between the ages of four and ten, far exceeding adult levels. During this period of synaptic growth, there is a concurrent pruning process as connections that do not get used die off. This process may help to explain the neurological bases of sensitive or critical periods in development. If, for instance, an infant does not hear language or does not establish an emotional bond with an adult, the neural connections that underlie language and emotion may be weakened. By the age of fifteen or sixteen the number of synapses has returned to adult levels.

Special Characteristics

In examining the attempts to teach language to apes, we saw that language is probably species unique; the specialized areas of the brain contribute to that uniqueness. Human beings, of course, also have unique cognitive abilities and unique social settings in which to acquire language. These are discussed in subsequent chapters—the intent here is to describe briefly the neuroanatomical foundations that make language acquisition possible. As Eric Lenneberg (1967) pointed out, language development in humans is associated with other maturational events. The appearance of language is a developmental milestone, roughly correlated with the onset of walking.

In addition to possessing specialized brain structures, humans, unlike other creatures, have a long list of adaptations in such things as the development of their vocal cords and larynxes and the ability to coordinate making speech sounds with breathing and swallowing. Humans perform a remarkably complex (and dangerous) set of actions when they engage in everyday activities, such as having a talk over lunch. As we noted earlier, our ape relatives do not have the capacity for speech; vocal tract reconstructions have also shown that even Neanderthal men and women had quite limited vocalizing capacity. With the evolution of *homo sapiens,* the larynx was lowered, and rapid, clear speech became a physical possibility, an advantage gained along with an increased risk of choking while eating (Lieberman, 1991).

Lenneberg (1967) cited a number of additional features as evidence that language is specific to our species and uniform across the species in its major characteristics.

1. *The onset of speech is regular.* The order of appearance of developmental milestones, including speech, is regular in the species—it is not affected by culture or the language to be learned.

2. *Speech is not suppressible.* Normal children learn to talk if they are in contact with older speakers. The wide variations that exist within and across cultures have all provided suitable environments for children to learn language.

3. *Language cannot be taught to other species.* Lenneberg made this claim in the 1960s, before there were results from the chimpanzee (and parrot) studies, and time may have proven him right. However, it is also clear that chimpanzees can be taught sign language comparable to the language of young children; and thus this claim depends on only one definition of language.

4. *Languages everywhere have certain universals.* They are structured in accordance with principles of human cognition, and any human can learn any language. At the same time, there are universal constraints on the kinds of rules that children can learn. The universals that are found in all languages include phonology, grammar, and semantics. These systematic aspects of language, along with another universal, the existence of social rules for language use, provide the research arena for developmental psycholinguistics.

The Structure of Language: Learning the System

Competence and Performance

A speaker who knows the syntactic rules of a language is said to have *linguistic competence.* Competence in this case refers to the inner (and unconscious) knowledge of the rules, not to the way the person speaks on any particular occasion. The expression of the rules in everyday speech is *performance.* In the normal course of events, speakers produce errors, false starts, slips of the tongue, and utterances flawed in various other ways. These are performance errors and are not thought to reflect the speakers' underlying competence. There is also a general assumption among linguists that within a given linguistic community, all adults who are native speakers of the language, and not neurologically impaired in some way, share linguistic competence; this claim, however, has never been substantiated. It is possible to find out a great deal about adults' syntax by asking them to judge the grammatical acceptability of a sentence. However, in studying children, researchers must either rely on performance for clues to competence or design clever experiments to probe inner knowledge, since young children do not have the metalinguistic ability required to discuss questions of "grammaticality."

When children learn language, what is it that they must learn? Language has many subsystems having to do with sound, grammar, meaning, vocabulary, and knowing the right way to say something on a particular occasion in order to accomplish a specific purpose. Knowing the language entails knowing its **phonology, morphology, syntax,** and **semantics,** as well as its social rules, or *pragmatics.* The speaker who knows all this has acquired *communicative competence* (Hymes, 1972).

Phonology

What are the sounds of English? Although we all speak the language, without specific training it would be difficult to list all of the sounds we make when we speak, and even more difficult to list the rules for their combination. Phonology includes all of the important sounds, the rules for combining them to make words, and such things as the stress and intonation patterns that accompany them. If you have studied foreign languages, you know that there are many different sounds used in the languages of the world and that any given language uses only a subset of the possibilities. Each language has its own set of important sounds, which are actually categories of sounds that include a number of variations. For instance, in English we pronounce the sound /t/ many different ways: At the beginning of a word like *top* it is pronounced with a strong aspiration, or puff of air (you can check this by holding the back of your hand near your mouth and vigorously saying *top*). We pronounce a word like *stop* without the puff of air, unaspirated. Some speakers produce a different, unreleased /t/ when they say a word like *hat* at the end of a sentence: They leave their tongues in place at the point of articulation. Many speakers pronounce an even different kind of /t/ in a word like *Manhattan* by releasing the air through their noses at the end. A phonetician would hear these /t/ sounds as four different sounds: aspirated, unaspirated, unreleased, and nasally released. But for untrained English speakers, these are all just one sound. A group of similar sounds that are regarded as all the same by the speakers of a language are called phonemes. The different /t/ sounds just described are all part of one /t/ phoneme in English. In Hindi and many other Indian languages, the aspirated and unaspirated versions of /t/ are heard and treated as very different sounds, two different phonemes.

Children have to learn to recognize and produce the phonemes of their own language and to combine those phonemes into words and sentences with the right sorts of intonational patterns. Some parts of the system, such as consonant-vowel combinations, are acquired early on. Others are not acquired until well into the elementary school years: for instance, the ability to distinguish between the stress patterns of *hot dog* (frankfurter, with mustard) and *hot dog* (Rottweiler, with leash) when the words are presented without a context (Atkinson-King, 1973). The phonological tasks that face a young child can vary considerably from language to language. English and other Germanic languages, for instance, have quite complicated rules for the combination of consonants: We have many words like *desks* or *healthful* that pose a challenge to anyone learning English. By contrast, Japanese has very few consonant clusters.

English has some sounds rarely found in other languages of the world, such as the *th* sound in *this;* but Czech has an even rarer sound, the medial sound /ř/ in the name *Dvořak,* which is a combination of an /r/ trilled on the tip of the tongue and the /ž/ sound in *azure,* said at the same time. Many African languages contain phonemic clicks rather similar to the sounds we make in English when we say what is written as "tsk tsk" or when we encourage a horse to go faster. In some languages tone is a phoneme: In Chinese, a rising or falling tone on a word can change its meaning entirely. When the tones are produced correctly, the sentence "Mama ma ma ma?" means "Did mother chide the horse?"

Morphology

When a new word like *glitch* comes into the English language, adult speakers can immediately tell what its plural is; they do not have to look it up in a dictionary or consult with an expert. They are able to pluralize a word that they have never heard before because they know the English inflectional morphological system. A **morpheme** is the smallest unit of meaning in a language; it cannot be broken into any smaller parts that have meaning. Words can consist of one or more morphemes. The words *cat* and *danger* each consist of one morpheme, which is called a **free morpheme** because it can stand alone. **Bound morphemes,** on the other hand, cannot stand alone and are always found attached to free morphemes; they appear affixed to free morphemes as prefixes, suffixes, or within the word as infixes. *Happiness, unclear,* and *singing* contain the bound morphemes *-ness, -un,* and *-ing.* Bound morphemes can be used to change one word into another word that may be a different part of speech; for instance, *-ness* turns the adjective *happy* into the noun *happiness.* In this case, they are called **derivational morphemes** because they can be used to derive new words.

Other bound morphemes do not change the basic word's meaning so much as they modify it to indicate such things as tense, person, number, case, and gender.

These variations on a basic word are inflections, and the morphemes that accomplish these changes are inflectional morphemes. Languages like Latin, Russian, and Hungarian are highly inflected. The verb *to love* (*amare*) in Latin has six separate forms in the present tense: the singular forms *amo, amas,* and *amat* (I love, you love, he loves) and the plural forms *amamus, amatis,* and *amant* (we love, you love, they love).

Compared with Latin, English has few verb inflections in the present tense: an added *-s* for the third person (he *loves*) and no inflection for other persons (I, we, you, they *love*). Latin indicates the subject and object of its sentences using case inflections—*agricola amat puellam* and *puellam amat agricola* both mean "the farmer loves the girl." The endings of the words mark the subject and the object. English does not have case endings on its nouns: Whether the girl loves the farmer or the farmer loves the girl is indicated entirely by word order. Grammar teachers, perhaps influenced by their knowledge of Latin, have tended to confuse the issue in English by referring to nouns as being in the subjective or objective case when, in fact, there are no separate noun case forms in English. Pronouns, on the other hand, have subjective, objective, and possessive forms: *I, me,* and *my.*

English inflectional morphology includes the progressive of the verb (e.g., *singing*); the past, pronounced with /d/, /t/ or /əd/ (*played, hopped, landed*); and the third person singular verb and the noun plural and possessive, all of which use /z/, /s/, or /əz/ in spoken language (*dogs, cats, watches*). Whether one says, "He dogs my steps" (verb), "It's the dog's dish" (possessive), or, "I have ten dogs" (plural), the inflected form is pronounced in exactly the same way. The forms of the inflections vary depending on the last sound of the word being inflected, and, as stated earlier, there is a complex set of rules that adult speakers know (at some level) that enables them to make a plural or past tense of a word that they have never heard before.

One task for the student of language development is to determine whether children have knowledge of morphology and, if so, how it is acquired and to what extent it resembles the rule system that adults follow.

Syntax

The syntactic system contains the rules for how to combine words into phrases and sentences and how to transform sentences into other sentences. A competent speaker can take a basic sentence like "The cat bites the dog" and make a number of transformations of it: "The cat bit the dog," "The cat didn't bite the dog," "Did the cat bite the dog?" and "Wasn't the dog bitten by the cat?" Knowledge of the syntactic system allows the speaker to generate an almost endless number of new sentences and to recognize those that are not grammatically acceptable. If you heard a nonsense sentence like "The gorpy wug wasn't miggled by the mimsy zibber," you could not know what happened because the vocabulary is strange. On the other hand, the morphology and syntax of the sentence convey a great deal of information, and with this information you could make a number of new, perfectly grammatical sentences: "The wug is gorpy," "The zibber did not miggle the wug," and "The zibber is mimsy."

There is a great deal of controversy among researchers as to whether young children just learning language are acquiring syntactic structures, that is, grammatical rules, or whether it is more reasonable to characterize their early utterances in terms of the semantic relations they are trying to express. The child who says, "Doggie eat lunch," can be said to have learned to produce subject-verb-object constructions and to be following English syntactic rules specifying that the subject comes first in active sentences. (Even very young children do not say, "Lunch eat doggie.") To describe the language of young children, however, it is probably more useful to note the kinds of semantic relations the children are using. In this case the child is expressing her knowledge that an action is taking place and that there is an agent and an object.

Once children begin to produce longer sentences, however, they add the grammatical words of the language and begin to build sentences according to syntactic rules. They learn how to make *negatives, questions, compound sentences, passives,* and *imperatives.* Later, they add very complex structures, including embedded forms. The child who early on was limited to sentences like "Doggie eat lunch" can eventually comprehend and produce "The lunch that Grandpa cooked the cleaning lady was eaten by the dog" in full confidence that the household helper was neither cooked by Grandpa nor eaten by Scout.

Semantics

Semantic acquisition refers to the acquisition of vocabulary and the meanings associated with words. Word meanings are complicated to learn; words are related to one another in complex networks, and awareness of words comes later than does word use. A very young child may use a word that occurs in adult language, but that word does not mean exactly the same thing, nor does it have the same internal status for the child as it does for the adult (Clark, 1993). Two-year-olds who say "doggie," for instance, may call sheep, cows, cats, and horses "doggie," or they may use the word in reference to a particular dog, without knowing that it refers to a whole class of animals. Vocabulary is structured hierarchically, and words are attached to one another in semantic networks. Dogs are a class of animals, and the adult who knows the meaning of *dog* also knows, for instance, that it belongs to a group known as domestic animals, it is a pet, it is related to wolves, it is animate, and so on. Studying semantic development in children involves examining how they acquire the semantic system, beginning with simple vocabulary. Ultimately, it includes studying their metalinguistic knowledge, which enables them to notice the words in their language and comment on them. A young child does not know what a word is, but by the time children are in the primary grades, they not only notice words, they can provide definitions and tell us what their favorite words are.

Language in Social Context: Pragmatics

Linguistic competence resides in knowing how to construct grammatically acceptable sentences. Language, however, must be used in a social setting, to accomplish various ends. Speakers who know how to use language *appropriately* have more than linguistic competence; they have communicative competence, a term first used by Dell Hymes (1972). *Pragmatics* refers to the use of language to express one's intentions and get things done in the world. Even children at the one-word stage use language to accomplish various pragmatic ends; John Dore (1978), for instance, found that such children used their single words to ask, demand, and label. Adult pragmatics may include such additional functions as denying, refusing, blaming, offering condolences, flattering, and a host of others.

Communicative competence includes being able to express one's intent appropriately in varying social situations. The importance of knowing the right forms becomes obvious when social rules are violated. Consider the use of directives. If you are seated in the aisle seat of a bus, next to a stranger, and you are cold because the window is open, you can express your intent in a syntactically correct sentence: "Shut that window." This could lead to an angry reaction or, at the very least, to the impression that you are a rude person. If, instead, you said, "I wonder if you would mind shutting the window?" compliance and the beginning of a pleasant conversation would probably follow. Knowing the politeness rules of language is part of communicative competence.

Research on pragmatics examines the way that children learn to use language appropriately in various social situations as they attain communicative competence. Pragmatics includes important topics, such as the ability to make conversation. Pellegrini, Brody, and Stoneman (1987) studied the ways that children learn to make appropriate conversations with their parents. These researchers used a model provided by the philosopher Herbert Grice.

Grice (1975) provided a framework for the study of conversations by setting forth a number of cooperative principles or maxims that successful conversationalists must obey. These *conversational principles* include:

1. *Quantity.* Say as much as you need to, but not too much. For instance, if someone asks a child what she would like to drink with dinner, she must know that it suffices to say, "Orange juice, please," and that it would be inappropriate to say, "Approximately eight ounces of juice squeezed from several oranges and placed in a clean glass here on the table at the right of my plate." Young children are, of course, likely to give too little rather than too much information.

2. *Quality.* The quality referred to by this maxim is truthfulness. Children must learn that their interlocutors expect them not to lie or confabulate.

3. *Relevance.* Contributions to the conversation are expected to be relevant. If a child responds to the question "What do you like for lunch?" by saying, "I

like my kitty," she is violating the relevance principle (or exhibiting serious antisocial tendencies).

4. *Manner.* Speakers are expected to take their turns in a timely fashion and to present their propositions in a logical order. It is a violation of this principle, for instance, to say, "We put on our pajamas and took a bath," since presumably bathing precedes putting on pajamas.

Adults, of course, violate these principles in order to achieve certain very human ends: to be ironic, for instance, or to make a joke, or perhaps to be deceptive or insulting. Every type of interaction between individuals requires observance of pragmatic conventions, and adults do not leave children's development of these rules to chance—whereas they may not correct syntactic violations except in the most superficial cases (see Chapter 5), they are active participants in their children's pragmatic socialization (Becker, 1994).

Just as there are phonological and grammatical rules, there are also rules for the use of language in social context. They are governed by such variables as the topic, the channel of communication (e.g., face-to-face, on the telephone, or over a CB radio), and the social situation—one might speak quite differently about the same topic at a funeral than at a wedding. There are also a number of speaker/hearer characteristics that affect the form of the communication; these include gender, age, rank, social class, and degree of familiarity. Mature language users have all of these variables under control. They know how to speak like men or women, to conduct discourse, to speak in appropriate ways to different people. They can talk baby talk to babies and be formal and deferential when appearing in court. All of these are part of communicative competence, which is the goal of language development.

The Study of Language Development

Historical Trends in Child Language Study

Probably the first recorded account of a language acquisition study is found in the work of the Greek historian Herodotus, who was a contemporary of the playwright Sophocles. Herodotus, sometimes called the father of history, lived from about 484 to 425 B.C. In Book 11 of his *History,* he relates the story of the ancient Egyptian king Psammetichus, who wanted to prove that the Egyptians were the original human race.

In order to do this, Psammetichus ordered a shepherd to raise two children, caring for their needs but not speaking to them. "His object herein was to know, after the indistinct babblings of infancy were over, what word they would first articulate." Presumably, Psammetichus believed that the children would develop the language of the oldest group of humans all by themselves. This is perhaps the strongest version of an innatist theory of language development that one could have: Babies arrive in the world with a specific language wired into their brains.

When the two children were about two years old, the shepherd went to their quarters one day. They ran up to him, with their hands outstretched, saying "Becos." Unfortunately for the Egyptians, *becos* was not a word that anyone recognized. The king, according to Herodotus, asked around the kingdom and eventually was told that *becos* meant "bread" in the Phrygian language, whereupon the Egyptians gave up their claim to being the oldest race of humans and decided that they were in *second* place, behind the Phrygians.

Even though interest in language development has ancient roots, the systematic study of children's language is new to our times, in part because the science of linguistics, with its special analytic techniques, came of age in the twentieth century. In earlier times, the structural nature of language was not well understood, and what studies there were tended to concentrate on the kinds of things that children said rather than on their acquisition of productive linguistic subsystems.

Studies in the Late Nineteenth and Early Twentieth Century

There were many studies of children, including notes on their language, published in Germany, France, and England during the latter half of the nineteenth century and the early years of the twentieth century. One of the main early figures in the United States in the field of developmental psychology, G. Stanley Hall, taught at Clark University in Worcester, Massachusetts. Hall (1907) was interested in "the content of children's minds," and he had been led to study children's language by the German philosopher Wilhelm Wundt. Hall, in turn, inspired a school of American students of child language (Bar-Adon & Leopold, 1971).

The kinds of questions that child language researchers asked during this period were primarily related to philosophical inquiries into human nature. (This was true of Charles Darwin, 1877, who kept careful diaries on the language development of one of his sons.) Many of these early investigations included valuable insights into language. (A number of such studies are summarized in Bar-Adon & Leopold, 1971.) The early studies were almost invariably in the form of diaries and were typically observations of the authors' own children. Notable exceptions were studies of feral or isolated children who had failed to acquire language. Just as in antiquity, there was philosophical interest in the effects of isolation on language development; that interest has been sustained to the present day: *The Wild Boy of Aveyron,* a landmark study of a feral child, Victor, was written in the eighteenth century (Lane, 1979), and the study of Genie, an American girl who was kept isolated from other humans, was published not long ago (Curtiss, 1977; Rymer, 1993).

During the first half of the twentieth century, many psychologists still kept diary records of their children. In the educational world, children's language was studied in order to arrive at norms, to describe gender and social class differences, and to search for the causes and cures of developmental difficulties. Educational psychologists frequently used group tests with large numbers of children, and there was a great interest in such things as the average sentence length used by children at different grade levels, or the kinds of errors they made in grammar or pronunciation (McCarthy, 1954).

Contemporary Research

The mid-1950s saw a revolution in child language studies. Work on descriptive linguistics (Gleason, 1955) and the early work of Noam Chomsky (1957) provided new models of language for researchers to explore. At the same time, a behaviorist theory of language put forth by B. F. Skinner (1957) inspired other groups of investigators to design studies aimed at testing this learning theory.

Psycholinguistics came into being as a field when linguists and psychologists combined the techniques of their disciplines to investigate whether the systems described by the linguist had psychological reality in the minds of speakers. The linguistic description of English might, for instance, point out that the plural of words ending in /s/ or /z/ is formed by adding /əz/, for example, *kiss* and *kisses*. A task for the psycholinguist was to demonstrate that the linguistic description matched what speakers actually do, that speakers have a "rule" for the formation of the plural that is isomorphic (i.e., identical in form) with the linguist's descriptive rule. If speakers merely memorized the plural of each new word in their lexicon or vocabulary, there would be no evidence of internal rules.

In the decade of the 1960s, after the powerful grammatical model of Chomsky became widely known, there was an explosion of research into children's acquisition of syntax. The 1960s were characterized by studies of grammar; many projects studied a small number of children over a period of time, writing grammars of the children's developing language. At Harvard University, for instance, a group of researchers, many of whom were to become prominent individually, worked with Roger Brown (1973) on a project that studied the language development of three children called Adam, Eve, and Sarah (not their real names!) These children were visited once a month in their homes by researchers who made tape recordings of their speech. The recordings were brought back to the laboratory and transcribed, and the resulting transcriptions were studied by a team of faculty and graduate students that met in a weekly seminar (DeCuevas, 1990).

As the 1960s drew to a close, the dominance of syntax in research gave way to a broadening interest that included the context in which children's language emerges and an emphasis on the kinds of semantic relations children are trying to express in their early utterances. The early 1970s saw a spate of studies on the language addressed to children; many of these were conducted to shed light on the innateness controversy. Researchers wanted to know whether children were innately programmed to discover the rules of language all by themselves, or whether adults provided them with help or even with language learning lessons.

Studies of the 1980s and 1990s included all of the traditional linguistic topics: phonology, morphology, syntax, semantics, and pragmatics. As the twenty-first century begins, there is growing interest in cross-cultural research in language development, and in understanding how language development interfaces with other aspects of children's social and psychological development; in acquiring a language, children become members of a society, with all of its unique cultural practices and belief systems. Cross-cultural work has shown, for instance, that in a nonliterate society such as that of Gypsies in Hungary, parents' speech to children has special features that serve to preserve traditions and inculcate cultural values—for example, parents tell even infants detailed stories about what their future life will be like (Réger & Berko Gleason, 1991).

Social class and gender differences in language, stylistic variation in acquisition and use, the use of language in poetry and metaphor and in jokes and games, and the language addressed to children are examples of topics found in current journals devoted to the various branches of linguistics. Many of these topics are also explored in later chapters of this book.

Research Methods

Equipment

Modern technology has made it possible to collect accurate data on children's everyday use of language and for researchers around the world to share data and data analysis programs. When developmental psycholinguistics was born in the 1950s, technology was very limited, and researchers had to rely on large reel-to-reel tape recorders and handwritten notes when they collected their data. There were no photocopy machines. Cassette audio recorders and small video cameras have greatly simplified data collection, and computers have made analysis easier.

Studies of phonology require especially sensitive recording equipment and must frequently use sophisticated laboratory hardware, which is now often computerized as well. Other studies, however, can usually be conducted with easily acquired equipment. A good cassette recorder is sufficient for most work, and if there is a great deal of data, a cassette transcriber is an invaluable aid. Some studies require a visual record; if, for instance, the researcher is interested in the gestural accompaniments of early language or the gaze behavior of subjects, excellent video equipment is now widely available. This equipment makes it possible to film in subjects' homes with a minimum of intrusion. Video makes it easier to study the context of language acquisition. Most researchers use a back-up tape recorder in addition to their video equipment. Because the presence of equipment and observers will invariably have some effect on the behavior of subjects, it is possible in some naturalistic studies to leave a recorder with the subjects, instructing them (or their parents) to turn it on at specified times, such as when the family is at dinner.

Regardless of the method of recording, it is necessary to make a transcription of the data for analysis. This involves writing out as exactly as possible everything that is said on the tape. Transcripts can then be prepared in such a way that computer analyses are possible (see Figure 1.2).

One of the most significant developments in child language research has been the creation of a computerized child language data base available to researchers. The Child Language Data Exchange System (CHILDES) was put into operation in 1984 at Carnegie Mellon University under the direction of Brian MacWhinney and Catherine Snow. Many powerful computer programs (CLAN, or Child Language ANalysis programs) are available, along with data, from CHILDES (MacWhinney, 1995). The advantages of such a system are that it allows (1) data sharing among researchers, who can test their hypotheses on many more subjects; (2) increased precision and standardization in coding; and (3) automation of many coding procedures. CLAN programs can operate on any or all speakers' output and can automatically derive the mean length of utterance (see Chapter 5), a total list of words used, as well as their frequency, and other data of immense value to the language researcher. Data from many studies in English and other languages are available; even older studies, such as Brown's famous work on Adam, Eve, and Sarah from the 1960s, have been optically scanned and entered, thus making these data available to anyone who wants them.

CHILDES continues to collect data from researchers all over the world and to evolve in remarkable ways. The entire database and the CLAN programs are now available for download from the Carnegie Mellon web site, as well as from mirror sites in Belgium and Japan. Since the electronic address is subject to change, the easiest way to find and access these sites is to enter the key word CHILDES into any web-based search engine. The newest development in progress as a part of CHILDES is called TalkBank. When completed, TalkBank will be an interactive internet resource that links transcripts with digitized video and audio data: It will be possible to read the transcript, view the subject, and hear the actual speech, all at the same time (MacWhinney, 1999).

Methods

Language development studies can be either *cross-sectional* or *longitudinal* in their design. Cross-sectional studies use two or more groups of subjects. If, for instance, you wanted to study the development of the negative between the ages of two and four, you could study a group of two-year-olds and a group of four-year-olds and then describe the differences in the two groups' use of negation.

Longitudinal studies follow individual subjects over time; one might study the same child's use of negatives at specified periods between the ages of two and four. Unless the researcher has ample funding, it is usually impossible to follow more than a few subjects in a longitudinal study.

Cross-sectional studies have the advantage of obtaining a great deal of data in a short time; one doesn't have to wait two years to get results. Having a sizable number of subjects also makes it more likely that the results of the study are generalizable to other children and not a reflection of the idiosyncratic behavior of a few. Longitudinal designs are used to study individuals over time when questions such as the persistence

```
@Begin
@Participants: CHI Charlie Child, MOT Mother, FAT Father
@Date: 7-JUL-1996
@Filename: CHARLIE.CHA
@Situation: Home Dinner Conversation.
*MOT: did you tell Dad what we did today?
*MOT: who'd we see?
*CHI: who?
*MOT: remember?
*CHI: Judy and my friend.
*MOT: did we see Michael?
*CHI: yes.
*FAT: was Mike at the beach?
*CHI: no.
*FAT: that's because he had work to do.
*FAT: do you remember the name of the beach you went to?
*CHI: not this time.
*FAT: you don't remember it this time?
*FAT: it was Winger-: what?
*FAT: Winger-Beach?
*CHI: yes.
*FAT: Winger Sheek Beach.
*CHI: Winger Sheek Beach.
*FAT: that's the one.
*CHI: Winger Beach.
*MOT: did you go swimming, Charlie?
*CHI: I went swimming, Dad.
*FAT: you did?
*FAT: did you wear water wings?
*CHI: no.
*FAT: no?
@End
```

Figure 1.2

Sample transcript. *This excerpt from CHILDES can be analyzed by a number of CLAN programs that can automatically compute MLU, list all vocabulary by speaker, and derive many standardized measures.*

of traits or the effects of early experience are relevant. If, for instance, you wanted to know whether children who talk early also become early readers, you would have to use a longitudinal design. Longitudinal studies are expensive and time-consuming, and they depend on the willingness of subjects to be available for a period of weeks, months, or years. Their advantage is that they can provide fine and accurate data about what happens to individuals during the course of language development.

Both cross-sectional and longitudinal studies can be either *observational* or *experimental.* Observational studies involve a minimum of intrusion by the researcher. Naturalistic observational studies attempt to capture behavior as it occurs in real life; for instance, one might record and analyze family speech at the dinner table. Controlled observational studies can be carried out in various settings, including the laboratory, where the researcher provides certain constants for all subjects. Fathers might come to the laboratory with their daughters and be observed reading them a book provided by the researcher. Observational research can indicate what kinds of behaviors correlate with one another, but it cannot reveal which behavior might cause another.

In experimental research, the researcher has some control and can manipulate variables. Typical experimental research includes:

- Hypotheses about what will happen
- An experimental group of subjects that receives the treatment (training, for instance) and a control group that receives no special treatment
- Independent variables, manipulated by the experimenter (training, exposure to a TV program, etc.)
- Dependent variables: the behaviors that are measured (for instance, the subjects' use of a particular grammatical form)
- Randomization: assignment of subjects at random to control or experimental conditions
- Standardization of procedures (all subjects receive the same instructions, etc.)

If you wanted to see whether training makes a difference in the acquisition of the passive voice, for instance, you might take a group of thirty three-year-olds and randomly assign them to two groups, a control group and an experimental group of fifteen children each. The experimental group would receive training in the passive; the control group, no special treatment. Finally, both groups could be asked to describe some pictures they had never seen before, and differential use of the passive would be recorded. If the trained group used passives and the control group did not, there would be evidence that training causes accelerated acquisition of one aspect of grammar. Experimental research can easily be replicated in the laboratory, but it may not be easily generalized to the outside world.

In addition to clear-cut observational and experimental methods, language development researchers use a variety of research techniques. These include *standard assessment measures,* in which subjects can be compared or evaluated on the basis of their responses to published standardized language tests. These are useful for indicating whether a subject's language is developing at a typical rate or whether some facet of development is out of line with the others.

Imitation is a technique used by many researchers—you simply ask the child to say what you say. Imitation reveals a great deal about children's language, since they typically cannot imitate sentences that are beyond their stage of development (Slobin, 1979). This is true of adults as well—try imitating a few sentences in Bulgarian the next time you meet someone from Sofia who is willing to say them to you.

Elicitation is a technique that works well when a particular language form is the target, and you want to give your subjects all the help they need (short of the answer itself). In investigating the plural through elicitation, you might show your subjects a picture, first of one and then of two birdlike creatures, and say, "This is a wug. Now there is another one. There are two of them. There are two…?" The subject obligingly fills in "wugs." This technique works well with aphasic patients, especially severe Broca's aphasics who have very little voluntary speech.

The *interview* is an old technique, but one that can be very effective if the researcher has the time to do more than ask a list of questions and fill in a form. Researchers of the Piagetian school frequently use an interview type called the *clinical method.* This is an open-ended interview in which the sequence of questions depends on the answers the subject has given. In studying metalinguistic awareness, the investigator might ask a series of questions, such as "Is *horse* a word? Why? (Or why not?) What is a word? How do you know? What is your favorite word? Why?" The choice of method depends very much on the theoretical inclination of the investigator. Since without some sort of intervention on the part of the researcher it might take a very long time before subjects said the kinds of things that interest us, many ingenious methods for studying language production have been designed (Menn & Bernstein Ratner, 2000). Every method that has been mentioned here, as well as a few that have not, appears in the pages that follow.

Summary

Babies seek the love and attention of their caregivers. Before they are even one year old, they are able to make fine discriminations among the speech sounds they hear, and they begin to communicate nonverbally with those around them. Young children acquire the basic components of their native language in just a few years: *phonology, morphology, semantics, syntax,* and the social rules for language use, often called *pragmatics.* By the time they are of school age, children control all of the major grammatical and semantic features. Language development, however, proceeds throughout the life cycle; as individuals grow older, they acquire new skills at every stage of their lives, and in the declining years they are vulnerable to a specific set of language disabilities. To elucidate both the scope and the nature of language development, this book is written from a life-span perspective.

Babies begin to acquire language during their first months, long before they say their first words; language is built upon an earlier affective communicative base. Midway through the first year, infants begin to babble, an event seen by many researchers as evidence of linguistic capacity. Near their first birthdays, infants say their first words. Early words, word meanings, and word combinations have universal characteristics, since toddlers' language is similar across cultures. Children's progress toward learning the particular grammatical structure of their own language follows a predictable order that is common to all children learning that language.

Although there are universal characteristics, there are also patterns of individual variation in language development. Different theories of language development emphasize *innate mechanisms, learning principles, cognitive prerequisites, information processing,* and *social interaction.*

During the school years, children perfect their knowledge of complex grammar, and they learn to use language in many different social situations. The develop *metalinguistic awareness,* the ability to consider language as an object. At the same time, they learn another major linguistic system: the written language. The demands of literacy remove a child's language from the here and now and emphasize *decontextualized language.* Not all children learn to read with ease.

Teenagers develop a distinct personal linguistic style, and young adults must acquire the linguistic register common to their occupations. With advancing age, numerous linguistic changes take place; there is some inevitable loss of word-finding ability, but vocabulary and narrative skill may improve.

Human language has special properties that have led many researchers to conclude that it is *species specific* and *species uniform.* Insects may have an elaborate communication system but their conversational topics are very limited, whereas humans can talk about any part of their experience. Sea mammals employ communicative systems of whistles and grunts, and many birds have been shown to have a variety of meaningful calls. None of these systems equals human language, however, which is *productive,* has *semanticity,* and offers the possibility of *displacement.*

During the past half-century, many researchers have turned their attention to primates in an attempt to discover whether language is really unique to humans or if it can be learned by other species. The early studies, which tried to teach spoken language to chimpanzees, showed conclusively that primates cannot speak as humans do. More recent studies have attempted to teach American Sign Language (ASL) to chimpanzees and have met with mixed results. The signing chimps may be responding at least in part to subtle cues from their trainers, but the question of the apes' potential is not completely settled. These studies have indicated that there are substantial similarities between very young children's and chimpanzees' abilities to engage in symbolic communication, and there is the possibility that the bonobo (pygmy chimpanzee) will reach new heights of linguistic achievement.

Language development requires social interaction, but spoken language in humans is possible only because we have evolved with specialized neural mechanisms that subserve language. These include special areas in the brain, such as *Broca's area,*

Wernicke's area, and the *arcuate fasciculus.* Other evidence of humans' biological disposition for language includes the regular onset of speech and the facts that speech is not suppressible, language cannot be taught to other species, and languages everywhere have universals.

The study of language development includes research into major linguistic subsystems. The *phonological system* is composed of the significant sounds of the language and the rules for their combination, the *morphological system* includes the minimal units that carry meaning, *syntax* refers to the rules by which sentences are constructed in a given language, and the *semantic systems* contain the meanings of words and the relationships between them. Finally, to function in society, speakers must know the social or *pragmatic rules* for language use. Individuals must be able to comprehend and produce all of these systems in order to attain *communicative competence.*

Although interest in language development has ancient roots, the scientific study of this subject began in the 1950s, with the appearance of new linguistic and psychological theories of language that gave birth to the combined discipline now known as *developmental psycholinguistics.* Developmental psycholinguists use all of the research techniques, designs, and resources employed by psychologists and linguists, as well as a few that are unique, such as a shared computerized data bank of child language materials.

Key Words

American Sign Language (ASL)
aphasia
arcuate fasciculus
autism
bound morpheme
Broca's area
child-directed speech (CDS)
communicative competence
comprehension
conduction aphasia
decontextualized language
derivational morpheme
Down syndrome
dyslexia
free morpheme
innate
internalized representation
lateralized
linguistic competence

metalinguistic awareness
morpheme
morphology
neologisms
overlaid function
overregularized
phonology
pragmatics
production
semantic development
semantics
species specific
species uniform
specific language impairment
speech acts
syntax
telegraphic
Wernicke's area

Suggested Projects

1. Choose three related articles on language development from the *Journal of Child Language,* or from another journal, such as *Child Development.* Write an introduction, explaining what the major questions of the research are, and then, for each article, describe the methods used by the authors, the subject population, any special equipment that was needed, and the nature of the results. In a separate discussion section, compare the results of the studies, and suggest other ways that the same question could be explored.

2. Tape-record a half-hour sample of a mother or father interacting with a one- or two-year-old child who does not yet combine words. At the end of the session, have a brief discussion with the parent about the child for about five minutes. Transcribe the entire tape. Analyze and compare the parent's speech to the child and speech to you in terms of (a) the average length of sentence, (b) repetitions, (c) the vocabulary used by the parent. Describe and categorize the vocabulary used by the child.

3. Read papers by Patterson, Premack & Premack, the Rumbaughs, and Terrace on their studies with the gorilla Koko and the various chimps. Summarize the claims that are made for these apes, and provide a critique.

Suggested Readings

Brown, R. W. (1970). The first sentences of child and chimpanzee. In R. W. Brown (Ed.), *Psycholinguistics.* New York: Macmillan.

Curtiss, S. (1977). *Genie: A psycholinguistic study of a modern day "wild" child.* New York: Academic Press.

Diamond, J. (1992). *The third chimpanzee: The evolution and future of the human animal.* New York: Basic Books.

Gardner, R. A., & Gardner, B. T. (1980). Two comparative psychologists look at language acquisition. In K. E. Nelson (Ed.), *Children's language* (Vol. 2). New York: Gardner Press.

Geschwind, N. (1982). Specializations of the human brain. In W. S. -Y. Wang (Ed.), *Human communication: Language and its psychobiological bases.* San Francisco: W. H. Freeman.

Greenfield, P. M., & Savage-Rumbaugh, E. S. (1991). Imitation, grammatical development, and the invention of protogrammar by an ape. In N. Krasnegor, D. M. Rumbaugh, M. Studdert-Kennedy, & R. L. Schiefelbusch (Eds.), *Biological and behavioral determinants of language development.* Hillsdale, NJ: Lawrence Erlbaum.

Lane, H. (1979). *The wild boy of Aveyron.* Cambridge, MA: Harvard University Press.

Terrace, H. S. (1980). *Nim: A chimpanzee who learned sign language.* New York: Knopf.

References

Atkinson-King, K. (1973). Children's acquisition of phonological stress contrasts. UCLA Working Papers in Phonetics (Department of Linguistics), 25.

Bar-Adon, A., & Leopold, W. (1971). *Child language: A book of readings.* Englewood Cliffs, NJ: Prentice-Hall.

Becker, J. A. (1994). Pragmatic socialization: Parental input to preschoolers. *Discourse Processes, 17,* 131–148.

Berko, J. (1958). The child's learning of English morphology. *Word, 14,* 150–177.

Berko Gleason, J., & Goodglass, H. (1984). Some neurological and linguistic accompaniments of the fluent and nonfluent aphasias. *Topics in Language Disorders, 4,* 71–81.

Blake, J., & de Boysson-Bardies, B. (1992). Patterns in babbling: A cross linguistic study. *Journal of Child Language, 19,* 51–75.

Bloom, L. (1970). *Language development. Form and function in emerging grammars.* Cambridge, MA: MIT Press.

Bonvillian, J. D., & Patterson, F. G. (1997). Sign language acquisition and the development of meaning in a lowland gorilla. In Mandell, C. & McCabe, A. (Eds.). *The problem of meaning: Behavioral and cognitive perspectives. Advances in psychology* (pp. 181–219). Amsterdam, Netherlands: North-Holland/Elsevier Science Publishers.

Brown, R. W. (1958). *Words and things.* Glencoe, IL: The Free Press.

Brown, R. W. (1970). The first sentences of child and chimpanzee. In R. Brown (Ed.), *Psycholinguistics.* New York: Macmillan.

Brown, R. W. (1973). *A first language.* Cambridge, MA: Harvard University Press.

Caplan, D., Lecours, A., & Smith, A. (Eds.). (1984). *Biological perspectives on language.* Cambridge, MA: MIT Press.

Clark, E. V. (1973). What's in a word? On the child's acquisition of semantics in his first language. In T. E. Moore (Ed.), *Cognitive development and the acquisition of language.* New York: Academic Press.

Clark, E. V. (1993). *The lexicon in acquisition.* Cambridge, UK: Cambridge University Press.

Chomsky, N. (1957). *Syntactic structures.* The Hague: Mouton.

Chomsky, N. (1965). *Aspects of the theory of syntax.* Cambridge, MA: MIT Press.

Curtiss, S. (1977). *Genie: A psycholinguistic study of a modern day "wild" child.* New York: Academic Press.

Darwin, C. (1877). A biographical sketch of an infant. *Mind, 2,* 285–294.

de Boysson-Bardies, B., & Vihman, M. M. (1991). Adaptation to language: Evidence from babbling and first words in four languages. *Language, 67,* 297–319.

DeCuevas, J. (1990, September-October). "No, she holded them loosely." *Harvard Magazine,* 61–67.

Diamond, J. 1992. *The third chimpanzee: The evolution and future of the human animal.* New York: Basic Books.

Dore, J. (1978). Variation in preschool children's conversational performances. In K. Nelson (Ed.), *Children's language* (Vol. 1). New York: Gardner Press.

Dromi, E., & Berman, R. (1982). A morphemic measure of early language development: Data from modern Hebrew. *Journal of Child Language, 2,* 403–424.

Eimas, P. D. (1975). Auditory and phonetic coding of the cues for speech: Discrimination of the /r-l/ distinction by young infants. *Perception and Psychophysics, 18,* 341–347.

Erikson, E. (1959). Identity and the life cycle. *Psychological Issues, 1,* 1–171.

Fenson, L., Dale, P. S., Reznick, J. S., Bates, E., Thal, D. J., & Pethick, S. J. (1994). Variability in early communicative development. *Monographs of the Society for Research in Child Development, 59* (Serial No. 242).

Fischer, S. (1993). The study of sign languages and linguistic theory. In C. Otero (Ed.), *Noam Chomsky: Critical assessments.* London: Routledge.

Gardner, R. A., & Gardner, B. T. (1969). Teaching sign language to a chimpanzee. *Science, 165,* 664–672.

Gardner, R. A., & Gardner, B. T. (1980). Two comparative psychologists look at language acquisition. In K. E. Nelson (Ed.), *Children's language* (Vol. 2). New York: Gardner Press.

Gardner, R. A., & Gardner, B. T. (1984a). A vocabulary test for chimpanzees. *Journal of Comparative Psychology, 98* (4), 381–404.

Gardner, R. A., & Gardner, B. T. (1984b). Signs of intelligence in cross fostered chimpanzees, *Philosophical Transactions in the Royal Society of London, B,* 1–34.

Geschwind, N. (1982). Specializations of the brain. In W. S. -Y. Wang (Ed.), *Human communication: Language and its psychobiological bases.* San Francisco: W. H. Freeman.

Gleason, H. A. (1955). *An introduction to descriptive linguistics.* New York: Henry Holt.

Goodglass, H. (1993). *Understanding aphasia.* San Diego, CA: Academic Press.

Greenfield, P. M., & Savage-Rumbaugh, E. S. (1991). Imitation, grammatical development, and the invention of protogrammar by an ape. In N. Krasnegor, D. M. Rumbaugh, M. Studdert-Kennedy, & R. L. Schiefelbusch (Eds.), *Biological and behavioral determinants of language development.* Hillsdale, NJ: Lawrence Erlbaum.

Grice, H. P. (1975). Logic and conversation. In P. Cole & J. Morgan (Eds.), *Syntax and semantics* (Vol. 3). New York: Academic Press.

Hall, G. S. (1907). *Aspects of child life and education.* New York: Appleton.

Hayes, C. (1951). *The ape in our house.* New York: Harper.

Herman, L. (1981). Cognitive characteristics of dolphins. In L. Herman (Ed.), *Cetacean behavior.* New York: Wiley.

Hymes, D. (1972). On communicative competence. In J. Pride & J. Holmes (Eds.), *Sociolinguistics.* Hammondsworth, G. B.: Penguin.

Jakobson, R. (1968). *Child language, aphasia, and phonological universals.* The Hague: Mouton.

Kellogg, W. N. (1980). Communication and language in the home raised chimpanzee. In T. Sebeok & J. Umiker Sebeok (Eds.), *Speaking of apes.* New York: Plenum Press.

Klima, E. S., & Bellugi, U. (1972). The signs of language in child and chimpanzee. In R. Alloway, L. Krames, & P. Pliner (Eds.), *Communication and affect. A comparative approach.* New York: Academic Press.

Klima, E. S., & Bellugi, U. (1979). *The signs of language.* Cambridge, MA: Harvard University Press.

Kuhl, P. K., Williams, K. A., Lacerda, F., Stevens, K. N., & Lindblom, B. (1992). Linguistic experience alters phonetic perception in infants by 6 months of age. *Science, 255,* 606–608.

Lane, H. (1979). *The wild boy of Aveyron.* Cambridge, MA: Harvard University Press.

Lenneberg, E. (1967). *The biological foundations of language.* New York: Wiley.

Lieberman, P. (1991). *Uniquely human: The evolution of speech, thought and selfless behavior.* Cambridge, MA: Harvard University Press.

Lieven, E. (1978). Conversations between mothers and young children: Individual differences and their possible implications for the study of language learning. In N. Waterson & C. E. Snow (Eds.), *The development of communication.* New York: Wiley.

Locke, J. L. (1990). Structure and stimulation in the ontogeny of spoken language. *Developmental Psychobiology, 23*(7), 621–644.

Locke, J. L. (1993). *The child's path to spoken language.* Cambridge, MA: Harvard University Press.

Lorenz, K. (1971). *Studies in animal behavior.* Cambridge, MA: Harvard University Press.

MacWhinney, B. (1995). *The CHILDES project: Tools for analyzing talk, 2nd edition.* Hillsdale, NJ: Erlbaum.

MacWhinney, B. (1999). From CHILDES to TalkBank: New systems for studying human communication. Paper presented at the VIIIth International Congress for the Study of Child Language, San Sebastian, Spain, 12–16 July.

Maple, T. L., & Cone, S. G. (1981). Aged apes at the Yerkes Regional Primate Research Center. *Laboratory Primate Newsletter, 20,* 10–12.

Marler, P. (1990). Innate learning preferences: Signals for communication. *Developmental Psychobiology, 23* (7), 557–569.

Masataka, N. (1993). Effects of contingent and noncontingent maternal stimulation on the vocal behavior of three- to-four-month-old Japanese infants. *Journal of Child Language, 20,* 303–312.

McCarthy, D. (1954). Language development in children. In P. Mussen (Ed.), *Carmichael's manual of child psychology.* New York: Wiley.

Menn, L., & Bernstein Ratner, N. (Eds.). (2000). *Methods for studying language production.* Mahway, NJ: Lawrence Erlbaum Associates.

Miles, H. L. (1983). Apes and language: The search for communicative competence. In J. deLuce & H. T. Wilder (Eds.), *Language in primates: Perspectives and implications.* New York: Springer-Verlag.

Nelson, K., & Lucariello, J. (1985). The development of meaning in first words. In M. Barrett (Ed.), *Children's single word speech.* Chichester, England: Wiley.

Papandropoulou, I., & Sinclair, H. (1974). What is a word? *Human Development, 17,* 241–258.

Patterson, F. G. P., & Cohn, R. H. (1990). Language acquisition by a lowland gorilla: Koko's first ten years of vocabulary development. *Word, 41,* 97–143.

Pellegrini, A. D., Brody, G. H., & Stoneman, Z. (1987). Children's conversational competence with their parents. *Discourse Processes, 10,* 93–106.

Pepperberg, I. M. (1991, Spring). Referential communication with an African grey parrot. *Harvard Graduate Society Newsletter,* 1–4.

Pepperberg, I. M. (1994) Vocal learning in grey parrots (psittacus erithacus): Effects of social interaction, reference, and context. *The Auk, 111,* 300–314.

Pinker, S. (1995). *The language instinct.* New York: Harper Perennial.

Premack, A. J. (1976). *Why chimps can read.* New York: Harper and Row.

Réger, Z., & Berko Gleason, J. (1991). Romani child-directed speech and children's language among Gypsies in Hungary. *Language in Society, 20,* 601–617.

Rumbaugh, D. M. (1977). *Language learning by a chimpanzee: The Lana project*. New York: Academic Press.

Rymer, R. (1993). *Genie: An abused child's flight from silence*. New York: Harper Collins.

Savage-Rumbaugh, E. S. (1990). Language acquisition in a nonhuman species: Implications for the innateness debate. *Developmental Psychobiology, 23* (7), 599–620.

Savage-Rumbaugh, E. S. (1993). Language learnability in man, ape, and dolphin. In H. L. Roitblat, L. M. Herman, & P. E. Nachtigall (Eds.), *Language and communication: Comparative perspectives. Comparative cognition and neuroscience* (pp. 457–484). Hillsdale, NJ: Lawrence Erlbaum.

Savage-Rumbaugh, S., Shanker, S. G., & Taylor, T. J. (1998). *Ape language and the human mind*. New York: Oxford University Press.

Shaywitz, B. A., Shaywitz, S. E., Pugh, K. R., Constable, R. T., Skudlarski, P., Fulbright, R. K., Bronen, R. A., Fletcher, J. M., Shankweiler, D. P., Katz, L. & Gore, J. C. (1995). Sex differences in the functional organization of the brain for language. *Nature, 6515,* 607–610.

Skinner, B. F. (1957). *Verbal behavior*. Englewood, NJ: Prentice-Hall.

Slobin, D. (1979). *Psycholinguistics* (2nd ed.). Glenview, IL: Scott, Foresman.

Snow, C. E. (1977). The development of conversation between mothers and babies. *Journal of Child Language, 4,* 1–22.

Snow, C. E. (1983). Literacy and language: Relationships during the preschool years. *Harvard Educational Review, 55,* 165–189.

Snow, C. E. (1990). The development of definitional skill. *Journal of Child Language, 17,* 697–710.

Snow, C. E., Perlmann, R. Y., Berko Gleason, J., & Hooshyar, N. (1990). Developmental perspectives on politeness: Sources of children's knowledge. *Journal of Pragmatics, 14,* 289–305.

Stoel-Gammon, C. (1998). The role of babbling and phonology in early linguistic development. In A. M. Wetherby, S. F. Warren, & J. Reichle (Eds.), *Transitions in prelinguistic communication: Preintentional to intentional and presymbolic to symbolic* (pp. 87–110). Baltimore: Brookes.

Stoel-Gammon, C., & Cooper, J. (1984). Patterns of early lexical and phonological development. *Journal of Child Language, 2,* 247–271.

Tager-Flusberg, H. (1999). The challenge of studying language development in children with autism. In L. Menn & N. Bernstein Ratner (Eds.), *Methods for studying language production*. Mahwah, NJ: Lawrence Erlbaum Associates.

Terrace, H. S. (1980). *Nim: A chimpanzee who learned sign language*. New York: Knopf.

Van Cantfort, T. E., & Rimpau, J. G. (1982). Sign language studies with children and chimpanzees. *Sign Language Studies, 34,* 15–72.

von Frisch, K. (1950). *Bees, their vision, chemical senses, and language*. Ithaca, NY: Cornell University Press.

Werker, J. F., & Tees, R. C. (1984). Cross-language speech perception: Evidence for perceptual reorganization during the first year of life. *Infant Behavior and Development, 7,* 49–64.

Chapter *2*

Communication Development in Infancy

Jacqueline Sachs
University of Connecticut

Most infants do not use their first word until around one year of age, and that first word is so special to their parents that the date is often noted in the "baby book" as "when baby started to talk." However, before that exciting event, much has happened that establishes the foundation for later stages in the acquisition of language. In this chapter we will discuss communication development in the period before the use of words. Although this stage is **preverbal** (sometimes called **prelinguistic**), the infant is responsive to language, vocalizes in a variety of ways, and, usually toward the end of the first year, discovers the possibility of communication through nonword vocalizations and gestures.

In the first chapter, we saw that there is a biological basis for language. Even before birth, the infant's brain and sensory systems are preparing for the task of acquiring a language. The fetus can hear sounds generated outside the mother's abdomen (Querleu & Renard, 1981), and newborn infants are affected by what they have heard before birth. They have heard their mothers' voices best, and at birth are already more responsive to their mothers' voices than they are to strangers' voices (DeCasper & Fifer, 1980). They even prefer the sound of the language they have been exposed to over the sound of a language they have not heard, probably responding primarily to the intonation patterns of the languages. For example, when French babies were played samples of French and Japanese speech, they listened more attentively to the French (Mehler, Jusczyk, Lambertz, Halsted, Bertoncini, & Amiel-Tison, 1988; Nazzi, Bertoncini, & Mehler, 1998).

Though those newborn French babies preferred French, if they had suddenly started hearing Japanese they would have been ready to start learning it, too. Most of the sounds that are used in speech (including those in languages to which the infant has never been exposed) are well discriminated by young infants (see Jusczyk, 1997, for a review of this area). Some research suggests that these discrimination abilities reflect special mechanisms for the processing of speech that are unique to humans (Eimas, 1974; Mehler & Christophe, 1995). However, already during the first year of life, infants' speech perception abilities gradually become shaped by the language heard, so that the ability to discriminate many of the sounds that are not used in their language is lost by about one year of age (Kuhl, Williams, Lacerda, Stevens, & Lindblom, 1992; Werker & Tees, 1984). If the French babies have not heard any Japanese, by the time they begin to say words they would not hear Japanese sounds in exactly the same way that the Japanese infant does.

As infants develop and experience their language, they build up an expectation of what their language sounds like. By late in the first year, certain familiar words become linked with objects or experiences, and infants begin to comprehend the meaning of some words well before they begin to speak (Fenson, Dale, Reznick, Bates, Thal, & Pethick, 1994). By that time they will normally have had a great deal of experience listening to speech. Table 2.1 shows the typical pattern of responses to sounds and speech in the first year of life. There are, however, large individual differences in the exact ages at which babies achieve these milestones.

The infants' ability to vocalize also changes dramatically in the first year of life. At birth, infants can only cry, but this is the first of many signals that inform caregivers about their needs. By the end of the first year, most babies will make sounds that reflect the sound patterns in the language heard. Table 2.2 shows the typical order of emergence of various types of vocalizations in the first year, with approximate ages. As with responses to sounds, there are individual differences in the ages at which infants achieve milestones in development, but the pattern appears to be the same across a wide variety of environmental and developmental conditions (Fenson et al., 1994;

Table 2.1	**Examples of the Typical Order of Emergence of Responses to Sounds and Speech in the First Year, with Approximate Ages**
Newborn	Is startled by a loud noise
	Turns head to look in the direction of sound
	Is calmed by the sound of a voice
	Prefers mother's voice to a stranger's
	Discriminates many of the sounds used in speech
1–2 mos.	Smiles when spoken to
3–7 mos.	Responds differently to different intonations (e.g., friendly, angry)
8–12 mos.	Responds to name
	Responds to "no"
	Recognizes phrases from games (e.g., "Peekaboo," "How big is baby?")
	Recognizes words from routines (e.g., waves to "bye-bye")
	Recognizes some words

$\mathcal{T}able$ 2.2	Examples of the Typical Order of Emergence of Types of Nonword Vocalizations in the First Year, with Approximate Ages
Newborn	Cries
1–3 mos.	Makes cooing sounds in response to speech ("oo," "goo")
	Laughs
	Cries in different ways when hungry, angry, or hurt
	Makes more speechlike sounds in response to speech
4–6 mos.	Plays with some sounds, usually single syllables (e.g., "ba," "ga")
6–8 mos.	Babbles with duplicated sounds (e.g., "bababa")
	Attempts to imitate some sounds
8–12 mos.	Babbles with consonant or vowel changes (e.g., "badaga," "babu")
	Babbles with sentencelike intonation (expressive jargon/conversational babble)
	Produces protowords

Oller, Eilers, Steffens, Lynch, & Urbano, 1994). Chapter 3 will provide more detail on sound production during this period as it relates to the development of the ability to produce speech sounds.

In this chapter, we will focus on the role that sounds made by infants play in the relationship between infants and their caregivers. With that first cry begins an amazingly complex interactive process, the success of which depends both on the ability of the infant to signal messages clearly, and the ability of the caregiver to interpret those signals. While cries will alert the caregiver to the infant's physical needs, other vocalizations such as cooing, laughing, and babbling are evidence of the infant's inherent interest in social contact.

In recent years, there has been great interest in the caregiver-infant dyad. (We will use the term **caregiver** because, even though many studies have looked at mothers and their infants, other communicative partners, including older children, also play a role in the infant's development.) Infants seem helpless and, indeed, are completely dependent on their caregivers. However, human infants have biologically given attributes and behaviors that draw caregivers to them. They are not simply passive recipients of stimulation, but instead are active interactional partners who are equipped to obtain the experiences that they need to develop. How the infant acts affects the subsequent behavior of the caregiver (Lewis & Rosenblum, 1974; Worobey, 1989), as has been shown in studies of various aspects of communication, such as eye contact. For example, it has been found that eye contact is very important to caregivers in establishing the original affective bond with the infant. Fraiberg (1974) discovered that parents of congenitally blind children often had difficulty in relating to their infants for this reason. Similarly, the parent of an autistic infant often will notice eye aversion as the very first sign of abnormality (Stern, 1971). In contrast, the normally interacting infant and caregiver form a mutual admiration society, engaging in "**gaze coupling**" that very much resembles conversational turn-taking (Jaffe, Stern, & Perry, 1973).

In vocal interaction, too, the caregiver is affected by the child's behavior. For example, in the course of carrying out research on young babies' vocalizations, Bloom (1990) noticed that occasionally students and staff members who overheard a tape made remarks like "That baby is really talking up a storm!" (p. 131). Suspecting that perhaps the adults were responding to specific sorts of infant vocalizations, Bloom and Lo (1990) had adults rate videotapes of three-month-old babies who were making sounds that were more speechlike or less speechlike. The adults preferred the babies who produced sounds that were more like speech, rating them "cuddlier," "more fun," and generally more likable.

The cooing and babbling sounds that infants make also draw caregivers into "conversations" with them. By even three months of age, if an adult responds vocally to a baby's sounds, the baby in turn will begin to produce more speechlike sounds. Furthermore, babies learn to wait for the adult's response after they have vocalized.

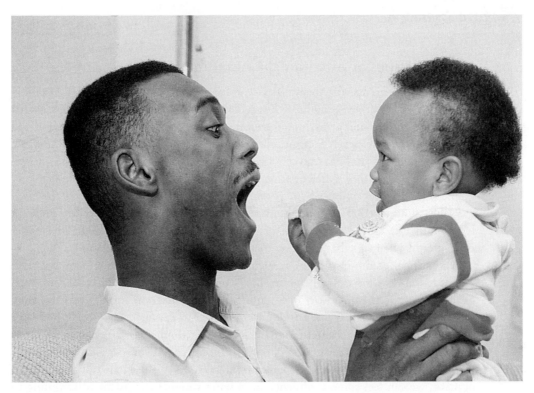

Gaze coupling in infancy is an important part of early communication development.

Thus, both the adult and the infant are constantly influencing one another in establishing conversation-like vocal interactions during a period well before the child uses words (Masataka, 1993).

From the beginning, the crying, cooing, and babbling of young infants are communicative in the sense that the infant is a member of a social species and caregivers are alert to those signals. However, in the latter part of the first year of life, the normally developing infant makes a very important discovery that provides a transition to language: that one can intentionally make a signal (a vocalization or a gesture) and expect that it will have a specific effect on the caregiver. Thus signals begin to have meanings arising out of the shared experiences of the child and the caregiver. In the next section, we will look in more detail at what typically occurs in the emergence of **intentional communication**. After that, we will look at some aspects of the social context of the emergence of these behaviors. Although we have divided what the infants do and what caregivers do into two sections for organizational purposes, keep in mind that the behaviors of infants and their caregivers are always mutually affecting one another.

The Expression of Communicative Intent Before Speech

Characteristics of Intentional Communication

Although most parents view their infants' vocalizations as communicative and meaningful from as early as three months of age (Miller, 1988), there is little indication at that age that the child is doing anything *intentionally* to obtain the caregiver's attention and help. In contrast, at eleven months, an infant might point to an object out of reach, make eye contact with the caregiver, look at the object again, and make a sound. How is this sequence of actions different from merely crying or fussing? Is it an example of intentional communication?

Deciding whether any one instance of behavior is intentionally communicative is very difficult. Think, for example, of a dog barking by the kitchen door. The owner may interpret that signal as meaning that the animal wants to be let out. Is the barking intentional communication or a behavior that simply is repeated because in the past it has lead to the desired event? How would one decide? There has been much debate about the characteristics of intentional communication and the issue of when the infant deliberately vocalizes or gestures in order to get the caregiver's help. Trying to establish a single crucial criterion for deciding whether a particular behavior is intentionally communicative seems hopeless. However, if we use a set of criteria, applying them to the infant's entire behavioral repertoire at a particular point in development, we can feel some confidence in judging whether the infant is beginning to communicate with intentionality (Bakeman & Adamson, 1984; Bates, 1979; Bruner,

1973; Harding & Golinkoff, 1979; Scoville, 1983; Sugarman, 1984). The following are among the criteria that are often applied:

1. The child makes eye contact with the partner while gesturing or vocalizing, often alternating his or her gaze between an object and the partner.

2. The child's gestures and vocalizations have become consistent and ritualized. For example, a child named Annie used a gesture of opening and closing her hand when she wanted something, rather than attempting to reach the object herself. The vocalization she used, "eh eh," was one that she consistently used in situations in which she wanted something. Another child would probably use a different sound in the same situation, because this sound was not copied from adult speech but rather was a communicative signal invented by Annie.

3. After a gesture or vocalization, the child pauses to wait for a response from the partner.

4. The child persists in attempting to communicate if he or she is not understood and sometimes even modifies behavior to communicate more clearly.

When an infant's behaviors are viewed in terms of such criteria, there is not a distinct boundary between behavior without communicative intent and intentional communication, or an exact age at which we classify the infant as intentionally communicative. Rather, the child moves gradually toward an understanding of goals and the potential role of others in achieving them (Harding, 1983a, 1983b). For example, in one study (Mosier & Rogoff, 1994) the mothers of infants ranging from six to thirteen months of age held a desirable toy out of reach. Observers videotaped and scored the infants' gaze, gestures, and vocalizations for signs that the infants were trying to influence their mothers, rather than simply attempting to get the toy or expressing frustration. In this situation, even some six-month-old infants were judged as deliberately using their mothers to meet their goals. For the average baby, we expect that the first signs of intentional communication will emerge between eight to ten months of age (Bates, Camaioni, & Volterra, 1975; Harding & Golinkoff, 1979). When we try to determine whether an infant has begun to communicate intentionally, even small differences in the situations observed or the criteria used to classify gestures or vocalizations as intentional will affect our judgments, but certainly the transition from inadvertent communicator to intentional communicator is a major one for both the child and that child's caregivers (Carpenter, Nagell, & Tomasello, 1998).

This is not to say that the infant who is not yet even using words understands the communicative process in the same way an older child does. A full realization of how words or gestures affect the knowledge and beliefs of others is a much later development, and even a talkative four-year-old is still learning about how communication takes place. Other aspects of the emergence of communicative intent will be discussed in Chapter 6. (Also, see Bloom, 1993; Golinkoff, 1993; Shatz & O'Reilly, 1990; Shwe & Markman, 1997.)

The Functions of Early Communicative Behaviors

Analyses of the functions of early communication stem from detailed observations of children's behaviors in various situations. For example, Halliday (1975) studied his son Nigel's progress in attempting to communicate between nine and sixteen months and found that several consistent nonword vocalizations seemed to convey meanings. Bates and her colleagues (Bates, 1979; Bates et al., 1975) reported on the gestures as well as preverbal vocalizations of the children they studied.

A number of different terms and systems of classification for early **communicative functions** have been proposed (e.g., Bates et al., 1975; Bruner, 1981; Chapman, 1981; Dore, 1974; Seibert & Hogan, 1982; Sugarman, 1984). Most systems distinguish at least between vocalizations or gestures that influence the listener to do something and vocalizations or gestures that direct the listener's attention, often with further subcategories, as shown here with examples of typical behaviors:

1. **Imperative Communicative Function** or **Behavioral Modification**

    A. *Rejection.* Consistent gestures or vocalizations are used to terminate an interaction. For example, the child pushes away an offered object and vocalizes, or uses a gesture or vocalization to end an action.

    B. *Request.* Consistent gestures or vocalizations are used to get the partner to do something or to help the child achieve a goal.

        1. **Request for social interaction.** Used to attract and maintain the partner's attention. For example, a child who is being ignored might use a vocalization or gesture to get the caregiver's attention.

        2. **Request for an object.** Used to indicate desire for an object. In our earlier example, Annie tried to obtain something she could not get herself by her abbreviated reaching gesture and vocalization.

        3. **Request for action.** Used to initiate an action by the listener. For example, the infant might lift her arms and use a vocalization when she wants to be picked up.

2. **Declarative Communicative Function** or **Comment.**

    Consistent gestures or vocalizations are used to direct the partner's attention for the purpose of jointly noticing an object or event. For example, the infant might "show" an object to the caregiver by holding it out and vocalizing, or the infant might give an object to the caregiver. Pointing might be used not for the purpose of obtaining an object, but for directing the partner's attention to an object. (This function is also referred to as **joint attention.**)

All of these communicative functions are expressed by normally developing infants before they begin to use words (Wetherby, Cain, Yonclas, & Walker, 1988). When children begin to talk using real words from their language, these words emerge within a rich framework of communicative functions that have been established toward the end of their first year of life.

The Forms of Early Communicative Behaviors

Early communication takes place using both gestures and sounds. As an example of a communicative gesture, consider pointing. Pointing is unlike reaching for something. When you reach, your fingers are open, but when you point, the index finger is extended while the other fingers are curled. Most infants begin pointing at objects or pictures around ten months of age (Murphy, 1978; Zinober & Martlew, 1985). By twelve months, many infants point at an object and then shift their gaze to make eye contact with the listener (Bates, 1979; Masur, 1983).

The infant also learns that the appropriate response to a caregiver's point is to look in the direction indicated by the finger, not at the end of the finger itself. (When you have a chance, observe the response of a dog or cat to pointing.) Babies usually begin responding appropriately to points by others a little later than they begin to use pointing themselves.

You may wonder why a book about *language* development even includes a discussion of pointing. For an adult speaker, although gestures typically accompany speech, they do not seem a part of "language" in the same way sounds, words, or sentences are. However, for the infant, both gestures and sounds can, and normally do, serve as symbols. The emergence of both types of symbols reflects an important developmental change in the child's mental ability. For example, babies who discover early how to communicate by pointing tend to be early in other aspects of language development as well, such as beginning to understand words (Butterworth & Morissette, 1996). Whether a child will eventually use predominantly sounds or gestures in communicating depends on the linguistic environment: spoken language or a gesture-based system such as American Sign Language. The hearing baby in a spoken-language environment will typically use more and more spoken words, but the child exposed to sign language will learn it just as easily as a deaf baby will.

While pointing continues to be a part of nonverbal communication throughout life, there are other communicative gestures used for a time by infants that may not even be noticed by their caregivers. Such gestures were first described by Goldin-Meadow and her colleagues (e.g., Goldin-Meadow, 1979; Goldin-Meadow & Morford, 1985) as they carried out studies of the communicative development of profoundly deaf children. Most deaf infants are born to hearing parents, and some families decide not to expose their deaf children to sign language in order to motivate the child to learn speech (following an oral approach to education of the deaf). The researchers found that these deaf children spontaneously developed gestures that were not based on gestures used by the parents. The babies actually invented a way to attempt to communicate. What about hearing babies? Acredolo and Goodwyn (1988) observed the behavior of normally hearing infants and found that they also attempted to convey a whole range of communicative functions using gestures. Since the babies' caregivers were not typically watching for gestural communication, many times they did not even realize that consistent gestures were being used. Acredolo and Goodwyn (1998) have written a book for caregivers in which they suggest that responding to an infant's gestures and even teaching the infant some signs is beneficial for communicative development. Whether or not that proves to be the case, recognizing that babies do try to communicate with gestures may make life easier for caregivers who are trying to figure out what their babies want! Of course, as hearing infants begin to pick up words, they come to depend increasingly on vocal communication to get their ideas across, and spontaneously some of the invented gestures fade away (Messinger & Fogel, 1998).

The vocalizations used by children shortly before they begin learning conventional words have also received much attention, because they form an interesting link between preverbal communication and speech. Preverbal vocalizations that contain consistent sound patterns and are used in consistent situations, but are unique to the child rather than based on the adult language, are referred to as **protowords.** For example, intonation patterns in nonword vocalizations can be used communicatively. Halliday (1975) discovered that his child used vocalizations with rising intonation contours for requests and falling contours for comments. Similar patterns have been found in other children (Flax, Lahey, Harris, & Boothroyd, 1991; Menn, 1976).

Children sometimes use vowel sounds consistently to convey certain emotions. One baby used the sound "eee" when he wanted an object, but used "uuu" for expressing disapproval (von Raffler Engel, 1973). Consonant sounds can also appear in protowords. For example, an infant might start using some vocalization (let us imagine that it sounds like "lala") when he is rubbing his blanket against his cheek, and then at a later time use "lala" when he wants his blanket. Sometimes the family even adopts the baby's "word" for a while, saying things that would be a mystery to strangers, like "I think he wants his lala."

Carter (1979) studied a child named David over several months as he began to communicate intentionally, and noted that his preverbal vocalizations were initially quite variable in their pronunciation but were always linked with particular gestures. For example, several sounds similar to "ba" accompanied by waving hands seemed to signal that he did not want something, whereas sounds incorporating "mmm" accompanied by reaching meant that he did want it. Over time, the vocalizations became more phonetically stable and less tied to a particular action. Other investigators have also noticed that vocalizations and gestures are originally linked together, but become more independent over time (e.g., Greenfield & Smith, 1976).

Some terms other than *protoword* that you may come across in reading about these interesting early language inventions are **phonetically consistent form (PCF)** (Dore, Franklin, Miller, & Ramer, 1976) and **vocable** (Ferguson, 1978). As we noted above for communicative gestures, it can be very helpful (and fun) for caregivers to listen for protowords and try to understand what the infant means. (See also Chapter 3 for further discussion of protowords.)

The Assessment of Communicative Intent

One might wish to assess a child's communicative abilities as a part of carrying out research on communication development, or in a clinical evaluation, in order to find out whether that child is progressing as expected compared with other children of the same age. In research, a method called **low-structured observation** is sometimes used (Coggins, Olswang, & Guthrie, 1987). The caregiver is instructed to play with the child in a natural way, and a trained observer scores the child's behavior either during the session or from a videotape. For example, the observer would look for instances of commenting, as indicated by the child's pointing at, showing, or giving objects (sometimes accompanied by consistent vocalizations).

In a **structured observation**, one manipulates the situation somewhat to increase the likelihood of observing the behavior of interest. For example, a **communicative temptation task** could be used to entice the child to produce requests (Casby & Cumpata, 1986; Dale, 1980; Snyder, 1984; Sugarman, 1978). The child might be presented with an attractive toy inside a tightly covered plastic container. An infant who is not yet communicating intentionally might bang the container and fuss or cry in frustration, while another preverbal infant might hand the container to an adult, make eye contact, point to the toy and/or vocalize, and persist in such behaviors that seem to be directed toward the adult. Similarly, one could see how the child expresses rejection by having some less desirable toys along. If such a toy is given to the child while more desirable toys are in view, the child may potentially produce rejection gestures and/or vocalizations (Olswang, Bain, Dunn, & Cooper, 1983).

To aid in a clinical evaluation, there are norms available for various aspects of language development, including the period before words are used, based on a large study that collected mothers' reports on their children's communicative behaviors (Fenson et al., 1994). The questions used in the study are available as two scales called the **MacArthur Communicative Development Inventories (CDI)**, one used for infants eight to sixteen months of age and the other for toddlers sixteen to thirty months of age (Fenson, Dale, Reznick, Thal, Bates, Hartung, Pethick, & Reilly, 1993). Typically, the child's mother is asked to report on words comprehended or said and is asked specific questions about her child's communicative behavior.

Although the MacArthur project and others have revealed that there are wide variations in the ages at which children learn language, a continuing goal in research is to find reliable early clues that would predict whether a child is having difficulty acquiring language. For example, if a baby seems somewhat slow in beginning to speak, but is understanding language and attempting to communicate with protowords or gestures, there would be less concern than there would be for a baby the same age who showed no interest in communication (McCathren, Warren, & Yoder, 1996; Tamis-Lemonda, Bornstein, Kahana-Kalman, Baumwell, & Cyphers, 1998). (See also Chapter 9 regarding atypical language development, and Cole, Dale, & Thal, 1996, for more information on assessment procedures.)

Cognition, Social Cognition, and Intentional Communication

Why does intentional communication emerge when it does? Can we identify some other underlying changes in the infant's mental processes or social abilities that appear at the same time and might be related to this development?

The developmental theory of the Swiss psychologist Jean Piaget (e.g., Piaget, 1952) has been one source of hypotheses about the cognitive changes that support the emergence of intentional communication. Piaget was interested in how the child's ability to solve problems concerning objects in the world changes over time. He argued that the infant is innately endowed with certain reflexes and with basic processes for learning from its interaction with objects in the environment. Thus, the infant's knowledge is constructed through a series of predictable stages in cognitive development.

The period from birth until about eighteen to twenty-four months is called the **sensorimotor stage.** In this stage, the infant is beginning the process of learning how to think. Piaget argued that the infant can experience objects through his or her senses and through actions with the objects, but does not yet have functional mental representations of them. For instance, a young infant might reach out to grasp an attractive toy, but when the toy is moved out of view, the infant stops reaching and appears not to remember his or her interest in the toy. Such behavior was taken as an indication that the infant did not hold a mental image of the toy in mind that would provide the basis for a continued effort to obtain the toy.

However, there are changes in the infant's cognitive abilities within the sensorimotor stage, and one of these changes has been viewed as possibly related to the changes in the infant's communicative abilities in the latter part of the first year of life. Between the ages of four and eight months, infants learn that they can make something happen again by repeating an activity that has led to the event, but they do not yet have a real sense of how to obtain the desired effect. Between eight and twelve months (called **Piagetian Stage** 4), infants begin to understand the relation between actions and outcomes. For example, the baby may pull on a cloth to bring an object into reach (an example of primitive tool using). She will begin to experiment with actions to see what the result will be, and start to be able to think ahead about what the result of an action might be. Also during this period, the infant will begin to anticipate what typically happens. For example, Piaget reported that at nine months his daughter would cry when someone stood up, because she had noticed that standing up was often followed by leaving. This change can be summarized by saying that the infant is attaining a **means–ends concept,** understanding that problems can be solved mentally so that a goal can be attained by methods other than trial-and-error.

It has been found that the emergence of the ability to express communicative intent corresponds, at least temporally, with Stage 4 cognitive changes such as those described above. Babies begin to communicate intentionally when they have learned that there are causes for events. As they learn that it is possible to bring about changes through various means, they discover that one of these means is to use another person to carry out one's goal. Thus the child is motivated to communicate to another person, rather than simply to attempt to achieve the goal himself (Bates, 1976; Harding & Golinkoff, 1979).

Piaget's descriptions of stages in development have been very influential and form the basis for much research about the relation between nonlinguistic thinking and language, as well as the basis for some clinical assessment of infants and children. However, other theorists have pointed out that Piaget's primary interest was in the child's understanding of the material world and that this focus may have led Piaget to ignore the importance of the child's social nature. Trevarthen and Hubley (1978) argued that the infant is from birth a social creature, able to share himself with others (a characteristic they called "primary intersubjectivity"), but that a major maturational change takes place in the infant's **social cognition** around nine to ten months as the infant becomes able to share *experiences* with others. Now the infant manages a three-term interaction consisting of the speaker, the listener, and the referent. This change, called the attainment of **secondary intersubjectivity,** is the basis of intentional communication, in their view. Sugarman (1978, 1984) used a similar framework in her description of the emergence of intentional communication: Before approximately ten months of age, infants can relate to *either* a person or an object, but after that they can relate to a person *about* an object.

The Social Context of the Preverbal Infant

Here we will look at some aspects of early communicative interaction between caregivers and preverbal infants. We will see that caregivers speak to infants in special ways, that they create situations in which their babies will have an opportunity to take their turns at talking, and that they behave in other ways that may be supportive of infants' attempts to communicate. We will not be able to describe all of the ways in which adults and infants communicate, but we will concentrate on those aspects of communication that seem most closely related to later language development. In describing the social context in which communication emerges, we are not arguing that social interaction *causes* the child to begin to communicate or that adults *teach* their infants to communicate. Think, for example, of trying to be supportive of communicative development with your cat or dog. Clearly, one cannot teach a cat or a dog to react like a baby! The infant has the **biological capacity** for certain sorts of behaviors and abilities to develop. However, that biological capacity will not be realized without certain kinds of environmental supports. An important goal of research concerning the social context of communicative development is to find out what kinds of experiences are sufficient to allow normal development and how variations in experiences ultimately affect the language abilities of the child.

The Sound of the Caregiver's Speech: "Listen to Me!"

Speech addressed to babies is typically quite unlike the speech directed to adults. We even have a name for it—**baby talk.** You will also see the terms **infant-directed speech (IDS)** and **child-directed speech (CDS)** used to refer to this speech style. The term *baby talk,* in particular, may merely bring to mind adult imitations of childlike speech ("Is ooo my tweetie-pie?") and special vocabulary words like *choo-choo* and *pottie,* along with strong denials that *you* would ever "use baby talk." However, as we will see here and in later chapters, there are actually many very interesting aspects of speech and language that are modified when we talk to infants and young children, and we make most of these modifications without even being aware of them. One of the most dramatic characteristics of talk to preverbal babies is that "the **prosodic features** or 'music' appears to be more important than the words or 'lyrics'" (Stern & Wasserman, 1979, p. 3). Special intonation patterns with higher pitch, more variable pitch, and exaggerated stress have been found in baby talk in a variety of languages.

Fernald and her colleagues (Fernald, 1989, 1992; Fernald, Taeschner, Dunn, Papousek, de Boysson-Bardies, & Fukui, 1989) have suggested that special intonation patterns may be a universal characteristic of baby talk. However, there are some differences in baby talk across cultures. Higher pitch and exaggerated intonation to infants were not found to be characteristic of rural African American families in North Carolina (Heath, 1983), Kaluli families in New Guinea (Schieffelin, 1979, 1990), and Quiche-Mayan families in Guatemala (Bernstein Ratner & Pye, 1984). Perhaps there are some general tendencies, such as using higher pitch, but these tendencies can be affected by other aspects of the way language is used in a particular culture. For example, Quiche-Mayan speakers use higher pitch as a sign of respect and thus might find higher pitch socially inappropriate for use with a baby. Baby talk speech modifications such as higher pitch may reflect social conventions that can vary from culture to culture (Ingram, 1995).

Next we will look in a little more detail at some of the possible reasons for the baby-talk characteristics that have been found in many cultures. Since certain prosodic features in speech to babies are common across many languages, it may be that these characteristics are used because they are especially appropriate. We can find out about babies' perceptual abilities and preferences by devising experiments in which they can "tell" us what they want to listen to. Infants cannot talk or press buttons, but they can turn their heads and control their eye movements, so a researcher might set up a situation in which a message plays only when the baby's head turns in a certain direction or when the eyes are fixated on a pattern and measure the amount of time the baby thereby "chooses" to listen to one message or another. (A very important application of such techniques is for the testing of hearing in young infants.) A number of studies have shown that babies prefer baby-talk patterns (Fernald, 1985; Fernald & Kuhl, 1987; Sullivan & Horowitz, 1983; Werker & McLeod, 1989), even when only two days old (Cooper & Aslin, 1990).

If babies are naturally responsive to speech that has certain features, adults may use these characteristics because they discover or know intuitively that infants pay more attention to them when they do. By holding the infant's attention, the adult may help to cement the emotional bond between caregiver and child (Sachs, 1977). The attentive infant becomes quiet, faces the speaker, establishes eye contact, and responds to the adult. Children, of course, can learn language even if they are not in loving interactions, given their resilient biologically based language abilities, but adult–infant attachment may be involved in the optimal development of communication. For example, Cicchetti (1989) has reported significant language delays in maltreated toddlers. (For further discussion of the relation between affective development and communicative development, see Prizant & Wetherby, 1990.)

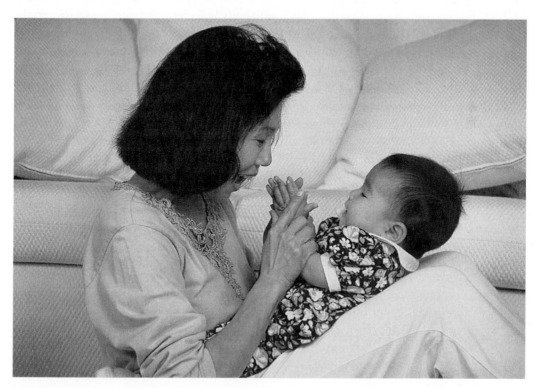

Infants are responsive to the prosodic features of baby talk.

As the infant attends carefully to the sound of the caregiver's speech, opportunities arise for processing and comprehending some aspects of speech considerably before the emergence of the first word. Locke (1993, 1994) suggested that the sound of the caregiver's voice provides the foundation for the child's entry into language learning: "Spoken language piggybacks on this open channel, taking advantage of mother–infant attachment by embedding new information in the same stream of cues" (Locke, 1994, p. 441). The voice will continue to carry information about emotional state, but the child will eventually discover that it also consists of sounds, that these sounds create meaningful words, and that the words combine to convey even more complex messages. For example, the exaggerated prosodic patterns of baby talk may help the infant become aware of the general intent of a message, such as praising, prohibiting, playing, or comforting, before individual linguistic elements are understood (Fernald, 1989).

Word learning could also be facilitated. There is a tendency to pronounce labels for objects more distinctly in baby talk, with less variability than one finds in speech to adults (Kuhl et al., 1997). Labels are also spoken with exaggerated stress and higher, more variable pitch (Fernald & Mazzie, 1991), perhaps encouraging the infant's attention to these words. In a study in which depressed mothers and nondepressed mothers were given passages to say to their four-month-old infants, it was found that the depressed mothers used less pitch variability (a flatter intonation) in saying certain words. This result is not surprising since flatness of affect is a common symptom of depression, but, interestingly, the infants of the depressed mothers showed poorer associative learning of the words they had just heard than did the infants of the normal mothers (Kaplan, Bachorowski, & Zarlengo-Strouse, 1999).

Baby-talk characteristics may even make it easier for infants to begin to segment larger units of speech. In one study, when preverbal seven- to nine-month-old babies heard samples of baby talk, they preferred to listen to messages in which the timing matched the natural clause structure of English rather than samples with altered clause structure. However, when the researchers played adult-directed speech to the babies, the babies did not discriminate between samples with natural and altered clause structure. This finding suggests that whether the samples had baby-talk features certainly made a difference for the babies processing abilities (Kemler-Nelson, Hirsh-Pasek, Jusczyk, & Wright-Cassidy, 1989).

A word of caution: Most studies to date have been carried out in the United States with babies of urban, middle-class families. Since babies everywhere learn to speak, one must be hesitant about concluding that some particular feature of baby talk is necessary (or even very useful) for babies. We do not know enough yet to tell caregivers how they *should* talk to babies. Research on language learning environments in a wide variety of cultures is needed (Blount, 1990), as is research to discover whether there are causal links between certain features of the linguistic environment and language learning.

The Conversational Nature of the Caregiver's Speech: "Talk to Me!"

Caregivers talk to infants in a way that is not simply engaging, but in a way that encourages the baby to participate. Based on her observations of mothers interacting with babies in England, Snow (1977) argued that the mothers' primary goal in talking with their infants seemed to be to have a "conversation" with them. Even at an early stage when the adult knows that the infant does not yet understand language, the adult behaves as if the child's response is a turn in the conversation. Here is a little "conversation" between a mother and her three-month-old daughter, Ann (p. 12):

Mother	**Ann**
	(smiles)
Oh what a nice little smile.	
Yes, isn't that nice?	
There. There's a nice little smile.	
	(burps)
What a nice wind as well!	
Yes, that's better, isn't it?	
Yes.	
Yes.	
Yes!	
	(vocalizes)
There's a nice noise.	

In this example, the mother spoke in short, simple utterances, although of course the three-month-old could not understand the content of the speech. The mother responded to whatever her infant did, commenting on the various nonverbal and vocal behaviors that occurred and incorporating them into the conversation. It is as if she allowed the infant's behaviors to stand for a turn in the interaction and treated the behavior, whether a vocalization or a burp, as if it were intentional communication on the part of the infant.

Snow also noticed that the mothers devoted many of their utterances to attempting to elicit some kind of behavior from the infant, such as coos and smiles. In contrast to adult–adult conversations, where we often must try very hard to get our own turn, each mother seemed intent on giving her child many turns in the conversation. Often the mothers' utterances were followed by pauses, providing the opportunity for responses from the infant, as in this example (Snow, 1977, p. 13):

Oh you are a funny little one, aren't you, hmm? (pause)

Aren't you a funny little one? (pause)

Hmm? (pause)

Although the mothers had accepted almost any behavior on the part of their three-month-olds as if it were an attempt to communicate, as the infants grew older, the mothers changed in what they accepted as a turn in the conversation. By seven months, when the babies had begun to be more active partners in the interactions, the mothers responded only to higher-quality vocalizations, such as a babbled sound, and not to sounds such as burps. At twelve months the mothers' criteria for a turn had changed again, and they began to interpret their children's vocalizations as words, as in the following example (Snow, 1977, p. 17):

Mother	Ann
	abaabaa
Baba.	
Yes that's you, what you are.	

Having seen that adults interact conversationally in certain ways with infants in the first year of life, we now consider the effect of this interaction.

The adult's linguistic behavior has an effect on the infant's behavior in the immediate situation. When mothers speak to three-month-old infants, the most common infant response is a vocalization (Lewis & Freedle, 1973). Furthermore, if the caregiver uses a conversational pattern of interaction, where the adult responds in a turn-taking manner to infant vocalizations, the type of sound a three-month-old baby will produce becomes more speechlike in response (Bloom, 1988).

It has also been suggested that the adult's interpretation of the infant's vocalizations may help the child get the idea that communication is possible (Harding, 1983a, 1983b). Adults interpret infants' behaviors as communicative long before the children have an intention to communicate. A two-month-old baby who is crying may be described by her mother as "wanting her diaper changed." The infant at this age is not actually intending a particular message but is crying because of discomfort. However, the fact that the mother accepts the cry as conveying a particular message creates the possibility for the child to begin to communicate different messages with different cries, and eventually perhaps notice the correspondence between the vocalizations and the effect they have on others.

What about the long-term effects of the caregiver's interactive style? We cannot yet conclude that any particular style of caregiver–infant interaction is necessary for language development. Children learn to talk with a wide range of linguistic experiences. For example, Ochs (1988) observed childrearing in Samoa and found that infants were typically not spoken to until they began to speak themselves (although, of course, they heard the speech going on around them). However, some research carried out on American families suggests that caregivers' language usage does at least affect the rate of language learning. For example, looking at the nine-to-eighteen-month period, Clarke-Stewart (1973) found that the amount of talking that a mother did directly with her child (but not the amount of speech to others) was highly correlated with measures of the child's later linguistic competence. This result would suggest that the overall quantity of speech that the child overhears is not so important for the rate of language development, but the quantity of direct adult-to-child talk is. Furthermore, infants whose mothers talk to them frequently using short utterances at nine months perform better on tests of receptive language abilities at eighteen months than do infants of less vocally responsive mothers (Murray, Johnson, & Peters, 1990). Since lower socioeconomic-status mothers within the United States talk less to their infants than do middle-class mothers (Richman, LeVine, New, Howrigan, Wells-Nystrom, Levine, 1988), one important question for future research is whether their less verbally interactive style, while sufficient for eventual language acquisition, slows the acquisition process and ultimately puts their children at a disadvantage in terms of some aspects of broader communicative abilities. If that is the case, it may be possible to improve children's communicative abilities by teaching mothers to interact with them in a more responsive manner. (See Spiker, Ferguson, & Brooks-Gunn, 1993, for an example of one such early intervention project, and Bornstein, 1989, for a discussion of maternal responsiveness.)

Contexts for the Emergence of Object Reference: "Look at That!"

At about six months, infants begin to show a great interest in objects, perhaps reflecting both advances in their visual ability to scan their environment and their motor ability to grasp and manipulate objects. While earlier infants were entertained by face-to-face social interactions, they now are drawn to investigate their surroundings. At this point, the caregivers will usually change the strategy of interacting with their infants, encouraging them to continue interpersonal interactions by jointly exploring objects and their potential (Adamson & Bakeman, 1984). For example, one might see a playful interaction in which a mother dramatically wiggles a toy cow, saying "Look at the *cow*! What does the cow say? The cow says 'mooooo.'" Caregivers label objects (and also the actions or characteristics of objects) in contexts of joint attention. These contexts can to be found in any activity: playing, looking at pictures in books, and carrying out everyday routines such as bathing and feeding.

Research has shown, not surprisingly, that children whose mothers encourage joint attention to objects and supply labels for them increase their vocabularies faster in the early language acquisition period (e.g., Smith, Adamson, & Bakeman, 1988). Again, one could ask whether we can at this point tell caregivers what they *should* do. For example, it probably would not be a good idea to tell moms "Go around the house and label everything in sight." Tomasello and his colleagues (Tomasello, 1988; Tomasello & Farrar, 1986) have shown that words are most likely to be learned if the caregiver focuses on what the child is interested in, providing a word at that moment, rather than trying to direct the child's attention and actively teach the child vocabulary.

When the caregiver follows the child's interest and bases the next utterances on what the child is focusing on, the interactional style is called verbally **sensitive** or **responsive,** as contrasted with a style that is constantly redirecting the child's attention (verbally **intrusive** or **controlling**). For example, if the baby points at his bottle and the mother says "bottle," her utterance would be coded as responsive. If she tried to redirect the child's attention, saying "Look at your book" in the same situation, the utterance would be coded as intrusive. Some studies have found that verbal sensitivity in mothers of preverbal infants predicts better language skills later (e.g., Baumwell, Tamis-Lemonda, & Bornstein, 1997; Carpenter et al., 1998), particularly among low-birthweight infants at risk for developmental delays (Landry, Smith, & Miller-Loncar, 1997).

Of course, as in other areas we have considered, there can be cultural differences in the pattern of joint attention involving objects. For instance, one set of studies revealed differences between mothers in the United States and Japan in the way they interacted with babies, even though both cultures are similar in paying a great deal of attention to infants and children. The American mothers encouraged their young infants when they looked away from them with comments such as "Want to look around? There you go," whereas Japanese mothers discouraged such looking away by saying things like "Say, look at me," and "What's wrong with you?" (Morikawa, Shand, & Kosawa, 1988, pp. 248–249). Also, American mothers often provided a name when the infants looked at objects, whereas Japanese mothers used those objects to engage their infants in social routines (Fernald & Morikawa, 1993). The authors of these reports noted that Americans tend to encourage independence in their children more than the Japanese do. Cultural values may begin to be transmitted by mother–infant interaction at a very early age, affecting subtle aspects of the child's socialization.

In another observation in a different culture, it was found that !Kung San caregivers in Botswana were more likely to interact with an infant when he or she was not focusing on an object. If the infant was attending to an object, the caregivers did not try to join in that interaction in the way seen in many studies of American mothers (Bakeman, Adamson, Konner, & Barr, 1990). (For additional information on the development of joint attention during infancy and the implications of variations in the environment for our understanding of this aspect of development, see Adamson & Bakeman, 1991, and Adamson, 1991.)

Joint attention to objects accompanied by labeling by the caregiver provides an opportunity for the infant to begin to learn names for things. Studies in the United States have found that infants generally comprehend many words before they begin to say words themselves. For most children, the first evidence of word understanding occurs between eight and ten months. At eight months, more than half of a large sample of infants were reported to respond to three words that referred to people ("mommy," "daddy," and their own names), to some words from games and routines, such as "peekaboo," and to "bottle." By eleven months a child typically responded to about fifty words, including many names for common objects (Fenson et al., 1994).

Talk in Structured Situations: "Here's What We Say"

Bruner and his colleagues (e.g., Bruner, 1983; Ratner & Bruner, 1978) have described the way early communication signals develop in structured situations. Bruner has used the term **format** (also called **scaffold**) to refer to such potential learning situations. One such context would be games that are often played with babies. Suppose that in playing a game such as riding "horsie" on daddy's knee, the infant is completely passive initially; he simply hears the words of the game and is moved about. Gradually, however, as the child learns what happens in the game, the father's expectations change. He comes to expect the infant to take a part in the game. Over time the father "raises the ante" so that more and more ritualized or conventional means of expression are demanded at various points in the game. Where the baby was jiggled, he now bounces up and down. Where the father said all of the words, perhaps a word is omitted to be filled in by a vocalization by the child. Eventually, within the game context, both father and child are truly communicating with each other. Such interactions may help the child get the idea that it is possible to communicate, and eventually know what is said in particular communicative situations.

Structured situations need not be games, of course. For example, Heath (1983) has pointed out that even within the United States there are speech communities in which games like pat-a-cake and peekaboo are not played. In some other cultures, play itself is not a normally occurring activity between mother and child (Ochs & Schieffelin, 1984; Schieffelin, 1990). Bruner (1982) has argued that though not all cultures will have play formats, they will have formats of some kind that facilitate the acquisition of language and culture. There may be certain things that are typically said in a feeding situation or when the infant is being dressed. Such routine events that occur frequently provide another way for the infant to begin noticing correspondences between sounds and meaning, initially leading to comprehension of words or phrases in the period just before the child will begin to say words.

The explanation of development that Bruner and other researchers who study the social context of language acquisition propose is similar to that of Lev Vygotsky (1978). Vygotsky was a Russian psychologist who criticized Piaget's theory that cognition developed primarily through the child's learning about the physical world. Vygotsky argued that infants are innately social beings and that one must include the role of the caregiver, who serves as a support for the child's acquisition of knowledge and skills, in any study of development. One concept that has influenced many contemporary researchers is the **zone of proximal development**. The zone of proximal development refers to the difference between what the child can do acting alone and what she can do when acting with the guidance of a caregiver. In terms of the emergence of intentional communication, the caregiver who is sensitive to an infant's current level of functioning cooperates with the child in a way that fosters growth. (For more information about Vygotsky's theory and its application to children's development, see Rogoff & Wertsch, 1984.)

A complete explanation of the emergence of intentional communication in the infant undoubtedly will have to consider the interaction of many factors, including at least the following: (1) the biological basis for language and changes that take place because of maturation of the central nervous system and peripheral structures, (2) the nonlinguistic cognitive development of the child, and (3) the types of experiences the child has had with caregivers. (See Hardy-Brown, 1983, for a discussion of the problems in disentangling maturational and experiential influences in development.) It is likely that there is both an inborn predisposition toward symbolic communication in the human infant and particular environmental experiences that normally interact with this predisposition to help bring about this important milestone in language development.

In this section on the social context of the infant, we have seen that caregivers typically speak in special ways to preverbal infants, behave as if infants are conversational partners well before they begin using language, and establish object and situationally focused contexts in which the correspondences between vocalizations and meaning can be discovered. Language normally has its beginning in a social communicative context, and patterns are established early that will continue to be used when a child's own speech emerges. There is some evidence that the specific characteristics of speech to prelinguistic infants play some role in the child's development. As one researcher in mother–infant communication put it, "The shared understandings which are built up between an infant and his familiars constitute the indispensable basic contexts for all his later interpersonal transactions, including the ones utilizing verbal language" (Bullowa, 1979, p. 12).

Summary

The first year of life—though the infant may not say a single word—is a very important period for communicative development. The infant is inherently social, responsive to caregivers, and draws caregivers into communicational interaction.

Perhaps one reason that children enter so naturally into communication is that they are well equipped for perceiving speech sounds. Already at birth, infants appear to hear and discriminate speech sounds very well and are thus prepared to begin the process of acquiring language. Because infants can also discriminate sounds that they have not heard before, it seems likely that they are born with the ability to hear many sound categories that are used in different languages. Whether this perceptual ability has evolved in humans especially for speech or reflects a general characteristic of the auditory system is still unresolved.

In the first year of life, there are dramatic changes in the ability of infants to produce sounds, reflecting physical growth, neurological maturation, and experiences with speech sounds. As infants develop control over their articulatory structures, they progress from simple cries to babbling to expressive jargon.

Finally, toward the end of the first year, children begin to behave in ways that seem intentionally communicative. They make gestures and vocalizations in a consistent and persistent manner to achieve goals. These early gestures and vocalizations are not learned from adults but are the child's own inventions. Through such means a child can express various communicative functions, such as rejecting, requesting, or commenting. It seems likely that children achieve the milestone of intentional communication through maturation, changes in their underlying cognitive abilities, and through their experience with others.

Caregivers in many cultures talk to infants in special ways, typically with higher pitch and more variable intonation patterns. Such speech provides one source of affectionate stimulation for the young child, and babies are responsive to such stimulation. This attention-holding speech may also help the child to become aware of the linguistic function of vocalizations. The caregiver, in turn, accepts the child's responses to speech as early attempts at communication. Thus, the caregiver and infant can engage in "conversations" that provide a rich social context for the child's learning about language. Talking while jointly attending to objects and actions, and talking in frequently repeated situations, also exposes the infant to language in a way that may support language acquisition. Through research in this culture and others, we are coming to understand the ways in which parents and other caregivers naturally provide a setting for their children's acquisition of communicative competence.

At the end of the first year, the child is finally ready for the accomplishment that caregivers view as the beginning of language—the first word—but the child has been preparing for that day from the very beginning.

Key Words

baby talk
behavioral modification
biological capacity
caregiver
child-directed speech (CDS)
comment
communicative functions
communicative temptation task
controlling interactional style
declarative communicative function
format
gaze coupling
imperative communicative function
infant-directed speech (IDS)
intentional communication

intrusive interactional style
joint attention
low-structured observation
MacArthur Communicative Development Inventories (CDI)
means–ends concept
phonetically consistent form (PCF)
Piagetian Stage 4
prelinguistic
preverbal
prosodic features
protoword
rejection
request
responsive interactional style

scaffold   social cognition
secondary intersubjectivity   structured observation
sensitive interactional style   vocable
sensorimotor stage   zone of proximal development

Suggested Projects

1. Locate infants of several ages (for example, four, eight, and twelve months) and observe the speech of the parents or caregivers to them. It is preferable to make tape recordings, so that transcripts can be made and segments can be heard repeatedly. (It is difficult to listen for a number of features of speech at one time in a live observation session.) Choose particular features such as pitch, intonation patterns, rhythmic patterns, or repetition, and compare them in the tapes made at different ages. You might also want to compare caregivers—for example, observe both the mother and the father playing with the infant.

2. Locate babies at several ages, such as one, four, eight, and twelve months. Make tape recordings of the infants' vocalization in social settings with a caregiver. It is difficult to make transcriptions of infants' sounds even if you have had training in phonetic transcription. If you have had such training, attempt to transcribe some samples and see what problems you encounter. If you have not had such training, listen to the tapes and attempt to compare the sounds the babies make with the sounds used in your language. Do you hear changes in the types of sounds from age to age?

3. Locate two babies, one about seven months and one about eleven months but not yet talking in words. Observe these babies interacting with caregivers in a relatively unstructured, playful situation. Take notes on each baby's vocalizations and behaviors, watching for signs of intentional communication (described on pages 44–45). Do you notice any differences between the two ages?

4. The notions of "communication," "intentionality" in communication, and "language" make very interesting topics for discussion. Think of various ways in which information is transmitted, within and across species. For example, wilted leaves on a plant might indicate to its caregiver that the plant needs water, and we often say things like "Ferns like to be kept moist," but we would not ordinarily think of the plant as communicating to us. If an animal or baby is shivering, we might infer that it is cold, without calling the shivering "communication." What counts as communicative behaviors? Is a cat meowing by its food bowl an example of intentional communication? Is an infant's vocable *eh-eh* different from the cat's meow? How is using the word *blanket* different from using an invented form such as *lala*?

Suggested Readings

Adamson, L. (1995). *Communication development during infancy.* Madison, WI: Brown & Benchmark.

Anisfeld, M. (1984). *Language development from birth to three.* Hillsdale, NJ: Erlbaum.

Bates, E. (1979). *The emergence of symbols: Cognition and communication in infancy.* New York: Academic Press.

Bruner, J. (1983). *Child's talk: Learning to use language.* New York: Norton.

Bullowa, M. (Ed.). (1979). *Before speech.* New York: Cambridge University Press.

Feagans, L., Garvey, C., & Golinkoff, R. (Eds.). (1983). *The origins and growth of communication.* Norwood, NJ: Ablex.

Foster, S. (1990). *The communicative competence of young children: A modular approach.* New York: Longman (particularly Chapters 2 and 3).

Golinkoff, R. (Ed.). (1983). *The transition from prelinguistic to linguistic communication.* Hillsdale, NJ: Lawrence Erlbaum.

Halliday, M. A. K. (1975). *Learning how to mean: Explorations in the development of language.* London: Edward Arnold.

Jusczyk, P. W. (1997). *The discovery of spoken language.* Cambridge, MA: MIT Press.

Locke, J. L. (1993). *The child's path to spoken language.* Cambridge, MA: Harvard University Press.

MacWhinney, B. (Ed.). (1998). *The emergence of language.* Hillsdale, NJ: Erlbaum.

Nadel, J., & Camaioni, L. (Eds.). (1993). *New perspectives in early communication development.* London: Routledge.

References

Acredolo, L., & Goodwyn, S. (1988). Symbolic gesturing in normal infants. *Child Development, 59,* 450–466.

Acredolo, L, & Goodwyn, S. (1998). *Baby signs.* Chicago: Contemporary Books

Adamson, L. B. (1991). Variations in the early use of language. In L. T. Winegar & J. Valsiner (Eds.), *Children's development in social context: Vol. 1. Metatheory and theory.* Hillsdale, NJ: Lawrence Erlbaum.

Adamson, L. B., & Bakeman, R. (1984). Mothers' communicative acts: Changes during infancy. *Infant Behavior and Development, 7,* 467–478.

Adamson, L. B., & Bakeman, R. (1991). The development of shared attention during infancy. In R. Vasta (Ed.), *Annals of child development: Vol. 8.* London: Kingsley.

Bakeman, R., & Adamson, L. B. (1984). Coordinating attention to people and objects in mother–infant and peer–infant interaction. *Child Development, 55,* 1278–1289.

Bakeman, R., Adamson, L. B., Konner, M., & Barr, R. (1990). !Kung infancy: The social context of object exploration. *Child Development, 61,* 794–809.

Bates, E. (1976). *Language and context: The acquisition of pragmatics.* New York: Academic Press.

Bates, E. (1979). *The emergence of symbols: Cognition and communication in infancy.* New York: Academic Press.

Bates, E., Camaioni, L., & Volterra, V. (1975). The acquisition of performatives prior to speech. *Merrill-Palmer Quarterly, 21,* 205–224.

Baumwell, L., Tamis-LeMonda, C. S., & Bornstein, M. H. (1997). Maternal verbal sensitivity and child language comprehension. *Infant Behavior and Development, 20,* 247–258.

Bernstein Ratner, N., & Pye, C. (1984). Higher pitch in BT is not universal: Acoustic evidence from Quiche Mayan. *Journal of Child Language, 11,* 515–522.

Bloom, K. (1988). Quality of adult vocalizations affects the quality of infant vocalizations. *Journal of Child Language, 15,* 469–480.

Bloom, K. (1990). Selectivity and early infant vocalization. In J. R. Enns (Ed.), *The development of attention: Research and theory.* North-Holland: Elsevier Science Publishers.

Bloom, K., & Lo, E. (1990). Adult perceptions of vocalizing infants. *Infant Behavior and Development, 13,* 209–219.

Bloom, L. (1993). *The transition from infancy to language: Acquiring the power of expression.* Cambridge, UK: Cambridge University Press.

Blount, B. (1990). Parental speech and language acquisition: An anthropological perspective. *Pre- and Perinatal Psychology Journal, 4,* 319–337.

Bornstein, M. H. (1989). Between caretakers and their young: Two modes of interaction and their consequences for cognitive growth. In M. H. Bornstein & J. Bruner (Eds.), *Interaction in human development.* Hillsdale, NJ: Lawrence Erlbaum.

Bruner, J. (1973). Organization of early skilled action. *Child Development, 44,* 1–11.

Bruner, J. (1981). The social context of language acquisition. *Language and Communication, 1,* 155–178.

Bruner, J. (1982). The formats of language acquisition. *American Journal of Semiotics, 1,* 1–16.

Bruner, J. (1983). *Child's talk: Learning to use language.* New York: Norton.

Bullowa, M. (1979). Introduction: Prelinguistic communication: A field for scientific research. In M. Bullowa (Ed.), *Before speech.* New York: Cambridge University Press.

Butterworth, G., & Morissette, P. (1996). Onset of pointing and the acquisition of language in infancy. *Journal of Reproductive and Infant Psychology, 14,* 219–231.

Carpenter, M., Nagell, K., & Tomasello, M. (1998). Social cognition, joint attention, and communicative competence from 9 to 15 months of age. *Monographs of the Society for Research in Child Development, 63* (Serial No. 255).

Carter, A. (1979). Prespeech meaning relations: An outline of one infant's sensorimotor morpheme development. In P. Fletcher & M. Garman (Eds.), *Language acquisition.* Cambridge, UK: Cambridge University Press.

Casby, M. W., & Cumpata, J. F. (1986). A protocol for the assessment of prelinguistic intentional communication. *Journal of Communication Disorders, 19,* 251–260.

Chapman, R. S. (1981). Exploring children's communicative intents. In J. Miller (Ed.), *Assessing language production in children.* Austin, TX: PRO-ED.

Cicchetti, D. (1989). How research on child maltreatment has informed the study of child development: Perspectives from developmental psychopathology. In D. Cicchetti & V. Carlson (Eds.), *Child maltreatment. Theory and research on causes and consequences of child abuse and neglect.* New York: Cambridge University Press.

Clarke-Stewart, K. A. (1973). Interactions between mothers and their young children: Characteristics and consequences. *Monographs of the Society for Research in Child Development, 38* (Serial No. 153).

Coggins, T. E., Olswang, L. B., & Guthrie, J. (1987). Assessing communicative intents in young children: Low structured observation or elicitation tasks. *Journal of Speech and Hearing Disorders, 52,* 44–49.

Cole, K. N., Dale, P. S., & Thal, D. J. (Eds.). (1996). *Assessment of communication and language.* Baltimore, MD: Paul H. Brookes.

Cooper, R. P., & Aslin, R. N. (1990). Preference for infant-directed speech in the first month after birth. *Child Development, 61,* 1584–1595.

Dale, P. (1980). Is early pragmatic development measurable? *Journal of Child Language, 7,* 1–12.

DeCasper, A. J., & Fifer, W. P. (1980). Of human bonding: Newborns prefer their mothers' voices. *Science, 208,* 1174–1176.

Dore, J. (1974). A pragmatic description of early language development. *Journal of Psycholinguistic Research, 3,* 343–350.

Dore, J., Franklin, M. B., Miller, R. T., & Ramer, A. L. H. (1976). Transitional phenomena in early language acquisition. *Journal of Child Language, 3,* 343–350.

Eimas, P. D. (1974). Auditory and linguistic processing of cues for place of articulation by infants. *Perception and Psychophysics, 16,* 513–521.

Fenson, L., Dale, P. S., Reznick, J. S., Bates, E., Thal, D. J., & Pethick, S. J. (1994). Variability in early communicative development. *Monographs of the Society for Research in Child Development, 59* (Serial No. 242).

Fenson, L., Dale, P. S., Reznick, J. S., Thal, D., Bates, E., Hartung, J., Pethick, S., & Reilly, J. (1993). *The MacArthur Communicative Development Inventories: User's guide and technical manual.* San Diego: Singular Publishing Group.

Ferguson, C. A. (1978). Learning to pronounce: The earliest stages of phonological development in the child. In F. D. Minifie & L. L. Lloyd (Eds.), *Communication and cognitive abilities—Early behavioral assessment.* Baltimore: University Park Press.

Fernald, A. (1985). Four-month-old infants prefer to listen to motherese. *Infant Behavior and Development, 8,* 181–195.

Fernald, A. (1989). Intonation and communicative intent in mothers' speech to infants: Is the melody the message? *Child Development, 60,* 1497–1510.

Fernald, A. (1992). Human maternal vocalizations to infants as biologically relevant signals: An evolutionary perspective. In J. H. Barkov, L. Cosmides, & J. Tooby (Eds.), *The adapted mind: Evolutionary psychology and the generation of culture.* New York: Oxford University Press.

Fernald, A., & Kuhl, P. K. (1987). Acoustic determinants of infant preference for motherese speech. *Infant Behavior and Development, 10,* 279–293.

Fernald, A., & Mazzie, C. (1991). Prosody and focus in speech to infants and adults. *Developmental Psychology, 27,* 209–221.

Fernald, A., & Morikawa, H. (1993). Common themes and cultural variation in Japanese and American mothers' speech to infants. *Child Development, 64,* 637–656.

Fernald, A., Taeschner, T., Dunn, J., Papousek, M., de Boysson-Bardies, B., & Fukui, I. (1989). A cross-language study of prosodic modifications in mothers' and fathers' speech to pre-verbal infants. *Journal of Child Language, 16,* 477–501.

Flax, J., Lahey, M., Harris, K., & Boothroyd, A. (1991). Relations between prosodic variables and communicative functions. *Journal of Child Language, 18,* 3–19.

Fraiberg, S. (1974). Blind infants and their mothers: An examination of the sign system. In M. Lewis & L. A. Rosenblum (Eds.), *The effect of the infant on its caregiver.* New York: Wiley.

Goldin-Meadow, S. (1979). Structure in a manual communication system developed without a conventional language model: Language without a helping hand. In H. Whitaker & H. A. Whitaker (Eds.), *Studies in neurolinguistics: Vol. 4.* New York: Academic Press.

Goldin-Meadow, S., & Morford, M. (1985). Gesture in early child language: Studies of deaf and hearing children. *Merrill-Palmer Quarterly, 31,* 145–176.

Golinkoff, R. M. (1993). When is communication a "meeting of minds"? *Journal of Child Language, 20,* 199–207.

Greenfield, P., & Smith, J. (1976). *The structure of communication in early language development.* New York: Academic Press.

Halliday, M. A. K. (1975). *Learning how to mean: Explorations in the development of language.* London: Edward Arnold.

Harding, C. G. (1983a). Acting with intention: A framework for examining the development of intention. In L. Feagans, C. Garvey, & R. Golinkoff (Eds.), *The origins and growth of communication.* Norwood, NJ: Ablex.

Harding, C. G. (1983b). Setting the stage for language acquisition: Communication development in the first year. In R. M. Golinkoff (Ed.), *The transition from prelinguistic to linguistic communication.* Hillsdale, NJ: Erlbaum.

Harding, C. G., & Golinkoff, R. M. (1979). The origins of intentional vocalizations in pre-linguistic infants. *Child Development, 50,* 338–340.

Hardy-Brown, K. (1983). Universals and individual differences: Disentangling two approaches to the study of language acquisition. *Developmental Psychology, 19,* 610–624.

Heath, S. B. (1983). *Ways with words: Language, life and work in communities and classrooms.* Cambridge, UK: Cambridge University Press.

Ingram, D. (1995). The cultural basis of prosodic modifications to infants and children: A response to Fernald's universalist theory. *Journal of Child Language, 22,* 223–233.

Jaffe, J., Stern, D., & Perry, C. (1973). "Conversational" coupling of gaze behavior in prelinguistic human development. *Journal of Psycholinguistic Research, 2,* 321–330.

Jusczyk, P. W. (1997). *The discovery of spoken language.* Cambridge, MA: MIT Press.

Kaplan, P. S., Bachorowski, J. A., & Zarlengo-Strouse, P. (1999). Child-directed speech produced by mothers with symptoms of depression fails to promote associative learning in 4-month-old infants. *Child Development 70,* 560–570.

Kemler-Nelson, D. G., Hirsh-Pasek, K., Jusczyk, P. W., & Wright-Cassidy, K. (1989). How the prosodic cues in motherese might assist language learning. *Journal of Child Language, 16,* 53–68.

Kuhl, P. K., Andruski, J. E., Christovich, I. A., Christovich, L. A., Kozhevnikova, E. V., Ryskina, V. L., Stolyarova, E. I., Sundberg, U., & Lacerda, F. (1997). Cross language analysis of phonetic units in language addressed to infants. *Science, 277,* 684–686.

Kuhl, P. K., Williams, K. A., Lacerda, F., Stevens, K. N., & Lindblom, B. (1992). Linguistic experience alters phonetic perception in infants by 6 months of age. *Science, 255,* 606–608.

Landry, S. H., Smith, K. E., & Miller-Loncar, C. (1997). Predicting cognitive-language and social growth curves from early maternal behaviors in children at varying degrees of biological risk. *Developmental Psychology, 33,* 1040–1053.

Lewis, M., & Freedle, R. (1973). Mother-infant dyad: The cradle of meaning. In P. Pliner, L. Krames, & T. Alloway (Eds.), *Communication and affect, language and thought.* New York: Academic Press.

Lewis, M., & Rosenblum, L. A. (Eds.). (1974). *The effect of the infant on its caregiver.* New York: Wiley.

Locke, J. L. (1993). *The child's path to spoken language.* Cambridge, MA: Harvard University Press.

Locke, J. L. (1994). Phases in the child's development of language. *American Scientist, 82,* 436–445.

Masataka, N. (1993). Effects of contingent and noncontigent maternal stimulation on the vocal behavior of three- to four-month-old Japanese infants. *Journal of Child Language, 20,* 303–312.

Masur, E. F. (1983). Gestural development, dual-directional signaling and the transition to words. *Journal of Psycholinguistic Research, 12,* 93–109.

McCathren, R. B., Warren, S. F., & Yoder, P. J. (1996). Prelinguistic predictors of later language development. In K. N. Cole, P. S. Dale, & D. J. Thal (Eds.), *Assessment of communication and language.* Baltimore, MD: Paul H. Brookes.

Mehler, J., Jusczyk, P., Lambertz, G., Halsted, N., Bertoncini, J., & Amiel-Tison, C. (1988). A precursor of language acquisition in young infants. *Cognition, 29,* 143–178.

Mehler, J., & Christophe, A. (1995). Maturation and learning of language in the first year of life. In M. S. Gazzaniga (Ed.), *The cognitive neurosciences.* Cambridge, MA: MIT Press.

Menn, L. (1976). Pattern, control, and contrast in beginning speech: A case study in the acquisition of word form and function. Unpublished doctoral dissertation, University of Illinois.

Messinger D. S., & Fogel, A. (1998). Give and take: The development of conventional infant gestures. *Merrill-Palmer Quarterly, 44,* 566–590.

Miller, C. L. (1988). Parents' perceptions and attributions of infant vocal behaviour and development. *First Language, 8,* 125–142.

Morikawa, H., Shand, N., & Kosawa, Y. (1988). Maternal speech to prelingual infants in Japan and the United States: Relationships among functions, forms and referents. *Journal of Child Language, 15,* 237–256.

Mosier, C. E., & Rogoff, B. (1994). Infants' instrumental use of their mothers to achieve their goals. *Child Development, 65,* 70–79.

Murphy, C. M. (1978). Pointing in the context of a shared activity. *Child Development, 49,* 371–380.

Murray, A. D., Johnson, J., & Peters, J. (1990). Fine-tuning of utterance length to preverbal infants: Effects on later language development. *Journal of Child Language, 17,* 511–526.

Nazzi, T., Bertoncini, J., & Mehler, J. (1998). Language discrimination by newborns: Toward an understanding of the role of rhythm. *Journal of Experimental Psychology: Human Perception and Performance, 24,* 756–766.

Ochs, E. (1988). *Culture and language development. Language acquisition and language social-ization in a Samoan village.* New York: Cambridge University Press.

Ochs, E., & Schieffelin, B. (1984). Language acquisition and socialization: Three develop-mental stories and their implications. In R. Shweder & R. LeVine (Eds.), *Culture theory: Essays on mind, self and emotion.* New York: Cambridge University Press.

Oller, D. K., Eilers, R. E., Steffens, M. L., Lynch, M. P., & Urbano, R. (1994). Speech-like vocal-izations in infancy: An evaluation of potential risk factors. *Journal of Child Language, 21,* 33–58.

Olswang, L., Bain, B., Dunn, C., & Cooper, J. (1983). The effects of stimulus variation on lexical learning. *Journal of Speech and Hearing Disorders, 48,* 192–201.

Piaget, J. (1952). *The origins of intelligence in children.* New York: International Universities Press.

Prizant, B. M., & Wetherby, A. M. (1990). Toward an integrated view of early language and communicative development and socioemotional development. *Topics in Language Disorders, 10,* 1–16.

Querleu, D., & Renard, K. (1981). Les perceptions auditives du foetus humain. *Medicine et Hygiene, 39,* 2102–2110.

Ratner, N. K., & Bruner, J. S. (1978). Games, social exchange and the acquisition of language. *Journal of Child Language, 5,* 391–401.

Richman, A., LeVine, R., New, R., Howrigan, G., Wells-Nystrom, B., & LeVine, S. (1988). Maternal behavior to infants in five cultures. In R. LeVine, P. Miller, & M. West (Eds.), *Parental behavior in diverse societies. New Directions in Child Development (No. 40),* 81–98.

Rogoff, B., & Wertsch, J. V. (1984). *Children's learning in the "zone of proximal development."* San Francisco: Jossey-Bass.

Sachs, J. (1977). The adaptive significance of linguistic input to prelinguistic infants. In C. Snow & C. A. Ferguson (Eds.), *Talking to children.* New York: Cambridge University Press.

Schieffelin, B. B. (1979). Getting it together: An ethnographic approach to the study of the development of communicative competence. In E. Ochs & B. B. Schieffelin (Eds.), *Develop-mental pragmatics.* New York: Academic Press.

Schieffelin, B. B. (1990). *The give and take of everyday life: Language socialization of Kaluli chil-dren.* Cambridge, UK: Cambridge University Press.

Scoville, R. (1983). Development of the intention to communicate: The eye of the beholder. In L. Feagans, C. Garvey, & R. Golinkoff (Eds.), *The origins and growth of communication.* Norwood, NJ: Ablex.

Seibert, J., & Hogan, A. (1982). *Procedures manual for the early social-communication scales.* Miami, FL: University of Miami.

Shatz, M., & O'Reilly, A. (1990). Conversation or communicative skill? A reassessment of two-year-olds' behavior in miscommunication episodes. *Journal of Child Language, 17,* 131–146.

Shwe, H. I., & Markman, E. M. (1997). Young children's appreciation of the mental impact of their communicative signals. *Developmental Psychology, 33,* 630–636.

Smith, C. B., Adamson, L. B., & Bakeman, R. (1988). Interactional predictors of early lan-guage. *First Language, 8,* 143–156.

Snow, C. (1977). The development of conversation between mothers and babies. *Journal of Child Language, 4,* 1–22.

Snyder, L. (1984). Communicative and cognitive abilities and disabilities in the sensorimotor period. *Merrill-Palmer Quarterly, 24,* 161–180.

Spiker, D., Ferguson, J., & Brooks-Gunn, J. (1993). Enhancing maternal interactive behavior and child social competence in low birth weight, premature infants. *Child Development, 64,* 754–768.

Stern, D. N. (1971). A micro-analysis of mother-infant interaction. *Journal of the American Academy of Child Psychiatry, 10,* 501–517.

Stern, D. N., & Wasserman, G. A. (1979). Maternal language to infants. Paper presented at a meeting of the Society for Research in Child Development.

Sugarman, S. (1978). Some organizational aspects of pre-verbal communication. In I. Markova (Ed.), *The social context of language.* London: Wiley.

Sugarman, S. (1984). The development of preverbal communication. In R. Schiefelbusch & J. Pickar (Eds.), *The acquisition of communicative competence.* Baltimore: University Park Press.

Sullivan, J. W., & Horowitz, F. D. (1983). The effects of intonation on infant attention: The role of the rising intonation contour. *Journal of Child Language, 10,* 521–534.

Tamis-Lemonda, C. S., Bornstein, M. H., Kahana-Kalman, R., Baumwell, L., & Cyphers, L. (1998). Predicting variation in the timing of language milestones in the second year: an events history approach. *Journal of Child Language, 25,* 675–700.

Tomasello, M. (1988). The role of joint attentional processes in early language development. *Language Sciences, 10,* 69–88.

Tomasello, M., & Farrar, M. J. (1986). Joint attention and early language. *Child Development, 57,* 1454–1463.

Trevarthen, C., & Hubley, P. (1978). Secondary intersubjectivity: Confidence, confiding and acts of meaning in the first year. In A. Lock (Ed.), *Action, gesture, and symbol: The emergence of language.* New York: Academic Press.

von Raffler Engel, W. (1973). The development from sound to phoneme in child language. In C. A. Ferguson & D. Slobin (Eds.), *Studies of child language development.* New York: Holt, Rinehart & Winston.

Vygotsky, L. (1978). *Mind in society: The development of higher psychological processes.* Cambridge, MA: Harvard University Press.

Werker, J., & McLeod, P. J. (1989). Infant preference for both male and female infant-directed talk: A developmental study of attentional and affective responsiveness. *Canadian Journal of Psychology, 43,* 230–246.

Werker, J. F., & Tees, R. C. (1984). Cross-language speech perception: Evidence for perceptual reorganization during the first year of life. *Infant Behavior and Development, 7,* 49–64.

Wetherby, A., Cain, D., Yonclas, D., & Walker, V. (1988). Analysis of intentional communication of normal children from the prelinguistic to the multi-word stage. *Journal of Speech and Hearing Research, 31,* 240–252.

Worobey, J. (1989). Mother-infant interaction: Protocommunication in the developing dyad. In J. F. Nussbaum (Ed.), *Life-span communication: Normative processes.* Hillsdale, NJ: Erlbaum.

Zinober, B., & Martlew, M. (1985). Developmental changes in four types of gesture in relation to acts and vocalization from 10 to 21 months. *British Journal of Developmental Psychology, 3,* 293–306.

Chapter 3

Phonological Development: Learning Sounds and Sound Patterns

Lise Menn
University of Colorado

Carol Stoel-Gammon
University of Washington

Children's early attempts at words often sound quite different from adult pronunciations, and people feel that the children's versions are somehow simplified—though it is not obvious why *wed* should be easier to say than *red,* or *tat* easier than *cat.* However, there are many other types of early pronunciations that adults are generally not aware of, such as *sore* for *store,* or *gig* for *pig.* Theories of phonetic and phonological development must explain both why the familiar early word forms are so common and why some children nevertheless use the less common forms.

In this chapter, we describe the transition from babble to speech and explain children's pronunciation in the first year or so after they begin to use words; then we look at some research on the later aspects of phonological development. But first, we must study the speech sounds themselves, so that we see the enormous amount of coordination that is involved in learning to produce them; pronunciation of words is an incredible skill, but adults tend to take it for granted.

English Speech Sounds and Sound Patterns

An important step in describing children's pronunciation is to establish a way of referring to speech sounds that will avoid the ambiguities of the English spelling system. Descriptions of sounds in terms like *hard* and *soft, long* and *short* rapidly become too cumbersome. The ambiguity of the letter *c* (is it an s-sound? a k-sound?) is only one kind of mismatch between English spelling and English speech sounds. Another kind arises when English uses two letters to spell a unitary sound, like *sh.* A third comes about because there are multiple ways of spelling almost any given sound—for example, the *f* in *fat* can also be spelled *ff*, *ph*, and even *gh* (as in *cough*).

Because sounds and letters match up so poorly, we will never refer to spoken words as being composed of letters. Instead, this chapter, like much of the literature on language development and linguistics, will refer to speech sounds or to segments; technical terms for the elements that compose spoken words will be defined. For written reference to speech sounds, we will use a system called the International Phonetic Alphabet (IPA). The IPA symbols presented in Table 3.1 represent the basic speech sounds of general American English.

Phonetics: The Production and Description of Speech Sounds

The sounds of any language are cross-classified in a web of similarities and differences of pronunciation, and understanding the reasons for these similarities and differences is the key to understanding young children's speech patterns. One of these classifications, the division into vowel and consonant, is part of school grammar, and many of the others are reasonably straightforward. For example, the sounds [p], [b], and [m] have in common the property that they are all produced with the lips closed.

Descriptive Features: Classifying Sounds by How They Are Produced

Descriptive features, as the name implies, are used to describe and classify each speech sound in terms of the *source* of the sound in the vocal tract and the *shape* of the vocal tract during sound production. Speech sounds are created as air passes through the

Table 3.1 **Phoneme Symbols for Speech Sounds of General American English**

Symbol	Example	Symbol	Example	Symbol	Example	Symbol	Example	Symbol	Example
	Vowels					Consonants			
/i/	b*ea*d	/ʊ/	p*u*t	/p/	*p*ill	/f/	*f*ie	/h/	*h*i
/ɪ/	b*i*d	/uw/	b*oo*t	/t/	*t*ill	/θ/	*th*igh	/m/	ra*m*
/ej/	b*ai*t	/ʌ/	p*u*tt	/k/	*k*ill	/s/	*s*igh	/n/	ra*n*
/ɛ/	b*e*t	/ɝ/	b*ir*d	/b/	*b*ill	/ʃ/	*sh*y	/ŋ/	ra*ng*
/æ/	b*a*t	/aj/	b*i*te	/d/	*d*ill	/v/	*v*at	/l/	*l*ed
/a/	t*o*t	/æw/	b*ou*t	/g/	*g*ill	/ð/	*th*at	/r/	*r*ed
/ɔ/	t*au*ght	/ɔj/	b*oy*	/tʃ/	*ch*ill	/z/	Cae*s*ar	/j/	*y*et
/ow/	t*o*te	/ə/	*a*bout[1]	/dʒ/	*J*ill	/ʒ/	sei*z*ure	/w/	*w*et

[1]This vowel occurs in unstressed syllables only.

vocal tract (larynx, pharynx, mouth, and nose); the shape is varied by moving the lips, tongue, and lower jaw. The sound waves that we hear are set in motion either by vocal cord vibration or by the friction of airstream turbulence. (Kissing and clucking mouth noises are examples of other oral sound sources.) Although they are not incorporated into English words, some other languages, such as Zulu and Xhosa (spoken in South Africa), do use such sound sources for their "click" consonants.

If the source of a speech sound is partly or entirely vocal cord vibration, it is called a **voiced** sound. It is easy to tell whether a sound is voiced: Voiced sounds can be hummed or sung, at least for a fraction of a second, but unvoiced sounds cannot, since it takes vocal cord vibration to produce a singing tone.

Turbulence (airstream friction) has the sound of air hissing slowly out of a tire; we hear it in speech sounds like [s] and [f]. Turbulence occurs when air is forced through a narrow opening. In the vocal tract, the narrow opening is usually made by bringing the lower articulators (lower lip, teeth, and tongue) close to the upper articulators (upper lip, teeth, and roof of the mouth). The sound produced by the vocal cords or airstream friction takes on different qualities depending on the exact position of the lips, jaws, and tongue; thus, [f] sounds different from [s] even though both have friction as their source, and [a] sounds different from [i] even though both have the vibration of vocal cords as their source. The study of how the shape of the vocal tract gives sounds their distinct identities is **articulatory phonetics.**

The Major Sound Classes

Vowel sounds are made with the vocal tract relatively unobstructed so that air moves through it smoothly; vocal cord vibration is the only sound source. Different vowel sounds result from varying the positions of the articulators: how wide the jaw opening is, whether the bulk of the tongue is held toward the front or the back of the mouth, and whether the lips are pursed, relaxed, or pulled out into a smile position. (Photographers ask their subjects to say "cheese" because the sounds of this word shape the mouth into a smile.)

Consonant sounds are made with a more constricted vocal tract and are classified on the basis of three aspects of their production: *place of articulation* (that is, which articulators are involved), *manner of articulation* (how the speech sound is produced), and *voicing* (presence or absence of vocal cord vibration during production). Table 3.2 provides a classification of the consonants of American English using these three features. We have already mentioned some of the consonants whose sound source is airstream friction produced in the mouth; these are called **fricatives.** Besides [f] and [s], the class of fricatives includes [θ] (as in *thigh*) and [ʃ] (as in *shy*); these four fricatives are produced without vocal cord vibration and are thus unvoiced fricatives. English has four other speech sounds made with turbulence in the mouth—[v], [z], [ð] (as in *the*) and [ʒ] (the second consonant of the word *seizure*); these four are produced with vocal cord vibration in addition to friction, and are subclassified as voiced fricatives. Another fric-

Table 3.2	Classification of Consonants						
Place	*Bilabial*	*Labiodental*	*Interdental*	*Alveolar*	*Palatal*	*Velar*	*Glottal*
Manner							
Stop	p b			t d		k g	
Fricative		f v	θ ð	s z	ʃ ʒ		h
Affricate					tʃ dʒ		
Nasal	m			n		ŋ	
Liquid				l	r		
Glide	w				j		

tion sound is [h], a voiceless consonant usually produced with friction in the **glottis** (the space between the vocal cords); [h] is called a glottal fricative.

The consonants made with the tightest vocal tract constriction are the **stops,** which are produced with upper and lower articulators pressed together so tightly that no air can escape from the mouth. The class of unvoiced stops is composed of [p], [t], and [k]; the set of voiced stops includes [b], [d], and [g]. Consonants classified as **affricates** begin like a stop and end like a fricative; [tʃ], the first sound of *chill,* is a voiceless affricate; [dʒ], as in *Jill,* is a voiced affricate. Together, stop, fricative, and affricate consonants are referred to as **obstruents** because they fully or partially obstruct the oral airflow.

During normal breathing, air from the lungs exits from the nose. In the production of most speech sounds, however, including the ones already described, the passage from the pharynx to the nose is closed off by raising the **velum** (soft palate), a soft tissue extension of the roof of the mouth (hard palate), as shown in Figure 3.1. However, three speech sounds of English, the **nasal stops,** [m], [n], and [ŋ], are made with the velum lowered so that air can escape through the nose; you can check that it does so by humming [m] or [n]. English speakers are often unaware of the third nasal stop listed here, the [ŋ], partly because it does not have its own symbol in the alphabet. It is the sound spelled *n* in *finger* and in *sink* (verify for yourself that this sound is not an [n]); it is also the final sound in words that end with the letters *ng,* such as *sing;* in most varieties of English, there is no [g] pronounced at the end of these words.

The **glides** [j] and [w] are made with a little more vocal tract constriction than the vowels and are often called **semivowels.** Traditional English grammar groups the glides with the consonants, but phonologically they are usually considered as lying in between the true consonants and the vowels.

The **liquids** [r] and [l] are made with a little more constriction in the vocal tract than the glides, but still not enough to cause friction; they also have characteristics intermediate between vowels and obstruent consonants. One important vowel-like characteristic is the role that liquids can play in syllable structure; we usually think of

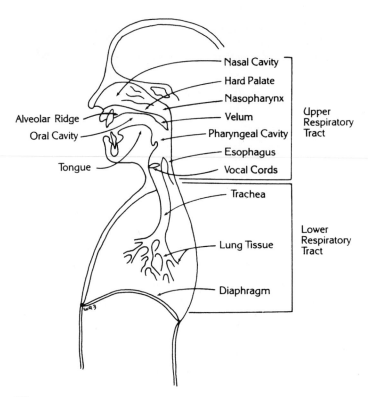

Figure 3.1
The vocal tract.

a syllable as having to contain a vowel, but there are syllables in which a liquid is used as if it were a vowel. The second syllable of *legal* is spelled with an *a,* but what we say is /li-gl/ or /lig-l/; and in most varieties of American English, the noun *record* is /rɛ-krd/. The nasal sounds also have this capacity to serve in place of vowels in certain syllables: consider *random* /ræn-dm/ and *season* /si-zn/.

The Shape of the Vocal Tract: Position of Articulation

The point at which the upper and lower articulators (upper lip, upper teeth, roof of the mouth; lower lip, lower teeth, tongue) touch or approach each other most closely is usually called the place or position of articulation. As mentioned, the sounds [p], [b], and [m] are all produced with the same mouth position; the lips are closed. They, therefore, are labeled as **labial** (or *bilabial*). Moving from the lips toward the back of the mouth, the other positions usually used in describing English sounds are:

Labiodental. This term is used to describe sounds articulated with the lower lip resting lightly against the upper teeth. A slight space is left between the lip and teeth for the air to escape. This is the position of articulation for [f] and [v].

Interdental. This term describes sounds made with the tongue lightly touching the upper teeth, perhaps projecting out slightly beyond them. This is the position of articulation for [θ], as in *thigh,* and [ð], as in *thy.*

Alveolar. This term refers to sounds made with the tongue in contact with the alveolar ridge. This is the point behind the upper teeth where the front of the tongue makes contact in producing [t], [d], or [n] in English. The [s] and [z] sounds are also alveolar; they are made with the tongue in essentially the same position as [t], [d], and [n], but not quite in contact with the alveolar ridge since [s] and [z] are fricatives. The sound [l] (at the beginnings of syllables) is also made with the front of the tongue touching the alveolar ridge, but [l] is not a stop; in making [l], air escapes from the mouth by passing out between the side of the tongue and the upper teeth.

Palatal. This term is used to refer to sounds articulated with the tongue near or contacting the hard palate and/or the slope leading up to it from the alveolar ridge. The tongue makes contact in the palatal area for production of the fricatives [ʃ] and [ʒ] and the affricates [tʃ] and [dʒ]. The tongue is positioned near the hard palate for the glide [j] and the liquid [r].

Velar. This term refers to sounds made when the back of the tongue touches the velum, as in the production of [k], [g], or [ŋ].

Glottal. This term refers to sounds produced in the area of the glottis, and denotes the usual place of articulation of the fricative [h].

English has no velar fricatives, but many other languages do, including German and Russian. There are many other descriptive features; some additional ones are needed for describing English, and even more are needed for sounds found in other languages of the world, and in children's babbling and speech. We will not attempt a larger catalog here but will define additional features as we need them.[1]

Variability in Production: Phonetic Detail

Laboratory measurements show that instances of "the same sound," like repetitions of any other natural event, are not completely identical. Instead, there is a range of tolerance for instances of, say, [d], which will all be taken as that sound. Outside this range of tolerance lie sounds that may be taken for a /d/ pronounced with some kind of foreign accent.

The range of acceptability is affected by many factors. Among them are the nearby sounds in the word and a sound's position at the beginning, middle, or end of a word. For example, measurements show that a voiced stop or fricative in the middle of an English word generally has vocal cord vibration extending throughout the whole period of oral closure. However, the voicing for an initial voiced stop need not begin

---

1. A primary object of linguistic research is to describe the precise minimal set of features sufficient to characterize all language sounds in a way that will bring out phonological patterns optimally; such a minimal set is called a set of *distinctive features.* In this chapter we are not concerned with whether a convenient descriptive feature is distinctive.

until about a fiftieth of a second after the closure has actually been released, and the voicing for a final voiced stop or fricative may die away well before the end of the oral closure. Some of these fine details are audible to the trained ear, but many of them are not, and instrumental analysis is required to study them.

Contrast: The Phoneme

On what grounds do we say that two audibly different sounds are both kinds of [t] but that another sound, objectively similar to them, is a [d] or a [k]? Native speakers of a language find such a question odd; we are normally quite sure that certain sounds are the same and others are different. Temporary confusion, however, may arise because of spelling, as in the two sounds [θ] and [ð], both spelled *th*. What we do to clear up that confusion is instructive. To show that there are two different sounds involved, we note that there are pairs of words, such as *thigh* and *thy*, that are kept distinct merely by the difference in pronunciation of the sounds in question. Such a pair of words, differing only with respect to one pair of sounds, is called a minimal pair, and two sounds are said to *contrast* if there is a **minimal pair** of words that displays the fact that simply changing from one sound to the other produces a change in meaning.

A linguist studying an unknown language looks for minimal pairs to try to establish whether two similar sounds should be treated as variants of the same speech sound or as separate sounds. All the contrasting sounds in a language constitute its set of **phonemes.** The unvoiced [θ] and the voiced [ð] are separate phonemes in English, but there are other pairs of sounds differing in exactly the same way that are not in contrast and therefore do not represent separate phonemes. For example, the sound spelled *r* in *truck* or *cream*—more generally, *r* after any syllable-initial unvoiced stop— can be shown by instrumental analysis to be completely or largely unvoiced, although this is extremely difficult to hear. The voiced and unvoiced *r* do not contrast—there is no pair of words that is kept distinct by virtue of the fact that one contains a voiced *r* and the other contains its unvoiced variant, written with the symbol ṛ. We speak of the two variants of *r* as being different phones but as representing the same phoneme, which we denote as /r/, using slanted lines. Square brackets are used to refer to phones; thus, the variants [r] and [ṛ] are phones that represent the phoneme /r/. Think of it this way: [Clark Kent] and [Superman] are variants of the same person; that person is generally referred to as /Superman/.

The distinction between **phone** and phoneme is just one instance of the basic idea that some elements of culture are two examples of one more abstract, socially defined unit. A dollar coin and a dollar bill are equivalent representations of a dollar value, but contrast in value with coins and bills of other denominations; the black queen on a chessboard contrasts with all the other pieces on the board, but it plays the same role whether it is stamped of plastic or carved of ebony.

If any of several phones may be used to represent the same phoneme in a particular context, those phones are said to be in **free variation.** For example, in English, initial voiced stops may really have vocal cord vibration extending through their period of closure, but the voicing may also begin anywhere within about a fiftieth of a second after closure is relaxed. It makes no difference to the English listener whether the first (fully voiced) or the second (short-lag) phone is used.

However, most linguistic variation is not free; some is stylistic and some is controlled by the linguistic context. The unvoiced [r] version of the phoneme /r/ is used only after unvoiced stops, and English speakers have no control over whether they will use it. In general, speakers find it difficult to learn to hear the difference between two (or more) phones that belong to the same phoneme in their language or to learn to override the automatic choice of which one to use in a given context. On the other hand, choice between separate phonemes is in general under voluntary control (with exceptions to be discussed in the next section); an English speaker can choose to say "red" or to say "led." This is one of the reasons that the phoneme is taken as a basic behavioral unit of language and that many central questions in developmental phonology have been raised in terms of the phoneme.

Phonotactics: Possible and Impossible Words

So far we have talked about properties, such as voicing and the place of articulation, which are intrinsic characteristics of how each speech sound is made. Now we will consider the various sequences of English sounds that can be found and the positions of these sequences at the beginning, middle, or end of a word. This topic is called **phonotactics.**

Not every sequence of English sounds is a possible English word. No English word begins with the sound /ŋ/, which is why a set like *ram, ran, rang* had to be used to present the nasals in Table 3.1. If a new product were to be called Ngicekreem, it might be pronounced /nəgajskrim/ or /ɛŋgajskrim/, but only a few English speakers would be able to master the pronunciation /ŋajskrim/. We have the same problem with African names like Nkomo /ŋkomo/; this name is usually turned into /n-komo/ or /ɛnkomo/. And while English words frequently end with consonant clusters such as *lp* or *rt,* no English word can begin with either of these sound sequences. We can say *plot* and *true,* but we cannot have a word like *lpot* or *rtue.* Similarly, English words can begin with *pl* or *tr* but cannot end with those sequences, unless the *l* or *r* is used as a vowel as in *example* /ɛg-zæm-pl/. In French, however, words can end in such consonant clusters; the word *exemple* is pronounced /ɛk-sãmpl/ with the *l* an unvoiced consonant.

Phoneme sequence and position restrictions such as these are by no means random. Instead of just listing permissible and impermissible sequences, we can make general statements with some notes of exception. In English, the major restriction on initial consonant clusters is that a word cannot begin with two stop consonants in a row. Most initial sequences of a stop followed by a liquid, /s/ followed by a stop, and /s/ plus stop plus liquid are pronounceable, as in *true, stew,* and *strew* respectively.

In learning a second language, mastering a new cluster or a new word position for a familiar sound may require quite as much work as mastering an entirely new sound. English speakers learning Russian usually have problems with monosyllabic words like *rta* (mouth) and *lba* (forehead) as well as *vzglyad* (glance). It turns out, similarly, that learning new phonotactic arrangements is as central a part of the child's acquisition of phonology as is the learning of individual phonemes.

Relationships Among Phonetic Properties

Linguists have tried various notations for describing the relationships among the properties or features that describe speech sounds. These relationships result from the way the vocal tract is constructed and from the way our minds categorize sounds, and they are useful for understanding the patterns of children's attempts to approximate adult sounds. For example, fricative and affricate are qualities that can only apply to consonants. They cannot apply to vowels, by definition, since vowels are among the sounds that are made without obstructing the airflow. Position of articulation features like "bilabial" and "interdental" also only describe consonants; if the mouth is far enough open to make a vowel like /a/, position of articulation—the point of closest contact between the upper and lower articulators—is hard to define and acoustically meaningless. However, "nasal" can apply to both consonants and vowels, since air can be released through the nose (by lowering the velum) independently of whether it is also being released through the mouth. *Autosegmental phonology* is one theory that represents such relationships among phonetic properties by using three-dimensional diagrams (Barnhardt & Stemberger, 1998; Goldsmith, 1990).

Some combinations of features and some sequences of phonemes are much more frequent across languages than others; *optimality theory* is a recent attempt to capture these general preferences (Barnhardt & Stemberger, 1998; Stemberger & Barnhart, 1999). This theory sets up a list of typical preferences as constraints that words "prefer" not to violate; for example, constraints like "every syllable should begin with one consonant followed by a vowel" (true for a fair number of human languages, and also a preference for most young children) or "stop consonants within a cluster should have the same position of articulation" (true for many adult languages and again, a preference for children).

Infant Speech Perception

To determine what infants perceive, researchers first needed to figure out a way of measuring babies' perceptual abilities. A number of ingenious techniques have been devised based on observations of the infant's physiological or behavioral responses to various sorts of auditory stimuli. One of the most successful techniques for studying the abilities of infants in the first few months after birth is **high amplitude sucking**

(HAS). In this method, the infant is given a pacifier to suck on that is connected to a sound generating system. Each suck causes a noise to be generated and the infant learns quickly that sucking brings about this noise. At first, babies suck frequently and the noise occurs often; then, gradually, they lose interest in hearing repetitions of the same noise and begin to suck less frequently. At this point, the experimenter changes the sound that is being generated. If the babies renew vigorous sucking, it can be inferred that they have discriminated the sound change and are sucking more in response to their interest in a new and different sound.

With this technique, researchers have been able to gain information about perceptual abilities of very young infants. We now know that even in the first few months, infants can discriminate many fine distinctions between speech sounds. For example, Eimas and colleagues (Eimas, Siqueland, Jusczyk, & Vigorito, 1971) demonstrated that infants as young as one month of age are capable of perceiving the distinction between /b/ and /p/ in the syllables /ba/ and /pa/, although /b/ differs from /p/ only in that vocal cord vibration starts sometime less than about one twenty-fifth of a second after the lips are opened for /b/, but sometime more than after one twenty-fifth of a second after the lips are opened for /p/. Interestingly, the infants' discrimination of these sounds was **categorical,** as it is in adults; that is, the infants discriminated the difference in vocal cord vibration delay (**voice onset time** between /b/ and /p/, but ignored similar-sized timing differences involving different tokens within the categories of /b/ or /p/ (e.g., they did not start sucking more frequently when the sound changed from /ba/ with a through-voiced [b] to /ba/ with a short-lag [b]).

It has also been shown that infants under three months can detect differences in place and manner of articulation of consonants and in contrasting intonational patterns (see Jusczyk [1997] for a review of these studies). The fact that infants can discriminate between very similar speech sounds at one month of age would suggest either that they have a built-in ability to make such distinctions or that they learn them very quickly. One way to test between these two alternative explanations is to look at a sound discrimination that infants could never have learned—that is, one that is not used in the language to which they have been exposed. Trehub (1976) ran such a study, testing Canadian infants who had not been exposed to any eastern European language for their discrimination of two fairly similar sounds used in Czech, [ʒa] and [řa]. Adult Canadian subjects were also tested for their ability to differentiate the two unfamiliar sounds. Although infants could discriminate [ʒa] and [řa] as well as they could English language contrasts such as [ba] and [pa], the English-speaking adults readily confused the Czech sounds.

The results of Trehub's study suggest not only that infants are born with the ability to hear the difference between the Czech phonemes, but that language experience may result in the loss of the ability to discriminate categories that are not functional in one's language. This possibility is supported by the results of another study of English-learning infants. Werker and Tees (1984) found that between six and eight months the infants could discriminate sounds that are used in Hindi or Nthlakapmx (a Salish language spoken in Canada) but not in English. By ten to twelve months, this discrimination ability had disappeared, and the infants' performance was as poor as that of English-speaking adults.

In a series of cross-linguistic studies on the perception of vowels, Kuhl (1992) has demonstrated that infants reared in different linguistic environments show an effect of language experience by six months of age. Specifically, infants begin to group vowels differently, reflecting language-specific characteristics of the ambient language input.

It appears, then, that infants start out the language-acquisition process with the capacity to discriminate the phonetic contrasts of any of the world's languages. With exposure to their own language, they begin to focus on those contrasts that are relevant for that particular language, and to lose the ability to perceive certain contrasts not found in their native language. However, this does not mean that infants (or adults) fail to distinguish among all nonnative contrasts; for instance, both English-learning babies of fourteen months and English-speaking adults can perceive differences among clicks in Zulu, even though these sounds do not occur in English (Best, McRoberts, & Sithole, 1988). It appears, then, that the decline in discrimination abilities affects primarily those foreign sounds that are phonetically similar, though not identical, to sounds of the native language.

Some of the most intriguing findings in the field of infant speech perception involve studies of infants' abilities in the first week of life. DeCasper and Fifer (1980), for example, showed that three-day-old infants can identify their own mothers' voices when presented with voices of various mothers; moreover, there was evidence that they prefer listening to their own mother than to another mother. Mehler and his colleagues (Mehler, Jusczyk, Lambertz, Halsted, Bertoncini, & Amiel-Tisson, 1988) demonstrated that four-day-old infants can distinguish between utterances in their maternal language and those of another language. In both cases, it appears likely that the discrimination abilities are based primarily on prosodic cues in the utterances (such cues could be perceived in the uterus) rather than phonetic features of particular sounds.

Infants also must learn words, which means they must learn to recognize sequences of sounds. The first word a child learns to recognize may be her own name; Mandel, Jusczyk, and Pisoni (1994) showed that four-and-a-half-month-old infants preferred to hear the sound of their names rather than other words with similar stress patterns. In addition to learning specific words, infants also learn the characteristic phoneme sequences of their languages, on a statistical basis; in fact, this ability, which is present before nine months (Aslin, Saffran, & Newport, 1999; Juszcyk, 1992), is critical to learning words. For further examples and discussion, see Chapters 3 and 4 of Vihman (1996), and for a complete treatment of perceptual development, Juszcyk (1997).

Production: The Prelinguistic Period

In Chapter 2, Table 2.2 introduced the development of children's vocalizations during the first year of life. Infants begin with simple cries at birth and progress through an ordered sequence of stages to complex babbling with identifiable syllables and adultlike intonation patterns. From quite early on, vocalizations can be divided into two categories, according to their function: (1) **reflexive vocalizations**—cries, coughs, and involuntary grunts that seem to be automatic responses reflecting the physical state of the infant—and (2) **nonreflexive vocalizations**, like *cooing* or *jargon babbling*—non-automatic productions containing many phonetic features found in adult languages.

Regardless of the linguistic community in which they are being raised, all infants seem to pass through the same stages of vocal development. In this section, we will describe these stages and the approximate ages associated with each, using the frameworks of Oller (1980) and Stark (1980), which are slightly more elaborate than the list presented in Chapter 2. (For a deeper and more comprehensive survey, see Chapter 5 of Vihman, 1996).

Although commonly referred to as "stages," the periods described here are not discrete; that is, vocalization types typically overlap from one stage to another. A new stage is marked by the appearance of vocal behaviors not observed in the preceding period.

> **Stage 1.** *Reflexive vocalizations (birth to two months).* This stage is characterized by a majority of reflexive vocalizations, such as crying and fussing, and vegetative sounds like coughing, burping, and sneezing. In addition, some vowel-like sounds may occur. The vocalizations of this period are partially determined by the infant's anatomical structure. In newborn babies, the vocal tract resembles that of a non-human primate in that the oral cavity is small and almost totally filled by the tongue, and the larynx is high in the neck, with little separation of the oral and nasal cavities (Lieberman, Crelin, & Klatt, 1972). This configuration limits the range of sound types that can be produced. Rapid growth of the head and neck area in the stages that follow allows production of a greater variety of sounds.
>
> **Stage 2.** *Cooing and laughter (two to four months).* During this stage, infants begin to make some comfort-state vocalizations, often called *cooing* or *gooing* sounds. As indicated by this label, these vocalizations seem to be made in the back of the mouth, with velar consonants and back vowels. Crying typically becomes less frequent and, much to parents' delight, sustained laughter and infant chuckles appear.
>
> **Stage 3.** *Vocal play (four to six months).* In this period it seems as though babies are testing their vocal apparatus to determine the range of vocal qualities they can produce. The period is characterized by the appearance of very loud and very soft sounds (yells and whispers), and very high and very low sounds (squeals and growls). Some babies produce long series of raspberries (bilabial trills) and sustained vowels, and occasionally some rudimentary syllables of consonants and vowels occur.
>
> **Stage 4.** *Canonical babbling (six months and older).* The prime feature of this period is the appearance of sequences of consonant–vowel syllables with adultlike timing. For the first time, babies sound as though they are actually trying to produce words. Upon hearing a sequence such as [mama] or [dada], parents often report with delight that their baby has begun to call them by name. To be sure, it does sound

as though the baby is saying *mama* or *daddy;* in most cases, however, there is no evidence that the productions are semantically linked to an identifiable referent, so for this reason these forms would not be considered words. Multisyllabic utterances in this period are often categorized as **reduplicated babbles** (i.e., strings of identical syllables like [bababa]) or **variegated babbles** (syllable strings with varying consonants and vowels, like [bagidabu]). While both types of utterances occur in the canonical stage, reduplicated babbles predominate initially; around twelve or thirteen months, variegated babbles emerge as the more frequent type.

The infant's hearing of his own vocalizations and the vocalizations of those around him takes on increased importance during this period. We know this because although deaf infants engage in the earlier forms of vocalization, they fail to enter the canonical babbling stage at the appropriate time (Oller & Eilers, 1988). Moreover, during this period the variety of consonants in the vocalizations of deaf infants decreases with age, whereas the variety increases with age in the vocalizations of hearing babies (Stoel-Gammon & Otomo, 1986).

Stage 5. *Jargon stage (ten months and older).* The last stage of babbling generally overlaps with the early period of meaningful speech and is characterized by strings of sounds and syllables uttered with a rich variety of stress and intonational patterns. This kind of output, also described in the section of Chapter 2 on The Forms of Early Communicative Behaviors, is known by such names as *conversational babble, modulated babble,* or *jargon.*

Some vocalizations appear to be made for their own sake. The child does not appear to be "talking" to anyone, and there seems to be no connection between the sounds and any other ongoing activity. Such **sound play** may contain recurring favorite sound sequences, or even early words. However, many vocalizations are delivered with eye contact, gesture, and intonation so rich and appropriate that the person addressed typically feels compelled to respond, at least with a friendly "That's nice." A child producing conversational babble seems to grasp the social nature of conversation and has merely missed the fact that the sounds in it have particular meanings. In fact, the gestures and the context often make it clear that the intonation—the rise and fall of the pitch of the voice—is indeed carrying meaning even if the articulated sounds are not. Thus, the term **modulated babble** is also used to refer to these conversational vocalizations. Sometimes, however, the child is apparently not conveying any meaning by this eloquent use of pitch modulation; instead, she appears to be simply imitating the outward form of adult conversation—for example, in pretended telephone conversations.

Sounds of Babbling

The speechlike sounds used by infants change dramatically during the first year of life. In the first six months, vowel articulations tend to predominate; as mentioned above, most of the consonantal sounds are produced in the back of the mouth (i.e., sounds like [k] or [g]). With the onset of the canonical babbling stage, there is a marked shift toward front consonants, particularly [m], [b], and [d].

Between six and twelve months, the sound repertoire expands considerably, and in a way that is similar across languages. Studies examining whether listeners or spectrographic analyses could distinguish the babbled sounds of babies who have been exposed to different languages have consistently shown that the sounds are very similar, even with input languages as different as English, Arabic, Spanish, Japanese, and Chinese (Atkinson, MacWhinney, & Stoel, 1970; Locke, 1983).

A relatively small set of consonants accounts for the great majority of consonantal sounds produced. In his review of babbling data from 129 infants aged eleven to twelve months, Locke (1983) showed that twelve of the twenty-four consonantal sounds of English accounted for nearly 95 percent of the consonants produced. In terms of articulatory features, this set of sounds is characterized by particular manner classes, namely the stops [p, b, t, d, k, g], the nasals [m, n], and the glides [w, j]; in addition, the fricative [s] and the glottal [h] are included in the list. Interestingly, the sound classes that are missing from babble—fricatives like [v] or [ð], affricates like [tʃ], and liquids [l] and [r]—are precisely those classes of sounds that are mastered relatively late in the production of *real words;* in contrast, the consonants that are frequent in late babbling (the stops, nasals, and glides) are nearly identical to those that appear in the first adult-based words (Stoel-Gammon, 1985). Thus, it seems that the sounds of late babbling may serve as the building blocks for the production of words. Although there is a fair amount of individual variation, on average, stops, nasals, and glides appear in children's words before fricatives, affricates, and liquids.

The Relationship Between Babbling and Speech

At one time, it was suggested that early attempts at speech grew directly out of babbling, in response to adult language teaching. There was a belief that infants babbled all possible sounds, and theory held that adults selectively reinforced those sounds that occurred in the input language and ignored sounds that did not (Mowrer, 1954; Winitz, 1969). There are several problems with this view. First, babies do not start out producing all possible sounds; they produce only a relatively small subset of them (Oller, 1980). Second, even though studies have shown that adult attention can increase the amount of babbling, it does not change the type of sounds that are produced (Dodd, 1972; Todd & Palmer, 1968; Wahler, 1969). Thus, reinforcement by adults is unlikely to be a major factor in the development of specific speech sounds, although it probably aids development by increasing the amount of practice that children get (Stoel-Gammon, 1998a).

A contrasting theory about the relationship between babbling and speech was that the two stages were essentially discontinuous. Jesperson (1925) proposed that babbling consisted of the playful exploration of the sounds that the baby could make, whereas speech involved the "planful" execution of particular sounds. Jakobson (1941/1968), impressed by the fact that some children have a "silent period" between babble and speech, developed this idea into the claim that babble and speech were essentially unrelated, since he was still under the misimpression that in babbling the infant randomly produces a wide range of sounds.

More recently, three kinds of evidence have suggested that the best way to characterize the relationship between babbling and speech is the *continuity* view, at least for normally hearing children. First, children in the late stages of babble apparently prefer to sound like the people around them. They make at least two kinds of changes in their babbling: They gradually stop using sounds that they do not hear being used, such as /h/ in French, and their babbled syllables start to acquire the timing and pitch contour of the language around them. Thus, while children acquiring French, English, Swedish, or Japanese tend to use the same types of sounds, there are systematic differences in the frequency of occurrence of particular sound classes (Boysson-Bardies & Vihman, 1991; Vihman, 1992). These differences in proportional occurrence mirror the proportional use of sounds in the children's early words. Also, when judges listened to long sequences of babbling that contained intonational cues, they could recognize babies from their own speech communities (de Boysson-Bardies, Sagart, & Durand, 1984), even though they could not identify differences in the babbled segments. When syllable lengths are actually measured, French infants' babble shows more lengthening of the final syllable of a babble sequence than American infants' babble does, the same pattern that is found when the adult languages are contrasted (Levitt & Wang 1991).

Second, longitudinal studies of prelinguistic vocalizations have shown that children's phonological patterns in early meaningful speech are directly linked to the patterns that they use in babbling, which Vihman calls **vocal motor schemes.** Specifically, some children have individual preferences in babbling, and these same preferences appear in the child's first words (Vihman, 1993; Vihman, Macken, Miller, Simmons, & Miller, 1985). Presumably, the early words tend to use the same sounds and sound sequences that the child has preferred in babbling because these are the vocal motor schemes that she has managed to bring under voluntary control (see Stoel-Gammon, 1998a).

Third, early speech usually coexists with babbling for several months at least, and some children have utterances that fall between speech and babble, either because they contain mixtures of babble and words, or because they consist of noncommunicative sound play that is based on the sounds of real adult words.

However, some individual children may have a silent period between babble and speech, and some late talkers seem not to make use of their babble patterns. Recent work from Yoshinaga-Itano's laboratory indicates that in deaf children, whose babble is very impoverished, babble does not develop into speech (which is also generally impoverished). Those deaf children who do learn to speak are not necessarily those who babble. Therefore, in children without audition to provide the feedback link between articulatory gestures and the output sound, babble and speech seem to be disconnected.

The Beginning of Phonological Development: Protowords

The beginning of speech seems easy to identify for some children. One day they make a sound that resembles an adult word, and they do it when that word would be appropriate. These first recognizable words are often greetings, farewells, or other social phrases, like "peek-a-boo." The situation is more problematic when the child has a recurrent form that doesn't resemble any appropriate adult word; for example, Halliday's (1975) subject Nigel created several of his own forms, such as "na" used to indicate that he wanted an object. Does a word that the child has made up—a **protoword**—"count"?

It does, in at least two respects. First, the child who uses such a form has demonstrated an important level of voluntary control over his vocalizations, a level that is necessary (though perhaps not sufficient) for starting to say words that do have adult models. Second, a child using one or two invented words has acquired the difficult concept that sounds have meaning and is unclear only about the fact that you are supposed to find out what words exist instead of making them up for yourself.

The term protoword is often used for the invented words that may occur during the transition from prespeech to speech; it is also sometimes used for carry words that have adult models but lack important semantic properties of those models. However, consideration of that topic will take us too far away from the acquisition of phonology. [The Halliday (1975) and Painter (1984) case studies are recommended for those who wish to explore this area further.]

Protowords (with or without adult models) often differ in another way from our usual notion of a word; although the sound sequences must be stable enough so that one can identify their recurrences (otherwise an adult would never realize that a child intended the sounds to have a particular meaning), they may be very poorly controlled, and individual instances may vary much more than repeated uses of a word do in adult usage. For example, Menn's (1976) subject Jacob had an identifiable protoword that he used to accompany the action of rotating anything that would turn (a wheel, a knob, a page of a book); the form of this "spinning song" varied from "io-ioio" to "weeaweeaweea."

Theories of the Acquisition of Phonology

Until about 1970, two kinds of theories of phonological development existed in sharp conflict, one nativist and the other behaviorist. A nativist theory of development holds that normal development proceeds like the development of an embryo; the environment provides raw materials that are assimilated and structured by the child according to an inborn program. The opposite theoretical pole is a behaviorist theory, which holds that the biological heritage is only anatomical—it determines, for example, the shape of the vocal tract, the auditory processing mechanism, and other physical characteristics that support language. All language behavior is held to be learned by stimulus-reward experience; children's word approximations are supposed to be shaped by the reward of getting what they ask for until their forms match adult models.

Nativist Theory

The best-known **nativist** theory was put forward by the late Roman Jakobson (1941/1968). Jakobson's theory was based on theoretical considerations drawn from adult language and from the few then-available reports of children's carry words, and it is now known to be inadequate in several important respects. However, his work was of great importance because of the interest it aroused in child phonology, especially his claim that sounds that are acquired late in any given language are those that are relatively rare in the languages of the world.

Jakobson's theory was really rather limited in scope; it dealt only with the order of phonemic contrasts developed by children, and it does, indeed, appear to describe this in broad outline. His notion was that all children should show essentially the same order of acquisition of phonemic contrasts and that the earliest contrasts developed by the individual should be those that are most common in the languages of the world. Therefore, children would first learn to produce the consonant–vowel contrast since that is found in all languages—syllables like "pa" and "ma," which of course many children do say. He proposed that children would then proceed to subdivide both vowels and consonants, making finer and finer distinctions until they reached the full set of contrasts demanded by the language around them. The subdivision of consonants was supposed to begin either by distinguishing nasal from nonnasal stops or labial from nonlabial stops; after the labial-nonlabial contrast had been acquired, a child could learn to distinguish back (usually velar) consonants from dental or alveolar ones.

While this order of development is fairly common, counterexamples have been published. Menn's (1976) subject Jacob, who was audiotaped three times per week from age twelve to twenty-one months, acquired a contrast between dental and velar stops before learning to produce labials. Other children who have been studied—for example, Hildegard (Leopold, 1970)—have produced a word without any vowel, like "mmm" or "shhh," as a first word. This contradicts the mama-papa prediction. We note again that Jakobson's theory says nothing about phones in themselves but only as they represent phonemes, so the development of phonetic accuracy simply falls outside the scope of his theory.

Behaviorist Theory

The **behaviorist** approach to the acquisition of phonology is best exemplified by the work of Olmsted (1971). Olmsted was concerned with phones, not phonemic contrasts, and he tried to show that children tended to begin acquisition with the most frequent phones of their language and then proceed to the least frequent ones. It seems to have been assumed that the reward for improved approximation of each phone should be roughly equal. This theory, like Jakobson's, doesn't account for the degree of individual variation that children show in the order of acquisition of phones; in addition, it is contradicted by the fact that the very frequent phone [ð] is among the last to be acquired. Clearly, some phones, like [ð], are harder to learn to say than others, either for perceptual or articulatory reasons.

Regression: Key Evidence Against Both Nativist and Behaviorist Theories

There is a counterargument that works against both nativist and behaviorist types of theories, at least in the forms in which they have been advocated. Both nativist and behaviorist theories predict that development will follow a course of smooth, regular improvement toward an adult model, without any regression. But in fact, there are cases of regression in the acquisition of phonology.

Menn's (1971) study of the acquisition of phonology provides an example of a child who clearly showed **regression;** the pronunciation of two frequently used words actually got worse over time. Daniel established the words *down* and *stone* as [dæwn] (correct) and [don] ("doan"). Then, however, when he tried to say other words beginning with oral stops and ending in nasals, he produced them with nasals in both positions. For example, he produced *beans* as [minz] ("means") and *dance* as [næns] ("nance"). After a few weeks this nasal assimilation began to take over the established forms for *down* and *stone;* soon he was saying [næwn] ("noun") and [non] ("noan"). Behaviorist theories must assume that correct forms are rewarded more than incorrect ones; therefore, they cannot deal with the replacement of correct forms with incorrect ones.

Another type of regression doesn't involve a particular word getting worse, but rather the apparent loss of the ability to say a sound in new words, coupled with retention of the correct pronunciation in older words. This variability is also in itself evidence against a strong nativist theory. For example, many children acquire a word or two whose pronunciation is much closer to the adult model than that of their other words. These words were called **progressive phonological idioms** by Moskowitz (1980). Menn's Daniel had initial [h] only on his second and third words, *hi* and *hello;* all other adult words beginning with /h/, for example *horse, hose, hat*—indeed, all adult words beginning with glides, liquids, or fricatives—were produced without the initial semivowel or consonant. The ability to begin words with [h] appears to have been acquired and maintained for the two words *hi* and *hello* but to have been absent in all other cases. It would be impossible to speak of Daniel either as having learned to produce [h] or as not having done so. No strictly nativist model can be flexible enough to deal with this kind of word-to-word variation. There is no linguistic way to predict which words will become progressive phonological idioms and which words will not.

Cognitive Approaches to the Acquisition of Phonology

The sort of theory of phonological development that seems to deal best with the data reported here is called a *cognitive* or *problem-solving* theory, for in it the child is seen as a somewhat intelligent creature actively trying to solve a difficult problem: how to talk like the people around her do (Macken & Ferguson, 1983). She may adopt several general strategies that can provide temporary solutions: avoidance of difficult sounds or sound sequences, exploitation of favorite sounds, systematic replacement or less systematic rearrangement of the sounds in the target word. She may also have a general one-word-at-a-time approach or instead try to approximate whole phrases (Peters, 1977).

Within a child's general strategy, one can see characteristic components of problem solving: first, trial-and-error articulation attempts, but then the use of existing solutions to deal with new problems (generalization), and the temporary extension of these behaviors to situations where they are not quite the needed response (overgeneralization), like Daniel's use of "noun" for *down*. This sequence of events is typical of all areas of linguistic development and is a major reason for considering language development to be a part of general cognitive development.

Before leaving the discussion of the older theories, let us see what they do have of continuing value. Both contain elements that must be incorporated into any adequate approach. Nativist theories highlight the fact that the raw materials—the brain and the perceptual and motor systems, including their patterns of postnatal maturation—are biologically given. These put limits, some absolute and some probabilistic, on behavior, and many of the similarities among children are surely to be accounted for by this biological "substrate" for language. For example, the perceptual system will respond to the acoustic similarities between the fricatives /s/ and /ʃ/; a child learning to say them by trial and error may therefore be satisfied temporarily by the same sound for both of them. Another example: Stops in general seem easier to produce than fricatives—perhaps because a stop can be produced by a fairly clumsy lip or tongue gesture since what is needed is a complete closure of the oral passage. However, the production of a fricative needs more delicate motor control: Just the right distance to cause airstream turbulence must be maintained between the upper and lower articulators, and the right airstream speed as well. All this is a matter of physiology and physics.

Such considerations of innate predispositions and abilities are most often helpful when we look for explanations of what children tend to have in common. We need to modify the old absolute statements, however, giving them a probabilistic cast (e.g., "It is more likely that a child will use a stop for a fricative than vice versa" rather than "Stops are mastered before fricatives"). General statements about the order of acquisition of particular segments also have to be made in probabilistic terms; the order varies across children, and the actual ages of acquisition vary even more.

When we look for explanations of how children differ from each other, it is also not surprising to find that there is a useful role for behaviorist notions of trial-and-error shaped by reward. But again, the problem-solving theory gives the behaviorist idea an important new twist, for the notion of where rewards come from has changed. Traditional behaviorism assumes that the reward for correct behavior is external. The successful communication of a demand is rewarded when the child gets what he wants and thus learns to say the word(s) the same way the next time.

The real-life problems in the traditional reward theory become obvious in any kitchen where a semi-intelligible child is trying to get a cookie; a child at this stage gets most of what she wants by whine, gaze, and gesture; adult commands to "say *cookie*" are seldom heeded by the child who really wants one. This gives little occasion for differential reinforcement of any kind of articulatory improvement; any version of "cookie" that the child produces will be rewarded, and quite likely, a cookie will also be obtained by continued inarticulate fussing.

There is also a stronger counterargument to the external-reward theory. If external reward were the principal shaper of behavior, prelingually deaf children would not have such a terribly difficult time learning to use spoken language. A deaf child in an oral training program is given intensive feedback from teachers, and yet many never learn to produce a useful amount of intelligible speech. In contrast, fully effective communication through manual sign language can be learned rapidly if the child has parents and companions who communicate with one of the sign languages used by the deaf community.

What is lacking in the deaf child's learning of speech but present in his acquisition of sign language? Clearly, because he cannot hear, he cannot monitor his speech performance and match it against the models provided by others. A deaf child can see his hands and the hands of others in order to judge the accuracy of his signs, but he cannot hear his words or compare them to the words of others and so he cannot judge the accuracy of his sounds. What he is missing is *internal feedback:* a way of assessing his own performance. Learning the intricate motor skill of speaking (like any other fine motor skill—see Kent, 1993 and Stoel-Gammon, 1992) requires internal feedback. Imagine learning to play tennis if you had to rely on someone else to tell you where the ball went!

Why is there such a difference in effectiveness between internal and external feedback? Probably because there are literally dozens—even hundreds—of phonetic details that must fall within narrow tolerances for production of an adult-sounding word. The language learner must be able to tell, consciously or unconsciously, what part of a word is wrong and to play around with it, listening to it until she gets it better. (For evidence that children practice their words and sounds, see Ferguson & Macken, 1980; Weir, 1962; for discussion of the relationship between practice and feedback, see Stoel-Gammon, 1992.) So, if learning depends on internal feedback, then the reward for a closer approximation of the adult form must be the child's own pleasure that she has managed to sound more like her family or her friends; it must be an internal reward, not an external one.

The problem-solving theory, in summary, assumes that most of the reward is internal; the child is innately disposed to feel pleasure with behavior that he apprehends as successful emulation of adult or peer models. One current research endeavor is the attempt to construct computer models of the **self-organizing system** type, using internal feedback, to see if they can indeed simulate early phonological development (Gupta & Dell, 1999; Leonard, 1992; Lindblom, 1992; Markey, 1994; Menn & Matthei, 1992; Stemberger, 1992).

Learning to Pronounce

How do very young children really pronounce words? Consider the examples from published literature found in Table 3.3. Some productions are quite accurate, others show overall resemblances between the target and the attempt, and some seem a little farfetched. Is there some order behind this variety? How can we discover what it is?

Regularity in Children's Renditions of Adult Words

One of the most important findings from the study of the acquisition of phonology is that most of the young children who have been studied have developed rather systematic approaches to the reproduction of adult target words.[2]

Feature Changes

For most children's early speech we can find a core of words that show very clear patterns. Let us begin with two hypothetical examples, simplified for the sake of clarity. One might find a child who gives these pronunciations:

Child A

pot [bat] ("bot")	back [bæk] (correct)
top [dap] ("dop")	day [dej] (correct)
cat [gæt] ("gat")	game [gejm] (correct)

Child A seems to use voiced stops in word-initial position both when they are appropriate (in the righthand column) and when the corresponding unvoiced stop is required (in the lefthand column). The place of articulation in all of these words is correct, however.

Another hypothetical child might pronounce the same words this way:

Child B

pot [pat] (correct)	back [bæt] ("bat")
top [tap] (correct)	day [dej] (correct)
cat [tæt] ("tat")	game [dejm] ("dame")

---

[2]Sometimes a particular word does seem to evoke an unsystematic series of potshots, and the difference between these words and others can be very striking. Ferguson and Farwell (1975) recorded a little girl's repeated attempts to say the word *pen* over the course of half an hour; they included the forms [mã⁹], [dɛᵈⁿ], [hɪn], [ᵐbō], [pɪn], [tntntn], [baʰ], [dʰauᵐ], and [buã]. (Transcription is simplified from the original; raised symbols indicate weak sounds, and the tilde [˜] over a vowel indicates a nasalized pronunciation.)

Table 3.3	Examples of Early Pronunciations of Common Words				
	Jacob (approx. 19 months)	*Hildegard (approx. 24 months)*	*Daniel (approx. 25 months)*	*Amahl (A) (approx. 25 months)*	*Amahl (B) (approx. 32 months)*
apple /æpl/	æpw	ʔapa	æpu[1]	ɛbu	æpəl
bottle /badl/	gʌgʌ	balu	baw	bɔgu	bɔkəl
water /wɔdr/[2]	—	walu	ɔərs	wɔ:də	wɔ:tə
house /hæws/	—	haws	æws	aut	haut
dog/doggie /dɔg/ /dɔgi/	dadi	doti	gɔg	gɔgi	dɔg
cookie /kʊki/	kikʌ kʌki	tuti	guki	—	—
shoe /ʃu/	du ʃɪw	ʒu	u	du:	tu:
sock /sak/	sʌk	—	ak	gɔk	tɔk
stone /ston/	—	doɪʃ	non	du:n	—

Note: ʔ is the glottal closure phone heard between the syllables of the expression "uh-oh" /ʌʔow/.
  : indicates lengthening of preceding vowel.

[1]Young children sometimes pronounce the vowels [u] and [o] without the [w] "off-glide" characteristic of adult pronunciation.

[2]Amahl's model was British "Received Pronunciation" /wɔtə/.

Source: Amahl's data in this chapter are from Smith, 1973; Hildegard's are from Leopold, 1970, and may also be found in Moskowitz, 1970.

Child B has voicing correct but is unable to manage the velar place of articulation; attempts at adult words containing /k/ come up with a [t] instead, and a [d] for /g/.

These hypothetical examples make it clear that there are two important benefits to be derived from descriptions in terms of features as well as in terms of segments. First, instead of saying that the child uses this sound instead of that one, we can see that the child's attempt may be partly right and partly wrong. For example, hypothetical Child A gets position of articulation right but voicing wrong for unvoiced stops. Children in general get things partly right before they get them correct, so it is valuable to have a way of describing their attempts that deals with some of the attributes of a segment individually. In fact, even features can prove to be too crude a tool for some needs, as we shall see.

The second benefit of using features is that it allows one to see what several different-looking errors may have in common. Using a feature description, it is evident that the three mistakes of Child A were essentially identical. All were errors in which word-initial unvoiced stops were replaced by voiced stops. Similarly, the three mistakes of Child B were all cases of using an alveolar articulation when the target word required a velar. Patterns or families of errors like this are very common in child language (and also in second language acquisition).

Patterns are not always so regular, however. Sometimes a child may learn to get voicing correct for, say, /t/ and /d/, and yet still use [b] for /p/; another child may follow the general pattern of using voiced stops for unvoiced stops at the beginnings of words but have one or two words in which a word-initial /t/ appears to be produced correctly. An adequate theory of the acquisition of phonology must be able to accommodate both the regular and irregular relations between the child's attempt and the target word. We can thus rule out theories that try to describe the acquisition of phonology only in terms of the acquisition of features. The individual phonemes, and even individual words, often must be taken into account.

Cluster Reductions

Let's consider some other typical patterns of early pronunciation. **Consonant clusters** (sequences of two consonants) appear to cause problems for most young speakers, and there are several patterns that children follow in dealing with them. Many children simply leave out one of the sounds. In English /s/ + stop consonant clusters are very common, and children often omit the /s/. Daniel, for example, would have produced the forms given in the first column of examples.

	Daniel	**Stephen**
spill	[pɪl] ("pill")	[fɪl] ("fill")
store	[tɔr] ("tore")	[sɔr] ("sore")
school	[kul] ("cool")	[sul] ("sool")

A less-common pattern, found perhaps in 10 percent of children learning English, is to leave out the stop consonant, as we see in the treatment of *store* and *school* in the second column. Frequently, the children like Stephen, who omit alveolar and velar stops in these clusters, do something a little different with /sp/ clusters. They use [f], not /s/. This [f] appears to be an attempt to match the sound of the whole cluster within a single consonant. It has the fricative character of the /s/ but the labial character of the /p/. (English has no bilabial fricative; the labiodental /f/ is the closest a child can come to the bilabial fricative sound [ɸ] unless he teaches himself to make a segment that he has never heard, and some children do just this, using [ɸ] for /sp/ and also the non-English velar fricative [x] for /sk/.)

Other kinds of clusters may also be treated by omission of one of the sounds, as in column 1 of the example that follows. However, these stop + liquid clusters are sometimes broken up by an unstressed vowel, as in column 2. We also find the use of [w] for the liquid, as in column 3.

	1	2	3
bread	[bɛd] ("bed")	[bərɛ́d] ("buh-RED")	[bwɛd] ("bwed")
blue	[bu] ("boo")	[bəlú] ("buh-LOO")	[bwu] ("bwoo")

Writing Rules

We can write down abbreviated, explicit statements for regular patterns of correspondence between child and adult sound patterns when they occur; such statements are usually called *child phonology* rules. Rules become particularly useful when we are trying to understand a child's form in which several different correspondence patterns are superimposed. For example, a child who has a pattern or rule of replacing velar stops with alveolars and another rule of approximating initial /sp/ with [f] would probably say the word *speak* as [fit] ("feet"); two separate rules have been applied independently.

Accuracy of Perception

Sometimes it is suggested that children who fail to pronounce particular sounds correctly have failed to perceive them accurately. Wholesale confusion of two similar adult phonemes may happen. Children learning English do appear to have some problems distinguishing between words that begin with a few pairs of extremely similar sounds, such as [f] and [θ], and this may contribute to the generally late acquisition of [θ] (Velleman, 1988). But usually, children with normal hearing are able to perform such discrimination tasks quite well, provided they are thoroughly familiar with both test words in a pair (Barton, 1980). Hence, hypothetical Child A described earlier might well be able to point correctly to a coat and a goat even while calling them both "goat."

Although complete fusion of two similar adult phonemes appears to be relatively uncommon for children who have begun to speak, misidentification of one segment in an individual word does occur (Macken, 1980; see also Butler Platt & MacWhinney, 1983). This is usually discovered in the following way: A child who has been producing [f] for both /f/ and /s/ at last begins to get an [s]-like sound for almost all adult words that begin with /s/, including those that she used to say with [f]. However, there are still one or two words that begin with /s/ that she continues to pronounce with the old [f]. The usual explanation of this phenomenon is that in those one or two lagging words, the child had misidentified the initial segments; she really thought they began with /f/, either on first hearing them or after listening to her own erroneous renditions.

Suprasegmental-Segmental Interactions

In the early period of development, word pronunciations are often affected by *length of the word* and *stress patterns.* For example, it is quite common for young children to omit the initial syllable of a multisyllabic word when that syllable is unstressed. Thus, we have forms like "mato" for *tomato,* "zert" for *dessert,* and "posed" for *supposed.* Unstressed syllables in medial position may also be omitted in words like *telephone* [tɛfon] and *elephant* [ɛfənt]. In final position, however, it is much less common for unstressed syllables to be omitted.

Pronunciations of this type do not appear to be due to difficulties with production of particular sounds, but rather to problems with the stress patterns of the words. Since weakly stressed syllables are harder to perceive, the errors may be due to perception rather than production. However, since final unstressed syllables are usually not omitted, most such perceptual problems cannot simply be a matter of not hearing the unstressed syllable; they must instead have to do with selective attention—perhaps the child who makes such errors only "tunes in" to the word when the stressed syllable starts. Another pattern is found in children who use **dummy syllables,** such as [tə] or [rɪ], to take the place of many or all initial unstressed syllables (Smith, 1973). Obviously, in such cases the child knows that the initial unstressed syllable is present. In some instances, perhaps his knowledge of the sounds in the adult syllable may be incomplete; in others, the problem may be organizing the production of the sounds using this less-common stress pattern. Suprasegmental patterns are also involved in the acquisition of grammatical morphemes (see Gerken & McIntosh, 1993; Peters & Menn, 1993).

Assimilation

So far we have talked about the ways in which children approximate the sounds of segments or clusters. However, many of the ways in which children adapt adult words cannot be explained without taking the sounds of the whole target word into account. Daniel (Menn, 1971) showed the following pattern:

- Initial voiced stops usually showed correct position of stop articulation and correct voicing.

    Set 1

bump	[bʌmp]	(correct)
down	[dæwn]	(correct)
gone	[gɔn]	(correct)

- Initial unvoiced stops usually showed correct position but incorrect voicing.

    Set 2

pipe	[bajp]	("bipe")
toad	[dowd]	("dode")
car	[gar]	("gar")

However, when Daniel attempted to say a word that begins with a stop in one place of articulation and ends with a stop in a different place of articulation, a very striking kind of error occurred:

- Initial labial stops became [g] when the target word ended with a velar stop.

  Set 3
bug	[gʌg]	("gug")
big	[gɪg]	("gig")
book	[guk]	("gook")
bike	[gajk]	("gike")
pig	[gɪg]	("gig")

- Initial alveolar stops and *s* + stop clusters also became [g] when the target word ended with a velar stop.

  Set 4
dog	[gɔg]	("gawg")
Doug	[gʌg]	("gug")
duck	[gʌk]	("guck")
stick	[gɪk]	("gick")

- Initial alveolar stops and *s* + stop clusters became [b] when the target word ended with a labial stop.

  Set 5
tub	[bʌb]	("bub")
top	[bap]	("bop")
step	[bɛp]	("bep")
stop	[bap]	("bop")

We cannot explain Daniel's changes in the initial consonants as an inability to pronounce the stops since he was able to get all three places of articulation correct individually (i.e., when there was only one stop in a word or two stops that shared the same place of articulation, as in *bump* or *pipe* in sets 1 and 2). However, when an adult word contained two stops with different places of articulation, he could only get one of the places right, and the place of the other stop was changed to match.

A change in one sound to make it more like another is called **assimilation.** (An example of nasal assimilation was given on p. 87.) One can see how rapidly a simple assimilation pattern like this one renders a child unintelligible to a person who is not familiar with the child's speech. What stranger would know that to decode *gig,* one must consider whether the context called for *big, pig,* or *dig*? And of course, there are many frustrating times when such a child's utterances remain unintelligible because the context does not give enough cues.

Assimilation may also involve manner rather than place of articulation, with similar effects on intelligibility. As was mentioned in the section on regression, Daniel later made initial consonants nasal if the final consonant or consonant cluster contained a nasal (he had almost no medial consonants at the time).

bump	[mʌmp]	("mump")
beans	[minz]	("means")
dance	[næns]	("nance")
going	[ŋowɪŋ]	(cannot be spelled with English orthography)

In the terminology of autosegmental phonology, the feature nasal spread from the final consonant of the word to the initial consonant (and probably to the intervening vowel); in articulatory terms, Daniel let his velum drop at the beginning of a word if the word had a nasal consonant anywhere in it.

Examples like these make it clear that tests or speech samples used for study of articulation must consider all the sounds in a target word. It would have been incorrect to say that Daniel, at either of the two stages just described, could not pronounce word-initial /b/ or /d/, which one might conclude from looking at his versions of *big, dog, duck, beans,* and *dance.* It is very important to use words with only one position and one manner of stop articulation—like *pipe, bib, daddy, papa, do, go, cake*—to assess stop production. Texts on functional articulation disorders (phonological disability) in children (Grunwell, 1987; Ingram, 1989; Stoel-Gammon & Dunn, 1985) make this point clearly. This quite normal two-year-old child's problem was in managing certain sound sequences, not in articulating the sounds themselves.

Rule Origin

Discovery of Rules

We have seen that many children have regular ways of replacing sounds in adult words; and if there is a regularity, we can write a rule to describe it. If the child has mastered accurate productions of adult sounds, these are also to be counted among the child's regularities, and rules (trivial-sounding but often useful) like "adult /t/ becomes child [t]" can be written for them as well.

So far, we have discussed several error patterns that are regular enough to be abbreviated as rules: for example, a rule making all initial stops voiced (hypothetical Child A), a rule replacing all velar stops by alveolar ones (hypothetical Child B), a rule omitting [s] in word-initial consonant clusters, a rule changing initial stops to nasals if there is a nasal at the end of the word, and a more complex pattern involving rules of velar and labial assimilation (Menn, 1971). In general, it appears to be the case, as common sense would suggest, that children produce these patterns because they can-

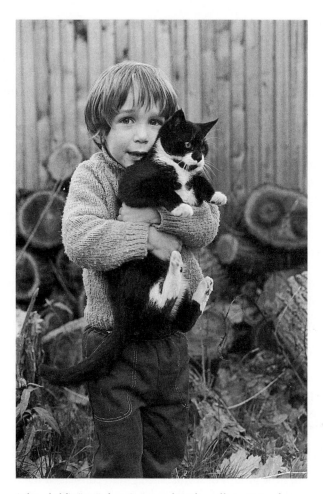

This child's "tat" doesn't care what she calls it. But what would you have to know in order to tell whether she says "tat" because of assimilation or because of difficulty with velars in general, like Child B in the text?

not yet produce any more accurate match to the adult target sound or sound sequence (except perhaps transiently during imitation). There are exceptions to this common-sense view, however; a child who has finally learned to say a sound or sound sequence in some new words may continue in her habit of changing that sound or sequence to something else in old words and in new words that very closely resemble the old words. Rules, once acquired, appear to have a life of their own.

Many phonological error patterns that children use can be explained as fairly natural outcomes of imperfectly coordinated articulatory movements. For example, trouble in delaying the start of vocal cord vibration after the release of a stop would mean a tendency to produce all stops as voiced. The assorted errors that we see in early attempts at producing consonant clusters could be due to various ways of compensating for trouble producing rapid shifts in manner and/or place of articulation. Such natural error patterns and the rules describing them are usually referred to as **natural processes** (Edwards & Shriberg, 1983; Ingram, 1989). However, individual children sometimes have error patterns that do not seem very "natural," such as use of [h] for a large number of different adult consonants.

Errors in a child's first handful of words are often not regular enough for rule writing. Early words typically include a few (progressive) phonological idioms and also a few grossly variable and inaccurate forms (e.g., "bye-bye" produced as [bæ-bæ], [ga-ga], and [ɣæ-ɣæ]; the symbol [ɣ] (gamma) denotes a voiced velar fricative). Apparently, it generally takes a child some time to develop regular ways—accurate or inaccurate— of dealing with adult sounds. This suggests that rules, even natural ones, are discovered by trial and error rather than coming into play automatically as the child starts to speak. This view is basic to the cognitive problem-solving approach to developmental phonology, but it is at odds with the most strongly nativist versions of the "natural phonology" approach, which predict that natural processes will operate most generally at the beginning of speech and then gradually be overcome (e.g., Stampe, 1969).

Canonical Forms

We concluded earlier that children learn sound sequences, not just sounds. The beginning speaker appears to discover how to say certain word-length sequences of sounds and then to attempt similar approaches to other adult words that he perceives as being similar to his initial conquests. In cognitive terms the solution of a problem—how to say a particular word—is generalized to similar problems. This procedure, first described in exquisite detail in a diary study by Waterson (1971), results in the development of little groups of words; each group consists of the child's renditions of adult words that are somewhat similar and have usually become even more similar in the child's versions. Consider the following sets of words from Waterson's work:

Set 1		Set 2	
Randall	[ɲaɲo]	fish	[ɪʃ]
window	[ɲeːɲeː]	dish	[dɪʃ]
finger	[ɲeːɲeː] or [ɲiːɲɪ]	vest	[uʃ]
another	[ɲaɲa]	brush	[byʃ]
		fetch	[ɪʃ]

Note. [ɲ] represents a palatal nasal, roughly the sound of *ny* in *canyon*.

[e] is used without [j] "off-glide."

[y] is the front rounded vowel spelled *u* in French and *ü* in German.

ː indicates that the preceding phone was of relatively long duration.

Each little group can be described by abstracting out what the child's renditions have in common. The words in the first column are disyllables consisting of two palatal nasals [ɲ] and two vowels. The words in the second column all end with the palatal fricative [ʃ], contain a short vowel made with the tongue relatively high in the mouth, and begin with either a stop or that vowel. Using V to stand for any vowel and C to stand for any stop consonant, we can abbreviate the two patterns just presented; the first is [ɲVɲV], and the second is [(C)Vʃ]. (Putting the C in parentheses is a standard way of indicating that it is sometimes omitted.)

Such abstracted patterns for sets of words are called **canonical forms,** and each word that conforms to that pattern is then an instance of that canonical form. The output of children who have more than about five but fewer than perhaps a hundred words can generally be described as several sets of canonical forms plus a handful of other words, usually phonological idioms, that are relatively isolated.

This organization of children's early vocabulary is currently seen as the key to understanding most of their ways of dealing with adult words. A child's canonical forms represent the kinds of sound sequences that she has learned to produce at will up to that point; her rules are representations of the regular ways that she adjusts adult words to fit into those available sequences. Not all children arrive at regular ways to make these adjustments; Daniel did but Waterson's subject did not, and neither did the children reported by Macken (1979) and Priestly (1977).

Children who do use rules may start to do so at different points in their development. Some researchers distinguish a prerule period, "the stage of the first fifty words," from a later rule-governed period, but we must be careful to bear in mind the great amount of individual variation across children and the fact that some aspects of a child's phonology can be quite rule-governed while other aspects remain irregular. A strength of a constraint-based approach like optimality theory is that it allows us to see how a variety of different rules (e.g., deletion of one consonant in a cluster and co-alescence of features of two adjacent consonants in a cluster) are all means to the same end; it also allows us to see that unruly processes, like those discussed for Waterson's subject, are related to rule-governed ones like those found in Smith's subject.

Instrumental Analyses of Children's Speech

Is the transcriber's ear really adequate to evaluate children's speech? And should children's words really be transcribed with the same symbols that we use for adult phones and phonemes? Macken and Barton (1980) have shown that some degree of caution is necessary in transcribing a child's speech on the basis of adult perceptions. Some children who appear to be using voiced stops for initial unvoiced stops are actually trying to make the correct distinction, but they have not learned to do so in a way that is audible to the unaided ear. Their use of longer voicing onset timing for their unvoiced stops than for their voiced ones is detectable only by laboratory measurements of the sound waves they produce. This is a case where a description of the child's language in terms of features is too crude to give an accurate reflection of what is happening. A child who is making an inaudible but correct distinction between voiced and unvoiced stops has the correct phonological distinction but an inadequate version of the phonetic distinction; it would not be correct to describe him either as having mastered or as not having understood the voicing distinction for initial stops. He is at an intermediate stage.

Strategies in Learning to Pronounce

A major focus of research in child phonology, as in developmental psychology, has been the study of differences among children. The data presented so far have shown several differences in the rules describing the forms that various children use. If we look at the overall strategies that children adopt to deal with the problem of producing words, another type of difference becomes apparent. Some children might be thought of as relatively conservative; they seem not to use a word if they cannot produce at least the beginning sounds fairly accurately. In a list of the words such a child recognizes compared to the words she uses, there may be a very striking imbalance; for example, Jacob, who has been cited several times in this chapter, understood and responded to many words beginning with /b/, /k/, and /d/ but only attempted to say those beginning with /d/ (with the exception of "bye-bye," which he said under social pressure and which came out [da-da]). This state of affairs lasted for several months; then a group of /k/-initial words were observed, all produced with a correct first segment, and then initial /b/ was finally mastered.

Clearly, Jacob was sticking to what he knew how to pronounce and avoiding other words until he had figured out how to produce them to his own satisfaction. Other children have also been observed to avoid certain sounds (Ferguson & Farwell, 1975), although until quite recently few people thought it was possible for a child of, say, fifteen months to have such a degree of phonological awareness. This skepticism was reinforced by the fact that many other children, often two years old or older, seem blissfully unaware of the discrepancy between what they are saying and the adult target. Most children probably fall between the extremes of selecting only what they can say, on the one hand, and casually adapting any adult word to fit their output repertoire on the other hand (see Schwartz & Leonard, 1982).

Another dimension of acquisition strategy seems closely related to Katherine Nelson's (1973) referential/expressive dimension (see Chapters 4 and 8). Some children attempt one word at a time, and these words generally have relatively clear and consistent (although possibly quite incorrect) pronunciation. Others use a more global approach to speech, approximating whole phrases with much less clear or consistent articulation (Branigan, 1979; Peters, 1977). The child's meaning may be understandable from context and tone of voice, and there may be enough recognizable phonetic material in the utterance to make it clear that particular words are intended; yet the phrase may be reduced to a virtually untranscribable mess.

There are other children who combine these approaches; for example, some embed one or two clear words in long, otherwise unintelligible strings. We know very little about why such differences among children exist or whether they correlate with any other developmental phenomena. However, as the selectors and the adaptors learn more sounds and as the one-worders start to put words together and the phrase-approximators become more precise in their articulation, the distinctions in strategy eventually blur and seem to disappear.

Children learning languages with different adult sound patterns—for example, children learning Spanish, Finnish, Japanese, and other languages that have very few one-syllable words—may have different strategies and patterns from children learning English, which has so many monosyllables. The frequency of sounds in the ambient language may also have an effect; children learning languages that have more /l/s (Quiche Mayan) tend to learn them earlier than do children learning English (Pye, Ingram, & List, 1987).

Change over Time: The Increasing Importance of Child-Phonology Rules

Let's review the developmental changes that we have seen up to now. A child's acquisition of phonology begins with trial-and-error attempts at isolated words, especially ones that match her favorite babble patterns. Some of these may be produced quite accurately, and these will become notable as progressive phonological idioms; others may be very loosely and variably approximated. Eventually, the child will be able to generalize some of his successes; thus, little groups of similar-sounding words form in his output repertoire. Canonical forms can be written to describe what the words in each group have in common; these help to capture the severe restrictions on what sounds can co-occur in the child's output.

A way of dealing with a group of adult words may be extended to a similar word that the child has already been pronouncing; if the old form was a closer approximation to the adult model than the new one, the change is a regressive one, as in Daniel's change from "down" to "noun" described earlier. If the adult words have regular correspondences to the child's words, rules can be written abstracting those regularities, and regression will be appropriately considered as a case of rule overgeneralization. This is the picture that we have described up to this point.

Now, gradually, an important change occurs. The child becomes able to combine a greater variety of sounds in a word. He no longer appears to be operating with little families of similar words but with segments, and so description in terms of canonical forms loses its usefulness. In psycholinguistic terms this development would reflect the ability to analyze a perceived word into segments and to pronounce those segments relatively independently. This development toward word segmentation is never complete, even in an adult, but the child moves toward whatever degree of combinatorial freedom the surrounding adults possess.

The developing ability to deal with individual segments increases the value of writing explicit rules to describe the child's renditions of those segments. N. V. Smith's child Amahl (Smith, 1973) gives a splendid example of this level of developing ability, and we will conclude this section with an account of his development of an initial [tʃ] ("ch"). This portion of Smith's study is particularly interesting because it shows that one needs to consider the range of variation in a child's renditions of adult segments in order to decide which ones the child is treating as "the same" and which ones she is treating as distinct. The clinical and research importance of this example cannot be overemphasized; several elicitations of each test word are required to establish a child's ways of rendering the sounds in it. Gradual replacement of one way of saying a word with a new way of saying it, as illustrated here, is the norm, not the exception. However, if only a single sample of a word is obtained in a given observation, these orderly but gradual changes can be mistaken for wildly random variation.

At a certain point late in his second year, referred to as stage 19 in Smith's (1973) book, Amahl used a *t*-like phone correctly for the stop /t/ and incorrectly for the fricative /s/ and the affricate stop /tʃ/. The following data are taken (in simplified notation) from a table that summarizes the changes in the renditions of three words beginning with these sounds (p. 154).

Target:	toe	say	chair
	/tow/	/sej/	[tʃeʌ]
Output:			
Stage 19	[to]	[tej]	[teʌ]
20	[to]	[tej], [tsej]	[teʌ], [tseʌ]
21	[to]	[tsej], [sej]	[tseʌ], [seʌ]
22	[to]	[sej]	[seʌ]
26	[to]	[sej]	[seʌ], [tseʌ]
29	[to]	[sej]	[tseʌ]
			[tʃeʌ]

Note: The target dialect, British "Received Pronunciation," has no [r] in word-final position.

We see that Amahl said these three beginning sounds all as [t] at stage 19. At stage 20, however, he had separated the target /t/ from the other sounds and had begun to use [ts] for the friction sounds of /s/ and /tʃ/ in some productions of *say* and *chair.* He was at this point capable of *making* the output distinction between /t/ and the other two sounds but not of *maintaining* it.

At stage 21 he had clearly severed the connection of /s/ and /tʃ/ with /t/; for now the friction sound was always present in his renditions of the first two sounds. However, it becomes increasingly clear that as far as output is concerned, there is no distinction between /s/ and /tʃ/, for the sound [s] is appearing for both of these. By stage 22 and for the next three stages (not shown), [s] is used reliably for them both. Note that although this is fine for the true /s/ sound, it is an overcorrection for the target /tʃ/; [ts] was a more accurate rendition of this sound.

Finally, at stage 26 Amahl's productions start to represent the phonemic distinction between /s/ and /tʃ/; he starts to use [ts] again in *chair,* and by stage 29 the use of [s] for /tʃ/ has disappeared. The final phonetic detail of replacing the [ts] (which we may consider an alveolar affricate) with the palatal affricate /tʃ/ comes later.

Development After Three Years

Although children's pronunciation patterns are not fully adultlike by three years of age, the basic features of the adult phonological system are present. Studies of groups of children tested at different ages (e.g., Prather, Hedrick, & Kern, 1975; Templin, 1957) provide a general picture of the acquisition of English during the period of *mastery*. These studies are important because they provide guidelines that speech therapists can use in identifying children whose phonological system is not developing normally (see Chapter 9). By three, most children can produce all the vowel sounds and nearly all the consonant sounds. This does not mean that their productions are 100 percent accurate, but rather that the sounds are produced correctly in at least a few words. Consonants that are likely to be in error, even at the age of four or five, are the liquids /r/ and /l/ and

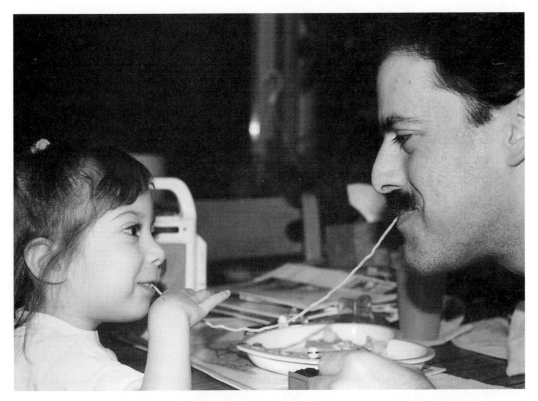

Initial consonant clusters can make a word like "spaghetti" difficult for preschoolers to pronounce.

the fricatives /v/, /θ/ as in *thin,* and /ð/ as in *the.* As might be expected, correct pronunciation patterns are often more accurate in short words, like the /v/ of *vase,* while longer words like *vacuum cleaner* may cause mispronunciations. In most cases, correct production of all sounds is achieved by around seven years of age.

Consonant clusters such as [spr-] at the beginning of the word *spring* and [-lps] at the end of *helps* are usually acquired relatively late. In some cases, the child is capable of producing the individual phonemes within the cluster, but not of putting them together in a sequence. Thus, the /s/ of *see* and the /n/ of *no* could be pronounced correctly whereas the /sn-/ combination in *snow* would be produced with omission of the /s/. (Examples of this pattern of "cluster of reduction" were presented earlier; see page 92.) Smit and colleagues (Smit, 1993; Smit, Hand, Freilinger, Bernthal, & Bird, 1990) report that some clusters in word-initial position are not mastered until the age of seven or eight years.

The Acquisition of English Morphophonology

Morphophonology concerns the kind of variation that we see when we compare the pronunciation of the *nat-* in sets of related words like *nation, native, nativity, nationality,* or the pronunciation of the "th" in *path* as compared to *paths.* Some languages have many more such patterns than English does. How do children master these sound-variation patterns?

Morphemes

To understand morphophonology, we must first consider the important concepts of **morpheme** and **allomorph.** Words often can be seen to consist of smaller meaningful parts; the smallest units that carry meaning are called *morphemes.* Any word that cannot be subdivided into smaller parts with meaning is therefore one morpheme: *hat, run, big, how. Hatband, runner, biggest,* and *however* consist of two morphemes each. The *-er* of *runner* and the *-est* of *biggest* are separable, meaningful elements; *-er* here means "one who," and *-est* means "most." The inflectional endings, like the *-s* that signals plural and the *-d* that indicates past tense, are also morphemes that cannot stand alone. English has a much smaller set of these endings than languages like Latin, German, or French.

Allomorphy in Inflectional Endings

Some inflectional endings have the same shape regardless of the words they are attached to, like the progressive *-ing* of verbs like *giving;* others, however, have different shapes depending on the sound of the word or stem that they are attached to.

These different shapes are called the *allomorphs* of the morpheme, and *morphophonology* describes the way that the choice among allomorphs is determined. The plural morpheme, for example, sounds like /s/ when it follows unvoiced stops: *cats, rocks.* When the plural morpheme follows a vowel or most voiced stops, its sound is /z/: *days, kids, dogs.* There is one group of final sounds that requires still a third variant of this morpheme. Words ending in the hissing or sibilant sounds /s/, /z/, /ʃ/, /ʒ/, /tʃ/, or /dʒ/ take the variant [əz]—*kisses, sneezes, fishes, garages, churches,* and *judges.* These three variants of the plural morpheme are referred to as its *regular allomorphs;* regular, in this case, means that if one knows the sound of the singular noun, the choice among the three plural endings is automatic. There are also some irregular plural allomorphs, which have to be separately learned: for example, the *-en* of *oxen,* the *-ren* of *children,* and the internal vowel changes that signal the plural of words like *man.* (*Men,* therefore, consists of two morphemes, *man* and the plural, even though it can't be separated into stem and ending as *cats* can.) There are also some words like *sheep* and *deer* that are unchanged in the plural; such words are said to have a zero plural allomorph when they are used with plural meaning.

Allomorphy in Other Morphemes

English has other morphemes that are found almost entirely in words inherited or derived from Greek and Latin origins. Some of these also exhibit allomorphy; that is, the same morpheme will have several allomorphs. For example, the adjective ending -*ic* (*electric, toxic*) is found in the form /ɪk/ when it stands at the end of a word or before certain other endings, but in the allomorph /ɪs/ when the noun-forming -*ity* is added to it, as in *electricity* or *toxicity.*

The form variations that we have discussed so far have all involved forms of word endings. The inflections (plural, past) showed different allomorphs depending on what base word (stem) they were attached to, and the adjective ending -*ic* showed up as /ɪs/ when the additional noun-forming ending -*ity* was attached to it. The stem of a word may also vary when an ending is attached. Consider the pronunciation (not the spelling) of the following verb–noun pairs, which show **stem allomorphy.**

Verb	Noun	Verb	Noun
inflate	inflation	abrade	abrasion
relate	relation	invade	invasion
pollute	pollution	delude	delusion
promote	promotion	corrode	corrosion

There seems to be an ending spelled -*ion* that turns these verbs into nouns, but the final consonant in the verb also changes in pronunciation when -*ion* is added. The morphemes ending in /t/, such as *promote,* show alternate forms with /ʃ/ in the related nouns; the morphemes ending in /d/, like *corrode,* show alternates ending in /ʒ/. We might try to link what happens to /t/ and what happens to /d/ by saying that alveolar consonants before -*ion* become palatal fricatives but do not change their voicing.

As we explore the English lexicon, however, we run into problems with formulating an explicit rule connecting a verb with its allomorph in an *-ion* noun. *Insert* gives *insertion,* with /ʃ/, but *invert* gives *inversion,* with /ʒ/; *degrade* gives *degradation,* not *degrasion; collect* gives *collection,* but *suspect* gives *suspicion,* not *suspection.* Many verbs have no *-ion* form at all (although one could imagine what such a related noun ought to be like): there is no *debation* or *debasion* to correspond to *debate.* Finally, there are many *-ion* nouns with no corresponding English verb: There is *vision* but not *vide, occasion* but not *occade.*

Recognition of Allomorphic Relations

In English, stem allomorphy involves many more irregularities and gaps than affix allomorphy. The question is often raised (Braine, 1974) as to whether English speakers apprehend these relationships at all since they have to memorize the proper noun and verb forms anyway. Furthermore, if speakers do sense correspondence between such pairs of words, can they be said to know rules expressing that correspondence in anything like the way they know rules linking the regular /s/, /z/, and /əz/ allomorphs of the plural?

Research (Jaeger, 1980; Myerson, 1975; Wilbur & Menn, 1975) indicates that speakers may indeed apprehend many of the less regular relationships between allomorphs, especially with the help of hints embodied in English spelling (the orthographic resemblance between *native* and *national* may make it easier to recognize that they are related words; if they were spelled phonetically, they wouldn't look so much alike). However, speakers do not have to extract the intricate patterns that we have just surveyed in order to become competent users of English: One does not have to make up new *-ion* words. In fact, one must refrain from doing so, since spiting someone is not *spition,* nor is avoiding *avoision.* Because *-ion* cannot be added freely to make new words, we say that it is not a **productive** ending in English. In contrast, the regular plural, past, and possessive endings are productive; that is, they can be added to almost any word, including new words, if the semantics of the occasion demand, so speakers must master the rules for choosing the right allomorph.

Stress in Morphophonology

The **stress** or accent pattern within a word is intimately related to the sounds in it, especially to the vowel sounds. In English, vowels are longer, louder, and often higher in pitch when they are in stressed (accented) syllables than when they are in unstressed syllables. In addition, if adding an ending to a word causes the stress to shift from one syllable to another, some of the vowels in the word may change more drastically and actually become different phonemes. These changes are often not reflected in spelling. For example, when the word *declare* /də-klɛ́r/ is used to make *declaration* /dɛ-klə-réj-ʃn/, the stress changes: /klɛ́jr/ loses its stress, /də/ gains a little, and the strongest accent goes to the third syllable. Other examples of stress shifting when an ending is added can be seen in pairs like *méthod–methódical* and *nórmal–normálity;* in each case the vowels are affected. Endings may also trigger changes in vowels even when the stress does not shift; consider pairs like *vain–vánity* or *south–soúthern.*

Development of Morphophonology

Children begin learning some of the regularities governing the choice among English allomorphs fairly early. However, some aspects of English stress appear not to be mastered until age twelve or so, and some nonproductive regularities are still being learned well into adolescence. Much work remains to be done in this area, but we will discuss two pioneering experimental studies.

Myerson (1975) carried out a study that showed an increasing ability over the ages eight through seventeen to deal with three types of allomorphy: (1) the change from alveolar stop to palatal fricative when *-ion* is added, as in *explode–explosion;* (2) the shift in stress when *-ity* or *-ical* are added to words like *stupid (stupidity)* or *method (methodical);* and (3) the changes in vowels associated with such shifts in stress.

It had been known for some time (Krohn, Steinberg, & Kobayashi, 1972) that adults do not reliably make these changes in consonants, stress, and vowels when they are simply asked to tack on endings like *-ion* or *-ity* to nonsense words or to existing words that do not occur with these endings. This situation holds true for children as well. However, Myerson showed that older children and adolescents do gradually learn to make use of these relationships, which apparently reduce the load on long-term memory storage of words. Myerson taught seventy-two children (eighteen each from grades three, six, nine, and twelve) ten pairs of made-up words presented as meaningful. Each subject was presented with the same base "word" and one of two versions of that base word with an ending (*-ion, -ical,* or *-ity*) attached. One of those two versions followed an English pattern; for example, a base that rhymed with *distort* was paired with a derived form rhyming with *distortion.* The other version of the derived form just tacked the ending onto the base without change so that the subject was taught a base rhyming with *distort,* and a derived form that was rhymed with "distortean" (rather like what one would call a native of a place called Distortea). Each subject learned five pairs of words made up according to the English pattern and five pairs of words with the same endings just tacked on. The pairs were thoroughly taught in the first session and then tested for recall one day, one week, and six weeks later. The teaching procedure went according to the following example:

> A picture of a lion about to pounce on a pig is presented while the following paragraph is read aloud: "*Delort.* To delort means to attack. The lion is about to delort the pig. The lion is about to attack the pig. Now add *i-o-n* to *delort* to make a new word meaning an attack. The lion is about to delort the pig. Whenever a lion delorts a pig, he makes a (*version 1*) /dəlɔrtiʌn/ (*version 2*) /dəlorʒn/. What does a lion do when he delorts a pig? He makes a _____. Whenever a lion delorts a pig, he makes a _____." Any errors are corrected. (Appendix p. xxix)

Similar presentations were used for pairs like *glane–glanity* (/gléjnəti/, /glǽnəti/) and *gathod–gathodical* (/ˈgǽθədɪkl/, /gəˈθádɪkl/).

Myerson found that the forms with the tacked-on endings were harder to recall for all children. Furthermore, there was an overwhelming tendency for a child who had been taught a tacked-on form like *delortean* to recall it incorrectly as *delortion,* a form that had the appropriate allomorphic base change, whereas the opposite error of recalling a *delortion* form as *delortean* rarely occurred.

Atkinson-King (1973) studied an aspect of word stress, the acquisition of the word-stress difference that distinguishes the noun *record* from the verb *record.* She found that kindergartners, the youngest children in her study, were able to listen to pairs of sentences like "I put the record (/rékrd/) on the shelf" and "I put the record (/rekórd/) on the shelf" and judge correctly that the first was better.

Acquisition of Compound and Phrase Stress

Stress has many uses in construction phrases and sentences that are beyond the scope of this chapter. The most familiar kind of stress is probably contrastive or emphatic stress, as when one says, "I want the bláck book, not the greén book," with the strongest stresses on *black* and *green.* Compare this sentence with "I want the black book, not the black notebook"; in the latter the strongest stresses are on the first *book* and on *note.* Another use of stress in English is to distinguish compounds from phrases: *greénhouse* (transparent structure for growing plants) is a compound and is stressed on the word *green,* but a *green hoúse* is any house painted green, and when there is no occasion for emphasis on the color, the word *house* bears greater or at least equal stress— "At the end of this road there's a green hoúse and then a pond."

In this particular pair spelling distinguishes the compound *greenhouse* from the phrase *green house;* however, orthography is not reliable since, for example, the compound *hót dog* (frankfurter) is spelled the same as the phrase *hot dóg* (a very warm canine pet). There are also some items, like *apple pie* and *chocolate cake,* that can be thought of either as compounds or as phrases; some speakers stress these on the first word and some on the second.

Atkinson-King (1973) found that kindergartners were able to produce emphatic stress correctly, as in "I want the réd book, not the green book." The major portion of her study, however, was a large set of imitation, judgment, and production tests of children's ability to distinguish phrases like "a green hoúse" or "the red sócks" from compounds like "a greénhouse" or "the Réd Sox" (the name of the baseball team from Boston, where the study was carried out).

For example, in one test the children were given pairs of pictures and asked to show which was the greenhouse and which was the green house. In a second task the children were given pairs of sentences, such as "I put mustard on my hót dog" and "I put mustard on my hot dóg," and asked which one was better. In a third task the children were given the pictures singly and asked to label them; adults heard tapes of their productions and attempted to decide which of the pair each child had intended. In a fourth test the children were given the pair of pictures together and asked to describe them so that the investigator could tell which was which. This one gave some curious results, for Atkinson-King found that

> some children knew that there was a difference between members of a pair but could not consistently and correctly signal that difference. For example, some used the same stress pattern on both members of a pair but said the entire first member very rapidly and the second extremely slowly (in this presentation, half the time the first member of the pair was the phrase and half the time it was the compound). A number of others were able to produce the two stress patterns correctly but always produced the compound and then the phrasal pattern, regardless of the order in which the pictures they were looking at appeared. (p. 111)

Note that this confusion did not indicate a general inability to control stress, since all of the children had been shown able to produce emphatic stress accurately.

All the children, even the kindergartners, could imitate each pair accurately, but the ability to deal with the other tasks at an adult level of performance (essentially perfect) developed gradually from first grade to sixth grade. Preference judgments were 80 percent correct by third grade; the ability to choose between two pictures given the label for one of them was acquired next, then the ability to produce the two labels accurately when presented with the paired pictures, and finally the ability to produce the label distinguishably when given only one of the pictures. The first two tasks (imitation and preference) may be seen as testing phonetic ability—can the child get the sound right and know how it should sound in context? The others require the ability to make a choice between stress patterns without the support of linguistic context; this can be considered a phonemic skill.

Parental Role in Phonological Development

It is often said that overt correction by adults plays no role in the acquisition of language, at least with respect to phonology and syntax. Certainly it can fail to have any noticeable effect, and the arguments against external-reward behaviorist models of acquisition show that, in any case, the child's own self-monitoring, quite possibly taking place below the level of consciousness, must be responsible for the bulk of the acquisition of phonology. The general (but not total) resistance of phonological errors to overt correction appears to reflect the difficulty of modifying any aspect of habitual or automatic behavior, including slouching at the table and allowing the screen door to slam. Conscious efforts trickle down to automatic behavior slowly, if at all. Yet learning—in the case of phonology, incredibly precise learning—does take place over time; children adjust their production of words so that it approaches some composite of their parents and their peers (Deser, 1990; Payne, 1976).

Regional Variants

Most of us have lived only in a few areas of our native countries, and so we tend to have a very limited idea of the variations of English spoken in other regions, let alone in other English-speaking countries. Advertisement and entertainment media may give us a superficial acquaintance with stereotypes of the American southern, New York, Australian, or Cockney varieties of English, but such stereotypes represent only a few of the most striking differences between these varieties of English and what may be called the broadcasting network standard of the United States. A few rough regional characteristics are listed below, but the best way to learn how people of a region really speak is to go there, tape, and listen to the fine details of their speech production. Study of such variations is an important branch of the field of **sociolinguistics.**

A Few Regional Characteristics of American English

In the Midwest and West, the vowels [a] and [ɔ] contrast before [r]—*car* and *core* are distinct—but before sounds other than [r], these vowels are both produced as [a]: *cot* and *caught* are both [kat].

In the Middle Atlantic states, *cot* has the vowel [a] and *caught* has pretty much the same vowel [ɔ] as *core.*

In much of the Northeast, the vowels of *Mary, merry,* and *marry* are differentiated from one another as [meri], [mɛri], and [mæri], but in most of the rest of the country, two or all three of these words are homonyms, that is, are pronounced exactly the same way.

In much of the central part of the United States, the vowels [ɪ] and [ɛ] are not distinguished before nasal consonants; *pin* and *pen,* for example, are homonyms, so that one may be asked, "Do you mean a [pɪən] to write with or a [pɪən] to fasten something with?"

In New York and New England, as well as much of the South, [r] is not pronounced at the ends of phrases nor before consonants. The [r] is often replaced by a lengthening, off-glide, or change of quality on the vowel preceding the position that it would have appeared in—for example, in some Boston-area speakers, the pronunciation of *shark* is [ʃaːk]. The vowel written [aː] is a long low front vowel, lower than the [æ] of *shack* [ʃæk] and farther front than the [a] of *shock* [ʃak].

In the New York area, a [g] is pronounced where it is written after [ŋ], but in the rest of the United States, there is no [g] after [ŋ] at the ends of words, nor in nouns (e.g., *singer*) derived from verbs ending in [ŋ].

In the East, many words written with *or* (e.g., *orange, horrible*) are pronounced with [ar] rather than [ɔr]; however this is not true for all such words—*orchid* has [ɔr], for example.

In most of the United States, [e], [i], [o], and [u] are **diphthongized,** that is, produced with a following off-glide as approximately [ej, ij, ow, uw], while [ɪ], [ɛ], and [ʊ] are **monophthongs;** however, in much of the South and Texas, the vowels in the first group are generally less diphthongized, while the vowels in the second set all tend to have a [ə] off-glide: *pan* is roughly [pæən].

In and near the large northern cities, the low vowels [æ] and [ɔ] are becoming more and more diphthongized, and the first part of the diphthong is becoming higher than it is in the rest of the United States, so that they are approximately [eə] (or even [iə]) and [uə]. The names *Ann* and *Ian* are homophonous for many speakers in this region.

Children acquire the regional and stylistic variants that they hear—which of course has major clinical and research implications. We often cannot tell whether a child's form that differs from our own is correct or incorrect until we compare it with how the child's parents and/or slightly older friends would say the same word in the same setting. A child with parents from New York who pronounces *bang* as [bĭəŋg] or one from the West who says it as [beŋ] is just as correct as one from the Middle Atlantic who says [bæŋ].

Pronunciation in Conversational Speech

A given person's pronunciation of a word also depends on the speech style being used at a given time. There is usually considerable variation between the highly self-monitored speech styles used for reading word lists aloud and presenting a new word to a young child, on the one hand, and the very unmonitored style used in a deeply involving conversation among family members or old friends, on the other hand. It is in the less monitored style that the most distinctive regional variations are most likely to be heard.

In conversational speech, the pronunciation of words may differ very strongly from the way the same words are produced when they are read aloud carefully from a list, but speakers are generally quite unaware of this fact. For example, in the phrase "I have to leave now," the *have* and *to* are always run together as a single word, pronounced [hæftə]; *want to* and *going to* are rendered as *wanna* or *wannu* and *gonna* or *gonnu,* except when they are being specially emphasized. In the conversational insert phrase *y'know,* many speakers reduce the sounds to something like [jõ]; the word *no* has a huge set of variants, which we sometimes try to write in English orthography as *naw, nah,* and the like.

Other common casual speech rules or processes in English include simplification of various word-final consonant clusters depending on how the next word begins ("George an' Mary"; "cann' peaches"), omission of vowels in unstressed syllables, partial devoicing of phrase-final voiced stops and fricatives, omission of /ð/ and /h/ in unstressed object pronouns ("I see 'er"; "Push 'em over here"), and so on.

Although young children are often given the opportunity to hear nouns in isolation in naming routines, they usually hear most other words in phrases, and the "targets" that they are trying to pronounce must be considered to be these phrasal forms (i.e., forms like *hafta, wan'em, couldja,* and so on).

Parents do seem to improve the precision of their articulation above normal conversational levels to help their children learn to speak, however. Two researchers, Malsheen (1980) and Bernstein Ratner (1984a, 1984b), have carried out major studies of this phenomenon using acoustic measurements to show that parents increase the articulatory precision of their speech to children in the first few years of their children's learning to speak. This adult behavior is probably not conscious either, except as an attempt to assure understanding; but there seems to be more to it than that, according to Bernstein Ratner.

Malsheen tape-recorded mothers of two children who had not yet produced any recognizable words (six and eight months old), two children who had produced one-word utterances (fifteen and sixteen months old), and two children (two-and-a-half and five years old) who had used an average of several words per utterance. She compared the word-initial consonants (*b, d, g, p, t, k*) used by each woman in speaking to her child and in speaking to an adult, and she found that mothers clarified their pronunciation of initial consonants in speech to the children at the one-word stage but not to the prelingual children or to the older ones. She measured this clarification in terms of the same parameter used by Macken and Barton, the voice onset time (the period between the release of the oral closure and the onset of vocal cord vibration). Recall that voiced word-initial stops in English are not necessarily produced with concurrent vocal cord vibration but that voicing begins, on the average, well within two hundredths of a second after the release of closure (when a vowel follows); in the production of unvoiced stops, vocal cord vibration usually begins more than four hundredths of a second after the release. However, in normal adult–adult conversation consonant production is quite sloppy; for example, in Malsheen's adult–adult conversations as many as half of the instances of word-initial /t/ had voice onset time of less than two hundredths of a second, which means that they would have been heard as /d/ if they had been taken out of context. The same kind of sloppy control was also found in the mothers' speech to the prelingual children and to the children who were using multiword utterances. However, speech to the children in the one-word stage showed very few sloppy unvoiced stops; almost all were produced with a voice onset time of four hundredths of a second or more, and many were hyperdistinct with voice onset time of over a tenth of a second.

Bernstein Ratner studied vowel production of nine mothers speaking to their children (some at the one-word stage and some using an average of two to four words per utterance) as compared with the vowels in the same words excerpted from speech to other adults. Her findings indicate that mothers' clarification of vowel production is best seen as modeling words of the type that the child is currently learning to use, rather than increasing the distinctness of overall speech. What she found was that speech directed to children at the one-word stage showed clarification of vowels in nouns, verbs, and adjectives—that is, the sort of words being used most by the children themselves. Speech directed to children using several-word utterances showed clarification not only in nouns, verbs, and adjectives, but also in the function words that these children were just beginning to use: pronouns, prepositions, and conjunctions.

Intonation Contour

The pitch or melody of the voice rises and falls during speaking, and the pattern of pitch changes accompanying a phrase or sentence is called its **intonation contour.** Strong final rises in pitch are found in many (but not all!) types of questions, and smaller rises are often found in tentative polite statements. A rise in pitch corresponds to an increase in frequency of vocal cord vibration, and this can easily be measured in the laboratory.

Although children begin to use intonation contour meaningfully while they are still babbling, learning the details of the adult language system may take many years (Cruttenden, 1985).

Summary

Phonology concerns the relations among the speech sounds of a language: their phonetic resemblances due to the way they are produced, their distributions as shown by minimal-pair contrasts, the possible phonotactic sequences in which they occur, and the way that distinct phonemes correspond to one another in the several allomorphs that a morpheme can have. The child learning to talk must learn to produce the right sounds, to put them in the sequences demanded by the ambient language, to recognize variant phones as representative of the same phoneme, and to learn at least the productive allomorphic relationships.

Humans have an innate, biological basis for hearing and producing speech sounds; this is then shaped by language experience, including cognitive reactions to articulatory challenges. There is strong evidence to suggest that normal infants are born with the ability to hear many distinctions between speech sounds, but that around age ten to twelve months their auditory perceptions become adultlike—that is, they become less sensitive to those differences that are subphonemic in whatever language is around them. Infants also appear to progress through the early months of sound production in a biologically determined way, for the detrimental effects of deafness on production only start to appear after babbling has begun. Individual differences and ambient language effects gradually appear in later babbling. The transition from babbling to speech is gradual; early words tend to utilize sounds that the child has been favoring in late babbling.

Nativist theories of phonological development emphasize the similarities among children; they have difficulty dealing with individual differences and with irregularities. In addition, the best-known nativist theory, that of Jakobson, deals only with the acquisition of phonemic contrast, not with phonetic targets or phonotactic patterns. Behaviorist theories that depend on external reward for improved pronunciation are inadequate; external reward is too crude to guide mastery of the myriad fine details of phonetics. Neither nativist nor behaviorist theories can deal with regression in accuracy of production; here, as elsewhere in language acquisition, the data require a cognitive problem-solving theory since only this type of theory predicts that there will be overgeneralizations.

With the aid of descriptive features, we can assess children's partial successes in pronunciation and see similarities linking their attempts at related sounds. Rendering all initial stops as voiced, using alveolar place of articulation for both alveolar and velar consonants, and assimilating nasality and/or place of articulation are common patterns in early child phonology, as are several varieties of cluster simplification. When such patterns occur regularly in a given child's speech, rules can be written to describe the relation between the adult word and the child's form, for both correct and incorrect renditions. Even when the adult–child correspondences are not regular enough to be called rules, early child words typically occur in little groups whose common properties can be abstracted and written in formulas called canonical forms. Often there are a few words whose pronunciation is much more adultlike than others; these isolated progressive phonological idioms do not, by definition, come under any of the child's canonical forms but are exceptions to the child's rules. They are usually among the child's earliest words; this supports the claim that rules for rendering adult words are discovered by the child through trial and error.

Not all of a child's progress is correctly assessed by the unaided ear; instrumental studies of tape recordings show that children's earliest steps toward mastering adult phonemic distinctions may be inaudible to adults.

Individual variation among children is found in the strategies they adopt as well as in their individual rules and canonical forms. Some children attempt whole phrases, others try words singly; some avoid (public) attempts at words they cannot pronounce, others rearrange adult words freely to fit them into their existing repertoire.

Eventually, as the child learns to put more different kinds of speech sounds together within one word, the small groups expand and merge; canonical forms become less useful as descriptors, while rules become more useful.

In the elementary school years, children learn to distinguish certain aspects of the English stress system, and in the later school years they become acquainted with some of the nonproductive relationships that prevail among words in the Latin-based portion of the English lexicon. These relationships strongly affect recall and presumably reduce the memory load required for learning new words.

Overt parental correction of pronunciation has perhaps the same effect on children as correction of any other habitual behavior. Yet mothers have been shown to increase the accuracy of their production of word-initial consonants just as children are learning to pronounce single words and to enhance the clarity of their vowels in content words during the same period. Furthermore, they later increase the clarity of function word production slightly, when their children are beginning to express the grammatical relations that adult grammar encodes in function words.

Key Words

articulatory phonetics	nativist
affricates	natural processes
allomorph	nonreflexive vocalizations
alveolar	obstruents
assimilation	palatal
behaviorist	phone
canonical form	phoneme
categorical perception	phonotactics
consonant	productive
consonant clusters	progressive phonological idioms
diphthongized	protoword
dummy syllable	reduplicated babble
free variation	reflexive vocalizations
fricative	regression
glide	self-organizing system
glottal	semivowels
glottis	sociolinguistics
high amplitude sucking	sound play
interdental	stem allomorphy
intonation contour	stop
labial	stress
labiodental	variegated babble
liquid	velar
minimal pair	velum
modulated babble	vocal motor scheme
monophthongs	voicing
morpheme	voice onset time
morphophonology	vowel
nasal stop	

Suggested Projects

The first three activities are time-consuming and, if carried out in full detail, might well take several weeks to complete.

1. Tape-record the babbling or speech of a child between the ages of twelve and thirty months, keeping notes of the child's accompanying activities. As soon as possible after this session, transcribe the sounds the child made and try to classify

them into the types of vocalizations discussed in the chapter: sound play, conversational babble, protowords, and words. What problems, if any, do you face in making these distinctions? What additional information do you need? Are there any utterances about which you could never be sure? Are there any utterances that are none of the above? If yes, what keeps them from fitting into each of the four major categories? What would you call them?

2.   Find a child whose speech is somewhat intelligible but whose pronunciation of words is still babyish. Tape-record and transcribe a half-hour of the child's speech during a play session. (A good-quality tape recorder will be needed for the best results; it will also help if you can get the child to wear a good external lavalier microphone.) Can you find regularities in the way the child renders adult words? If not, can you find canonical output forms that the child seems to rely on? Are any adult sounds or sequences of sounds especially variable in the way the child produces them? If you do find some regularities, write rules to describe them. Do these rules have exceptions? Are the forms of these exceptions closer to the adult word or farther from it?

3.   If you have no access to a child of the appropriate age for activities 1 or 2, go over the examples presented in this chapter and write explicit rules to describe what the child is doing to the adult words. Which rules can be written simply as "Adult (target) segment X becomes child (output) segment Y"? Which ones must also mention other sounds in the target word? Which ones must mention whether the sound in the adult word is in initial, medial, or final position? If you can't answer the last question from the small number of cases presented for a given real or hypothetical child in this chapter, give two formulations: a general one, assuming that what you see is broadly representative of what the child does, and a narrow one, allowing for the possibility that the child does something quite different if the segments are not in the given word position. Consider formulating your rules in terms of features or in terms of phonemes. For each rule indicate which mode of formulation is more helpful in understanding what the child is doing and explain why.

4.   Consider the development of /s/ and /tʃ/ by N. V. Smith's child, as described on pages 101–103. Suppose you had only one sample of each word per stage. Show how you might get rather different ideas of what the child was doing, depending on which rendition of each word appeared in your data.

Suggested Readings

Barton, D. P. (1980). Phonemic perception in children. In G. Yeni-Komshian, J. F. Kavanagh, & C. A. Ferguson (Eds.), *Child phonology: Vol. 2. Perception.* New York: Academic Press.

Braine, M. D. S. (1974). On what might constitute a learnable phonology. *Language, 50,* 270–299.

Clumeck, H. (1980). The acquisition of tone. In G. Yeni-Komshian, J. F. Kavanagh, & C. A. Ferguson (Eds.), *Child phonology. Vol. 1. Production.* New York: Academic Press.

Demuth, K. (1996). The prosodic structure of early words. In J. Morgan & K. Demuth (Eds.), *Signal to syntax: Boot-strapping from speech to grammar in early acquisition* (pp. 171–184). Mahwah, NJ: Erlbaum.

Ferguson, C. A., & Farwell, C. B. (1975). Words and sounds in early language acquisition. *Language, 51,* 439–491.

Ferguson, C. A., & Macken, M. A. (1980). Phonological development in children's play and cognition. In K. E. Nelson (Ed.), *Children's language* (Vol. 4). New York: Gardner Press.

Ferguson, C. A., Menn, L., & Stoel-Gammon, C. (Eds.). (1992). *Phonological development: Models, research, implications.* Timonium, MD: York Press.

Fey, M., & Gandour, J. (1982). Rule discovery in early phonology acquisition. *Journal of Child Development, 9,* 71–82.

Grunwell, P. (1982). *Clinical phonology.* London: Croom Helm.

Grunwell, P. (1987). *The nature of phonological disability in children* (2nd ed.). London: Academic Press.

Halliday, M. A. K. (1975). *Learning how to mean: Explorations in the development of language.* London: Edward Arnold.

Hyman, L. M. (1975). *Phonology: Theory and analysis.* New York: Holt, Rinehart & Winston.

Ingram, D. (1986). Phonological patterns in the speech of young children. In P. Fletcher & M. Garman (Eds.), *Language acquisition* (2nd ed.). Cambridge, UK: Cambridge University Press.

Ingram, D. (1989). *Phonological disabilities in children.* London: Cole and Whurr.

Jakobson, R. (1968). *Child language, aphasia, and phonological universals* (A. Keiler, Trans.). The Hague: Mouton.

Jusczyk, P. W. (1997). *The discovery of spoken language.* Cambridge, MA: MIT Press.

Kent, R. D. (1992). The biology of phonological development. In Ferguson, C. A., Menn, L., & Stoel-Gammon, C. (Eds.), *Phonological development: Models, research, implications.* Timonium, MD: York Press.

Labov, William. (1972). *Sociolinguistic patterns.* Philadelphia: University of Pennsylvania Press.

Ladefoged, P. (1971). *A course in phonetics.* New York: Harcourt Brace Jovanovich.

Leonard, L. B., Newhoff, M., & Mesalam, L. (1980). Individual differences in early child phonology. *Applied Psycholinguistics, 1,* 7–30.

Leonard, L. B., Schwartz, R., Folger, M. K., & Wilcox, M. J. (1978). Some aspects of child phonology in imitative and spontaneous speech. *Journal of Child Language, 5,* 403–416.

Lindblom, B. (1992). Phonological units as adaptive emergents of lexical development. In Ferguson, C. A., Menn, L., & Stoel-Gammon, C. (Eds.), *Phonological development: Models, research, implications.* Timonium, MD: York Press.

Locke, J. L. (1983). *Phonological acquisition and change.* New York: Academic Press.

Macken, M. A. (1979). Developmental reorganization of phonology: A hierarchy of basic units of acquisition. *Lingua, 49,* 11–49.

Macken, M. A., & Barton, D. (1980). The acquisition of the voicing contrast in English: A study of voice onset time in word-initial stop consonants. *Journal of Child Language, 7,* 41–75.

Macken, M. A., & Ferguson, C. A. (1982). Cognitive aspects of phonological development: Model, evidence, and issues. In K. E. Nelson (Ed.), *Children's language* (Vol. 4). New York: Gardner Press.

MacNeilage, P., & Davis, B. (1990). Acquisition of speech production: The achievement of segmental independence. In W. J. Hardcastle & A. Marchal (Eds.), *Speech production and speech modelling.* Dordrecht: Kluwer Press.

MacWhinney, B. (1978). The acquisition of morphophonology. *Monographs of the Society for Research in Child Development, 43,* 1–2.

Malsheen, B. (1980). Two hypotheses for phonetic clarification in the speech of mothers to children. In G. Yeni-Komshian, J. F. Kavanagh, & C. A. Ferguson (Eds.), *Child phonology: Vol. 2. Perception.* New York: Academic Press.

Menn, L. (1983). Development of articulatory, phonetic, and phonological capabilities. In B. Butterworth (Ed.), *Language production* (Vol. 2). London: Academic Press.

Menyuk, P., Menn, L., & Silber, R. (1986). Early strategies for the perception and production of words and sounds. In P. Fletcher & M. Garman (Eds.), *Language acquisition* (2nd ed.). Cambridge, UK: Cambridge University Press.

Morgan, J. L., & Demuth, K. (1996). *Signal to syntax: Boot-strapping from speech to grammar in early acquisition.* Mahwah, NJ: Erlbaum.

Obenchain, P., Menn, L., & Yoshinaga-Itano, C. (1999). Can speech development at thirty-six months in children with hearing loss be predicted from information available in the second year of life? In C. Yoshinaga-Itano & A. Sedey (Eds.), *Language, speech, and social-emotional development of deaf and hard-of-hearing children: The early years.* Volta Review Research Monograph.

Oller, D. K. (1980). The emergence of the sounds of speech in infancy. In G. Yeni-Komshian, J. F. Kavanagh, & C. A. Ferguson (Eds.), *Child phonology: Vol. 1. Production.* New York: Academic Press.

Painter, C. (1984). *Into the mother tongue: A case study in early language development.* London: Frances Pinter.

Peters, A. M. (1977). Language learning strategies. *Language, 53,* 560–573.

Peters, A. M. (1983). *The units of language acquisition.* Cambridge, UK: Cambridge University Press.

Priestly, T. M. S. (1977). One idiosyncratic strategy in the acquisition of phonology. *Journal of Child Language, 4,* 45–66.

Smith, N. V. (1973). *The acquisition of phonology: A case study.* Cambridge, UK: Cambridge University Press.

Stoel-Gammon, C., & Dunn, C. (1985). *Normal and disordered phonology in children.* Austin, TX: Pro-Ed.

Velten, H. V. (1971). The growth of phonemic and lexical patterns in the infant. Reprinted in A. Bar-Adon & W. Leopold (Eds.), *Readings in child language.* Englewood Cliffs, NJ: Prentice-Hall. (Originally published in 1941 in *Language, 19,* 440–444.)

Vihman, M. M. (1992). Early syllables and the construction of phonology. In C. A. Ferguson, L. Menn, & C. Stoel-Gammon (Eds.), *Phonological development: Models, research, implications.* Timonium, MD: York Press.

Vihman, M. M. (1996). *Phonological development: The origins of language in the child.* Oxford: Basil Blackwell, Ltd.

Wallace, V., Menn, L., Yoshinaga-Itano, C. (1999). Is babble the gateway to speech for all children? A longitudinal study of deaf and hard-of-hearing infants. In C. Yoshinaga-Itano & A. Sedey (Eds.), *Language, speech, and social-emotional development of deaf and hard-of-hearing children: The early years.* Volta Review Research Monograph.

Waterson, N. 1987. *Prosodic phonology: The theory and its application to language acquisition and speech processing.* Newcastle upon Tyne: Grevatt and Grevatt.

Werker, J. F., & Pegg, J. E. (1992). Infant speech perception and phonological acquisition. In C. A. Ferguson, L. Menn, & C. Stoel-Gammon (Eds.), *Phonological development: Models, research, implications.* Timonium, MD: York Press.

References

Aslin, R. N., Saffran, J. R., & Newport, E. L. (1999). Statistical learning in linguistic and non-linguistic domains. In B. MacWhinney (Ed.), *The emergence of language* (pp. 358–380). Mahwah NJ: Lawrence Erlbaum Associates.

Atkinson, K. B., MacWhinney, B., & Stoel, C. (1970). An experiment in the recognition of babbling. *Papers and Reports in Child Language Development, 1,* 71–76.

Atkinson-King, K. (1973). Children's acquisition of phonological stress contrasts. *UCLA Working Papers in Phonetics, 25.*

Barnhardt, B., & Stemberger, J. P. (1998). *Handbook of phonological development: From the perspective of constraint-based non-linear phonology.* San Diego, CA: Academic Press.

Barton, D. P. (1980). Phonemic perception in children. In G. Yeni-Komshian, J. F. Kavanagh, & C. A. Ferguson (Eds.), *Child phonology: Vol. 2. Perception.* New York: Academic Press.

Bernstein Ratner, N. (1984a). Patterns of vowel modification in mother-child speech. *Journal of Child Language, 11,* 557–578.

Bernstein Ratner, N. (1984b). Cues to post-vocalic voicing in mother-child speech. *Journal of Phonetics, 12,* 285--289.

Best, C. T., McRoberts, G. W., & Sithole, N. M. (1988). Examination of the perceptual reorganization for speech contrasts: Zulu click discrimination. *Journal of Experimental Psychology: Perception and Performance, 14,* 245–360.

Braine, M. D. S. (1974). On what might constitute a learnable phonology. *Language, 50,* 270–299.

Branigan, G. (1979). *Sequences of words as structured units.* Unpublished doctoral dissertation, Boston University School of Education.

Butler Platt, C., & MacWhinney, B. (1983). Solving a problem vs. remembering a solution: Error assimilation as a strategy in language acquisition. *Journal of Child Language, 10,* 41–75.

Cruttenden, A. (1985). Intonation comprehension in ten year olds. *Journal of Child Language, 12,* 643–61.

de Boysson-Bardies, B., Sagart, L., & Durand, C. (1984). Discernible differences in the babbling of infants according to target language. *Journal of Child Language, 11,* 1–15.

de Boysson-Bardies, B., & Vihman, M. M. (1991). Adaptation to language: Evidence from babbling and first words in four languages. *Language, 67,* 297–319.

DeCasper, A. J., & Fifer, W. P. (1980). Of human bonding: Newborns prefer their mothers' voices. *Science, 208,* 1174–1176.

Deser, T. (1990). *Dialect transmission and variation: An acoustic analysis of vowels in six urban Detroit families.* Bloomington, IN: Indiana Linguistics Club Publications.

Dodd, B. J. (1972). Effects of social and vocal stimulation on infant babbling. *Developmental Psychology, 7,* 80–83.

Edwards, M. L., & Shriberg, L. D. (1983). *Phonology: Applications in communicative disorders* (pp. 123–199). San Diego, CA: College-Hill Press.

Eimas, P. D., Siqueland, E. R., Jusczyk, P., & Vigorito, J. (1971). Speech perception in infants. *Science, 171,* 303–306.

Ferguson, C. A., & Farwell, C. B. (1975). Words and sounds in early language acquisition. *Language, 51,* 439–491.

Ferguson, C. A., & Macken, M. A. (1980). Phonological development in children's play and cognition. In K. E. Nelson (Ed.), *Children's language* (Vol. 4). New York: Gardner Press.

Ferguson, C. A., Menn, L., & Stoel-Gammon, C. (Eds.). (1992). *Phonological development: Models, research, implications.* Timonium, MD: York Press.

Gerken, L., & McIntosh, B. (1993). The interplay of function morphemes and prosody in early language. D*evelopmental Psychology, 29,* 448–457.

Goldsmith, J. (1990). *Autosegmental and metrical phonology.* London: Blackwell.

Grunwell, P. (1987). *Clinical phonology* (2nd ed.). Baltimore: Williams and Wilkins.

Gupta, P., & Dell, G. S. (1999). The emergence of language from serial order and procedural memory. In B. MacWhinney (Ed.), *The emergence of language* (pp. 447–481). Mahwah, NJ: Erlbaum.

Halliday, M. A. K. (1975). *Learning how to mean: Explorations in the development of language.* London: Edward Arnold.

Ingram, D. (1989). *Phonological disabilities in children* (2nd ed.). London: Cole and Whurr.

Jaeger, J. J. (1980). *Categorization in phonology: An experimental approach.* Unpublished doctoral dissertation. Berkeley, CA: University of California.

Jakobson, R. (1941/1968). *Child language, aphasia, and phonological universals.*(A. Keiler, Trans.). The Hague: Mouton.

Jesperson, O. (1925). *Language.* New York: Holt, Rinehart & Winston.

Jusczyk, P. W. (1992). Developing phonological categories for the speech signal. In C. A. Ferguson, L. Menn, & C. Stoel-Gammon (Eds.), *Phonological development: Models, research, implications.* Timonium, MD: York Press.

Jusczyk, P. W. (1997). *The discovery of spoken language.* Cambridge, MA: MIT Press.

Kent, R. D. (1993). Infants and speech: Seeking patterns. *Journal of Phonetics, 21,* 117–123.

Kuhl, P. K. (1992). Speech prototypes: Studies on the nature, function, ontogeny and phylogeny of the "centers" of speech categories. In Y. Tohkura, E. Vatikiotis-Bateson, & Y. Sagiska (Eds.), *Speech perception, production and linguistic structure.* Tokyo: Ohmsha.

Krohn, R., Steinberg, D., & Kobayashi, L. (1972). The psychological validity of Chomsky and Halle's vowel shift rule. *20th International Congress of Psychology,* Tokyo (Abstract Guide, paragraph 1905).

Leonard, L. B. (1992). Models of phonological development and children with phonological disorders. In C. A. Ferguson, L. Menn, & C. Stoel-Gammon (Eds.), *Phonological development: Models, research, implications.* Timonium, MD: York Press.

Leopold, W. (1970). *Speech development of a bilingual child, 1–4.* New York: AMS Press.

Levitt, A., & Wang, Q. (1991). Evidence for language-specific rhythmic influences in the reduplicative babbling of French- and English-learning infants. *Language and Speech, 34,* 235–249.

Lieberman, P., Crelin, E. S., & Klatt, D. H. (1972). Phonetic ability and related anatomy of the newborn, adult human, Neanderthal man, and the chimpanzee. *American Anthropologist, 74,* 287–307.

Lindblom, B. (1992). Phonological units as adaptive emergents of lexical development. In C. A. Ferguson, L. Menn, & C. Stoel-Gammon (Eds.), *Phonological development: Models, research, implications.* Timonium, MD: York Press.

Locke, J. L. (1983). *Phonological acquisition and change.* New York: Academic Press.

Macken, M. A. (1979). Developmental reorganization of phonology: A hierarchy of basic units of acquisition. *Lingua, 49,* 11–49.

Macken, M. A. (1980). The child's lexical representation: The "puzzle-puddle-pickle" evidence. *Journal of Linguistics, 16,* 1–19.

Macken, M. A., & Barton, D. (1980). The acquisition of voicing contrast in English: A study of voice onset time in word-initial stop consonant. *Journal of Child language, 7,* 41–75.

Macken, M. A., & Ferguson, C. A. (1983). Cognitive aspects of phonological development: model, evidence, and issues. In K. E. Nelson (Ed.), *Children's language* (Vol. 4). Hillsdale, NJ: Lawrence Erlbaum Associates.

Malsheen, B. (1980). Two hypotheses for phonetic clarification in the speech of mothers to children. In G. Yeni-Komshian, J. F. Kavanagh, & C. A. Ferguson (Eds.), *Child phonology: Vol. 2. Perception.* New York: Academic Press.

Mandel, D. R., Jusczyk, P. W., & Pisoni, D. B. (1994). Do 4-½ month olds know their own names? Paper presented at the 127th meeting of the Acoustical Society of America, Cambridge, MA.

Markey, K. L. (1994). *The sensorimotor functions of phonology: A computational model of early childhood articulatory and phonetic development.* Unpublished doctoral dissertation, University of Colorado.

McCawley, J. D. (1977). Acquisition models as models of acquisition (pp. 51–64). In R. Fasold & R. Shuy (Eds.), *Studies in language variation.* Washington, DC: Georgetown University Press.

Mehler, J., Jusczyk, P. W., Lambertz, G., Halsted, N., Bertoncini, J., & Amiel-Tisson, C. (1988). A precursor of language acquisition in young infants. *Cognition, 29,* 143–178.

Menn, L. (1971). Phonotactic rules in beginning speech. *Lingua, 26,* 225–241.

Menn, L. (1976). *Pattern, control, and contrast in beginning speech: A case study in the acquisition of word form and function.* Unpublished doctoral dissertation, University of Illinois.

Menn, L., & Matthei, E. (1992). The "two-lexicon" account of child phonology: Looking back, looking ahead. In C. A. Ferguson, L. Menn, & C. Stoel-Gammon (Eds.), *Phonological development: Models, research, implications.* Timonium, MD: York Press.

Moskowitz, A. I. (1970). The two-year-old stage in the acquisition of English phonology. *Language, 46,* 426–441.

Moskowitz, B. A. (1980). Idioms in phonology acquisition and phonological change. *Journal of Phonetics, 8,* 69–83.

Mowrer, O. H. (1954). The psychologist looks at language. *American Psychologist, 9,* 660–694.

Myerson, R. (1975). *A developmental study of children's knowledge of complex derived words of English*. Unpublished doctoral dissertation, Harvard Graduate School of Education.

Nakazima, S. A. (1962). A comparative study of the speech developments of Japanese and American English in childhood (1): A comparison of the developments of voices at the prelinguistic period. *Studia Phonologica, 2*, 27–46.

Nelson, K. (1973). Structure and strategy in learning to talk. *Monographs of the Society for Research in Child Development, 38.*

Oller, D. K. (1980). The emergence of the sounds of speech in infancy. In G. Yeni-Komshian, J. F. Kavanagh, & C. A. Ferguson (Eds.), *Child phonology: (Vol. 1). Production.* New York: Academic Press.

Oller, D. K., & Eilers, R. (1988). The role of audition in babbling. *Child Development, 59*, 441–449.

Olmsted, D. L. (1971). *Out of the mouth of babes.* The Hague: Mouton.

Painter, C. (1984). *Into the mother tongue: A case study in early language development.* London: Frances Pinter.

Payne, A. (1976). *The acquisition of a phonological system of a second dialect.* Unpublished doctoral dissertation, University of Pennsylvania.

Peters, A. M. (1977). Language learning strategies. *Language, 53*, 560–573.

Peters, A., & Menn, L. (1993). False starts and filler syllables: Way to learn grammatical morphemes. *Language, 69*, 742–777.

Plaut, D. C., & Kello, C. T. (1999). The emergence of phonology from the interplay of speech comprehension and production: A distributed connectionist approach. In B. MacWhinney (Ed.), *The emergence of language* (pp. 381–416). Mahwah, NJ: Lawrence Erlbaum Associates.

Prather, E., Hedrick, D., & Kern, C. (1975). Articulation development in children aged two to four years. *Journal of Speech and Hearing Disorders, 40*, 179–191.

Priestly, T. M. S. (1977). One idiosyncratic strategy in the acquisition of phonology. *Journal of Child Language, 4*, 45–66.

Pye, C., Ingram, D., & List, H. (1987). A comparison of initial consonant acquisition in English and Quiché. In K. E. Nelson & A. Van Kleeck (Eds.), *Children's language, Vol. 6* (pp. 175–190). Hillsdale, NJ: Lawrence Erlbaum Associates.

Schwartz, R. G., & Leonard, L. B. (1982). Do children pick and choose? An examination of phonological selection and avoidance in early lexical acquisition. *Journal of Child Language, 9*, 319–336.

Smit, A. B. (1993). Phonological error distributions in the Iowa–Nebraska articulation norms project: Word-initial consonant clusters. *Journal of Speech and Hearing Research, 36*, 931–947.

Smit, A. B. Hand, L., Freilinger, F. F., Bernthal, J. E., & Bird, A. (1990). The Iowa articulation norms project and its Nebraska replication. *Journal of Speech and Hearing Disorders, 55*, 779–798.

Smith, N. V. (1973). *The acquisition of phonology: A case study.* Cambridge, UK: Cambridge University Press.

Stampe, D. (1969). The acquisition of phonemic representation. *Proceedings of the Fifth Regional Meeting, Chicago Linguistic Society*, pp. 433–444.

Stark, R. E. (1980). Stages of speech development in the first year. In G. Yeni-Komshian, J. A. Kavanagh, & C. A. Ferguson (Eds.), *Child phonology* (Vol. 1). New York: Academic Press.

Stemberger, J. P. (1992). A connectionist view of child phonology: Phonological processing without phonological processes. In C. A. Ferguson, L. Menn, & C. Stoel-Gammon (Eds.), *Phonological development: Models, research, implications.* Timonium, MD: York Press.

Stemberger, J. P., & Barnhart, B. H. (1999). The emergence of faithfulness. In B. MacWhinney (Ed.), *The emergence of language* (pp. 417–446). Mahwah NJ: Lawrence Erlbaum Associates.

Stoel-Gammon, C. (1985). Phonetic inventories, 15–24 months: A longitudinal study. *Journal of Speech and Hearing Research, 28,* 505–512.

Stoel-Gammon, C. (1992). Research on phonological development: Recent advances. In C. A. Ferguson, L. Menn, & C. Stoel-Gammon (Eds.), *Phonological development: Models, research, implications* (pp. 273–282). Timonium, MD: York Press.

Stoel-Gammon, C. (1998a). The role of babbling and phonology in early linguistic development. In A. M. Wetherby, S. F. Warren, & J. Reichle (Eds.), *Transitions in prelinguistic communication: Preintentional to intentional and presymbolic to symbolic* (pp. 87–110). Baltimore: Paul H. Brookes.

Stoel-Gammon, C. (1998b). Sounds and words in early language acquisition: The relationship between lexical and phonological development. In R. Paul (Ed.), *Exploring the speech-language connection* (pp. 25–52). Baltimore: Paul H. Brookes.

Stoel-Gammon, C., & Dunn, C. (1985). *Normal and disordered phonology in children.* Austin, TX: Pro-Ed.

Stoel-Gammon, C., & Otomo, K. (1986). Babbling development of hearing-impaired and normally hearing subjects. *Journal of Speech and Hearing Disorders, 51,* 33–41.

Templin, M. C. (1957). *Certain language skills in children: Their development and interrelationships.* Minneapolis: University of Minnesota Press.

Todd, G., & Palmer, B. (1968). Social reinforcement of infant babbling. *Child Development, 39,* 591–596.

Trehub, S. E. (1976). The discrimination of foreign speech contrasts by infants and children. *Child Development, 47,* 466–472.

Velleman, S. (1988). The role of linguistic perception in later phonological development. *Journal of Applied Psycholinguistic*s, *9,* 221–236.

Vihman, M. M. (1992). Early syllables and the construction of phonology. In C. A. Ferguson, L. Menn, & C. Stoel-Gammon (Eds.), *Phonological development: Models, research, implications.* Timonium, MD: York Press.

Vihman, M. M. (1993). Variable paths to early word production. *Journal of Phonetics* 21, 61–82.

Vihman, M. M. (1996). *Phonological development.* Oxford, UK: Blackwell.

Vihman, M. M., Macken, M. A., Miller, R., Simmons, H., & Miller, J. (1985). From babbling to speech: A re-assessment of the continuity issue. *Language, 61,* 397–445.

Wahler, R. G. (1969). Infant social development: Some experimental analyses of an infant-mother interaction during the first year of life. *Journal of Experimental Child Psychology, 7,* 101–113.

Waterson, N. (1971). Child phonology: A prosodic view. *Journal of Linguistics, 7,* 179–221.

Weir, R. (1962). *Language in the crib.* The Hague: Mouton.

Werker, J. F., & Tees, R. C. (1984). Cross-language speech perception: Evidence for perceptual reorganization during the first year of life. *Infant Behavior and Development, 7,* 49–64.

Wilbur, R., & Menn, L. (1975). *Towards a redefinition of psychological reality: The internal structure of the lexicon* (Occasional Papers in Linguistics). San Jose, CA: San Jose State College.

Winitz, H. (1969). *Articulatory acquisition and behavior.* New York: Appleton-Century-Crofts.

Chapter 4

Semantic Development: Learning the Meanings of Words

Barbara Alexander Pan
Harvard Graduate School of Education

Jean Berko Gleason
Boston University

Long before they know the meanings of any individual words, infants understand some of what is said to them. This earliest comprehension is at the emotional and social level: The exaggerated prosodic contours of their mothers' speech carry varied messages of comfort, happiness, or anger (Fernald, 1992; Locke, 1993). Very young children understand the pragmatic intent of adults' utterances before they can understand the words themselves. A toddler who begins to peel off his clothes on hearing his father say, "It's time for your bath now," may be responding to a variety of situational cues—it is a particular time of day, they are in a certain room, they are engaged in a familiar activity, or the parent may actually be pointing to the bathtub. Only very slowly do children come to understand and use words in adult fashion, to break them free of context and use them flexibly in a variety of situations. The acquisition of words, their meanings, and the links between them does not happen at once. During the course of this process, which is usually called **semantic development,** children's strategies for learning word meanings and relating them to one another change as their internal representation of language constantly grows and becomes reorganized.

In this chapter we will describe the relationship between words and their referents, and some of the theories that attempt to explain how children acquire and represent meaning. We will address what is known about early words and the ways in which contemporary researchers have attempted to interpret the data on children's early words and word meanings. We will also present research on later semantic development, which examines the ways that the semantic system is elaborated as words become related to one another in more complex semantic networks. Finally, we will describe children's growing awareness of words as physical entities independent of their meanings and discuss the implications of such metalinguistic development for a variety of nonliteral language uses.

The Relations Between Words and Their Referents

What does it mean to say that children acquire meaning? And what is it that adults have in common when they know the meaning of a word? First, it is important to note that the meaning of a word resides in the speakers of a common language, not in the world of objects. The word is a sign that signifies a **referent,** but the referent is not the meaning of the word. If, for example, you say to a child, "Look at the kitty," the referent, the actual cat, is not the meaning of *kitty*—if the cat ran away or were run over by a truck, the word would still have meaning because meaning is a cognitive construct.

Let us assume that a child learns that the word *kitty* refers to her cat; in this case, the actual cat is the referent of the word *kitty.* But what is the relationship between the word and the cat? Cats can be called *kitty, cat, koshka, macska, katze,* or *chat,* depending on whether one is speaking English, Russian, Hungarian, German, or French. There is nothing intrinsic to cats that makes one or another name more appropriate or fitting—the relationship between the name and the thing is thus *arbitrary,* and it is by social convention in a particular language that speakers agree to call the animal by a particular word (Morris, 1946). This arbitrary relationship between the referent (the cat) and the sign for it (the word *cat*) is *symbolic.* Nonverbal signs can also share this symbolic nature; the red light that means stop, for instance, is purely symbolic because there is no obvious connection between the color red and the action of stopping. We could agree to have blue lights or even green lights mean *stop,* as long as we all agreed on the meaning of the light.

For a few words, the relation between word and referent is not arbitrary. If one says, for example, "The book fell with a *thud,*" the relationship between the word *thud* and the actual sound referred to is not arbitrary, since the word resembles the sound. Nor is the name of the cuckoo bird arbitrary: It represents the sound that the bird actually makes. Although the study of semantic acquisition has concentrated on how children learn the meaning of symbols, we should not be surprised to learn that many of children's earliest words or protowords have a less-than-arbitrary relation to their referents; trains are called *choo-choos,* and dogs become *woof-woofs.* Some of these words are in the baby-talk lexicon that adults use when attempting to communicate with babies, and others are the children's own creations.

It is probably easier for children to learn a word that is obviously related to its referent than one that is totally arbitrary and symbolic, and, as some research has shown, young children believe that the name and the referent are intrinsically related.

They think that one cannot change the name of something without changing its nature as well; for instance, many children believe that if we decided to call a dog a *cow,* it would begin to moo (Vygotsky, 1962).

This belief in the essential appropriateness of names was a subject of argument among ancient philosophers as well. Plato, writing in the fourth century B.C., discussed the question of whether there is a natural relation between names and referents in his Cratylus dialogue. The Anomalists of Plato's day believed that the relation was inexplicable, but the Analogists believed that through careful etymology the essential nature of words could be revealed (Bloomfield, 1933). Using English examples, we might show that a blackberry is so called because it is a berry that is black, and a bedroom is so named because it is a room containing a bed. The ancient Greek Analogists would also claim that if we only looked hard enough, we would find the natural connections behind *gooseberry* and *mushroom* as well. This altogether human desire to produce order can be seen in many **folk etymologies** today and explains why college students as well as young children, when asked why Friday is called *Friday,* may respond, "Because it is the day you eat fried fish," or why they may hold that a handkerchief is so named "Because you hold it in your hand and go *kerchoo*" (Berko, 1958).

Mental Images

Although meaning is a mental event, we still have to specify what its exact nature is. One possibility is that meaning is a mental picture. As we have seen earlier (see Chapter 1), incoming language is processed in the part of the brain known as Wernicke's area, which is near the auditory association areas of the brain. The belief that the sound of a word evokes a mental picture of its referent and that the image is the meaning of the word has a long history (see Tichener, 1909). However, even though it is true that many people are able to visualize words, not everyone does so. Furthermore, many words, such as *happy* or *jealousy,* do not have picturable referents and still we know their meanings. Even if one has an image for a word, it is likely to be quite particularistic—*dog,* for instance, might evoke a picture of a black poodle you know. Yet anyone who knows the meaning of *dog* can recognize many hundreds of real dogs of all sizes and shapes, so the mental image would have to be a very complicated composite if it were it to account for all instances. Clearly, this is not the case. Finally, images tend to be quite idiosyncratic; speakers who share meaning may hold very different internal images. One speaker's mental house may look like a mansion, whereas another's may be a simple cottage, yet both speakers recognize new instances of houses when they encounter them.

Concepts

One of the child's primary tasks in semantic development is to acquire categorical concepts (e.g., to learn that the word *dog* refers to a whole class of animals) and to be able to extend the word to appropriate new instances of the category. Theorists differ as to how they characterize the nature of children's categorical concept acquisition. One view is that children acquire categories by learning the essential semantic features of the category; a second is that they first learn prototypical examples of a category, and yet another is that they use a probabilistic strategy in assigning category membership.

The **semantic feature** view is that children learn a set of distinguishing features for each categorical concept (Clark, 1974). At first the word *dog* may be understood to apply only to the child's own dog, but the child soon comes to understand that other creatures may also be called *dog* as long as they share a small set of critical features: Dogs are alive and warm-blooded, have four legs, bark, and are usually covered with hair. According to semantic feature theory, overextensions occur when the child infers category membership from a partial match of features. A toddler may, in this way, call a moose *doggie* because both animals have hair and four legs. The child in this case does not yet know that antlers disqualify an animal from membership in the dog category.

According to prototype theory (see Figure 4.1), children acquire **prototypes,** or core concepts, when they acquire meaning and only later come to recognize category

Category	Prototypical Member	Nonprototypical Member
Vegetable	Carrot 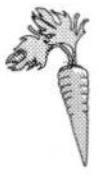	Eggplant 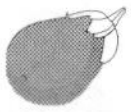
Dog	Collie 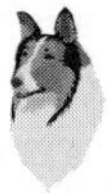	Chihuahua 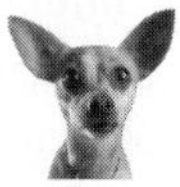
Fruit	Apple 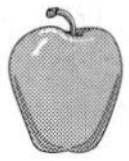	Tomato 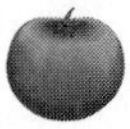
Bird	Robin 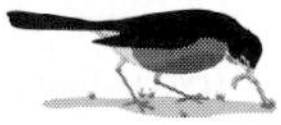	Penguin 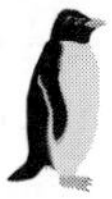
Flower	Rose 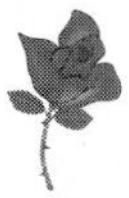	Gladiolus 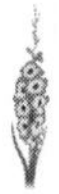
Chair	Armchair 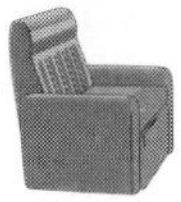	Throne 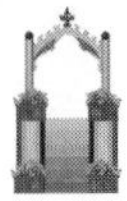

Figure 4.1

Prototypical and nonprototypical category members.

members that are distant from the prototypes. Apples, collies, and roses are examples of prototypical fruits, dogs, and flowers. Andrick and Tager-Flusberg (1986) found that **focal colors**—the bluest blue and the reddest red—were most easily named by children. For adults as well, prototypical members of a category are more accessible in memory (Rosch, 1973). A robin has more typical *bird* characteristics than does a penguin; therefore, people see robins as better examples of birds, and they also can classify them faster when asked if a robin is a bird.

A slightly different view is that children assign category membership not on the basis of essential features or on prototypes, but on probabilistic grounds. Upon first seeing a penguin, children (and adults) would decide that it is *probably* a bird, because it has many bird-like features, such as a beak and wings. Thus, even though it does not fly or chirp, it still qualifies for membership in the bird category.

Some researchers, notably Smith and Medin (1981), have pointed out that even if children are acquiring their concepts as categories, there are great differences in the nature of the concepts themselves. For instance, there are **classical concepts,** like *triangle*, which can be unambigously defined: All triangles must have three angles, or they are simply not triangles. *Bird,* on the other hand, is an example of a **probabilistic concept.** Most, but not all, birds have many features in common, but there is not a single set of essential features. Furthermore, some concepts have fairly sharp boundaries and are hierarchically organized, while others are not: For instance, most adults can agree on what is and is not a dog and know that dogs belong to the superordinate category of animals. By contrast, color concepts have fuzzy boundaries: Even adults find it difficult to agree on color names for nonfocal shades (Braisby & Dockrell, 1999). Given these differences among concepts, it is unlikely that any one theory can account for the nature of children's categorical concepts.

Next we consider behavioral and developmental theories of how children acquire words and their meanings.

Theoretical Perspectives on Semantic Development

Learning Theory

One of the simplest explanations of how children learn the meanings of their first words is that they do so through association. This behavioral model is very similar to the classical conditioning model proposed by learning theorists for any kind of associative learning (see Chapter 7 for further discussion of behavioral theory). In learning through association, there is first an unconditioned stimulus that produces a response. In Pavlov's famous experiments, dogs were first presented with meat powder (the unconditioned stimulus), which caused the quite natural response of salivating. Later, a bell was rung at the same time that the powder was presented. Eventually, the dogs salivated when the bell rang, even when there was no meat powder present. The dogs responded to the sound of the bell, at least in part, as they had responded to the meat powder. They had become conditioned to the bell, which had thus become the conditioned stimulus.

How might this model be extended to cover the acquisition of meaning? Research has shown that infants will make associative pairings between sounds (such as bells), gestures, or words and their possible referents. With age, infants become more discriminating and give words a special status. They no longer readily map referents to noises or gestures, unless these are part of the linguistic system used in their community (Namy & Waxman, 1998; Woodward & Hoyne, 1999). Learning theory predicts that if a parent points and says *kitty* every time the family cat appears, eventually the infant will react to the word alone, as if the cat were there—looking around for it or feeling pleased and ready for play. The cat, in this model, is the unconditioned stimulus that gives rise to certain predispositions or responses in the child. Eventually, the word *kitty* becomes the conditioned stimulus that evokes much the same set of responses.

It is important to remember that the conditioned response is similar to, but not really the same as, the original response to the unconditioned stimulus (Lashley, 1954). Pavlov's dogs may have salivated at the sound of the bell as they had salivated at the sight of the meat powder, but they did not try to eat the bell. The infant may respond somewhat to the word *kitty* as if it were the actual cat, but not to the extent of stroking the empty air. For learning to have taken place, it suffices that the word *kitty* and the actual cat have been associated so that they evoke at least some of the same responses. Learning theory may explain the earliest and simplest kinds of linking between words and objects. Many of children's early words, such as *bottle* and *blanket,* have concrete referents and could be learned through association. This kind of associative word learning by children may be facilitated by many factors: Not only do adults put special emphasis on new words and the things they refer to, but children themselves are especially sensitive to novelty in their environment and predisposed to apply new words to new objects (Samuelson & Smith, 1998).

Developmental Theories

In contrast to the behavioral model, developmental theories consider semantic development within the wider context of the child's unfolding social, cognitive, and linguistic skills. Developmental theories attempt to explain how the child may acquire first words, why the scope of reference of children's early words may not match that of adults, and how children's semantic systems become more adultlike over time. It is clear that young children first acquire meaning in a very context-bound way, as a part of their real-world expectations. Clark (1993) theorizes that before they start learning language, all children have developed a set of **ontological categories** (concepts about how the world is organized). These ontological categories include objects, actions, events, relations, states, and properties. These are the basic categories in all languages that speakers refer to when they use language.

In addition, over the course of their first year of life, children develop a rudimentary interpersonal understanding of other people's attentional states and how those states relate to what is likely to be communicated (Tomasello, 1995). In order to become efficient word learners, young children must come to understand, for example, that a novel word they hear probably relates to an object or event that the *speaker* is paying attention to. If the infant simply assumes that the word she hears relates to whatever is present or that it relates to whatever she herself is attending to, she will be relying solely on associative learning and no doubt make many mismappings. Baldwin (1995) has shown that by eighteen months, infants hearing an adult produce an unfamiliar label check to see whether the adult is attending to the same object or event they themselves are, and if not, adjust their own focus of attention to match the adult's. The ability to establish and maintain joint focus of attention with those around them is crucial for children's efficient word learning.

Even equipped with a set of ontological categories and some understanding of others' likely intentions, the infant's task is still quite daunting. Consider what an infant must understand about verbal communication in order to begin mapping words she hears to referents. Let us say, for instance, that the infant is in her home, and the family dog Rufus is lying nearby on a rug with a bone. The baby hears her mother say words such as *Rufus, dog, bone,* and *look.* An infant may assume that the word *dog* applies only to the family dog. Most theorists and researchers would agree, however, that young children must come to understand that a single label can be applied to more than one specific case (that is, *dog* refers not only to their own Rufus, but to many different dogs, seen in the park, pictured in books and on dog food boxes, etc.). Without this insight, infants cannot begin to understand the nature of reference, or to communicate about objects, actions, and properties (Clark, 1993). However, this understanding is only one step in cracking the mapping puzzle. Not only does the label *dog* refer to many different dogs, but a particular dog may be labeled in many different ways (*Rufus, dog, retriever, pet, puppy*). Moreover, when a child hears a new word, the word could refer to an action, a property, or even a part of an object.

Principles and Strategies

To explain how young children avoid this mapping nightmare, theorists have suggested some **principles** or strategies that children may use as working hypotheses about the meanings of new words:

- *Words refer to objects.* One basic hypothesis young children may have is that when they hear a new word, it probably refers to an object, that is, to a person, place, or thing (Golinkoff, Mervis, & Hirsh-Pasek, 1994). This working hypothesis could sometimes lead to inaccurate mappings (when, for example, the parent points at a bird and says "Look!", rather than "Birdie!"). It would probably more often result in correct mappings, however, given that adults talking to young children produce more nouns than verbs (Goldfield, 1993).

- *Words refer to whole objects.* A second, related, hypothesis children may have is that when they hear a new label it refers to a *whole* object, rather than to its parts (Macnamara, 1982; Markman & Wachtel, 1988). This principle would predispose the child to eliminate the family dog's floppy ears or his appealing expression as likely referents for the new label *bone.* Because young children seem to rely heavily on shape to identify whole objects, this hypothesis has also been referred to as a **shape bias** (Landau, Smith, & Jones, 1988).

- *New words can be extended to other members of the same category.* For instance, when extending a word like *cookie,* children assume it can be applied to other referents that are in the same category as cookies (cookie-like objects, such as crackers), rather than to referents that are thematically related to cookies, such as spatulas or cookie cutters. This is sometimes called the **taxonomic principle** (Markman, 1987), because it suggests that children form mental taxonomies or classifications of the objects in their world.

- *New words refer to categories that do not already have a name.* Golinkoff and her colleagues (1994) suggest that on hearing a new label, children will try to map the label to an as-yet-unlabeled object in the environment (**novel name-nameless category principle**). Thus, the child might assume that the new label *bone* referred to either the bone or the rug the dog is lying on (if the child did not yet know either of these words). As the child acquires more and more labels, the number of unlabeled referents in any given setting decreases, and the mapping task becomes easier.

- *No two words have exactly the same meaning.* Clark (1987) proposes a slightly different child principle, that is, that words contrast in meaning. According to this **principle of contrast,** the child would not completely eliminate Rufus as a possible referent for the new label *bone,* but would assume that the meaning of the word *bone* did not overlap perfectly with the meaning of the word *Rufus.*

- *Each object can have only one name.* Markman and her colleagues (Markman, 1987; Markman & Wachtel, 1988) propose a more stringent **constraint** than the one proposed by Clark, that is, that children assume an object can have only one name. According to this **principle of mutual exclusivity,** there is no overlap between words. In our example, this would lead the child to eliminate Rufus as a possible referent for *bone,* because Rufus already has a name.

Although children may rely in part on some or all of these principles, they also use linguistic and world knowledge in learning the meanings of words. Clark & Grossman (1998) suggest that children first make use of semantic and syntactic information or pragmatic information about the speaker's intent and only resort to lexical principles such as mutual exclusivity in the absence of other information. Au and Glusman (1990) found that children who heard the novel material term *rattan* linguistically contrasted with other material terms (*It's not paper, and it's not cloth; it's rattan.*) were more likely to learn the new material name than were children who simply heard rattan labeled. Hall (1994a) showed that three-year-olds assumed that *zav* was a proper name in a sentence such as *This dog is zav,* but interpreted it as an adjective in the sentence, *This caterpillar is zav.* Even three-year-olds had the real world knowledge that it was likely that a dog had a proper name, but that a caterpillar did not, and were able to use this knowledge to interpret the new word.

Regardless of what hypotheses children adopt, they will occasionally make incorrect initial mappings. As we will see later, children rely on input and feedback from mature speakers to test and revise their label-to-referent mappings.

Early Words

Early in their second year, most children have begun to produce some words themselves. They begin with words related to what is intellectually and socially most meaningful to them (Anglin, 1995), such as names for important people and objects in their lives. Thus *mommy, daddy, doggie,* and *blankie* are common early words, and *tree, vase,* and *policeman* are not. Subsequent patterns of word meaning and use reflect development not only within children's semantic systems, but also in other areas such as their cognition and memory, in addition to widened experience.

The Study of Vocabulary

Examination of children's vocabulary is probably the oldest approach to the study of language acquisition. Beginning word use signals that children have a new tool that will enable them to learn about and participate more fully in their societies. Furthermore, word use is thought to provide tangible indicators of the makeup and workings of children's minds. The first studies—some as early as the eighteenth century (e.g., Tiedemann, 1787)—were almost invariably based on observations of the authors' own children and were kept in the form of diaries. During the nineteenth century and the first half of the twentieth century, many psychologists kept diary records of their children's development. This remains a valuable way to trace the development of language in individual children. By themselves, however, diaries can be misleading, since the temptation to write what is unusual or interesting, rather than what is daily and ordinary, is hard to resist. More recently, a number of researchers have found ways to augment and improve diary studies by giving parents who are participating in a study checklists of the words that their children are likely to acquire during their first years (Dale, Bates, Reznick, & Morisset, 1989). The checklists help parents organize their observations and remind them of the more ordinary, but important, things their children understand and say that they might otherwise overlook.

What Are Early Words Like?

By the time children begin to acquire a vocabulary, they have already been exposed to a great deal of language and have had a wide range of individual experiences. It is interesting, therefore, that children's initial productive or expressive vocabularies have been found to be quite similar, despite differences in upbringing and environment.

The words children acquire in their early productive vocabularies are influenced by many factors. One of these factors is phonological composition. Researchers have analyzed the phonology of children's first fifty words (Ferguson & Farwell, 1975; Stoel-Gammon & Cooper, 1984), studied children's imitations of words (Leonard, Schwartz, Folger, Newhoff, & Wilcox, 1979), and tried to teach new words to one-year-olds (Leonard, Schwartz, Morris, & Chapman, 1981; Schwartz & Leonard, 1982). The results of these studies show that words that are easier for children to pronounce are more likely to be included in their early productive vocabularies, and that favored sound patterns may vary greatly across children. Moreover, phonological composition continues to play a role in vocabulary through the early school years. Unlike adults, children aged five to seven tend to use few words that sound very similar to one another (Charles-Luce & Luce, 1990).

From the beginning, children's vocabularies appear to include words from a variety of grammatical classes; their first fifty words represent all of the major grammatical classes found in adult language (see Table 4.1). Nonetheless, common nouns predominate in young English-speaking children's early speech; Mandarin-speaking children do not show this noun bias, so we cannot assume that it is universal (Tardif, Gelman, & Xu, 1999). Nearly 40 percent of the average English-speaking child's first fifty words are common nouns, while verbs, adjectives, and function words each account for less than 10 percent. By the time children's productive vocabularies exceed 600 words, about 40 percent are nouns, 25 percent verbs and adjectives, and about 15 percent function words (Bates, Marchman, Thal, Fenson, Dale, Reznick, Reilly, & Hartung, 1994). Of course, these proportions vary from child to child (see Chapter 8), and it becomes increasingly clear that context is an important variable. For instance, Tardif and her colleagues (1999) have shown that both English-speaking and Mandarin-speaking children produce larger proportions of nouns in book reading than while playing with toys. It is also possible that the numbers of nouns reported using checklists are somewhat inflated relative to children's actual use because mothers are more likely to notice nouns in their children's speech (Pine, Lieven, & Rowland, 1996).

Why should nouns initially be acquired more rapidly than other types of words? Several possible explanations have been suggested. One hypothesis holds that children's vocabularies reflect the input directed to them; studies have shown that in adult speech to English-speaking children, labels for different kinds of objects are more numerous than labels for actions, properties, or relations (Goldfield, 1993). An alternative explanation is that nouns are favored over verbs in acquisition because verbs are more linguistically complex. In addition, the concepts referred to by nouns are clearer, more concrete, and more readily identifiable than those of verbs (Gentner, 1983, 1988). Among nouns, those that are the easiest to distinguish from the surroundings, such as animate beings or things that move, are the earliest learned (Gentner, 1999). Nouns tend to refer to the same concepts in different languages, but the particular aspects of meaning covered by verbs are not identical in different languages. Learning a verb's meaning requires a child to find out which of the possible aspects are included and which are not. The linguistic and conceptual complexity of verbs may be one reason that children initially rely on general-purpose verbs such as *do, go, make,* and *get* (Clark, 1993). Comprehension and production of decontextualized verbs (those that do not refer to the here and now) appear to be particularly late to emerge (Smith & Sachs, 1990).

Although children's early vocabularies are quite varied, Bloom and Lahey (1978) found that children whose vocabularies are at the fifty-word level may actually use only eight or ten of those words very frequently and in a variety of contexts. Bloom and Lahey refer to this group of words as the **core group.** Children's vocabularies also

Table 4.1	**Children's Earliest Words: Examples from the Vocabularies of Children Younger than 20 Months**

Sound effects
   baa baa, meow, moo, ouch, uh-oh, woof, yum-yum

Food and drink
   apple, banana, cookie, cheese, cracker, juice, milk, water

Animals
   bear, bird, bunny, dog, cat, cow, duck, fish, kitty, horse, pig, puppy

Body parts and clothing
   diaper, ear, eye, foot, hair, hand, hat, mouth, nose, toe, tooth, shoe

House and outdoors
   blanket, chair, cup, door, flower, keys, outside, spoon, tree, tv

People
   baby, daddy, gramma, grampa, mommy, [child's own name]

Toys and vehicles
   ball, balloon, bike, boat, book, bubbles, plane, truck, toy

Actions
   down, eat, go, sit, up

Games and routines
   bath, bye, hi, night-night, no, peekaboo, please, shhh, thank you, yes

Adjectives and descriptives
   allgone, cold, dirty, hot

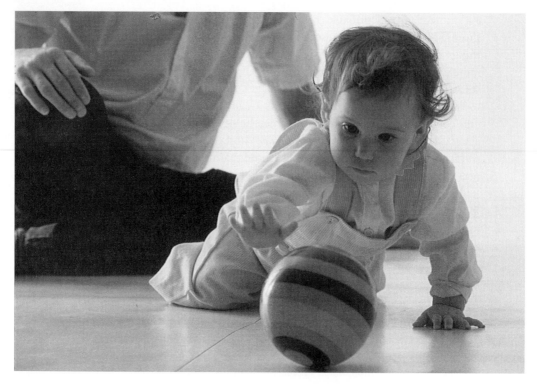

Words like "ball" that are easy to pronounce are likely to be in children's early vocabularies.

include another group of less-favored words, somewhat greater in number, that are used at least once every day or two. The remaining vocabulary words are used rarely, perhaps as infrequently as once in a few months. Rescorla (1980) found in a longitudinal study that by the time her subjects had produced 445 words, 5 percent of those words had not been used for two months. While most English-speaking children learn more *different* nouns than verbs or other relational words early on, they make more frequent and consistent *use* of relational words such as *that, there, no, more,* and *uh-oh* (Gopnik & Choi, 1995).

Unconventional Word/Meaning Mappings

An **overextension** is said to occur when a child uses a word in a context or manner that is inconsistent with, but in some way related to, the adult meaning of the word, as when a dog is called *kitty* or a cotton ball *snow,* or when a visitor is greeted with a hearty *bye-bye!* Thus, the term *overextension* derives from the fact that the child is extending the term beyond the adult word concept. An **underextension** is said to occur when a child uses a particular word for only a limited subset of the contexts allowed by the adult concept. A child who uses *duck* for birds that swim, *bird* for those that fly, and *chicken* for those that don't fly would appear to be using the term *bird* for a reduced set of referents (Clark, 1987). Both overextensions and underextensions are common in one- and two-year-old children's speech, accounting for up to one-third of their production vocabulary (Clark, 1993). Beyond age two-and-a-half, however, such unconventional mappings become less noticeable.

What do children's extensions of words tell us? At best, they reveal how children categorize the world and what aspects of their experiences they find relevant to certain words. Mervis and Mervis (1988) and others have pointed out that children's categories may not initially match those of adults. At the same time, some caution must be exercised. As some researchers (e.g., Hoek, Ingram, & Gibson, 1986) have noted, the extent to which the child's spoken word should be considered an accurate representation of her inner structuring of the world remains unclear. Although some of children's unconventional mappings occur because their underlying word concepts differ from those of adults, other plausible explanations for overextensions and underextensions exist:

- As noted earlier, not all categories have clear-cut boundaries. Carabine (1991) found that most of the inappropriate labeling by two- and three-year-old children he studied consisted of labels applied to objects that were not uniformly categorized by adults either.

- Some of children's overextensions may reflect retrieval problems, such that an older, better-known label (e.g., *dog*) may be inappropriately used in place of a more recently acquired, but more appropriate one such as *moose* (Hoek et al., 1986).

- At other times, children may not yet have acquired the proper label, even though their concepts match those of adults. They may then opt to use words as semantic stand-ins for the words they do not know. Gelman and her colleagues, for example, have shown that children are much more likely to overextend in production—when they must come up with the appropriate word themselves—than in comprehension—when they need only choose the appropriate referent for a given word (Gelman, Coley, Rosengran, Hartman, & Pappas, 1998).

- Children may use their single words analogically to comment on similarities they have noticed (Nelson, Benedict, Gruendel, & Rescorla, 1977). Thus, the child who points to a Saint Bernard and says "cow" may only mean that the dog is like a cow. Additional evidence that children are using analogy comes from the fact that they are seldom observed to use words in this fashion after they acquire syntax and can explain what they mean.

- In other situations, children seem to overextend words as a humorous gesture. When a two-year-old who routinely uses the word *hat* puts an overturned bowl on his head, giggles and says "hat," we can be fairly certain that he is making a joke.

Determining what a child's early words mean requires attention to the contexts in which they are spoken and understood, as well as information about how the child has referred to the concepts or used the words before. Recent research thus shows that children's unconventional mappings are not simply a reflection of incomplete categorization skills. Over- and underextensions may reflect the structure of the category; alternatively, they may be retrieval errors, semantic stand-ins, analogies, or even jokes.

Invented Words

In an early study, Berko (1958) found that preschoolers and first-graders were often able to invent words to refer to meanings that were specified by an experimenter. In this structured situation, children and adults were asked questions like "What would you call a man who 'zibs' for a living?" Although children only rarely employed the typical adult strategy of creating **derived words** by adding suffixes (a *zibber* zibs for a living), they were frequently able to create words by using alternative techniques (e.g., making **compound words** like *zib-man*).

Children also often invent or coin words spontaneously in their own speech. Sometimes invented words are used interchangeably with conventional words, as, for example, when a child uses *bee-house* and *bee-hive* in the same sentence (Becker, 1994). At other times, children may invent new words to fill gaps in their vocabularies (Clark, 1982). Clark found that these gaps occurred when the child had forgotten or did not know the usual word. Inventions such as *pourer* for *cup* and *plant-man* for *gardener* were common. Preschoolers frequently created needed verbs from nouns they knew, as when one child said, while putting crackers in her soup, "I'm crackering my soup" (Clark, 1981, p. 304).

Clark found that children's lexical innovations follow fairly regular principles. These are:

- *Simplicity.* Simplicity is reflected in children's use of a conventional word in an unconventional, but totally obvious, role (for example, *to pillow,* meaning *to throw a pillow at;* Clark, 1993, p. 120).
- *Semantic transparency.* Semantic transparency is evident in innovations such as *plant-man* for *gardener;* the meaning of the invented word is more apparent and more easily remembered than the conventional one.
- *Productivity.* Productivity is shown in children's use of forms that are frequently used by adults as the basis of new words. Many English words meaning *people who do something,* for instance, end in *-er* (*teacher, player*). Thus, children create agentival nouns such as *cooker* and *bicycler.*

Differences Between Comprehension and Production

According to Nelson and her colleagues (1977), comprehension of a word requires that a child, on hearing the word, anticipate or do something. Production of a word requires on its most basic level that the child speak the word at an appropriate time and place. Productive vocabularies typically lag behind receptive vocabularies. According to maternal reports, for example, most sixteen-month-olds comprehend between 100 and 200 different words, but produce fewer than fifty (Bates et al., 1994).

For many years, researchers interested in investigating young children's vocabulary comprehension relied on tasks requiring the child to select or point to an object or picture labeled by the researcher. This methodology was less than ideal for at least two reasons. First, referents for some words, such as action verbs, are often difficult to depict. Second, infants and young children often do not reliably touch or point to the referent requested, even when their looking behaviors suggest they recognize the referent being labeled. Recently, researchers have begun using a new method, called the **preferential looking paradigm,** to test infants' and toddlers' vocabulary comprehension (Golinkoff, Hirsh-Pasek, Cauley, & Gordon, 1987). In this paradigm, the infant is seated on his blindfolded mother's lap facing two video monitors (see Chapter 5). Words or sentences are played over a centrally located speaker. At the same time, brief segments of videotape are shown on the two monitors. The object or action sequence shown on one monitor matches the word or sentence the child hears, while that shown on the other screen does not. Because children prefer to gaze at video segments matching what they hear, they will look longer at the matching screen if they understand the word or sentence. Using this method, Naigles and Gelman (1995) showed that children who call *cow* "doggie" nonetheless look longer at the picture of a cow than the competing picture of a dog, suggesting that young children's underlying concepts may be more adult-like than their productive vocabulary would indicate. Receptive vocabulary, then, rather than productive vocabulary may be a more accurate reflection of children's conceptual knowledge (Gershkoff-Stowe, Thal, Smith, & Namy, 1997).

Clearly, then, the receptive and expressive systems do not overlap perfectly, and a clear understanding of the dimensions and features of each requires careful study.

How Adult Speech Influences Children's Semantic Development

Even before children begin using words themselves, adults' labeling and gaze behaviors serve to focus children's attention on objects. Much of adult speech addressed to young children deals with the here and now (Cross, 1977; Phillips, 1973; Shatz & Gelman, 1973; Snow, 1972). When adults look at and label objects that are visible to children, children assume the label refers to the adult focus of attention, and make an initial object-label mapping (Baldwin, 1991). This dovetailing of adults' and children's predispositions may help explain how children as young as thirteen months learn to comprehend new words after only a few exposures (Woodward, Markman, & Fitzsimmons, 1994). Adults also give children many opportunities to practice producing object labels themselves by engaging them in naming games (Ninio & Bruner,

1978). In these interactions, the parent points to and names specific objects for the child and then helps the child say the name. As children acquire language, parents' speech to them incorporates increasingly rich information about the categories they are acquiring. For instance, in book reading parents go beyond labeling ("That's a bat"), to explain that "Bats live in caves. Bats have big wings" (Gelman et al., 1998).

The labels adults provide for children are not always the ones they would use with adults or older children. Anglin (1977, 1978) showed that adults vary their object labeling according to the audience. When asked to label a set of pictures of objects for two-year-olds, adults used general names like *money* instead of *nickel,* and *dog* instead of *collie.* Anglin also gave the adults sets of words at different levels of generality and asked them to group them according to the way they thought two-year-olds would categorize them. The adults' picture labeling for the children had the same patterns as their ratings of two-year-olds' categorizations. Thus, it appears that adults have preconceived notions of the minds and activities of two-year-olds and use labels that reflect those notions.

Adults sometimes mislabel objects when speaking to very young children, teaching them in some cases to use labels that are incorrect by adult standards. Mervis and Mervis (1982) gave ten mothers and their thirteen-month-olds sets of toys to play with and recorded their speech. The mothers named almost all of the toys for their children and were observed quite often to misname some of them according to how their children might have categorized them. For example, a toy leopard was commonly referred to as *kitty-cat,* and a toy tow truck was referred to as *car.* Why would parents mislabel objects for their children? According to Mervis and Mervis, children provide their parents with signals indicating how they might categorize objects. Although babies first treat all objects in the same ways (mouthing, touching, shaking, and banging them), eventually they begin treating them differently. At this point a doll might be held and a toy car pushed on the floor. Children's differential treatment of objects indicates on a fundamental level how they are categorizing the objects. By labeling the objects for children according to the children's own categories, parents are probably showing how words are used. That is, objects that differ in minor ways but are of the same category share names.

The naming practices of mothers seem to be based on children's own ways of categorizing the world (Golinkoff, Shuff-Bailey, Olguin, & Ruan, 1995). The names chosen follow what Rosch and colleagues (Rosch, Mervis, Gray, Johnson, & Boyes-Braem, 1976) have called **basic level categories.** The first principle underlying such categories is that similarities within categories are emphasized, rather than similarities between categories. Thus, because leopards are more like cats than other objects, they are labeled *cats.* The second principle defining the basic level is that it is the most general level at which objects are similar because of their forms, functions, component parts (Poulin-Dubois, 1995), or motions. Thus, although an owl bank and a Christmas ornament share neither name nor function for adults, because they are round objects that would most likely be treated similarly (i.e., rolled) by very young children, they were grouped with balls and identified as "ball" by the mothers studied by the Mervises.

Mothers of young children use different strategies when teaching their children basic level terms than when they teach either more general or more specific terms (Callanan, 1985; Hall, 1994b). For basic level words, mothers use **ostension;** they may point and say, "That's a tractor." When asked to teach superordinates, however, they employ a strategy of *inclusion,* mentioning both basic level terms and the superordinate term. For instance, they say things such as "A car and a bus and a train. All of them are kinds of *vehicles.*" When teaching terms such as *passenger,* which are more specific than basic level terms, mothers provide an explanation that includes a basic level term as well as the new word. For example, they may say, "The pig is a passenger because he's riding in a car" or "A passenger is a person when he is riding in a car." Parents provide particular help with rare words by explaining them explicitly or embedding them in a context that calls on the child's prior knowledge or real world experience. For instance, at dinner four-year-old George's mother explained what *cramps* are: "Cramps are when your stomach feels all tight and it hurts 'cause you have food in it..." (Beals, 1997, p. 682).

Mothers' speech has also been shown to have an effect on the ways that children come to understand and use vocabulary relating to their own inner states (Beeghly, Bretherton, & Mervis, 1986; Tingley, Gleason, & Hooshyar, 1994). In a study conducted in Great Britain, Dunn, Bretherton, and Munn (1987) found that mothers talking with their young children routinely labeled a variety of the children's inner states, including quality of consciousness (e.g., *bored*), physiological states (*dizzy*), and emotional states (*happy*). By the age of two, the children used many of these inner-state words themselves, particularly those relating to sleep, distress, dislike, temperature, pain, and pleasure. An even more intriguing finding of this study was that mothers used more of these labels with daughters, and, by the age of two, girls themselves referred to feeling states significantly more frequently than boys did.

In addition to the special vocabulary directed to young children, adults and even older children (Shatz & Gelman, 1973) seem to tailor other aspects of their language to the child's ability level; some of the characteristics of input language may facilitate semantic development. Input language, especially when young children begin to understand and use words, is more clearly and slowly enunciated and is characterized by exaggerated intonation and clear pauses between utterances (Sachs, Brown, & Salerno, 1976). In addition, sentence elements are often uttered in an isolated fashion (Newport, 1975; Snow, 1972), and words that are being taught or focused on tend to be placed in sentence-final position with especially marked pitch and stress (Fernald & Mazzie, 1991). Thus, speech directed to young children tends to be better formed and more intelligible than speech to other adults, which tends to be fraught with sloppily pronounced words, false starts, and ill-formed or incomplete sentences with unclear boundaries between words. This clearer, more precise, and simpler input language could assist children in separating words from the flow of speech and in perceiving correct pronunciation. Similarly, the consistent pronunciation could aid them in becoming familiar with new words and in picking out those words that map meanings they wish to express.

Adults communicate with young children in order to share information about social, emotional, and physical topics, but in so doing, they provide children with feedback about their own language. Some feedback is nonverbal, as for example, when a mother appears when her child calls "mama" from the crib, or brings the child a saltine when he asks for a "cracker." If the child really wanted a cookie instead of a cracker, he will have made a useful (if disappointing) discovery. Corrective feedback can also be in verbal form. For example, when a child labels a yo-yo *ball,* the adult may provide the correct label, accompanied by a description of critical features (e.g., *That's a yo-yo. See? It goes up and down.*). Chapman, Leonard, and Mervis (1986) found that these types of corrections were the most effective in correcting children's overextensions.

Children's vocabulary development is also affected by the amount of speech that is directed to them. Children can quickly form an initial hypothesis about a word's meaning after hearing it only once or twice, often called **fast mapping,** but in-depth learning requires multiple exposures to the word in many different contexts (Hoff-Ginsberg & Naigles, 1999). It should not be surprising, then, that children exposed to larger amounts of adult input develop larger, richer vocabularies than children exposed to more limited input (Huttenlocher, Haight, Bryk, Seltzer, & Lysons, 1991).

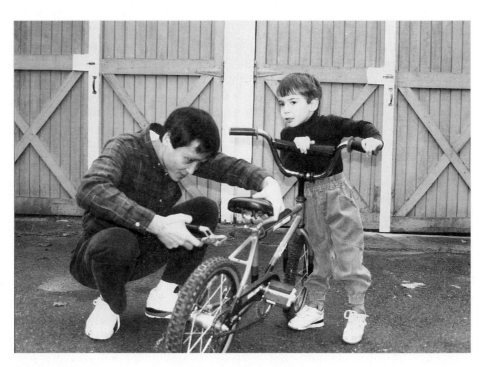

Much of adults' language to children focuses on shared activity.

Recent research has shown differences in the amount of input to children that are associated with social class (upper-middle-class families are the most talkative) and wide variation among families within a social class as well (Hart & Risley, 1995; Pan & Rowe, 1999).

Later Semantic Development

Complex Concepts

As we noted earlier, not all concepts are of comparable complexity; concrete object categories tend to be easier concepts to acquire than are action or affective categories, and superordinates are more difficult than are basic level categories. Clark's semantic feature hypothesis, discussed earlier in this chapter, would predict that terms whose meanings are defined by many features would be more difficult for children to master than terms that are semantically less complex. **Kinship terms** exemplify this situation since many of them, such as *aunt* and *uncle,* share all but one feature. To test this hypothesis, Haviland and Clark (1974) asked children between the ages of three and eight to define English kinship terms. They asked questions like "What is an uncle?" or "What is a grandfather?" Terms that have only one relational component (e.g., *father:* a parent who is male) were expected to be less difficult than terms defined by many features (e.g., *aunt*). As expected, children learned the less complex kinship terms earlier, regardless of whether they had experience with the particular relationship. Haviland and Clark found that children's order of acquisition could be described in terms of adding component features, and that acquisition proceeded through four stages (see also earlier work by Danziger, 1957, and Piaget, 1928). At the earliest stage, one typical child (at three years, five months) has no component features:

Stage 1.
Q: What's a cousin?
A: I have a cousin Daniel.
Q: Are cousins big or little?
A: No.

Stage 2.
In the second stage, a child describes some features of the term but not relational ones, as in this example from a child of five years, ten months:

Q: What's a father?
A: A father is somebody who goes to work every day except Saturday and Sunday and earns money.

Stage 3.

At the third stage, relational terms are used, but they are not yet reciprocal, as exemplified in this conversation with a child of six years, six months:

Q: What's a mother?
A: It's a mommy. I have a mommy. It's somebody in your family.

Stage 4.

Finally, as with this seven-year-old, the child knows that the term is both relational and reciprocal:

Q: What's a niece?
A: A niece is like a mother had a sister, and I'd be her niece.

Another type of complex concept that has received the attention of researchers is *deixis*. **Deictic terms** are pointers or contrasting relational terms that are used to indicate which of multiple objects is being referred to. The chief acquisitional challenge lies in the fact that the reference points for such terms depend upon who says them. Thus, for example, understanding the terms *I* and *you,* and *this* and *that,* requires that the speaker, rather than a fixed point, be assumed as the point of reference against which the meaning of the terms can be interpreted.

Some researchers have been interested in the acquisition of deictic terms for insights it might provide into the developmental relationship between cognition and language (deVilliers & deVilliers, 1974; Webb & Abrahamson, 1976). Comprehension of deictic terms would appear to require the type of multiple-perspective-taking ability that Piagetians maintain only becomes possible when children reach the stage of concrete operations, usually around seven years of age, However, deVilliers and deVilliers (1974) reported that three- and four-year-old preschoolers were able to use different points of view to employ deictic terms such as *here* and *there.* They also found that differences in perspective-taking demands made by different pairs of relative terms had acquisitional consequences. Their three-year-old subjects could comprehend terms that required them to assume the speaker's perspective; their four-year-old subjects could, in addition, correctly produce terms that required them to assume the listener's perspective. In addition, even though the meanings of terms that do not usually require a shift in perspective (e.g., *in front of* and *behind*) were acquired first, they became less well understood for a time when the children were beginning to take into account the effect of perspective on the meanings of other relational terms.

Another example of how children acquire concept-label mappings for complex concepts is their acquisition of **color terms.** The conceptual knowledge required to learn the meanings of color terms includes being able, for analytic purposes, to isolate color from objects, differentiate among hues, and notice similarities among related shades. Linguistically, the child must know that color words refer to the dimension of color rather than, for instance, size (Bartlett, 1977). Color terms are somewhat unusual in that they (like number terms) may be recognized by children before the terms are connected to their referents. For example, when asked to group similar objects, two-year-olds who know no color words can use color as the basis for grouping (Soja, 1994). Likewise, well before they correctly and reliably answer the question "What color is this?", most children supply *some* color term, rather than saying they don't know (Braisby & Dockrell, 1999). Once children begin to use color terms correctly, they generally do so in an order that some researchers say reflects a universal hierarchy (Berlin & Kay, 1969), but which others suggest may reflect parental patterns of use. Ely and Berko Gleason (1998) have shown that the colors referred to by parents overlap with the basic colors in the hierarchy proposed by Berlin and Kay: When talking with their young children, parents use *blue, red,* and *green* most frequently, and never use terms like *beige* and *fuchsia*.

Semantic Networks

As children's vocabularies grow, measuring vocabulary size and assessing children's word knowledge become very difficult (Miller & Wakefield, 1993). Should *cat* and *cats* be counted as two words? Should *walk, walks, walking,* and *walked* all be counted as a single word? Does a child who correctly uses the verb *run* and the noun *run* with reference to a baseball game also know how to refer appropriately to a *run* in her mother's stocking?

The difficulty of assessing children's semantic knowledge arises, of course, because children's semantic systems themselves are becoming more complex. Not only do children learn new words and new concepts, they also enrich and solidify their knowledge of known words by establishing multiple links among words and concepts. For example, children learn that the words *cat* and *cats* refer to the same category of animate object, but differ in number, while the words *cats* and *books* share the feature *number* even though they refer to quite different objects. The words *walk, walks, walking,* and *walked* refer to similar actions that differ in tense or duration, while *eat* and *devour* refer to actions that differ in manner. *Compete, win,* and *lose* share some semantic components, but differ in the outcome each conveys. *Pain* and *pane* are linked phonologically, as are *pane, mane,* and *lane,* though each has a different referent. *Oak, spruce,* and *birch* are linked by virtue of their co-membership in the superordinate category *tree*. These types of connections among words and concepts form what are called **semantic networks**.

Although formation of semantic networks continues throughout the life span, there is evidence that children begin forming rudimentary semantic networks very early in development. Clark (1993), for example, notes that children often add several new words for one semantic domain all at once, as when one-year-old Damon learned *ant, bug,* and *ladybug* all in one week, and *frog, snake,* and *alligator* the next.

According to Bowerman (1978), children seek links, relationships, and conceptual wholes in everything they experience, including language. As a result, they add to their vocabularies not only words that will give them new communicative possibilities, but also synonyms that do not increase their communicative abilities. Other semantic links are evident in young children's inappropriate use of certain words after they have learned the appropriate use. In such cases, Bowerman observed that there was some semantic overlap between the word used incorrectly and the correct word. An example of this phenomenon was when two-year-old Christy said, "Daddy take his pants on" (p. 986), after having previously used *put* correctly in similar circumstances. Both *put* and *take* refer to actions that result in a change of location for an object. Bowerman suggests that such substitutions can be interpreted most adequately as "incorrect choices among semantically related words that compete for selection in a particular speech context" (p. 979).

Another indication that words in children's vocabularies are becoming interconnected is developmental change that has been documented in children's **word associations.** Significantly, responses to such tasks have been shown to be indicative of other measures of linguistic sophistication (Brown & Berko, 1960). There are three general types of word association tasks that have been used. In **free-word-association** tasks, children are given a particular word and instructed to give the next word that comes to mind (see Palermo, 1971; Palermo & Jenkins, 1963). In **restricted-word-association** tasks, children are given additional semantic criteria for selecting responses; for example, the response must bear a particular relationship to the stimulus word, such as superordinate, opposite, or rhyming (see Riegel, Riegel, Quarterman, & Smith, 1968).

In **set tests,** children are given the name of a language category, such as "animals" or "furniture," and are asked to supply as many names of category members as they are able. On all three types of tasks, older individuals' responses represent a narrower, better-defined set than do those of younger children, and on set tests older children produce longer lists of group members. For example, Nelson (1974) found that eight-year-olds were able to supply nearly twice the number of responses of five-year-olds, and only the five-year-olds included "meat" and "ice cream" in the vegetable category and "wall" and "door" in the furniture category.

Young children respond to free-word-association tasks with words that are related in syntax to the stimulus word; that is, they give words that would typically follow the stimulus word in a normal sentence (Brown & Berko, 1960; Entwisle, 1966). For example, in response to the stimulus word *eat,* a child might say "lunch." In contrast, older individuals tend to respond with words that are of the same grammatical category as the stimulus word (e.g., *eat*—"drink"). Around age seven, children begin to respond with class-related words. While this trend in response pattern continues to evolve from first grade to college, it shows by far the greatest change between first and second grades. Explanations for the shift include general cognitive strategy shifts (Nelson, 1977), developmental changes in children's interpretation of the task, changes in knowledge of the features that define words (Lippman, 1971; McNeill, 1966), and cognitive reorganization that accompanies the acquisition of reading (Cronin, 1987).

Metalinguistic Development

The primary focus of this chapter is on children's development of semantic knowledge, in which words symbolize, or stand for, particular meanings. Once we know the meanings of words, we do not need to notice the words themselves in order to appreciate the information they carry. However, along with the development of semantic knowledge, children come to appreciate that language has potential greater than that of simple symbols. Children begin to notice words as objects, and later become able to manipulate them to learn to read and write and to accomplish a host of nonliteral ends such as using metaphors, creating puns, and using irony. These language uses depend on **metalinguistic awareness,** or knowledge of the nature of language as an object. Metalinguistic awareness develops gradually through the middle school years (see Chapter 10 for a further discussion).

Before children can engage in flexible uses of words, they must have an implicit understanding that words are separable from their referents. As noted earlier in the chapter, young children often consider the name of an object another of its intrinsic attributes. Later, children learn that words themselves are not inherent attributes of objects, which allows them to move beyond literal word use and adopt a metaphoric stance.

Once children understand that a word and its referent are separable, they can begin to reflect on the properties of words and objects separately. They learn that although words and their referents sometimes share properties, more often they do not. For example, *elephant* and *hippopotamus* are big words for big animals; however, other long words such as *mosquito* and *dragonfly* refer to very tiny insects. Similarly, while the sound of the words *slip, slide,* and *slink* convey a notion of smooth motion, the sounds of the words *crocus* and *sunset* suggest nothing of the beauty of their referents.

Children's ability to compare and contrast such properties *explicitly,* in a formal way, develops only gradually over a period of several years, but even very young children on occasion are able to appreciate and reflect upon the physical attributes of words (Chaney, 1992). For example, preschoolers can recognize and sometimes comment that different pronunciations of words do not alter their meanings (Leopold, 1948). Children as young as two or three also engage in spontaneous rhyming, which involves implicit comparison and matching of phonological sequences within words, and they recognize that some words include other words within them (e.g., *garden* includes *den*). Occasionally, children's awareness of phonological sequences, combined with their tendency to assume a relationship between form and meaning, may lead them to predict incorrect semantic correspondences between words that sound similar. Thus, at four years of age, Phoebe, on the basis of her knowledge of *tomato,* believed that *tornadoes* were whirling masses of red air; and Polly, who knew the word *eagle,* wondered whether *beagle* referred to a kind of dog that could fly (Pease, 1986).

Many studies that aim to examine children's developing metalinguistic notions of the concept of *word* require that the child be able to verbalize such concepts. For example, in a seminal study of word awareness, Papandropoulou and Sinclair (1974) presented preschool and elementary school children with a variety of metalinguistic tasks, including one in which children were read a list of words, asked whether each was a word, and asked to explain why or why not. The researchers observed improvement across the ages studied, both in children's recognition of words and in their ability to verbalize such concepts. Specifically, older children acknowledged both content and function words as words, while younger children sometimes rejected the latter; further, older children were more adept at articulating what constitutes a word.

It is likely, however, that well before children can demonstrate such explicit knowledge on demand, they have a rudimentary awareness of the nature of words. This view is supported, for instance, by a study by Pease (1986) that attempted to examine children's implicit awareness of the concept of *word*. Children between the ages of four-and-a-half and ten years were asked to tell the investigator their favorite words and favorite things. At the youngest ages, a few children failed to differentiate between the two questions, naming favorite things in response to both questions. For example, one child's favorite word was *toys* because "they are fun to play with" and her favorite thing was *car*, again because "it's fun to play with." In the kindergarten group, some children were able to articulate the reason why a particular word was their favorite (e.g., the word *ear* because "it sounds neat"). The ability to differentiate between the two questions and to articulate metalinguistic aspects of words was even clearer at older ages, with children reporting favorite objects or activities (e.g., swimming) for favorite things and giving words with interesting sound or spelling patterns (e.g., *petrified* or *Mississippi*) for favorite words. Furthermore, the oldest children reported that they and their friends had talked about words they liked, indicating that by the early school years children are actively and explicitly reflecting on and discussing words as objects.

Segmentation

Children's awareness of words in context has also been investigated. Researchers have studied the development of children's ability to segment a stream of speech into words, syllables, and phonemes. The ability to correctly segment at the word level (and eventually at the phoneme level) facilitates the mapping of spoken language onto written language. Although literate adults may find the identification of word units in spoken language a trivial task, in fact, boundaries between words in the speech stream are not identifiable on the basis of pauses or other acoustic features. Thus, children must depend on a variety of other cues and information about semantics and syntax in order to identify word boundaries. The age at which children are able to segment utterances into adult word units varies depending on how the task is presented and on what response is required of the child (cf. Ehri, 1975; Fox & Routh, 1975; Hardy, Stennet, & Smyth, 1973; Huttenlocher, 1964). Sometimes children are asked to count the words in a spoken utterance, tap out each word in a phrase or sentence, or represent each word with a token. Such tasks involve auditory memory and the coordination of a verbal or motoric response, as well as metalinguistic awareness. Coordinating the various elements of the task tends to be difficult for preschoolers. Tasks in which children are asked instead to repeat smaller and smaller bits of an utterance are somewhat easier (Fox & Routh, 1975).

A different technique was used by Huttenlocher (1964), who presented children with pairs of words and asked them either to reverse the members of the pair or to pause between them. The pairs of words that were least likely to occur together in normal speech (e.g., *peach-apple*) were the easiest for children to separate, while those that often occur together (e.g., *happy-birthday*) were more difficult. Huttenlocher concluded that children as young as four are aware of words, but that their awareness is strongly related to the context in which the words appear. It may be that successful accomplishment of such "simpler" segmentation tasks relies more on perceptual skills than on a conceptual awareness of words; alternatively, it may be that when extraneous task demands are reduced in this way, children are better able to demonstrate their awareness of words.

More recently, when Chaney (1989) looked at the developing metalinguistic awareness of word boundaries in children between the ages of four-and-a-half and six-and-a-half, she found that children first were able to recognize phrase boundaries, then syllable boundaries, and finally were able to segment according to word boundaries. When children were faced with unknown or more abstract words, they tended to revert to a phrase strategy or to substitute common, known words for the unknown ones. Some substitutions made in repeating the Pledge of Allegiance were "the night of states" instead of "the United States," "for witches stand" instead of "for which it stands," and "liver T" instead of "liberty." It is perhaps not surprising that children's first strategy is to segment at the phrasal level, since phrases are relatively self-contained units of meaning. Children's later segmenting at syllable and word boundaries may reflect their growing ability to attend to the physical, auditory properties of segments, rather than to semantic properties exclusively.

It is worth noting that most of these studies involved children who already had some experience with written language or who were in the process of learning to read. Because developmental change in children's word awareness tends to coincide with their beginning to read, researchers have been interested in exploring the role certain kinds of metalinguistic awareness may play in reading readiness and reading acquisition. Word segmentation skills in first-graders, for example, have been shown to be strong predictors of later reading success (Evans, Taylor, & Blum, 1979). Of course, the converse is also possible; experience with seeing words represented on paper may facilitate children's segmentation of the speech stream into adult word units. Tentative support for the latter is found in research by Kolinsky, Cary, and Morais (1987) with illiterate adults and adults who had only recently learned to read. When their subjects were asked to produce long and short words and to match spoken words of different lengths to written words, those with some reading experience were better able to perform the task than those without. Like young prereaders, adults without reading experience tended to produce long and short phrases, rather than words. This research suggests that literacy and experience with printed matter may promote awareness of certain physical aspects of words (see Chapter 10 for a discussion of the development of literacy).

Humor, Metaphor, and Irony

From very young ages, children can be observed to play with semantic elements in syntactic structures for humorous effect, as in: "Daddy's proud of you; Grandma's proud of you; Uncle David's proud of you; Hamburger not proud of you, ha ha!" (Horgan, 1981). Toddlers and preschoolers find word play such as rhyming and intentional nonsensical talk amusing and at times even hysterical, but delight in puns and riddles—like interest in favorite words—becomes particularly intense in the middle elementary school years. In fact, many humorous uses of language such as puns and riddles depend on the speaker's ability to separate different facets of language (Horgan, 1981; McGhee, 1979; Schultz, 1976; Slobin, 1978). Thus, what some elementary teachers have dubbed "third-grade humor" is an overt sign that children are actively practicing and consolidating their metalinguistic skills.

In addition to using language for humorous effect, children also learn to use language in other nonliteral ways, such as metaphor and irony. Winner (1988) has studied the development of **metaphor,** which she says generally serves to clarify meaning, and **irony,** which is usually used to evaluate or criticize. Initially, the ability to understand metaphoric uses of language is important because it offers children an additional strategy for clarifying communication, both in production and in comprehension. Even very young children spontaneously use and understand certain types of metaphor for communicative purposes, though their use becomes much more fluent and less context-specific with age (Pearson, 1990). Later, in addition to its clarifying function, metaphor also begins to be used as an important tool in grasping new concepts in relatively unfamiliar areas of knowledge. Winner (1988) cites examples from a variety of fields (art, science, medicine,) in which analogy and metaphoric thinking greatly facilitated the generation of solutions to difficult problems. Both the clarifying and the problem-solving functions of metaphoric language and thinking continue to be crucial throughout the life span.

Using and understanding irony involves appreciating that words and phrases not only can have meanings different from their literal ones, but that the meaning the speaker intends to convey can in fact be precisely the opposite of what the surface meaning would suggest. Irony is most commonly used to express **sarcasm** (that is, the intent to criticize or insult). Adults rely both on contextual cues and on intonational cues in interpreting sarcasm. Thus, if a speaker comments, "Nice catch," after a spectacularly clumsy miss, adult listeners will consider a nonliteral, or sarcastic, interpretation even if the comment is made in a neutral tone of voice. Children, on the other hand, appear to be much more sensitive to intonational than to contextual cues (Capelli, Nakagawa, & Madden, 1990). Thus, despite the blatant mismatch between context and literal meaning, they might fail to interpret the "Nice catch" comment as sarcastic if it were expressed without the typical mocking intonation. Children younger than about eight rarely understand sarcasm even when intonational cues are present. One first-grader we know got off the school bus with a big smile to report that a much-respected third-grader thought his new notebook was really neat. When asked how he knew the older child was so impressed with the new possession, the first-grader promptly replied, "because when I showed it to him he said, 'Big deal!'" Irony and sarcasm are probably other areas of metalinguistic awareness in which verbal interaction with peers provides the young language learner with important data and a forum in which to practice his developing communicative skills.

Word Definitions

Defining a word involves metalinguistic skills as well as semantic knowledge. Children's ability to use linguistic context to deduce the meanings of new words was studied by Werner and Kaplan (1950). In this landmark study, children were presented with a number of sentences with a nonsense word in the place of a key word (e.g., "The painter used a *corplum* to mix his paints" or "A wet *corplum* does not burn"). The children were to figure out the meanings of the nonsense words from their linguistic contexts. Werner and Kaplan found age-related differences in the strategies children used to perform the task. For instance, five-year-olds, who tended to fuse the meaning of the word with the meaning of the sentence, might define *corplum* by saying, "A corplum is wet and painters use it," whereas an eleven-year-old might say, "A corplum is a kind of stick!"

Defining a word involves metalinguistic skills as well as semantic knowledge. With development, children become better able to define words as semantically unique by including critical types of information and using different approaches to organize it. For example, during the early school years children's definitions are concrete (descriptions of the referent's appearance or function), personal, and incidental (Snow, 1990). Through the elementary school years, these are gradually joined by abstract types of responses: synonyms, explanations, and specifications of categorical relationships (Al-Issa, 1969; Kurland & Snow, 1997; Litowitz, 1977; Wolman & Baker, 1965). Swartz and Hall (1972) compared children's word definitions and their performance on a variety of tasks involving relational concepts. They found that children who were least able to consider relational concepts favored *functional* definitions, whereas older children (ages nine to eleven), who were most able to consider relational concepts, gave a majority of *abstract* definitions. Wehren, DeLisi, and Arnold (1981) found a developmental progression in word definitions among children aged five to eleven and college students, beginning with an emphasis on personal experience and moving toward information of a more general, socially shared nature. Snow (1990) has shown that knowledge of the conventional form for good definitions (the definitional genre), combined with frequent opportunities to practice hearing and giving definitions, are necessary for the development of adultlike definitional skills.

A Lifelong Enterprise

Semantic development continues apace throughout the life span. Not only do we as adults continue to add new words to our lexicons, but we also continue to fine-tune the extensions of old words in response to widening experience and to social and cultural changes in our linguistic community. Reflection on and analysis of language result in continual lexical reorganization, a flexibility that is essential if we are to use our language in the most adaptive and effective way to address a wide variety of communicative tasks throughout the life span.

Summary

Words are related to their referents in an arbitrary and symbolic way, defined by social convention. Thus, learning word meanings involves learning how one's own language community labels the physical and mental world. Developmental theorists suggest that very young children have a rudimentary understanding of others' intentions, and that they also have some predispositions, or principles, that help them quickly make initial word-to-referent mappings. For example, children may assume that words refer to whole objects, rather than to their parts. Feedback from more competent speakers allows children to confirm or disprove their initial hypotheses and gradually make their mappings conform to those of their speech community.

English-speaking children's early vocabularies typically include more nouns than verbs or function words, perhaps because the referents of nouns are more concrete and more easily identifiable, or perhaps because they are more common in the speech addressed to young children. Unconventional word-to-meaning mappings (overextensions and underextensions) in children's early speech may reflect processing limitations such as retrieval errors, underlying conceptual differences, or even analogical use of limited vocabulary. Even very young children use language creatively to draw analogies, make jokes, and to invent their own words in systematic ways.

Many features of adult speech to young children are thought to facilitate children's semantic development. Slow, clear enunciation and exaggerated intonation may help children segment the speech stream and identify new words. Talk about the here and now and labeling of objects at the basic level may also simplify the mapping task. Parents' speech provides children with rich information about the words they are acquiring, and children who hear more of this elaborated speech develop larger vocabularies.

As they get older, children not only continue to acquire new words and to learn new meanings for familiar words, but they also make connections among words. They learn, among other things, which words are similar in meaning, which contrast, which are subordinate to others, and which are phonologically related. In addition to semantic knowledge of words, children begin to develop the metalinguistic understanding that words themselves have properties that can be reflected on and discussed.

The development of semantic networks, along with the continual reorganization of our inner lexicon, is a lifelong process.

Key Words

basic level category	preferential looking paradigm
classical concept	principle of contrast
color term	principle of mutual exclusivity
compound word	principles
constraints	probabilistic concept
core group	productivity
deictic terms	prototypes
derived word	referent
fast mapping	restricted-word association
focal colors	sarcasm
folk etymology	semantic development
free-word association	semantic feature
irony	semantic network
kinship terms	semantic transparency
metalinguistic awareness	set test
metaphor	shape bias
novel name-nameless category principle	simplicity
ontological categories	taxonomic principle
ostension	underextension
overextension	word associations

Suggested Projects

1. Visit a parent who has a child who is two years old, or a bit younger. Take a tape recorder, a picture book, and an age-appropriate toy with you. Begin by asking the parent to tell you all the words that the child knows, and write these down. Then tape record the parent and child looking at the book together and playing with the toy. Transcribe your tape and compare the words the child produced in interaction with the parent with those reported to you earlier by the parent.

2. Choose a passage of very technical language (e.g., legal document or technical manual). Practice reading it aloud until you can do it smoothly; then tape-record yourself reading it. Have five friends listen to the tape and write down what they hear. Examine their dictation samples to see if there are any incorrect segmentations.

3. Tape-record half-hour speech samples of a three-year-old and a five-year-old at play. Compare the topics they include and the words they use. What similarities and differences do you note?

4. Find a children's picture book with few or no words. Ask a parent of a child eighteen to twenty-four months old to spend ten or fifteen minutes using the book with the child. Ask a parent of a three-and-a-half-year-old to four-year-old child to do the same thing. Record and compare the words the parents use with the two children.

5. Ask children of different ages to tell their favorite words and things, and explain their choices. Compare their choices and explanations.

6. Ask children of different ages to tell you what particular words mean. Include some words with multiple meanings, such as *cold*.

Suggested Readings

Anglin, J. (1993). Vocabulary development: A morphological analysis. *Monographs of the Society for Research in Child Development, 58* (10).

Au, T., & Laframboise, D. (1990). Acquiring color names via linguistic contrast: The influence of contrasting terms. *Child Development, 61,* 1808–1823.

Bates, E., Marchman, V. Thal, D., Fenson, L., Dale, P., Reznick, S., Reilly, J., & Hartung, J. (1994). Developmental and stylistic variation in the composition of early vocabulary. *Journal of Child Language, 21,* 85–123.

Clark, E. (1993). *The lexicon in acquisition.* Cambridge, UK: Cambridge University Press.

Golinkoff, R., Mervis, C., & Hirsh-Pasek, K. (1994). Early object labels: The case for a developmental lexical principles framework. *Journal of Child Language, 21,* 125–155.

Mervis, C. B., & Mervis, C. A. (1982). Leopards are kitty-cats: Object labeling by mothers for their thirteen-month-olds. *Child Development, 53,* 267–273.

Tomasello, M., & Merriman, W. (Eds.) *Beyond names for things: Young children's acquisition of verbs.* Hillsdale, NJ: Erlbaum.

Tunmer, W., Pratt, C., & Harriman, M. (1984). *Metalinguistic awareness in children.* Berlin: Springer-Verlag.

Winner, E. (1988). *The point of words: Children's understanding of metaphor and irony.* Cambridge, MA: Harvard University Press.

References

Aitchison, J. (1987). *Words in the mind: An introduction to the mental lexicon.* Oxford: Basil Blackwell.

Al-Issa, I. (1969). The development of word definitions in children. *Journal of Genetic Psychology, 114,* 25–28.

Andrick, G., & Tager-Flusberg, H. (1986). The acquisition of colour terms. *Journal of Child Language, 13,* 119–134.

Anglin, J. (1977). *Word, object, and conceptual development.* New York: Norton.

Anglin, J. (1978). From reference to meaning. *Child Development, 49,* 969–976.

Anglin, J. (1995). Classifying the world through language: Functional relevance, cultural significance, and category name learning. *International Journal of Intercultural Relations, 19,* 161–181.

Au, T., & Glusman, M. (1990). The principle of mutual exclusivity in word learning: to honor or not to honor? *Child Development, 61,* 1474–1490.

Baldwin, D. (1991). Infants' contribution to the achievement of joint reference. *Child Development, 62,* 875–890.

Baldwin, D. (1995). Understanding the link between joint attention and language. In C. Moore & P. Dunham (Eds.), *Joint attention: Its origins and role in development* (pp. 131–158). Hillsdale, NJ: Erlbaum.

Bartlett, E. (1977). The acquisition of the meaning of color terms: A study of lexical development. In R. Campbell & P. Smith (Eds.), *Recent advances in the psychology of language* (Vol. 4a, pp. 89–108). New York: Plenum Press.

Bates, E., Marchman, V., Thal, D., Fenson, L., Dale, P., Reznick, S., Reilly, J., & Hartung, J. (1994). Developmental and stylistic variation in the composition of early vocabulary. *Journal of Child Language, 21,* 85–123.

Beals, D. (1997). Sources of support for learning words in conversation: Evidence from mealtimes. *Journal of Child Language, 24,* 673–694.

Becker, J. (1994). Sneak-shoes, sworders, and nose-beards: A case study of lexical innovation. *First Language, 14,* 195–211.

Beeghly, M., Bretherton, I., & Mervis, C. (1986). Mothers' internal state language to toddlers: The socialization of psychological understanding. *British Journal of Developmental Psychology, 4,* 247–260.

Benedict, H. (1979). Early lexical development: Comprehension and production. *Journal of Child Language, 6,* 183–200.

Berko, J. (1958). The child's learning of English morphology. *Word, 14,* 150–177.

Berlin, B., & Kay, P. (1969). *Basic color terms: Their universality and evolution.* Berkeley: University of California Press.

Bloom, L., & Lahey, M. (1978). *Language development and language disorders.* New York: Wiley.

Bloomfield, L. (1933). *Language.* New York: Henry Holt.

Bowerman, M. (1978). Systematizing semantic knowledge: Changes over time in the child's organization of word meaning. *Child Development, 49,* 977–987.

Braisby, N., & Dockrell, J. (1999). Why is colour naming difficult? *Journal of Child Language, 26,* 23–48.

Brown, R., & Berko, J. (1960). Word association and the acquisition of grammar. *Child Development, 31,* 1–14.

Callanan, M. (1985). How parents label objects for young children: The role of input in the acquisition of category hierarchies. *Child Development, 56,* 508–523.

Capelli, C., Nakagawa, N., & Madden, C. (1990). How children understand sarcasm: The role of context and intonation. *Child Development, 61,* 1824–1841.

Carabine, B. (1991). Fuzzy boundaries and the extension of object words. *Journal of Child Language, 18,* 355–372.

Chaney, C. (1989). I pledge a legiance to the flag: Three studies in word segmentation. *Applied Psycholinguistics, 10,* 261–282.

Chaney, C. (1992). Language development, metalinguistic skills, and print awareness in three-year-old children. *Applied Psycholinguistics, 13,* 485–514.

Chapman, K., Leonard, L., & Mervis, C. (1986). The effect of feedback on young children's inappropriate word usage. *Journal of Child Language, 13,* 101–117.

Charles-Luce, J., & Luce, P. (1990). Similarity neighborhoods of words in young children's lexicons. *Journal of Child Language, 17,* 205–215.

Clark, E. (1974). Some aspects of the conceptual basis for first language acquisition. In R. L. Schiefelbusch & L. L. Lloyd (Eds.), *Language perspectives—Acquisition, retardation, and intervention.* Baltimore: University Park Press.

Clark, E. (1978). Strategies for communicating. *Child Development, 49,* 953–959.

Clark, E. (1981). Lexical innovations: How children learn to create new words. In W. Deutsch (Ed.), *The child's construction of language.* London: Academic Press.

Clark, E. (1982). The young word maker: A case study of innovations in the child's lexicon. In E. Wanner & L. Gleitman (Eds.), *Language acquisition: The state of the art.* New York: Cambridge University Press.

Clark, E. (1987). The principle of contrast: A constraint on language acquisition. In B. MacWhinney (Ed.), *Mechanisms of language acquisition.* Hillsdale, NJ: Lawrence Erlbaum.

Clark, E. (1993). *The lexicon in acquisition.* Cambridge, UK: Cambridge University Press.

Clark, E., & Grossman, J. (1998). Pragmatic directions and children's word learning. *Journal of Child Language, 25,* 1–18.

Cronin, V. (1987). Word association and reading. Paper presented at the meeting of the Society for Research in Child Development, Baltimore, MD.

Cross, T. (1977). Mothers' speech adjustments: The contributions of selected child listener variables. In C. Ferguson & C. Snow (Eds.), *Talking to children: Language input and acquisition.* Cambridge, UK: Cambridge University Press.

Dale, P., Bates, E., Reznick, J., & Morisset, C. (1989). The validity of a parent report instrument of child language at twenty months. *Journal of Child Language, 16,* 239–250.

Danziger, K. (1957). The child's understanding of kinship terms: A study in the development of relational concepts. *Journal of Genetic Psychology, 91,* 213–232.

deVilliers, P., & deVilliers, J. (1974). On this, that, and the other: Nonegocentrism in very young children. *Journal of Experimental Child Psychology, 18,* 438–447.

Dunn, J., Bretherton, I., & Munn, R. (1987). Conversations about feeling states between mothers and their young children. *Developmental Psychology, 23,* 132–139.

Ehri, L. (1975). Word consciousness in readers and prereaders. *Journal of Educational Psychology, 67,* 204–212.

Ely, R., & Berko Gleason, J. (1998). What color is the cat? Color words in parent-child conversations. In A. Aksu-Ko, E. Erguvanli-Taylan, A. Sumru Ozsoy, & A. Kuntay (Eds.), *Perspectives on language acquisition: Selected papers from the VIIth International Congress for the Study of Child Language.* Istanbul.

Entwisle, D. (1966). *Word association responses of young children.* Baltimore: Johns Hopkins University Press.

Evans, M., Taylor, N., & Blum, I. (1979). Children's written language awareness and its relationship to reading acquisition. *Journal of Reading Behavior, 11,* 7–19.

Ferguson, C., & Farwell, C. (1975). Words and sounds in early language acquisition: English initial consonants in the first 50 words. *Language, 51,* 419–439.

Fernald, A. (1992) Meaningful melodies in mothers' speech to infants. In H. Papousek, U. Jurgens, & M. Papousek (Eds.), *Origins and development of nonverbal vocal communication: Evolutionary, comparative, and methodological aspects.* Cambridge, UK: Cambridge University Press.

Fernald, A., & Mazzie, C. (1991). Prosody and focus in speech to infants and adults. *Developmental Psychology, 27,* 209–221.

Fox, F., & Routh, D. (1975). Analyzing spoken language into words, syllables, and phonemes: A developmental study. *Journal of Psycholinguistic Research, 4,* 331–342.

Gelman, S., Croft, W., Fu, P., Clausner, T., & Gottfried, G. (1998). Why is a pomegranate an *apple*? The role of shape, taxonomic relatedness, and prior lexical knowledge in children's overextensions of *apple* and *dog*. *Journal of Child Language, 25,* 267–291.

Gelman, S., Coley, J., Rosengran, K., Hartman, E., & Pappas, A. (1998). Beyond labeling: The role of maternal input in the acquisition of richly structured categories. *Monographs of the Society for Research in Child Development, 63,* (253).

Gentner, D. (1983, February). Nouns and verbs. Symposium presented at the meeting of the New England Child Language Association, Tufts University, Medford, MA.

Gentner, D. (1988). Cognitive determinism: Object reference and relational reference. Paper presented at the Boston University Child Language Conference, Boston, MA.

Gentner, D. (1999). Individuability and early word meaning. Paper presented at the VIIIth International Congress for the Study of Child Language, 12–16 July, San Sebastian, Spain.

Gershkoff-Stowe, L., Thal, D., Smith, L., & Namy, L. (1997). Categorization and its developmental relation to early language. *Child Development, 68,* 843–859.

Goldfield, B. (1993). Noun bias in maternal speech to one-year-olds. *Journal of Child Language, 20,* 85–99.

Golinkoff, R., Hirsh-Pasek, K., Cauley, K., & Gordon, P. (1987). The eyes have it: Lexical and syntactic comprehension in a new paradigm. *Journal of Child Language, 14,* 23–46.

Golinkoff, R., Mervis, C., & Hirsh-Pasek, K. (1994). Early object labels: The case for a developmental lexical principles framework. *Journal of Child Language, 21,* 125–155.

Golinkoff, R., Shuff-Bailey, M., Olguin, R., & Ruan, W. (1995). Young children extend novel words at the basic level: Evidence for the principle of categorical scope. *Developmental Psychology, 31,* 494–507.

Gopnik, A., & Choi, S. (1995). Names, relational words, and cognitive development in English and Korean speakers: Nouns are not always learned before verbs. In M. Tomasello & W. Merriman (Eds.), *Beyond names for things: Young children's acquisition of verbs.* Hillsdale, NJ: Erlbaum.

Hall, D. (1994a). Semantic constraints on word learning: Proper names and adjectives. *Child Development, 65,* 1299–1317.

Hall, D. (1994b). How mothers teach basic-level and situation-restricted count nouns. *Journal of Child Language, 21,* 391–414.

Hardy, M., Stennet, R., & Smyth, P. (1973). Auditory segmentation and auditory blending in relation to beginning reading. *The Alberta Journal of Educational Research, 19,* 144–158.

Hart, B., & Risley, T. (1995). *Meaningful differences in the everyday experience of young American children.* Baltimore: Paul H. Brookes.

Haviland, S., & Clark, E. (1974). "This man's father is my father's son": A study of the acquisition of English kin terms. *Journal of Child Language, 1,* 23–47.

Hoek, D., Ingram, D., & Gibson, D. (1986). Some possible causes of children's early word overextensions. *Journal of Child Language, 13,* 477–494.

Hoff-Ginsberg, E., & Naigles, L. (1999). Fast mapping is only the beginning: Complete word learning requires multiple exposures. Paper presented at the VIIIth International Congress for the Study of Child Language, 12–16 July, San Sebastian, Spain.

Horgan, D. (1981). Learning to tell jokes: A case study of metalinguistic abilities. *Journal of Child Language, 8,* 217–227.

Hudson, J., & Nelson, K. (1984). Play with language: Overextensions as analogies. *Journal of Child Language, 11,* 337–346.

Huttenlocher, J. (1964). Children's language: Word-phrase relationship. *Science, 143,* 264–265.

Huttenlocher, J., Haight, W., Bryk, A., Seltzer, M., & Lysons, T. (1991). Early vocabulary growth: Relation to language input and gender. *Developmental Psychology, 27,* 236–248.

Kolinsky, R., Cary, L., & Morais, J. (1987). Awareness of words as phonological entities: The role of literacy. *Applied Psycholinguistics, 8,* 223–232.

Kurland, B., & Snow, C. (1997). Longitudinal measurement of growth in definitional skill. *Journal of Child Language, 24,* 603–625.

Landau, B., Smith, L., & Jones, S. (1988). The importance of shape in early lexical learning. *Cognitive Development, 3,* 199–321.

Lashley, K. (1954). The problem of serial order in behavior. In L. Jeffress (Ed.), *Cerebral mechanisms in behavior.* New York: Wiley.

Leonard, L., Schwartz, R., Folger, M., Newhoff, M., & Wilcox, M. (1979). Children's imitations of lexical items. *Child Development, 50,* 19–27.

Leonard, L., Schwartz, R., Morris, B., & Chapman, K. (1981). Factors influencing early lexical acquisition: Lexical orientation and phonological composition. *Child Development, 52,* 882–887.

Leopold, W. (1948). Semantic learning in infant language. *Word, 4,* 179.

Lippman, M. (1971). Correlates of contrast word associations: Developmental trends. *Journal of Verbal Learning and Verbal Behavior, 10,* 392–399.

Litowitz, B. (1977). Learning to make definitions. *Journal of Child Language, 4,* 289–304.

Locke, J. (1993) *The child's path to spoken language.* Cambridge, MA: Harvard University Press.

Macnamara, J. (1982). *Names for things: A study of human learning.* Cambridge, MA: MIT/Bradford.

Markman, E. (1987). How children constrain the possible meanings of words. In U. Neisser (Ed.), *Concepts and conceptual development: Ecological and intellectual factors in categorization.* Cambridge, UK: Cambridge University Press.

Markman, E., & Wachtel, G. (1988). Children's use of mutual exclusivity to constrain the meanings of words. *Cognitive Psychology, 20,* 121–157.

McGhee, P. (1979). *Humor: Its origin and development.* San Francisco: Freeman.

McNeill, D. (1966). A study of word association. *Journal of Verbal Learning and Verbal Behavior, 5,* 548–557.

Mervis, C. B., & Mervis, C. A. (1982). Leopards are kitty-cats: Object labeling by mothers for their thirteen-month-olds. *Child Development, 53,* 267–273.

Mervis, C., & Mervis, C. (1988). Role of adult input in young children's category evolution. I. An observational study. *Journal of Child Language, 15,* 257–272.

Miller, G. & Wakefield, P. (1993). On Anglin's analysis of vocabulary growth. *Monographs of the Society for Research in Child Development, 58,* 167–175.

Morris, C. (1946). *Signs, language, and behavior.* New York: Prentice-Hall.

Naigles, L., & Gelman, S. (1995). Overextensions in comprehension and production revisited: Preferential looking in a study of dog, cat, and cow. *Journal of Child Language, 22,* 19–46.

Namy, L., & Waxman, S. (1998). Words and gestures: Infants' interpretations of different forms of symbolic reference. *Child Development, 69,* 295–306.

Nelson, K. (1974). Variations in children's concepts by age and category. *Child Development, 45,* 577–584.

Nelson, K. (1977). The syntagmatic-paradigmatic shift revisited: A review of research and theory. *Psychological Bulletin, 84,* 93–116.

Nelson, K., Benedict, H., Gruendel, J., & Rescorla, L. (1977). Lessons from early lexicons. Paper presented at the meeting of the Society for Research in Child Development, New Orleans.

Newport, E. (1975). *Motherese: The speech of mothers to young children* (Tech. Rep. No. 52). San Diego: University of California, Center for Human Information Processing.

Ninio, A., & Bruner, J. (1978). The achievement and antecedents of labeling. *Journal of Child Language, 5,* 1–14.

Palermo, D. (1971). Characteristics of word association responses obtained from children in grades one through four. *Developmental Psychology, 5,* 118–123.

Palermo, D., & Jenkins, J. (1963). *Word association norms: Grade school through college.* Minneapolis: University of Minnesota Press.

Pan, B., & Rowe, M. (1999). Sources of variation in the amount of mothers' talk and gesture in interaction with their 14 month old children. Paper presented at the VIIIth International Congress for the Study of Child Language, 12–16 July, San Sebastian, Spain.

Papandropoulou, I., & Sinclair, H. (1974). What is a word? *Human Development, 17,* 241–258.

Pearson, B. (1990). The comprehension of metaphor by preschool children. *Journal of Child Language, 17,* 185–203.

Pease, D. (1986). *The development of semantic and metalinguistic knowledge.* Unpublished doctoral dissertation, Boston University.

Phillips, J. (1973). Syntax and vocabulary of mothers' speech to young children: Age and sex comparisons. *Child Development, 44,* 182–185.

Piaget, J. (1928). *Judgment and reasoning in the child.* London: Routledge and Kegan Paul.

Pine, J., Lieven, E., & Rowland, C. (1996). Observational and checklist measures of vocabulary composition: What do they mean? *Journal of Child Language, 23,* 573–589.

Poulin-Dubois, D. (1995). Object parts and the acquisition of the meaning of names. In K. Nelson & Z. Réger (Eds.), *Children's language,* v.8. Hillsdale, NJ: Erlbaum.

Rescorla, L. (1980). Overextension in early language development. *Journal of Child Language, 7,* 321–335.

Riegel, K., Riegel, M., Quarterman, C., & Smith, H. (1968). An analysis of difference in word meaning and semantic structure between four educational levels. *Human Development, 11,* 92–106.

Rosch, E. (1973). Natural categories. *Cognitive Psychology, 4,* 328–350.

Rosch, E., Mervis, C., Gray, W., Johnson, D., & Boyes-Braem, P. (1976). Basic objects in natural categories. *Cognitive Psychology, 8,* 382–439.

Sachs, J., Brown, R., & Salerno, R. (1976). Adults' speech to children. In W. von Raffler Engel & Y. Lebrun (Eds.), *Baby talk and infant speech.* Lisse, The Netherlands: Swets and Zeitlinger.

Samuelson, L., & Smith, L. (1998). Memory and attention make smart word learning: An alternative account of Akhtar, Carpenter, & Tomasello. *Child Development, 69,* 94–104.

Schultz, T. (1976). A cognitive-developmental analysis of humor. In A. Chapman & M. Foot (Eds.), *Humor and laughter: Theory, research, and applications.* New York: Wiley.

Schwartz, R., & Leonard, L. (1982). Do children pick and choose? An examination of phonological selection and avoidance in early lexical acquisition. *Journal of Child Language, 9,* 319–336.

Shatz, M., & Gelman, R. (1973). The development of communication skills: Modifications in the speech of young children as a function of the listener. *Monographs of the Society for Research in Child Development, 38* (152).

Slobin, D. (1978). A case study of early language awareness. In A. Sinclair, R. Jarvella, & W. Levelt (Eds.), *The child's conception of language.* New York: Wiley.

Smith, C., & Sachs, J. (1990). Cognition and the verb lexicon in early lexical development. *Applied Psycholinguistics, 11,* 409–424.

Smith, E., & Medin, D. (1981). *Categories and concepts.* Cambridge, MA: Harvard University Press.

Snow, C. (1972). Mothers' speech to children learning language. *Child Development, 43,* 549–585.

Snow, C. (1990). The development of definitional skill. *Journal of Child Language, 17,* 697–710.

Soja, N. (1994). Young children's concept of color and its relation to the acquisition of color words. *Child Development, 65,* 918–937.

Stoel-Gammon, C., & Cooper, J. (1984). Patterns of early lexical and phonological development. *Journal of Child Language, 11,* 247–271.

Swartz, K., & Hall, A. (1972). Development of relational concepts and word definitions in children five through eleven. *Child Development, 43,* 239–244.

Tardif, T., Gelman, S., & Xu, F. (1999). Putting the "noun bias" in context: A comparison of English and Mandarin. *Child Development, 70,* 620–635.

Tichener, G. (1909). *Lectures on the experimental psychology of the thought processes.* New York: Macmillan.

Tiedemann, D. (1787). Über die Entwicklung der Seelenfähigkeiten bei Kindern. *Hessiche Bectragzur Gelehrsamkeit und Kunst.* Reprinted in English in A. Bar-Adon & W. Leopold (Eds.). (1971). *Child language: A Book of readings.* Englewood Cliffs, NJ: Prentice-Hall.

Tingley, E., Gleason, J., & Hooshyar, N. (1994). Mothers' lexicon of internal state words in speech to children with Down syndrome and to nonhandicapped children at mealtime. *Journal of Communication Disorders, 27,* 135–155.

Tomasello, M. (1995). Pragmatic contexts for early verb learning. In M. Tomasello & W. Merriman, (Eds.) *Beyond names for things: Young children's acquisition of verbs.* Hillsdale, NJ: Erlbaum.

Vygotsky, L. (1962). *Thought and language.* Cambridge, MA: MIT Press.

Webb, P., & Abrahamson, A. (1976). Stages of egocentrism in children's use of *this* and *that:* A different point of view. *Journal of Child Language, 3,* 349–367.

Wehren, A., DeLisi, R., & Arnold, M. (1981). The development of noun definition. *Journal of Child Language, 8,* 165–175.

Werner, H., & Kaplan, E. (1950). Development of word meaning through verbal context: An experiment study. *Journal of Psychology, 29,* 251–257.

Winner, E. (1988). *The point of words: Children's understanding of metaphor and irony.* Cambridge, MA: Harvard University Press.

Wolman, R., & Baker, E. (1965). A developmental study of word definitions. *Journal of Genetic Psychology, 107,* 159–166.

Woodward, A., & Hoyne, K. (1999). Infants' learning about words and sounds in relation to objects. *Child Development, 70,* 65–77.

Woodward, A., Markman, E., & Fitzsimmons, C. (1994). Rapid word learning in 13- and 18-month-olds. *Developmental Psychology, 30,* 553–566.

Chapter 5

Putting Words Together: Morphology and Syntax in the Preschool Years

Helen Tager-Flusberg
University of Massachusetts at Boston
and Eunice Kennedy Shriver Center

After months of coaxing and prompting the meaningless babbles of their babies, parents are finally rewarded when the first word is produced. Several weeks after this important milestone is duly recorded, vocabulary begins to grow quite rapidly, as new words are learned daily. At this initial stage young children use their words in a variety of contexts, most frequently to label objects or to interact socially, but they always limit their messages by speaking one word at a time. Still, parents and children together delight in showing off these earliest linguistic accomplishments that mark the beginning of the journey toward full mastery of language.

Within a few months, usually in the latter half of the second year, children reach the next important milestone: They begin putting words together to form the first "sentences." This new stage marks a crucial turning point, for even the simplest two-word utterances show evidence of **syntax;** that is, the child combines words in a systematic way to create sentences that appear to follow rules rather than combining words in random fashion. Recent research on the timing of first word combinations has found that it is related to several developmental factors. These include the timing of the child's first words, the time at which they understand about fifty words, and the responsiveness of mothers to their children's communications at around the first birthday (Tamis-Lemonda, Bornstein, Kahana-Kalman, Baumwell, & Cyphers, 1998).

According to Tomasello and Brooks (1999), the importance of syntax is that it allows the child to code and communicate about events in his or her environment, taking the child well beyond the communicative possibilities allowed by single words. One of the remarkable features about the development of syntactic rules is that it seems to take place almost unnoticed, with no explicit instruction. Parents who quite consciously and conscientiously teach their children new concepts and words never presume to teach syntax. They focus more on *what* the child is saying rather than *how* the child says it (Brown & Hanlon, 1970).

Even though parents and others have essentially ignored the child's use and occasional misuse of syntactic rules, child language researchers and linguists have studied that usage closely all over the world. Years of careful and painstaking research have yielded a detailed, descriptive picture of the course of syntactic development in English and other languages, although the mechanisms that account for these accomplishments are still being hotly debated (see Chapter 7). In this chapter, we describe the main stages of syntactic development that take place during the preschool years, focusing on the order in which various constructions are acquired. At each stage we are concerned with extracting the universal and invariant features of children's language and characterizing the underlying knowledge of linguistic rules and categories that fit the language at that point in development. Questions remain, however, whether children's early sentences are really based on linguistic categories at all, or whether they are fundamentally different from adult-based grammars and limited to lexically based combinations of words (e.g., Pine, Lieven, & Rowland, 1998)

The Nature of Syntactic Rules

Much of our understanding of the nature of syntactic rules has come from linguists who have been concerned primarily with characterizing the rules that underlie the well-formed sentences of adult language users—the natural end point of the acquisition process. The most influential linguistic framework is the one developed by Noam Chomsky, called the theory of **universal grammar,** or UG. Chomsky began developing this framework in 1957, but it has undergone several revisions since. One recent version is known as **government and binding theory,** or GB (Chomsky, 1981, 1982). Although an even newer theoretical program has been developed (Chomsky, 1995), in this chapter we focus on the GB version, because it has had such a significant influence on research on grammatical development. We shall first describe briefly some of the major concepts and characteristics of this linguistic approach.

According to Chomsky, the goals of any theory of grammar, such as universal grammar, are that it is compatible with the grammars of all the world's languages (the goal of **universality**), and that it must, in principle, be compatible with the fact that children worldwide acquire the grammar of their language within a few short years, usually with little or no explicit training or correction (the goal of **learnability**). GB theory is a theory of language knowledge; essentially, it is a theory of how we represent language as a set of principles in our mind. Chomsky believes that our mental representation of grammar is autonomous of other cognitive systems, which means that the principles and rules of grammar are not shared with other cognitive systems but are in fact unique and highly specialized.

The central tenet of GB theory is that there are several components of the grammar that are linked at different levels of representation. Figure 5.1 provides a simplified view of the main components. Of key interest are the two levels: **d-structure,** which captures the underlying relationships between subject and object in a sentence (the basic unit of grammar); and **s-structure,** which captures the surface linear arrangements of words in a sentence. In order to see why these two levels are necessary, consider the following sentences:

> John is easy to please.
> John is eager to please.

Both sentences have virtually the same s-structures:

> noun-verb-adjective-infinitive verb

However, they mean quite different things. The subject of the verb "to please" is John in the second sentence, but someone else in the first. This difference in the underlying grammatical relationships of subject, predicate, and so forth would be captured by very different d-structures. From a developmental point of view, we must ask the question of how children come to grasp the underlying grammatical relations of sentences they hear (d-structures) when they are only presented with s-structures.

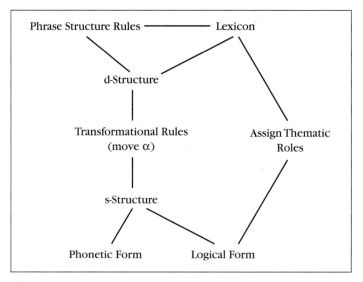

Figure 5.1
Main components of a grammar.

Figure 5.1 also shows that each level, s-structure and d-structure, has several components. The s-structure has two parts: **phonetic form,** which is the actual sound structure of the sentence; and **logical form,** which captures the meaning of sentences (this component connects the grammar to other aspects of cognition). The d-structure also has two parts: the **phrase structure rules,** which capture the basic subject/predicate structure of a sentence; and the *lexicon,* which specifies a number of important features (morphophonological, syntactic) for each lexical item in a sentence. Together, the lexicon and the phrase structure rules generate the d-structure of a sentence.

The phrase structures are often represented in "tree diagrams" of the sort you see in Figure 5.2. They capture the underlying relationships of parts or *phrases* of the sentence, including *noun phrases, verb phrases, adjectival phrases,* and so on. The phrase structure of a sentence also includes some additional syntactic elements, such as *complementizers (that, what),* which introduce each sentence, and an *inflectional* category, which holds the auxiliary verb *(do, will, may,* etc.) and carries information about tense. Thus the basic structure of the sentence is organized in the d-structure by the phrase structure rules. And within these phrases, we see that there are two important types of *categories.* One type is called a **lexical category,** headed by lexical forms such as nouns or verbs; the other is called a **functional category,** which is a grammatical category, such as inflectional (INFL) or complementizer (COMP), as shown in Figure 5.2. This distinction plays an important part in current theories of grammatical development (e.g., Radford, 1990).

The lexicon provides the specific "words" or lexical items that get inserted at the end of the phrase structure trees. The lexicon contains information for each item about its syntactic category (noun, verb, adjective, etc.), much like a dictionary. It also

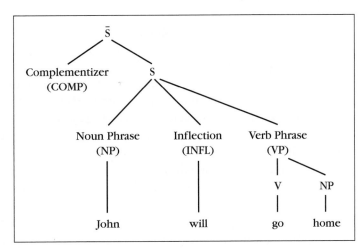

Figure 5.2
A simple tree diagram.

contains information about what kinds of sentence structures the item requires, which is especially important for verbs. Consider the following set of verbs:

> run
> see
> put

The lexicon would include different information for each verb because they all appear in different sentence structures, or *argument structure.* Thus the verb *run* only requires a subject; it does not require an object, but it could take a location as an optional argument:

> John runs (to the store).

The verb *see* requires both a subject and an object, and it can take as an object either a simple noun phrase or a complete sentence:

> John sees Mary (writing her book).

The verb *put* not only requires a subject and object, but also needs a location specified:

> John put the book on the shelf.

This information about the argument structure of different verbs is all contained in the lexicon and is critical in organizing appropriate phrase structures. In addition to required arguments, additional optional phrases may also be added to other phrases in a sentence. For example,

> John put the book on the shelf *last night.*

This optional phrase is referred to as an *adjunct.*

The d-structure is connected to the s-structure by a rule that reorders the elements of the phrase structure into the linear arrangement of the surface form. This rule, called the **transformational rule,** is extremely general—"move any category anywhere"—which allows elements to get moved around. This movement rule is important in English—for example, in creating questions (as in the example in Figure 5.3) or passive constructions. Because the transformational rule is so general, the grammar also needs to have a set of rules, or *constraints,* on which elements may be moved and which may not, as well as where they may be moved to. Many of these restrictions are included in the numerous subtheories that form a part of the GB framework, but we will not go into these here. Some constraints are universal and apply to all languages; some are specific to each language (e.g., the English question-formation rule that moves the *wh-* word to the beginning of the sentence).

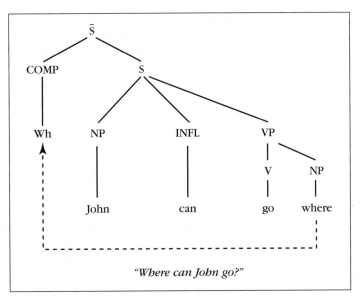

Figure 5.3
Formation of a question in English.

The lexicon is also connected to the logical form component of s-structure (see Figure 5.1) via the assignment of **thematic roles** (also called *semantic roles* in other linguistic systems). This assigns to each of the main noun phrases a role in the sentence like agent, patient, recipient, and location:

	John	gave	the book	to Mary	at school.
Thematic roles:	*agent*		*patient*	*recipient*	*location*

All these components and rule systems are considered to be universal in UG. The grammar also has a system for handling the kind of syntactic and morphological variations that exist across languages of the world. UG includes a set of principles that vary as **parameters.** They operate one way for some languages and another way for other languages. These parameters are conceived of as a set of switches, with several settings (typically two) on each switch. In theory, at least, each language's grammar is captured by a unique combination of switch settings on all the main parameters. This is one of the exciting new ideas in UG, because it addresses the goal of universality, but so far not many parameters have been well worked out. It is also an important idea for researchers of language development, because one hypothesis that has been proposed is that in each child UG starts off with its collection of parameters. As a child is exposed to her native language, the evidence from this input is used to guide which way the switches on each parameter should be set. Thus, the parameter setting hypothesis also addresses the goal of learnability (Meisel, 1995).

One example of a parameter is called the *null-subject parameter* (sometimes also called *pro-drop*). In English, every sentence is required to have an explicit subject; however, languages such as Italian or Spanish allow sentences to drop their subjects in the s-structure. So, for example, one can say in Italian:

Sta piovendo. (Is raining).

For this sentence to be grammatical in English, we must add an *It* as the subject, although the pronoun does not refer to anything at all. This kind of pronoun is called an *expletive,* and only languages that require subjects also have expletive pronouns. There are other differences between Italian and English that all covary under the null-subject parameter. In this way language variation is captured by an economical system that considers under a single parameter a range of correlated syntactic features. We shall see later in this chapter how this idea of parameters, especially the null-subject parameter, has motivated some interesting though not uncontroversial research into early child language.

Studying Syntactic Development

Much of what we know about the development of syntax comes, of course, from studying what children actually say. Longitudinal studies of children in their homes, talking with their mothers or fathers, have produced vast quantities of raw data in the form of transcripts. They have been an especially rich source of information about language development in children from many different cultures and language-learning environments, although many methodological issues must be considered when undertaking this kind of research (Demuth, 1996). In order to find out what the child knows of syntactic rules at any given stage, the researcher must examine the full corpus of speech, looking for patterns and regularities, searching through what is said for what is left unspoken, and contrasting the language at this stage with what came earlier and what will come later. Spontaneous speech data are an especially important source of information about the kinds of errors that children make at different stages of grammatical development; these errors are often the most interesting clues about the child's underlying linguistic knowledge (Stromswold, 1996). These studies of spontaneous speech can tell us a great deal about the language produced by the child, but they do not reveal much about what the child can or cannot understand. Nor do they tell us what the child might have been able to say but was never given the opportunity. Because of these limitations, spontaneous speech data need to be complemented with more controlled, experimental studies that are designed to test children's comprehension of various syntactic forms, or their ability to produce or judge particular constructions in less natural but more controlled situations. In recent years the use of a variety of creative ways for eliciting rare grammatical constructions, such as complex *wh*-questions or passives, have been introduced to child language research (Thornton, 1996).

In this chapter we utilize both sources of evidence—spontaneous speech and controlled experiments—in describing the course of syntactic development. However, we depend more on spontaneous speech, which has been most widely used by researchers studying a variety of languages and provides us with the least problematic source of child language data since it is elicited in naturalistic contexts.

Entering the Complex Linguistic System

One of the most difficult issues about acquiring language that the child faces is how to break into the system. How do children manage to break up the steady stream of sounds they hear into basic units like words and morphemes? How do they learn to map specific sound sequences onto meanings? And how do they learn to figure out the basic grammatical categories of their language such as nouns, verbs, and adjectives? These are some of the fundamental questions about language acquisition that child language researchers must also address in their theories, even though young children at the earliest stages of development provide us with few clues.

One interesting hypothesis that has received some empirical support has been suggested by Morgan (1986), among others. According to Morgan, if adults were providing information in their speech to children about where boundaries exist, not only between words but also between phrases, the task of acquiring language would become feasible and simplified.

There does appear to be evidence that mothers and fathers provide strong intonational or prosodic evidence about word and phrase boundaries, not only in English, but also in other languages, such as French and Japanese (Fernald, Taeschner, Dunn, Papousek, de Boysson-Bardies, & Fukui, 1989). More importantly, there is also evidence that infants are sensitive to the salience of the information sent in pauses (Jusczyk, 1997). Shady and Gerken (1999) found that very young English-speaking children are sensitive to prosodic cues as well as other cues provided by their caregivers in experiments that tested their ability to understand spoken language. Extending this research to children learning other languages, Shi, Morgan, and Allopenna (1998) found that caregivers' speech to infants acquiring both Turkish and Mandarin Chinese contained similar kinds of phonological and acoustic cues that allowed them to distinguish different lexical and grammatical categories.

Once the child has broken the stream of speech into words, he or she may use other "bootstraps" into the syntactic system. Some researchers have suggested that meaning, or *semantics,* plays a key bootstrapping role for the child (e.g., Pinker,

1984); others suggest that the functions of language, or *pragmatics,* provide the primary route into the abstract grammatical system (e.g., Bates & MacWhinney, 1982). A third alternative is that grammar provides its own bootstrapping operation, suggesting that it operates as an independent cognitive system. We will consider the role that semantics, pragmatics, and grammar play in facilitating grammatical development at each of the different stages of the process.

Measuring Syntactic Growth

As children get older, their sentences grow longer. Recent studies of large numbers of children have provided excellent normative data on the age at which English-speaking children make the transition to combining words and using simple sentences. These data come from a set of parental report measures called the *Communicative Development Inventories* (Fenson, Dale, Reznick, Bates, Thal, & Pethick, 1994; Fenson, Dale, Reznick, Thal, Bates, Hartung, Pethick, & Reilly, 1993), which provide highly reliable information about children's language abilities at the early stages. There is wide variability in the onset of combinatorial language. Some children begin as early as fifteen months, the average seems to be at about eighteen months, and by the age of two almost all children are producing some word combinations (Bates, Dale, & Thal, 1995). While age itself is not a good predictor of language development since children develop at vastly different rates, the length of a child's sentences is an excellent indicator of syntactic development; each new element of syntactic knowledge adds length to a child's utterances. Roger Brown (1973) introduced the major measure of syntactic development, the **mean length of utterance** or **MLU**, which is based on the average length of a child's sentences scored on transcripts of spontaneous speech. Length is determined by the number of meaningful units, or *morphemes,* rather than words. Morphemes include simple content words such as *cat, play, do, red;* function words such as *no, the, you, this;* and affixes or grammatical inflections such as *un-, -s, -ed.* The addition of each morpheme (or minimal unit carrying meaning) reflects the acquisition of new linguistic knowledge. So children who have similar MLUs are at the same level of linguistic maturity, and their language is at the same level of complexity.

In order to calculate the MLU of a particular child, one needs a transcript of a half-hour conversation. The child's language must be divided into separate utterances, and these utterances must be divided into morphemes. Brown (1973) provides detailed rules for judging what constitutes a morpheme for the child learning English (see Figure 5.4). For example, although compound words like *birthday* or *goodnight* contain two morphemes, they only count as one. The same is true for diminutives (e.g., *doggie, ducky*) and irregular past tense verbs (e.g., *got, did*). On the other hand, inflections (e.g., regular past tense *-ed,* plural *-s,* progressive *-ing*) and auxiliaries (e.g., *is, have, will*) count as separate morphemes. The number of morphemes in each of

1. Start with the second page of the transcription unless that page involves a recitation of some kind. In this latter case, start with the first recitation-free stretch. Count the first 100 utterances satisfying the following rules.

2. Only fully transcribed utterances are used; none with blanks. Portions of utterances, entered in parentheses to indicate doubtful transcription, are used.

3. Include all exact utterance repetitions (marked with a plus sign in records). Stuttering is marked as repeated efforts at a single word; count the word once in the most complete form produced. In the few cases where a word is produced for emphasis or the like (*no, no, no*) count each occurrence.

4. Do not count such fillers as *mm* or *oh,* but do count *no, yeah,* and *hi.*

5. All compound words (two or more free morphemes), proper names, and ritualized reduplications count as single words. Examples: *birthday, rackety-boom, choo-choo, quack-quack, night-night, pocketbook, see saw.* Justification is that no evidence that the constituent morphemes function as such for these children.

6. Count as one morpheme all irregular pasts of the verb (*got, did, went, saw*). Justification is that there is no evidence that the child relates these to present forms.

7. Count as one morpheme all diminutives (*doggie, mommie*) because these children at least do not seem to use the suffix productively. Diminutives are the standard forms used by the child.

8. Count as separate morphemes all auxiliaries (*is, have, will, can, must, would*). Also all catenatives: *gonna, wanna, hafta.* These latter counted as single morphemes rather than as *going to* or *want to* because evidence is that they function so for the children. Count as separate morphemes all inflections, for example, possessive {s}, plural {s}, third person singular {s}, regular past {d}, progressive {in}.

9. The range count follows the above rules but is always calculated for the total transcription rather than for 100 utterances.

Figure 5.4

Rules for calculating mean length of utterance. (Reprinted by permission of the publishers from *A First Language* by Roger Brown, Cambridge, MA: Harvard University Press, Copyright 1973 by the President and Fellows of Harvard College.)

the first 100 fully transcribed utterances is counted, and the total is then divided by 100 (see Figure 5.4).

In longitudinal studies, the MLUs calculated at successive points in time gradually increase. Figure 5.5 shows the MLU plotted against chronological age for the three children studied by Brown and his colleagues. Clearly, MLU grows at different rates in different children. Of the children followed by Brown, Eve's MLU rose most sharply, indicating very rapid language development, whereas Sarah and Adam showed more gradual and less consistent increments in their MLU. According to the MLU norms developed by Miller and Chapman (1981), based on a sample of over 100 middle-class children in Madison, Wisconsin (see Figure 5.6), Adam and Sarah

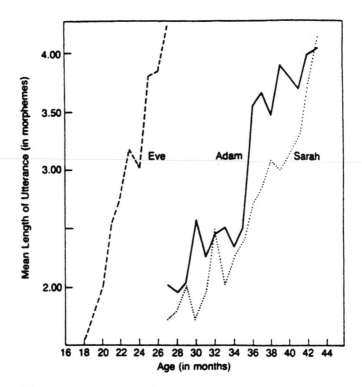

Figure 5.5

Mean length of utterance and chronological age of three children. (Reprinted by permission of the publishers from *A First Language* by R. Brown, Cambridge, MA: Harvard University Press. Copyright 1973 by the President and Fellows of Harvard College.)

are about average for their age, whereas Eve is very much advanced for her age. Using the MLU, Brown subdivided the major period of syntactic growth into five stages, beginning with Stage I when the MLU is between 1.0 and 2.0. Successive stages are marked by increments of .5; thus, Stage II goes from 2.0 to 2.5, Stage III is from 2.5 to 3.0, Stage IV is from 3.0 to 3.5, and Stage V is from 3.5 to 4.0. Beyond an MLU of about 4.0 some of the assumptions on which the measure is based are no longer valid, and longer sentences do not simply reflect what the child knows about language; so MLU loses value as an index of language development after this stage.

There are some questions that arise in calculating MLUs in foreign languages, especially highly inflected and synthetic languages such as German, Russian, or Hebrew. In these cases it becomes difficult to decide what functions as a morpheme in the child's speech, and it is easy to obtain inflated numbers. Still, there have been attempts to extend the concept of MLU to structurally varied languages (Bowerman, 1973) or

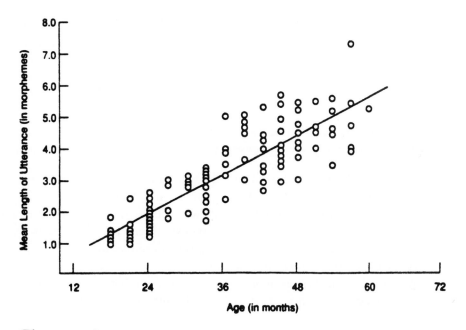

Figure 5.6

MLU norms. (From "The Relations between Age and Mean Length of Utterance" by J. F. Miller and R. S. Chapman, 1981, *Journal of Speech and Hearing Research, 24*, pp. 154–161. © American Speech-Language-Hearing Association. Reprinted by permission.)

to modify the measure to account for cross-linguistic differences (Dromi & Berman, 1982). In some languages, calculating the length of utterances in words, rather than morphemes, has proven to be quite useful. One example comes from a recent study on the acquisition of Irish (Hickey, 1991). It remains to be seen how well this or some other related measure would apply to other languages. By using a similar index to chart language growth across a range of languages, we can search for the universal and invariant features that characterize the main stages of syntactic development.

Other measures of syntactic development have also been developed. One example is the **Index of Productive Syntax,** or **IPSyn,** introduced by Hollis Scarborough (1989). For this measure one also needs a transcript of 100 spontaneous speech utterances from a child. Using the scoresheet provided by Scarborough, the researcher marks the use, up to a maximum of two very different uses, of a variety of structures in four categories: in noun phrases (e.g., nouns, pronouns, articles, plural endings, compound nouns), verb phrases (verbs, prepositions, verb endings, auxiliaries, modals, tense), questions and negation forms (at various levels of complexity), and sentence structure (simple, complex, complements, conjunctions, infinitive forms). The score received is simply the total number of points, with points awarded for each structure used. The IPSyn measure correlates very highly with MLU, demonstrating its validity as a measure of grammatical development. However, it has the advantage of providing a measure that remains useful far beyond the MLU limit of 4.0, at least until around five years of age, and it has the potential for being adapted to other languages.

Two-Word Utterances

The first stage defined by Brown follows children through their earliest attempts at multiword utterances, as the MLU grows from 1.0 to 2.0. Most of the child's sentences are two words long, although a few may be as long as three or even four words. Table 5.1 lists numerous examples of two-word sentences taken from separate children acquiring English as their first language. Examples from children learning other languages are very similar to these.

Looking at these examples, we can note a number of interesting features about children's early sentences. First, from the beginning the child's language is truly cre-

Table 5.1	Examples of Two-Word Utterances
Andrew	*Eve*
more car	bye-bye baby
more cereal	Daddy bear
more high	Daddy book
more read	Daddy honey
outside more	there Daddy
no more	there potty
no pee	more pudding
no wet	Mommy stair
all wet	Mommy dimple
all gone	Mommy do
bye-bye Calico	Mommy bear
bye-bye back	eat it
bye-bye car	read it
bye-bye Papa	see boy
Mama come	more cookie
see pretty	

Note: Terms in column 1 are from Braine, 1976; those in column 2 are from Eve's transcripts and from Brown and Fraser, 1963.

ative; many of these sentences would never have been spoken by an adult. The particular word combinations spoken by Stage I children are unique and novel rather than mere imitations of adult sentences. Second, these sentences are simple, compared to adult sentences, and simplicity is accomplished in a systematic way. Certain words called *content* or **open-class** words dominate the children's language. Thus, their sentences are composed primarily of nouns, verbs, and adjectives. These large word classes are called open since they freely admit new items and drop old ones as a language evolves. The most frequent open class words are nouns, which dominate most very young children's language at this stage (Imai & Gentner, 1997). In contrast, *function words* or **closed-class** words are usually missing at this stage of language development. The closed word classes (including prepositions, conjunctions, articles, pronouns, auxiliaries, and inflections) are much smaller and do not change their composition readily. The absence of these grammatical terms lends to the impression of simplicity. We can also notice that some words are very frequent in a particular child's corpus (Andrew uses *more* and *bye-bye* often and in combination with many different words), and the order of the words appears quite regular. Finally, if we look at what the children are talking about, we can see that certain topics (such as possession, location, recurrence) are very prevalent.

Investigators of child language have spent the last twenty years trying to come up with the best, most accurate way of characterizing Stage I language. There have been a number of changes in these characterizations as the focus shifted from one significant feature to another. However, these changes do not reflect differences in the data but in the kinds of categories imposed on the data by different researchers. The challenge is to ascribe neither too little nor too much knowledge of syntactic categories or rules to the child just beginning to acquire syntax.

Telegraphic Speech

The earliest characterizations of Stage I language focused on the contrast between the open-class and closed-class words. Brown and Fraser (1963) called these two-word utterances **telegraphic** because the omission of closed-class words makes them resemble telegrams. In fact, not all of the words used are from the open classes. A small handful of functors like *more, no, you,* and *off* are scattered throughout the transcripts and can be seen in the examples in Table 5.1. Miller and Ervin (1964) suggested that children choose just those words that are highly stressed in adult language and are thus perceptually more salient. These include nouns, adjectives, and verbs and also some closed-class words, especially those that are syllabic and express semantic information (Brown, 1973). Gleitman and Wanner (1982) have suggested that children, in fact, learn open- and closed-class words quite separately. The earlier acquisition of open-class words is based on their perceptual salience, according to Gleitman and Wanner, and thus represents a good example of prosodic features helping the child to discover basic language structure.

The idea that Stage I language consists almost exclusively of open-class words comes from research on the acquisition of English. More recent studies that have looked at children acquiring other languages, for example, Italian (Caselli, Casadio, & Bates, 1999), Turkish (Aksu-Koc, 1988), or Hebrew (Levy, 1988), which have much richer morphological systems and may be less reliant on words to express basic grammatical relations, have shown that even at the earliest stages children acquiring these kinds of languages are also beginning to acquire some of the closed-class morphology. Hung and Peters (1997) found that prosody helps children learning Mandarin and Taiwanese to acquire closed-class morphology at this developmental stage. Studies on the acquisition of other languages have also led some to question whether nouns really are acquired before verbs, as suggested by Imai and Gentner (1987). For examples, studies of both Korean (Gopnik & Choi, 1995) and Mandarin Chinese (Tardiff, 1996) indicate that in these Asian languages verbs do not emerge later than nouns.

Semantic Relations

Studies of children from around the world in Stage I, using two-word utterances, have shown that one universal feature of this stage is that only a small group of meanings, or **semantic relations,** is expressed in the children's language. Bloom (1970) first observed this in her study of three American children. Later, Brown (1973) extended her findings to children acquiring Finnish, Swedish, Samoan, Spanish, French, Russian, Korean, Japanese, and Hebrew. Table 5.2 lists the eight most prevalent combinatorial meanings found by Brown (pp. 193–197) along with some examples of each.

From these examples we see that during Stage I children talk a great deal about objects—they point them out and name them (demonstrative) and they talk about where the objects are (location), what they are like (attributive), who owns them (pos-

Table 5.2	Set of Prevalent Semantic Relations in Stage I
Semantic Relation	*Examples*
agent + action	mommy come; daddy sit
action + object	drive car; eat grape
agent + object	mommy sock; baby book
action + location	go park; sit chair
entity + location	cup table; toy floor
possessor + possession	my teddy; mommy dress
entity + attribute	box shiny; crayon big
demonstrative + entity	dat money; dis telephone

session), and who is doing things to them (agent–object). They also talk about actions performed by people (agent–action), performed on objects (action–object), and oriented toward certain locations (action–location). Objects, people, and actions and their interrelationships thus preoccupy the toddler universally, and, as Brown points out, these are precisely the concepts that the child has just completed differentiating during what Piaget has called the sensorimotor stage of cognitive development.

Early Grammar

Another important feature of children's two-word utterances is their consistent word order. In his study, Brown (1973) used the children's correct use of word order as evidence in support of the semantic relations approach to Stage I. Braine (1963, 1976)

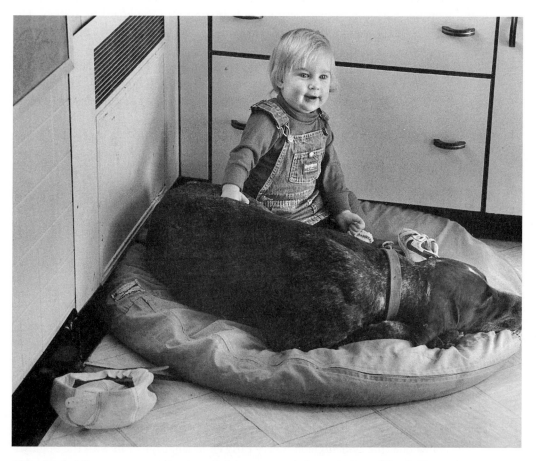

"My doggie." Possessor + possession is one of the semantic relations expressed by children who are just beginning to combine two words in Stage I speech.

also has documented the early productive use of word order rules for children acquiring a variety of languages. He noted, however, that early two-word combinations had more limited, lexical-specific scope than either Bloom or Brown had suggested, which he called **limited scope formulae.** Moreover, Braine (1976) showed that there were large individual differences in the order in which different semantic relations were acquired. In an interesting recent study, Tomasello and his colleagues taught novel nouns or verbs to very young children at this stage of language acquisition (Tomasello, Akhtar, Dodson, & Rekau, 1997). They found that while the children were able to combine the novel nouns with other words, they were not able to do so for novel verbs. This highlights the lag between the acquisition of nouns and verbs as grammatical categories, at least for English-speaking children. At a slightly later stage, children are able to learn new transitive verbs, especially if they are presented in sentence frames that include a noun actor (Dodson & Tomasello, 1998).

Pinker (1984, 1987) has taken the findings about Stage I speech to argue that children use semantics to provide the key bootstrap into the linguistic system. The child can use the correspondence between things and names to map onto the linguistic category of nouns. Names for physical attributes or changes of state are expressed as verbs. Because all sentence subjects at this stage are essentially semantic agents, children can use this syntactic-semantic correspondence to begin figuring out the abstract syntactic relations for more complex sentences that require the category of subject, but which are not clearly agents too.

Paul Bloom (1990a) provides some interesting evidence for this general idea that semantics may bootstrap the child directly into the grammatical system. He found that from the start children assign words to syntactic categories such as noun, verb, and adjective. Even in Stage I, children learning English know that pronouns and proper nouns are different from common nouns because adjectives can only come before the latter. Thus the first sentence below is grammatical, but the other sentences (marked with an *) are not:

> The *big dog* runs away.
> *Small *she* goes home.
> *Happy Fred is here.

Looking through the transcripts from children in Stage I, Bloom found that children almost never violated this word order rule of English and seemed therefore to know the difference between common nouns, pronouns, and proper nouns. At the same time, Gleitman (1990) argues that very young children also seem able to use syntax to provide them clues about semantics or the meanings of words, and there is some evidence for this hypothesis (Naigles, 1990).

How does the evidence about very early child language fit in with the linguistic theory proposed in GB theory? One answer to this question comes from a British linguist, Andrew Radford (1990), who argues that much of the linguistic system is absent in Stage I, but what the child does have at this stage is a lexicon and a limited set of phrase structure rules in d-structure. Specifically, Radford claims that English-speaking children at Stage I only have lexical categories; what is missing from their grammars are the functional categories such as INFL and COMP. There is also no transformational rule; however, the d-structure does get assigned thematic roles to yield the s-structure. These ideas are very similar to the other descriptions of Stage I language that we have discussed earlier, but Radford uses the terminology and framework of the GB theory.

Another use of the GB framework to explain Stage I grammar has been proposed by Hyams (1986a, 1989). If one looks at the examples of Stage I utterances listed in Table 5.1 that contain verbs (e.g., *eat it*), one notices that these utterances lack a subject. Hyams suggests that this is the result of the **null-subject parameter,** which starts off in all children in the position for languages, like Italian, that allow subjectless sentences. According to Hyams, all children begin with the parameter set one way (e.g., the Italian way), and so English-speaking children eventually have to switch the setting of the parameter to the other position. During Stage I, when English-speaking children often omit subjects and do not have any expletive pronouns in their language, their grammars conform to this setting.

Although Hyams's hypothesis is attractive because it is theoretically grounded, there have been some important criticisms raised by other researchers (O'Grady, Peters, & Masterson, 1989). Valian (1990) points out some logical problems with the claim that parameters start off in one particular setting. She also provides evidence that even though American children at the early stages of language development omit subjects, they do, in fact, include a sentence subject significantly more often than do Italian children at the same stage of development, suggesting that they know that subjects need to be expressed. But if they know that subjects must be included in a sentence, why do young children omit them frequently? Bloom (1990b) shows that the problem for young children is that they have a limited processing capacity—they can only cope with producing utterances of limited length, and this constrains which elements will be included in a sentence and which will be omitted. Subjects are omitted more frequently than objects (which are also occasionally absent) either because of processing limitations (since subjects come at the beginning of a sentence and this places a heavier processing load than do elements, like objects, which appear at ends of sentences) or for pragmatic reasons (the subject of a sentence is often provided by context, or has been established in prior discourse). Finally, Ingham (1992) reports a recent case study that found that the acquisition of obligatory sentence subjects in English was not tied to other developments in the child's grammar, as would be predicted on Hyams's theory.

Controversies about the nature of children's early grammars, the role of GB theory, and the best way to conceptualize the child's early linguistic system have yet to be resolved. This extensive look at one stage in the acquisition of grammar highlights the importance of both theories in motivating new research and a closer, more detailed look at children's language, for English as well as other languages.

Children's Early Comprehension of Syntax

Thus far we have presented a picture of early language development that is based entirely on studies of spontaneous speech production. These studies, however, leave unanswered a host of questions about young children's comprehension of syntax. We might ask, for example, when children begin to comprehend two or more word utterances. Is comprehension in advance of production or *vice versa*? What is the relationship between comprehension and production?

Parents generally believe that their children are understanding multiword utterances almost from the time they begin using their first words, and that comprehension is clearly in advance of production. Unfortunately, until very recently, research on this issue yielded conflicting results. For example, some studies supported the parents' view that children understand more than they can say (e.g., Fraser, Bellugi, & Brown, 1963; Huttenlocher, 1974; Sachs & Truswell, 1978), while others found that children could say more than they really understood (e.g., Chapman, 1977) or that the two abilities were at about the same level (e.g., Roberts, 1983). Of course, one difficulty in comparing different studies is that researchers have used very different methods for assessing comprehension while ensuring that children could not be relying on context to interpret the linguistic message (cf. Leonard, 1983). Different methods that have been used to assess comprehension include diary studies (which document conditions under which the child can or cannot understand), act-out tasks (in which the experimenter asks the child to act out a sentence using toys—e.g., "Make the girl kiss the duck"; see Goodluck, 1996), direction tasks (in which the child is asked to carry out a direction, such as "Tickle the duck" or answering questions; see de Villiers & Roeper, 1996), and picture-choice tasks (in which the child must select the picture that best represents the linguistic form being tested; see Gerken & Shady, 1996).

In recent years, Golinkoff and Hirsh-Pasek have pioneered the use of the **preferential looking paradigm** for assessing language comprehension in infants as young as twelve months old. Using this method, these researchers have found that even in the single-word stage, seventeen-month-old children can use word order to comprehend multiword utterances (Hirsh-Pasek & Golinkoff, 1996). Their method (illustrated in Figure 5.7) involves setting the child on its mother's lap equidistant from two video monitors. While the mother closes her eyes and makes no attempt to communicate with her child, the child watches two simultaneously presented color videos. The linguistic message, presented over a centrally placed loudspeaker in synchrony with the videotaped scenes, directs the child to attend to one of the monitors. A hidden experimenter directly observes the child's eye movements and records the amount of time spent watching the two videos on each trial.

Hirsh-Pasek and Golinkoff (1993) have used this paradigm to assess comprehension of various language features. For example, one key comparison they used to test comprehension of word order involved observing very young children while they heard the sentence "Cookie Monster is tickling Big Bird." One of the video scenes had Cookie

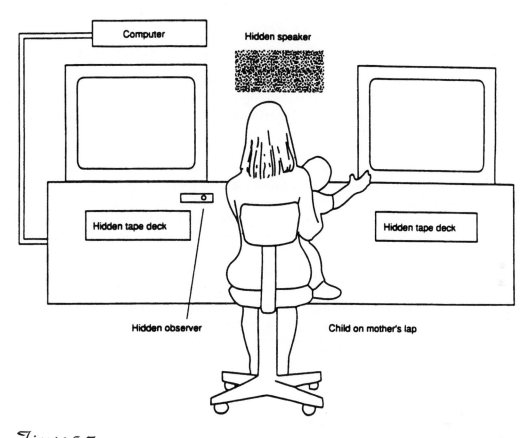

Figure 5.7

Experimental setup of the preferential looking paradigm. (From L. Naigles, Children use syntax to learn verb meanings. *Journal of Child Language* (1990), *17*, 357–374. Cambridge University Press. Reprinted with permission.)

Monster tickling Big Bird, while in the other scene, simultaneously presented, Big Bird was tickling Cookie Monster. Because children at seventeen months of age reliably spent longer looking at the former scene, Golinkoff and Hirsh-Pasek (1995) concluded that children can comprehend word order before they even begin using two-word sentences.

These findings suggest that comprehension is indeed in advance of production, as parents have always known. Hirsh-Pasek & Golinkoff (1996) propose that very young children use a number of cues to help them comprehend grammatical forms. These cues include prosody, semantics, syntax, as well as the environmental and social context in which they hear utterances. Children are thus able to exploit knowledge gained from listening to adult speech in context to guide the acquisition of grammatical forms. Future studies perhaps will tell us whether comprehension development follows the same stages that have been found in the development of spontaneous speech.

Developing Grammatical Morphemes

When we look at children's language as it develops beyond Stage I, we notice two important changes. One is that sentences get longer as children begin combining two or more basic semantic relations. For example, agent + action and action + object may be combined to yield agent + action + object, as in "Adam hit ball." In this way sentences also become progressively more complex in content. The second change is the gradual appearance of a few inflections and other closed-class terms that, "like an intricate sort of ivy, begin to grow up between and upon the major construction blocks, the nouns and verbs, to which Stage I is largely limited" (Brown, 1973, p. 249).

The process of acquiring the major *grammatical morphemes* in English is gradual and lengthy. Some are still not fully controlled until the child enters school (for example, certain irregular past-tense verbs). Nevertheless, the process begins early, as soon as the MLU approaches 2.0, and we will discuss the main research findings on the acquisition of a small subset of fourteen English grammatical morphemes.

The development of these morphemes was studied by Brown and his colleague Courtney Cazden (1968) using the longitudinal data from Adam, Eve, and Sarah (Brown, 1973). The fourteen morphemes were selected both because they were very frequent and because one can easily identify the contexts in which they are needed to produce a grammatically well-formed sentence.

The Fourteen Morphemes

Grammatical morphemes, even though they do not carry independent meaning, do subtly shade the meaning of sentences. The morpheme group studied by Brown included two prepositions (*in, on*), two articles (*a, the*), noun inflections marking possessive (*'s*) and plural (*-s*), verb inflections marking progressive (*-ing*), third-person present tense of regular verbs (e.g., he walk*s*) or irregular verbs (e.g., he *has*), past tense of regular verbs (e.g., he walk*ed*) and irregular verbs (e.g., *had*), and the main uses of the verb *to be*—as auxiliary, both when it can be contracted (e.g., I *am* walking or I'*m* walking) and when it cannot be contracted (e.g., I *was* walking), and as a main verb or *copula* in its contractible form (e.g., I *am* happy or I'*m* happy) and its uncontractible form (e.g., This *is* it).

In order to chart the development of these morphemes, Brown closely examined each child utterance to identify whether it required any of the morphemes to make it fully grammatical by adult standards. Both the linguistic context (the utterance itself) and the nonlinguistic context can be used to decide which morphemes are necessary. For example, when a child says "that book" while pointing out a book, we know that there should be a copula (*'s* or *is*) and an article (*a*). Or if a child says "two book table" when there are a couple of books lying on the table, we know that *book* should have a plural *-s* and the preposition *on* and article *the* are required before the word *table*. In this way Brown went through the transcripts of his three subjects from Stage I to Stage V and identified all of the obligatory contexts for each morpheme. Then he checked how many of these contexts were actually filled with the appropriate morphemes at the different stages of development. From this he calculated the percentage of each morpheme actually supplied in its obligatory context for each child for each sample of spontaneous speech. This measure has the advantage of being independent of actual frequency of use since frequency may vary considerably from one child to another and from one point in time to the next.

The process of acquiring each of these grammatical morphemes is a gradual one—they do not suddenly appear in their required contexts all of the time. Rather, their appearance fluctuates, sometimes quite sharply, during the period when they are being acquired until they are almost always present. After this point is reached, there is rarely any regression (see also Mervis & Johnson, 1987, for a detailed case study).

Order of Acquisition

The most important finding that Brown reports is the remarkable similarity among his three subjects in the order in which these morphemes were acquired. Acquisition is defined as the time when the morpheme was supplied in 90 percent of its obligatory contexts. The first set of morphemes to be acquired included the two prepositions, the plural, and the present progressive inflection. The last morphemes were the contractible copula and auxiliary, which had not yet reached the acquisition criterion by Stage V. Table 5.3 shows the average order of acquisition of all fourteen morphemes. This order was confirmed in a study of a larger sample of children by de Villiers and de Villiers (1973).

Explaining the Order of Acquisition

What accounts for this invariant sequence of development? Why do all children find the progressive inflection (*-ing*) easier than the past tense inflection (*-ed*) and articles (*a, the*) harder than the plural ending? One possible explanation is that the morphemes the children hear most often will be acquired earlier. Brown tested this *frequency hypothesis* in the following way. He examined the speech of each child's parents just before the child reached Stage II and began using the morphemes. He tallied the number of times each morpheme was used by each parent and compared these frequencies with the order in which the morphemes were acquired by the children. But there was no relationship between these figures. For example, the most frequent morphemes in the parents' speech were the articles, but these were not among the earliest to be acquired. And even though prepositions were not so frequent in the parents' samples, they were acquired very early by all the children. So overall, frequency does not account well for the particular order in which the fourteen morphemes develop,

Some more recent attempts to demonstrate that frequency can account for the order in which grammatical morphemes are acquired (e.g., Moerk, 1980) have been criticized and shown to be quite incorrect both in the methodologies used and in the conclusions drawn (Pinker, 1981).

On the other hand, Brown (1973) did find that *linguistic complexity* predicted the order of acquisition very well. Complexity can be defined in two ways: *semantic* (the number of meanings encoded in the morpheme) and *syntactic* (the number of rules required for the morpheme). Brown defined complexity in a conservative way that he called cumulative complexity. Only morphemes that share common meanings or rules can be fairly compared. A morpheme that requires knowledge of both *x* and *y* is defined as more complex than a morpheme requiring knowledge of only *x* or *y*, but it cannot be compared to a morpheme requiring knowledge of *w*. When complexity is defined like this, not all the morphemes can be ordered, but those that can be predict well the order of acquisition found by Brown and the de Villierses.

If we look at cumulative semantic complexity, the plural morpheme encodes only number, the past tense (regular or irregular) morphemes encode "earlierness," and the present progressive morpheme encodes temporary duration. Since the copula verb and the third-person singular morphemes encode both number and "earlierness," we would predict that these morphemes would be acquired later. This prediction is borne out by the order shown in Table 5.3. We would also predict that the auxiliary—which encodes number, "earlierness," and temporary duration—would be acquired after all of these since it entails all of these meanings. This prediction, too, is confirmed by the data. From a syntactic point of view it is interesting to note that the

Table 5.3	**Average Order of Acquisition of Fourteen Grammatical Morphemes by Three Children Studied by Brown**
1. present progressive	(sing*ing*; play*ing*)
2/3. prepositions	(*in* the cup; *on* the floor)
4. plural	(book*s*; doll*s*)
5. irregular past tense	(*broke*; *went*)
6. possessive	(Mommy*'s* chair; Susie*'s* teddy)
7. copula uncontractible	(This *is* my book)
8. articles	(*The* teddy; *A* table)
9. regular past tense	(walk*ed*; play*ed*)
10. third-person present tense regular	(he climb*s*; Mommy cook*s*)
11. third-person present tense irregular	(John *has* three cookies)
12. auxiliary uncontractible	(She *was* going to school; *Do* you like me?)
13. copula contractible	(I*'m* happy; you *are* special)
14. auxiliary contractible	(Mommy*'s* going shopping)

morphemes that are acquired early involve only lexical categories, whereas the later-acquired morphemes all involve functional categories, particularly INFL (present and past tense; auxiliary verbs).

Brown carried out a similar analysis for ordering the morphemes in terms of their cumulative syntactic complexity. In this case the rules needed to derive the morphemes were used to generate predicted orderings, which were also confirmed by the data in Table 5.3. Unfortunately, these two hypotheses—cumulative semantic complexity and cumulative syntactic complexity—cannot be teased apart; they make almost identical predictions for the set of English grammatical morphemes studied by Brown and his colleagues. Research on other languages provides further support for these hypotheses.

Productivity of Children's Morphology

Even though it is generally accepted that children cannot and do not learn the morphology of a language by repeating specific examples they have heard from others, some researchers suggest that at the initial stages, children use grammatical morphemes in a "constructivist" way, by combining them with particular lexical forms. Pine and Lieven (1997) showed that early use of determiners, such as "a" and "the" were learned in combination with specific vocabulary items, and tense endings (e.g., -ed) were also used in combination with particular verbs only (Pine, 1999). Nevertheless, by age three or four there is clear evidence that children are indeed acquiring a rule-governed system. To start with, there are the charming mistakes that children make—mistakes in applying a morphological rule when it should not be applied. For example, children frequently add the plural *-s* to exceptional nouns (man*s*, foot*s*, *teeths*, people*s*) or use the regular past tense *-ed* on irregular verbs (fall*ed*, go*ed*, brok*ed*), even when the correct irregular form has previously been used. **Overregularization errors** like these are an excellent source of evidence for the productivity and creativity of the child's morphology; these are the forms no child would have heard from an adult.

Other evidence for the productive use of morphological rules came from a pioneering study by Berko (1958). Berko designed an elicited production task in which children were shown novel creatures and actions that were given invented names. The children were then provided with the linguistic context for adding plural and possessive inflections to the novel nouns and progressive, third person present tense, and past tense endings to the novel verbs. Figure 5.8 shows two examples from this study. Overall, Berko found preschool and first-grade children performed well with the nonsense words, although their performance was clearly constrained by the controlled, somewhat artificial conditions of the experiment (cf. Levy, 1983). Nevertheless, the ability to supply correct morphemes on novel nouns and verbs demonstrates beyond doubt that children have internalized knowledge about English morphological rules and have not simply learned the morphemes in a rote fashion by imitating others.

Children's knowledge of both regular and irregular forms of English, particularly the past tense ending, has been the focus of a number of recent studies by Pinker

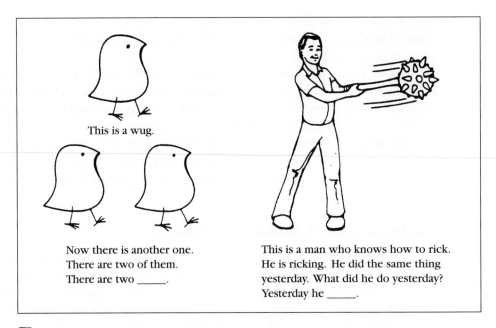

This is a wug.

Now there is another one.
There are two of them.
There are two _____.

This is a man who knows how to rick.
He is ricking. He did the same thing
yesterday. What did he do yesterday?
Yesterday he _____.

Figure 5.8
Two example items from the wug test. (From Berko, 1958.)

and his associates (Marcus, Pinker, Ullman, Hollander, Rosen, & Xu, 1992; Pinker &
Prince, 1992). Their findings, based on spontaneous speech analyses and experimental studies suggest that past tense overregularization errors are, in fact, relatively rare
(between 5 and 10 percent), but they persist well into middle childhood for particular
types of verbs. Based on these findings, Pinker (1991) argues that two different mechanisms are involved in acquiring regular and irregular forms. Regular forms involve a
rule-governed mechanism that applies the *-ed* ending in contexts requiring the expression of a past tense, while irregular forms are retrieved directly from the lexicon and
thus involve a memory storage system. This dual-mechanism hypothesis has come
under attack from models developed within a *connectionist* framework (see Chapter
7), in which only a single mechanism is needed to compute the correct past tense ending (Plunkett, 1995; Plunkett & Marchman, 1991, 1993; Rumelhart & McClelland,
1986). Connectionist models learn the verb endings based on the input they receive.
The debate between the dual mechanism and connectionist camps continues in a
lively fashion in the current psycholinguistic literature.

Cross-Linguistic Data

There is by now a growing literature on the acquisition of grammatical morphology in
other languages, though not all of these studies use Brown's exact methodology. Nev-

ertheless, some of his findings on English have been supported by data on children's acquisition of other languages. For example, records of children's acquisition of the morphology of Russian (Slobin, 1966), Hebrew (Berman, 1981), and many other languages all include abundant examples of overgeneralization errors (see the relevant chapters in Slobin, 1985).

Studies of other languages also yield some contrasting data. While English morphology is acquired slowly and in a piecemeal fashion, some aspects of Italian morphology, for example, may be acquired very rapidly (Hyams, 1986b). There is, in fact, some controversy in the literature about the ease and rate of development of morphology in Italian. Pizzuto and Casselli (1992) analyzed the spontaneous speech from three children from about eighteen months to thirty months of age. While many grammatical morphemes appeared very early in their speech, full mastery of these morphemes took much longer, with the developmental curves resembling data found for English-speaking children. A follow-up cross-sectional study of larger numbers of children confirmed these findings and showed that by age three-and-a-half to four, most morphemes had been acquired (Caselli, Leonard, Volterra, & Campagnoli, 1993).

There is also evidence that both semantic and syntactic complexity play significant roles in determining the order in which grammatical morphemes are acquired in some other languages. The best evidence for this comes from Slobin's monumental cross-linguistic project, in which the acquisition of Turkish, Italian, Serbo-Croatian, and English were studied with similar methods and in comparable groups of children. In one study (Johnston & Slobin, 1979) the acquisition of the morphology used to express location (such as the English prepositions *in* and *on*) was compared across these four languages, using an elicited production measure. There was some degree of similarity in the order of acquisition, which can be explained by the semantic complexity hypothesis.

However, there were also some interlanguage differences that could only be accounted for by the syntactic complexity hypothesis. For example, Levy (1997) showed that in Hebrew, which is a highly inflected language in which the morphology does not have simple semantic mappings, some aspects of morphology are acquired very early. She suggests that in languages like Hebrew where morphology can only be viewed as a set of formal paradigms, these forms are acquired very early. This is also true for languages such as Inuktitut, a polysynthetic language spoken by Canadian natives. Allen (1996) studied the acquisition of Inuktitut by four children and found they combined morphemes productively by the age of two, rarely making the kinds of omission or overgeneralization errors reported for English-speaking children.

Different Sentence Modalities

After Stage II, when the grammatical morphemes begin to appear, the major changes in the child's language are in the development of different types of sentences, such as negatives, questions, and imperatives. Although children most certainly say no, ask questions, and make demands at the very earliest stages of language development, it is not until about Stage III (when the MLU reaches 2.5) that they begin to acquire the adult forms for their expression. During earlier stages of language development children rely on different intonation patterns, closely matching those used by adults, to mark different sentence modalities (Bassano & Mendes-Maillochon, 1994). Gradually, children begin to master the morphosyntactic devices that mark **sentence modality,** and these come to complement the earlier acquired prosodic devices. In this section we will follow the course of development of two different sentence modalities—negatives and questions.

Negatives

Ursula Bellugi, one of Brown's students, undertook the analysis of the expression of **negation** in the longitudinal transcripts of Adam, Eve, and Sarah (Bellugi, 1967). Like most of the child language researchers during the 1960s, Bellugi focused exclusively on a syntactic analysis that was heavily influenced by the prevailing linguistic theories of the time. She identified three main periods in the acquisition of the full negative. In the first period a sentence was made negative by placing the negative marker, *no* or *not,* outside the sentence, usually preceding it. There were many utterances of this form:

> No go movies.
> No sit down.
> No Mommy do it.

In the next period, the negative word was moved inside the sentence and placed next to the main verb; however, there was no productive use of the auxiliary system. During this period Bellugi reports examples such as these:

> I no like it.
> Don't go.
> I no want book.

The final period (which is not usually reached until Stage V) was marked by the appearance of different auxiliaries, and the child's negative sentences then approximated the adult forms. Negatives such as these are produced during this final period:

> You can't have this.
> I don't have money.
> I'm not sad now.

Thus Bellugi's analysis of negation focused on the development of its syntactic form. Because of the complexity of the English auxiliary system, children take a long time to acquire full mastery over the expression of negation in English.

Bloom (1970) soon criticized Bellugi's approach. She argued that almost all of the sentences produced during the first period had no subjects anyway, and so, in fact, the negative marker was correctly placed next to the verb or predicate. In those few instances where there was a sentence subject and the *no* was outside the sentence (as in "No Mommy do it"), Bloom inferred that *no* was not negating the sentence but was *anaphoric;* that is, it referred back to a preceding utterance. In this example the meaning of the sentence would be "No, I want Mommy to do it." The thrust of Bloom's argument, then, was to question the existence of the first period of negative acquisition, even though some had claimed this was a universal first stage (see McNeill, 1970). But de Villiers and de Villiers (1979) pointed out that there were too few critical sentences in the existent literature on which to judge the issue. Fortunately, their own children had learned how to say *no* and, in the process, provided large numbers of these critical sentences (de Villiers & de Villiers, 1979).

The de Villierses found that their son, Nicholas, produced two kinds of negative sentences during the first period. One kind confirmed Bellugi's analysis of a *no* + sentence rule—where the *no* was not anaphoric but negated the sentence. However, at the same time he produced sentences that had the negative marker placed internally, next to the verb or predicate. Nicholas, therefore, appeared to use two different rules to generate negatives.

When these two groups of negatives were carefully analyzed, de Villiers and de Villiers saw that Nicholas used one form (*no* + sentence) to express one kind of negative meaning and the other form (internal *no*) to express a different negative meaning. Bloom herself had proposed that one could distinguish at least three semantic categories of negation in early speech. These categories include (1) nonexistence—when the child remarks on the absence of something, for example, "no cake" or "all gone cookie"; (2) rejection—when the child opposes something, for example, "no wash hair"; and (3) denial—when the child denies the truth of a statement made or implied by someone else, for example "that not Daddy." Both Bloom (1970) for English and McNeill and McNeill (1968) for Japanese found that these three semantic categories of negation appeared in children's speech in the order given here. De Villiers and de Villiers found that Nicholas used the *no* + sentence form to express rejection and the internal-*no* form to express denial. This same pattern was confirmed in their second child, Charlotte, and in Eve, but they did not find it in Adam's speech.

Where did this pattern come from? De Villiers and de Villiers suggest that the children picked it up from their parents' speech. Both Eve's parents and Nicholas and Charlotte's parents (but not Adam's) used a polite but indirect form to express rejection, which inadvertently modeled a *no* + sentence form. For example, they would say, "No, I don't think you should do that."

We see, then, that the development of negation reflects a complex interaction of syntactic, semantic, and input factors that may combine in different ways for different children learning various languages in the early stages. Clancy (1985) extended McNeill and McNeill's earlier work on the acquisition of the different negative markers in Japanese. She, too, found early acquisition of the negative marking nonexistence (*nai*) and rejection (*iya*), which was often overextended to include prohibition (*dame*). In the early stages *nai* and *iya* (but never *dame*) were overextended to express denial (*chigan*), which was a late-emerging negative morpheme.

The late development of negative forms to express denial, and prohibition, contrasting with early appearing expressions of rejection and nonexistence, has also been demonstrated in a study on the acquisition of Tamil, a language spoken on the subcontinent of India and Sri Lanka (Vaidyanathan, 1991).

Just as young children differentiate negative sentences according to their semantic function, there is also evidence that they are sensitive to the *pragmatic* or contextual factors influencing negation. This was demonstrated in an elicited production study conducted by de Villiers and Tager-Flusberg (1975). Their study showed that children made fewer errors and were faster responding to negative sentences expressing denial when the context for the sentences was plausible rather than implausible. Thus nonlinguistic context can also influence young children's processing of linguistic forms such as negation.

Questions

In English and other languages we can ask different kinds of questions for different purposes in a number of ways. For example, we can simply use rising intonation on a declarative sentence to signal that we are asking a question: "Mommy is tired?" Children seem to rely on rising intonation in the earliest stages (Klima & Bellugi, 1966). We can also ask this question, called a **yes/no question,** since these are the responses that are called for, by reversing the subject of the sentence (*Mommy*) and the auxiliary verb (*is*). This syntactic rule is much more complex, and children only begin to master it in Stage III.

A different group of questions is used for obtaining more than a simple *yes/no* answer. They are called the ***wh*-questions** in English since they begin with *what, where, which, who, whose, when, why,* and *how.* Answers to these questions will be more complex and contain more information. These questions also require the rule of inverting the subject and the auxiliary, as well as the correct placement of the appropriate *wh*-word at the beginning; for example, "When is dinner?" or "Why are we staying home?" Children initially ask *wh*-questions omitting the auxiliary altogether:

What that?
Where Daddy go?

They then include the auxiliary but do not consistently switch it around with the subject:

Where are you going?
What she is playing?

Wh-questions can also be formed from complex sentences, including two or more clauses. For example:

How did Jane think she could fix the shelf?

On one reading of this question, the answer might be:

Using a hammer and nails.

The *wh*-question, *how,* has moved *long-distance* from the end of the complex sentence (i.e., How could she fix the shelf?)

On a different reading of this question, the answer might be:

Because she took a course in woodworking (i.e., How could she *think* it?)

Not all verbs or sentence structure allow long-distance movement. For example:

How did Jane know she could fix the shelf?

Only the second reading is possible in this example (Because she took a course in woodworking). Different languages form *wh*-questions in different ways, and there are variations in the rules that allow long-distance movement across clauses. One key question in language acquisition is how children acquire these highly complex rules that are specific to their language (de Villiers, Roeper, & Vainikka, 1990; Weissenborn, Roeper, & de Villiers, 1991).

Finally, children are able to incorporate all of the syntactic rules necessary to produce well-formed *wh*-questions.

Klima and Bellugi (1966) hypothesized that since *yes/no* questions involved only one rule (inverting subject and auxiliary) and *wh*-questions required two rules (*wh*-word placement and subject-auxiliary inversion), one should find that children produce correctly inverted *yes/no* questions earlier than inverted *wh*-questions. Their analysis of questions asked by Adam, Eve, and Sarah confirmed this hypothesis; however, later studies, using larger groups of children, found no evidence for this (Erreich, 1980; Ingram & Tyack, 1979). Instead, many children employ the inversion rule for both kinds of questions at about the same time. A careful analysis of the emergence of the auxiliary verb in *wh*-questions has found that if it appears, it is generally inverted; otherwise it is most often absent from the question altogether (Stromswold, 1995; Valian, 1992). De Villiers and colleagues (1990) explored the spontaneous speech of a few children and found that for each child the presence of inverted auxiliaries in their *wh*-questions emerged at separate points for each *wh*-term (*what, how, why*), and that there was a close developmental relationship between inverting auxiliaries and expressing embedded *wh*-questions (e.g., *How did you know that? I saw how you played the game.*) De Villiers

(1991, 1995; see also Radford, 1994) argues that these developments reflect the acquisition of the functional category of COMP (or complementation). Rowland and Pine (2000) however, argue that questions emerge based on lexical combinations and there is no need to posit in the child's grammar abstract functional categories.

There is more agreement among researchers concerning the order in which children acquire the various *wh*-questions. Wootten, Merkin, Hood, and Bloom (1979) found that *what, where,* and *who* were the first questions asked by the children they followed longitudinally. Only later did their subjects ask questions about *when, how,* and *why*. And studies of children's comprehension of different *wh*-questions have found that *what, where,* and *who* are easier to understand and correctly respond to than *how, why,* and *when* (Ervin-Tripp, 1970; Tyack & Ingram, 1977; Winzemer, 1980). Erreich (1980) also found that her subjects inverted the subject and auxiliary more often in *what, where,* and *who* questions and less often in *how, why,* and *when* questions (but see Labov & Labov, 1978).

What factors account for this invariant acquisition order? One of the primary determinants appears to be semantic or cognitive complexity. The concepts that are required for encoding *how, when,* and *why* questions, including manner, time, and causality, are more abstract and develop later than the concepts encoded in *what, where,* and *who* questions, which are already incorporated into early Stage I speech. A second important factor is linguistic complexity. Wootten and colleagues (1979) point out that children begin by asking (and answering) questions concerning objects, people, and locations that can be answered with a single word or short phrase. The later questions typically need whole sentences for an adequate response and thus require more sophisticated linguistic capacity. De Villiers (1991, 2000) has also found that comprehension of complex *wh*-questions (e.g., How did Jane think she could fix the shelf?) is also closely related to some aspects of cognitive development in the preschool years.

Just as children are sensitive to the plausible contexts in which negatives are used, research has also shown that they are sensitive to the contexts in which various questions are plausible or implausible. Winzemer (1980) showed that children who were asked, "Where is the girl eating?" when shown a picture of a girl eating an apple made many more errors than they did when asked, "What is the girl eating?" The less plausible the question was in relation to the picture, the more frequent the errors. Thus, we find that the development of questions is determined not only by linguistic complexity, but also by semantic and contextual factors that interact with the acquisition of the requisite syntactic rules.

Later Developments in Preschoolers

By the time children begin school, they have acquired most of the morphological and syntactic rules of their language. They can use language in a variety of ways, and their simple sentences, questions, negatives, and imperatives are much like those of adults.

There are more complex grammatical constructions that children begin using and understanding during the preschool years, by early Stage IV, but their acquisition is not complete until some years later. In this section we will briefly consider three such constructions: passives, coordinations, and relative clauses.

Passives

The **passive** is a construction that is used relatively rarely in English for highlighting the object of a sentence or the recipient of an action. For example, one might say, "The window was broken by a dog," if the focus is on the window. Not surprisingly, passives are extremely rare in transcripts of children's spontaneous speech—too rare to study unless the researcher specifically tries to elicit them in an experimental situation. Nevertheless, a great deal of attention has been paid to how children handle passive sentences. Because the order of the agent and the object is reversed in passives in English, this particular construction can reveal a great deal about how children acquire word order rules that play a major rule in English syntax.

One of the few studies on children's production of passive sentences was carried out by Horgan (1978). She used a set of pictures to elicit passives from a group of children who ranged in age from two to thirteen. She found that the younger children produced full passives far less frequently than *truncated* passives, in which no agent is specified, as in "The window was broken." She also found that there were topic differences between the children's full and truncated passives. Full passives almost always had animate subjects (e.g., girl, boy, cat), whereas truncated passives almost always had inanimate subjects (e.g., lamp, windows). Because of these differences, Horgan argued that full and truncated passives develop quite separately and, at least for the young child, are unrelated. This contrasts with the typical grammar of adult language that considers truncated passives to be derived from full passives by deleting the agent. The child apparently relies on different syntactic rules to form truncated passives. One interpretation of the two different forms of the passive is given by Borer and Wexler (1987), who suggest that the early appearing truncating passives are really adjectival in form; whereas the later-appearing full forms are complete verbal passives.

Most of the experimental research has focused on children's comprehension of passive sentences. One of the earliest studies on passive sentence comprehension was conducted by Bever (1970). He compared children aged two, three, and four on their understanding of active and passive sentences. Some of the sentences were semantically reversible; that is, both nouns could plausibly act as agent or object—"The boy kissed the girl" (active) or "The boy was kissed by the girl" (passive), And some of the sentences were semantically irreversible; that is, only one of the nouns could plausibly act as agent—"The girl patted the dog" or "The dog was patted by the girl."

Not surprisingly, Bever found that children could understand the irreversible passives earlier than the reversible ones. It was not until children were about four or five that they could act out correctly the reversible passive sentences, making passives quite a late development for English-speaking children. The most interesting aspect of Bever's results were the systematic mistakes that the three- and some of the four-year-olds made on the reversible passive sentences. They consistently reversed the agent and object. When they were given a sentence like "The car was pushed by the truck," they made the car push the truck, as if they had heard an active sentence.

Bever proposed that children by three or four years of age have developed a generalized abstract rule that the order of words in English signals the main sentence relations. They know that English uses predominantly noun–verb–noun sequences that, in the active voice, mean agent–action–object. Consequently, when they hear a passive sentence, they ignore the *was* and *by* and infer the meaning of the passive noun–verb–noun sequence to be active.

Many subsequent experiments have confirmed Bever's findings, and the strategy that children use at about three or four is usually called the word-order strategy. However, research conducted on children learning languages other than English has shown that this is not a universal strategy. Studies of the development of some non–Indo-European languages have also found that children learning these languages in fact acquire the passive construction very much earlier than children learning languages like English (e.g., Demuth, 1990; Pye, 1988; Suzman, 1987). Thus, children acquiring Inuktitut use passive frequently by age three (Allen & Crago, 1996), and Demuth's study of children acquiring Sesotho, a language spoken in southern Africa, found that these children began using the passive in everyday conversation by the time they were two years old, and it was quite frequent by the time they were four. Demuth (1990) suggests this is because in Sesotho, where subjects always mark the topic of a sentence, the passive is a very basic and quite frequent construction since most verbs can be passivized. She argues that the typology of a language, and the importance of the passive to a particular language, will influence the timing of its development.

Coordinations

At very young ages, as early as two-and-a-half, children begin combining sentences to express complex or compound propositions. The simplest and most frequent way children combine sentences is to conjoin two propositions with *and.* Research on young children's development of **coordination** with *and* has demonstrated that, like many of the other constructions we have considered, its development depends not only on linguistic complexity, but also on semantic and contextual factors.

There have been a number of independent studies on the development of coordination in spontaneous speech. One of the questions that has interested researchers is the order in which different coordinations enter the child's speech. There are two main forms of coordination according to linguists: *sentential coordination,* in which two (or more) complete sentences are conjoined, as in "I'm pushing the wagon and I'm pulling the train," and *phrasal coordinations,* in which phrases within the sentence are conjoined, as in "I'm pushing the wagon and the train." There does not seem to be a strict sequence of acquisition for these two forms. Bloom and her colleagues (Bloom,

Lahey, Hood, Lifter, & Fiess, 1980) reported that for three of the children they studied longitudinally both forms entered the children's speech at the same time. Their fourth subject, as well as Adam, Eve, and Sarah, who were studied by de Villiers, Tager-Flusberg, and Hakuta (1976, 1977), all used phrasal coordinations before sentential coordinations. The only constraint on acquisition order is that sententials generally do not develop before phrasals.

From the beginning, children seem to be sensitive to the different contexts in which phrasal and sentential coordinations should be used. Jeremy (1978) examined the contexts in which children used these forms to describe events enacted by an experimenter. She found that sentential forms were used when the events took place at different times or in quite separate locations. But when the events occurred simultaneously and in the same location, phrasal forms were preferred at all ages.

In their longitudinal study Bloom and her colleagues (1980) found that the course of acquisition of coordination was also influenced by semantic factors. All four of their subjects used *and* to encode a variety of meanings, and these meanings developed in a fixed order. The earliest meaning to develop was additive (no dependency relation between the conjoined clauses), as in "Maybe you can carry this and I can carry that." Several months later children began using *and* to encode temporal relations (the two clauses were related by temporal sequence or simultaneity); for example, "Jocelyn's going home and take her sweater off." Later still, *and* was used to encode causal relations—for example, "She put a bandage on her shoe and it maked it feel better." Some of the children went on to use *and* to encode other meanings—for example, object specification, "It looks like a fishing thing and you fish with it," and adversative relation (expressing opposition), "Cause I was tired and now I'm not tired"—but these were less frequent and more variable among the children. This study is important since it highlights the variety of meanings encoded by the single connective *and.* Thus, at the early stage of coordination development, children use *and* in a semantically limited way; however, as they progress, children add greater semantic flexibility as well as syntactic complexity to their language. It would be most interesting to see whether children acquiring languages other than English develop the meanings encoded by conjunctions in the same order that Bloom has found in her American subjects.

Relative Clauses

Even though children begin producing and understanding some sentences with embedded **relative clauses** when they are about three years old, in Stage IV, they do not develop the full structural knowledge of this construction until long after they reach school. In their longitudinal study, Bloom and colleagues (1980) reported that relativization developed much later than coordination, and it was used exclusively to specify information about an object or person. Limber (1973) and Menyuk (1971) also examined the emergence of relative clauses in the spontaneous speech of preschool children. They both found that initially all the relative clauses specified information about the object of the sentence; there were no subject relative clauses. Thus, children would say, "Let's eat the cake what I baked," or "Give the chair you sitting on." Often children omitted a relative pronoun (e.g., *that, who, which*), or they substituted an incorrect pronoun, usually *what.* Yet in all three studies the authors found that the actual number of sentences with relative clauses was disappointingly small. It seems to be difficult to capture a sufficiently large number of examples of relative clause sentences. Perhaps children avoid them since they are syntactically complex, or they may lack the occasion to use them in a naturalistic setting, where knowledge about the context is shared by listener and speaker and need not be made explicit.

To get around these problems, research has attempted to use elicitation techniques, providing children with the opportunity to use relative clauses for describing scenes. Both Hamburger and Crain (1982) and Tager-Flusberg (1982) asked children to describe a scene with nearly identical objects to a blindfolded listener. If children are to communicate successfully in this situation, they must use a relative clause or similar construction to clearly specify the object. Hamburger and Crain (1982) confirmed the earlier research on spontaneous speech and found that four-year-olds could perform successfully by using object relatives, such as "Pick up the walrus that is tickling the zebra." These studies of elicited production of relative clauses have also been conducted with Italian-speaking children (Crain, McKee, & Emiliani, 1990).

Tager-Flusberg (1982) provided children with the opportunity to use both subject and object relative clauses and found that once they used relative clauses (at about age four) they could produce both types equally well. However, if the main sentence was more complex and included a direct object and an indirect object phrase, such as "The boy gave the dog to the bear," the four-year-olds could add a relative clause only to the final object (the bear) and not to the subject or direct object. So they would say, "The boy gave the dog to the bear who is holding the wagon." It seems that children initially find it easiest to add a clause at the end of a sentence rather than in the middle, since this minimizes constraints on processing (see Hakuta, de Villiers, & Tager-Flusberg, 1982; Slobin, 1973).

Tager-Flusberg also gave this task to younger, three-year-old children who relied mostly on prepositional phrases to express restriction and used hardly any relative clauses. They would describe the same scene like this: "The boy gave the dog to the bear with the wagon." Children may be using their knowledge of a simpler construction to guide the acquisition of more complex constructions. In this task both forms, prepositional phrases and relative clauses, fulfill the functions adequately, but younger children used primarily simpler prepositional phrases, whereas older children used primarily more complex relative clauses. Perhaps the developmental roots of relative clauses lie in simpler constructions. This study, using production data, suggests that prepositional phrases are one such possible origin, although Tavakolian (1981), relying on comprehension data, has proposed that children initially treat relative clauses as if they were structurally equivalent to coordinations.

There have been just a few studies on the acquisition of relative clauses in other languages. Perez-Leroux (1998) found that in Spanish, some aspects of relative clause usage was related to aspects of cognitive development. Jisa and Kern (1998) confirmed that in French, acquisition of the production of relative clauses in narratives extends well into later childhood.

It is safe to conclude from all of the research conducted thus far that preschoolers are just beginning to use and understand relative clauses. Their knowledge of the syntactic structure of this construction is fairly incomplete, and their actual performance with relative clause sentences is highly constrained by processing limitations.

Beyond the Preschool Years

Before we leave the topic of syntactic and morphological development, we should note that even during the school years, children continue to develop in this domain of language. Certain constructions are not yet fully controlled by children at the time they enter school. One area that has received much attention in recent years, because of its centrality to GB theory, is the child's knowledge of **anaphora**—how different pronoun forms link up with their referents in a sentence.

Anaphora

Consider the following sentences:

> John said that Robert hurt himself.
> John said that Robert hurt him.

We know that in the first sentence Robert was hurt—the reflexive pronoun *himself* is "bound" to the referent *Robert.* In the second sentence, Robert cannot be the one to get hurt; it must be John—here we note that the pronoun *him* is bound to the referent *John.* According to GB theory, this knowledge is encompassed in the **binding principles,** which are a part of our grammar. These sentences illustrate two of the binding principles (A and B), which are loosely defined here:

> *Principle A:* A reflexive is always bound to a referent that is within the same clause.
> *Principle B:* An anaphoric pronoun cannot be bound to a referent within the same clause.

These two principles explain our intuitions about the meanings of the two sentences above. The third binding principle (C) is concerned with "backwards" sentences, in which the pronoun comes before the referent. The following two sentences illustrate this principle:

> When he came home John made dinner.
> He made dinner when John came home.

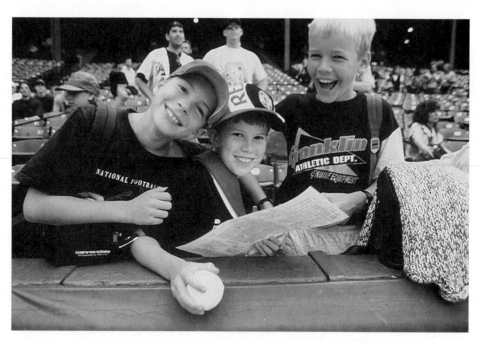

"When he's at a game, Charlie is happy." The principle that backward co-reference is possible only if the pronoun is in a subordinate clause is learned during the school years. Here "he" can refer to Charlie; but if the pronoun preceding the noun is in the main clause it refers to someone else: "He is happy when Charlie's at a game."

In the first sentence, *he* can refer to John, or we could say that the pronoun is bound to the referent in the same sentence (backward co-reference), but in the second sentence *he* cannot be John—here, backward co-reference is not allowed. These intuitions are explained by the third binding principle:

> *Principle C:* Backward co-reference is only allowed if the pronoun is in a subordinate clause to the main referent.

From a developmental perspective, we can ask the question about when children seem to know these principles. Dozens of experiments have been conducted on children's knowledge of all three principles, using a variety of tasks and paradigms. One example is a recent study by Chien and Wexler (1990), which looked at children's knowledge of Principles A and B. In one experiment, children were asked to judge the truth of sentences paired with pictures. (Some of the test pictures and sentences used are shown in Figure 5.9.) In this study, the researchers found that by age six children knew Principle A, but were still making errors on pronouns, for example saying "yes" to the sentence–picture illustrated in (46). Children's difficulties with Principle B have been confirmed in numerous other studies but they have been given different interpretations by different researchers. Some argue that the grammatical knowledge is absent until after the age of six or seven; others argue that children lack some important pragmatic knowledge (Foster-Cohen, 1994; Grodzinsky & Reinhart, 1993). Principle C also does not seem to be firmly controlled by children until the middle school years, which may be due either to grammatical limitations or to processing factors (Hsu, Cairns, Eisenberg, & Schlisselberg, 1991). Clearly, there is more research

The "Match" Cases   The "Mismatch" Cases

Name-Reflexive

(41) This is Goldilocks; this is Mama Bear. Is Mama Bear <u>touching</u> herself?

Name-Reflexive

(45) This is Goldilocks; this is Mama Bear. Is Mama Bear <u>touching</u> herself?

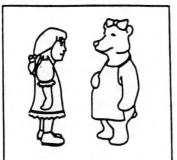
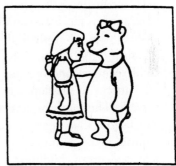

Name-Pronoun

(42) This is Mama Bear; this is Goldilocks. Is Mama Bear <u>touching</u> her?

Name-Pronoun

(46) This is Mama Bear; this is Goldilocks. Is Mama Bear <u>touching</u> her?

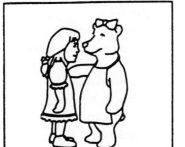
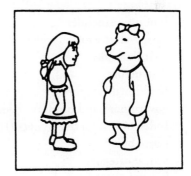

Figure 5.9

A test of anaphora—how pronouns must be used in a sentence. (From Y-C. Chien & K. Wexler, Children's knowledge of locality conditions in binding as evidence for the modularity of syntax and pragmatics. *Language Acquisition* (1990), *3*, 225–295. © Lawrence Erlbaum Associates. Reprinted with permission.)

to be done in this interesting and important area of language acquisition and linguistic theory.

Summary

We have followed the course of children's acquisition of syntax and morphology from its very beginnings in Stage I until the end of the preschool years. During these few years children develop an extremely rich and intricate linguistic system. They go from expressing just a few simple meanings in two words to expressing abstract and complex ideas in multiword sentences. Yet the journey is not quite complete—children continue in the early school years to acquire full structural knowledge of constructions such as passives, coordinations, and relative clauses. And all of this is accomplished with no formal instruction and little informal guidance or correction. Maratsos (1998) points out that grammar involves many different features, some are highly complex and opaque, others other more transparent. In order to account for the patterns of development for these different features, no single interpretation is possible. The course of development is influenced by linguistic, semantic, and contextual factors that together determine the order of grammatical development. The acquisition of grammar is, indeed, one of the most remarkable and mysterious achievements of childhood.

Key Words

anaphora
binding principles
closed-class word
coordinations
d-structure
functional category
government and binding theory (GB)
Index of Productive Syntax (IPSyn)
learnability
lexical category
limited scope formulae
logical form
mean length of utterance (MLU)
negation
null-subject parameter
open-class word
overregularization errors

parameter
passive
phonetic form
phrase structure rules
preferential looking paradigm
relative clause
semantic relations
sentence modalities
s-structure
syntax
telegraphic
thematic roles (semantic roles)
transformational rule
universal grammar
universality
wh-question
yes/no question

Suggested Projects

1. This project is highly recommended in order to appreciate fully the richness of a spontaneous speech sample and its utility as a source of data and insight into the child's linguistic system. First, you need to collect a speech sample. (Most researchers rely on tape recordings of naturalistic interactions between children and their mothers. About one hour is long enough to obtain a useful sample of child speech.) You should assemble a group of toys, such as a dollhouse with furniture and suitable occupants, a set of blocks, animals and a farmhouse, and play dough—toys that will elicit comment by both mother and child. After a few minutes warming up, during which the child can get used to your presence, turn on the tape and allow the child and mother to play naturally. Make sure that you are not intrusive. To facilitate coding later on, it is important to make detailed notes about the ongoing activity and context associated with the child's remarks.

   After the session is over, the tape should be transcribed as soon as possible, while your memories of the activities and the conversation are as fresh as possible. Divide the page down the middle into two halves. Keep the mother's speech on the right and the child's on the left. Contextual notes can be placed wherever relevant. Each new utterance should begin on a new line to make a transcript that is both easy to read and easy to code. It is not always simple to judge when a new utterance or sentence begins. Try using falling intonation and pauses to mark breaks between utterances.

   Once you have created the written transcript in this way, it is ready for analysis. First, you could compute the mean length of utterance (MLU) for the child in the sample. Just follow the rules set out in Figure 5.4. The MLU will provide some indication about the child's current stage. If the child speaks a language other than English, calculating the MLU will be much trickier. You will have to come up with a new set of rules, comparable to those for English, that will provide objective criteria for deciding what functions as a morpheme in the child's language.

   The transcript can be used to analyze any number of syntactic forms, depending on the child's stage. You could examine the child's use of different verbs, looking for example at which verbs the child uses, how verbs are combined with different nouns, to check whether their use of verbs is limited to only certain lexical combinations. You might also explore whether children are using verbs to talk about current events, past or future events, and the extent to which they mark tense on the verb.

   Any of the other forms described in this chapter can be similarly examined (i.e., grammatical morphemes, negatives, coordinations, relative clauses). If the child is a little older (four or more), other constructions not discussed here could also be analyzed—for example, pronouns, complements, past and future tenses.

2. It is becoming increasingly popular to use an elicited production technique to complement spontaneous speech samples as a source of production data. The main

advantage of this method is that the experimenter can control which forms the children should produce, so that one can test the children to their limits. One way of reliably eliciting forms is using a puppet that has to say things in a certain way. In this project it is suggested that you might introduce a puppet who is never quite sure about what has happened. This puppet, then, always needs to ask questions, which you can elicit from children aged two to five.

Select a sample of children between about two-and-a-half and five. You should see each child individually. Introduce the child to a hand puppet and explain that he is never sure about what he has heard.

Experimenter: Sally can drive.
Puppet: Can Sally drive?

Experimenter: Johnny likes spaghetti.
Puppet: What does Johnny like?

Experimenter: You may have some marbles.
Puppet: May I have some marbles?

Notice that each example is slightly different. The examples may be used to elicit yes/no or *wh*-questions; different kinds of *wh*-questions; simple or complex questions.

After the examples have been given, ask the child to take the puppet. At this point present your own test sentences, one at a time. After each test sentence, have the child produce the question in the role of the puppet. Provide the child with plenty of encouragement and praise. Present the test sentences in random order and tape-record what the child says.

You will need to transcribe your tapes before the data can be analyzed. Check which sentences the children get right and which ones have errors. Look for improvements with age. Examine the kinds of errors that children make at different age levels. Look for systematic patterns of correct and incorrect responses, both by subject and age group. What do your findings tell about the developmental course of the syntax of questions?

3. One of the most suitable ways for assessing children's understanding of language is to have them act out sentences or phrases, using toys. This project can be done with very young children (two- and early three-year-olds) who are still in the process of acquiring grammatical morphology. The purpose of this project is to find out whether children who omit inflections (such as articles, tense endings, and prepositions) understand equally well sentences that are presented with and without such inflections.

You will need to select subjects who are still in their early stages of language development and are still omitting inflections. Try taping several young two- and three-year-olds for about ten minutes and examine their speech for the presence or absence of the morphemes listed in Table 5.3. When you have your subjects picked out, you will need to demonstrate the procedure. You will need to see each child one at a time. First, give the child two toys and then tell the child that you will say something that she should show you with the toys. Then give a sample sentence: "The boy pats the dog." If the child doesn't know what to do, show her, and then have her repeat the action. Give several more examples using correct syntax.

Once the child understands the task, present your test sentences. Half of these should be presented normally, including all of the relevant morphology. Because your subjects will be very young, you will need to make the sentences simple, with only a single clause. The other half of the sentences should be presented without relevant morphology, but in other respects they should be like the normal sentences.

Normal: The boy puts the ball on the table.
No inflections: Girl put book chair.

Normal: The cow pushes the kangaroo.
No inflections: Dog hit horse.

Make up about eight sentences of each kind (complete and without inflections) and collect the toys you will need for all of them. Before giving the sentence, place the relevant toys in front of the child. Write down exactly what the child does with the toys.

Code the children's responses as correct/incorrect. Compare within and across ages the percentage correct on normal sentences and that on sentences without inflections. What do your results tell you about young children's use of morphology in comprehension before they can produce that morphology?

4. One interesting project to illustrate some of the errors that even older children still make in interpreting and judging sentences would be to test children's knowledge of the binding principles. Select children between the ages of four and eight. You can use the set of pictures in Figure 5.9 or make up some of your own. Code the children's responses as correct or incorrect and look at the percentage of children making errors at each age level.

You can also test children's knowledge of Principle C using an act-out procedure with some toy animals. Make up a set of suitable sentences (using the animals you have) of the following form:

After he touched the cow the horse ran away.
He ran away after the horse touched the cow.

Again, code children's responses as correct or incorrect and look at the percentage of errors at each age. Do children seem to control Principle B before or after Principle C? What kinds of performance factors (e.g., pragmatics, test factors, processing load) may be accounting for the younger children's errors?

Suggested Readings

Brown, R. (1973). *A first language*. Cambridge, MA: Harvard University Press. This classic in the field provides the most detailed discussions of Stages I and II.

Cook, V. J. (1988). *Chomsky's universal grammar: An introduction*. Oxford: Blackwell. An excellent introduction to Chomsky's theory (especially the GB framework), including some of the implications for first and second language acquisition.

Hirsh-Pasek, K., & Golinkoff, R. M. (1996). *The origins of grammar: Evidence from early language comprehension*. Cambridge, MA: MIT Press. Provides a summary of the authors' own research on language comprehension in infants and presents a model of the development of grammatical understanding at different stages.

Levy, Y., Schlesinger, I. M., & Braine, M. D. S. (Eds.). (1988). *Categories and processes in language acquisition*. Hillsdale, NJ: Lawrence Erlbaum Associates. Covers a range of theoretical perspectives on the central issue of the early categories in child language.

Lust, B. (Ed.). (1987). *Studies in the acquisition of anaphora* (Vol. I–II). Dordrecht: Reidel. A detailed look from several research groups on the acquisition of anaphora in different languages, including signed languages.

Maratsos, M. P. (1998). The acquisition of grammar. In W. Damon (Series Ed.), *Handbook of child psychology* (5th ed.): Vol. 2, D. Kuhn & R. Siegler (Volume Eds.), *Cognition, perception and language*. New York: Wiley. This is a thorough review of research and theories of syntactic development, with special reference to English.

McDaniel, D., McKee, C., & Cairns, H. S. (Eds.). (1996). *Methods for assessing children's syntax*. Cambridge, MA: MIT Press. An excellent detailed discussion of how to study grammatical development in young children.

Morgan, J., & Demuth, K. (1996). *Signal to syntax: Bootstrapping from speech to grammar in early acquisition*. Mahwah, NJ: Lawrence Erlbaum Associates. Extensive discussion of how infants can use information in the speech signal (e.g., acoustic factors, timing, etc.) to uncover basic grammatical categories and distributional rules.

Radford, A. (1990). *Syntactic theory and the acquisition of English syntax*. Oxford: Blackwell. A theoretical linguistics approach to the earliest stages of grammatical development.

Slobin, D. I. (Ed.). (1985–97). *A cross-linguistic study of language acquisition*. Hillsdale, NJ: Lawrence Erlbaum Associates. This five-volume work presents an excellent survey of morphological and syntactic development covering a broad range of languages.

References

Aksu-Koc, A. A. (1988). *The acquisition of aspect and modality*. Cambridge, UK: Cambridge University Press.

Allen, S. E. M. (1996). *Aspects of argument structure in Inuktitut*. Philadelphia: Benjamins.

Allen, S. E. M., & Crago, M. (1996). Early passive acquisition in Inuktitut. *Journal of Child Language, 23,* 129–156.

Bassano, D., & Mendes-Maillochon, I. (1994). Early grammatical and prosodic marking of utterance modality in French: A longitudinal case study. *Journal of Child Language, 21,* 649–675.

Bates, E., Dale, P., & Thal, D. (1995). Individual differences and their implications for theories of language development. In P. Fletcher & B. MacWhinney (Eds.), *The handbook of child language* (pp. 96–151). Oxford: Blackwell.

Bates, E., & MacWhinney, B. (1982). Functionalist approaches to grammar. In E. Wanner & L. Gleitman (Eds.), *Language acquisition: The state of the art*. New York: Cambridge University Press.

Bellugi, U. (1967). *The acquisition of negation*. Unpublished doctoral dissertation. Cambridge, MA: Harvard University.

Berko, J. (1958). The child's learning of English morphology. *Word, 14,* 150–177.

Berman, R. A. (1981). Regularity vs. anomaly: The acquisition of Hebrew inflectional morphology. *Journal of Child Language, 8,* 265–282.

Bever, T. G. (1970). The cognitive basis for linguistic structure. In J. R. Hayes (Ed.), *Cognition and the development of language*. New York: Wiley.

Bloom, L. (1970). *Language development: Form and function in emerging grammars*. Cambridge, MA: MIT Press.

Bloom, L., Lahey, J., Hood, L., Lifter, K., & Fiess, K. (1980). Complex sentences: Acquisition of syntactic connectives and the semantic relations they encode. *Journal of Child Language, 7,* 235–261.

Bloom, P. (1990a). Syntactic distinctions in child language. *Journal of Child Language, 17,* 343–355.

Bloom, P. (1990b). Subjectless sentences in child language. *Linguistic Inquiry, 21,* 491–504.

Borer, H., & Wexler, K. (1987). The maturation of syntax. In T. Roeper & E. Williams (Eds.), *Parameter setting*. Dordrecht, Holland: Reidel.

Bowerman, M. (1973). *Early syntactic development. A cross-linguistic study with special reference to Finnish*. Cambridge, UK: Cambridge University Press.

Braine, M. D. S. (1963). The ontogeny of English phrase structure: The first phase. *Language, 39,* 1–13.

Braine, M. D. S. (1976). Children's first word combinations. *Monographs of the Society for Research in Child Development, 41* (Serial No. 164).

Brown, R. (1973). *A first language*. Cambridge, MA: Harvard University Press.

Brown, R., & Fraser, C. (1963). The acquisition of syntax. In C. N. Cofer & B. Musgrave (Eds.), *Verbal behavior and learning: Problems and processes*. New York: McGraw-Hill.

Brown, R., & Hanlon, C. (1970). Derivational complexity and the order of acquisition in child speech. In J. R. Hayes (Ed.), *Cognition and the development of language*. New York: Wiley.

Caselli, M. C., Casadio, P., & Bates, E. (1999). A comparison of the transition from first words to grammar in English and Italian. *Journal of Child Language, 26,* 69–111.

Caselli, M. C., Leonard, L. B., Volterra, V., & Campagnoli, M. G. (1993). Toward mastery of Italian morphology: A cross-sectional study. *Journal of Child Language, 20,* 377–393.

Cazden, C. (1968). The acquisition of noun and verb inflections. *Child Development, 39,* 433–448.

Chapman, R. S. (1977). Comprehension strategies in children. In J. F. Kavanaugh & W. Strage (Eds.), *Speech and language in the lab, school, and clinic*. Cambridge, MA: MIT Press.

Chien, Y. -C., & Wexler, K. (1990) Children's knowledge of locality conditions in binding as evidence for the modularity of syntax and pragmatics. *Language Acquisition, 3,* 225–295.

Chomsky, N. (1981). *Lectures on government and binding.* Dordrecht: Foris.

Chomsky, N. (1982). *Some concepts and consequences of the theory of government and binding.* Cambridge, MA: MIT Press.

Chomsky, N. (1995). *The minimalist program.* Cambridge, MA: MIT Press.

Clancy, P. (1985). Acquisition of Japanese. In D. I. Slobin (Ed.), *The cross-linguistic study of language acquisition.* Hillsdale, NJ: Lawrence Erlbaum Associates.

Crain, S., McKee, C., & Emiliani, M. (1990). Visiting relatives in Italy. In L. Frazier & J. de Villiers (Eds.), *Language processing and language acquisition.* Dordrecht: Kluwer.

Demuth, K. (1990). Subject, topic and Sesotho passive. *Journal of Child Language, 17,* 67–84.

Demuth, K. (1996). Collecting spontaneous production data. In D. McDaniel, C. McKee, & H. S. Cairns (Eds.), *Methods for assessing children's syntax* (pp. 3–22). Cambridge, MA: MIT Press.

de Villiers, J. G. (1991). Why questions? In T. Maxfield & B. Plunkett (Eds.), *The acquisition of wh.* University of Massachusetts Occasional Papers in Linguistics. Amherst, MA: University of Massachusetts.

de Villiers, J. G. (1995). Empty categories and complex sentences: The case of *wh*-questions. In P. Fletcher & B. MacWhinney (Eds.), *The handbook of child language* (pp. 508–540). Oxford: Blackwell.

de Villiers, J. G. (2000). Language and theory of mind: What are the developmental relationships? In S. Baron-Cohen, H. Tager-Flusberg, & D. J. Cohen (Eds.), *Understanding other minds: Perspectives on developmental cognitive neuroscience* (2nd ed.). Oxford: Oxford University Press.

de Villiers, J. G., & de Villiers, P. A. (1973). A cross-sectional study of the acquisition of grammatical morphemes in child speech. *Journal of Psycholinguistic Research, 2,* 267–278.

de Villiers, J. G., & Roeper, T. (1996). Questions after stories: On supplying context and eliminating it as a variable. In D. McDaniel, C. McKee, & H. S. Cairns (Eds.), *Methods for assessing children's syntax* (pp. 163–187). Cambridge, MA: MIT Press.

de Villiers, J. G., Roeper, T., & Vainikka, A. (1990). The acquisition of long distance rules. In L. Frazier & J. G. de Villiers (Eds.), *Language processing and acquisition.* Dordrecht: Kluwer.

de Villiers, J. G., & Tager-Flusberg, H. (1975). Some facts one simply cannot deny. *Journal of Child Language, 2,* 279–286.

de Villiers, J. G., Tager-Flusberg, H., & Hakuta, K. (1976). *The roots of coordination in child speech.* Paper presented at the First Annual Boston University Conference on Language Development, Boston, MA.

de Villiers, J. G., Tager-Flusberg, H., & Hakuta, K. (1977). Deciding among theories of the development of coordination in child speech. *Papers and Reports on Child Language Development, 13,* 118–125.

de Villiers, P. A., & de Villiers, J. G. (1979). Form and function in the development of sentence negation. *Papers and Reports on Child Language Development, 17,* 56–64.

Dodson, K., & Tomasello, M. (1998). Acquiring the transitive construction in English: The role of animacy and pronouns. *Journal of Child Language, 25,* 605–622.

Dromi, E., & Berman, R. A. (1982). A morphemic measure of early language development: Data from modern Hebrew. *Journal of Child Language, 9,* 403–424.

Erreich, A. (1980) *The acquisition of inversion in wh-questions: What evidence the child uses?* Unpublished doctoral dissertation, City University of New York.

Ervin-Tripp, S. (1970). Discourse agreement: How children answer questions. In J. R. Hayes (Ed.), *Cognition and the development of language.* New York: Wiley.

Fenson, L., Dale, P., Reznick, S., Thal, D., Bates, E., Hartung, J. P., Pethick, S., & Reilly, J. S. (1993). *The MacArthur Communicative Development Inventories: User's guide and technical manual.* San Diego: Singular Publishing Group.

Fenson, L., Dale, P., Reznick, S., Bates, E., Thal, D., & Pethick, S. (1994). Variability in early communicative development. *Monographs of the Society for Research in Child Development, 59,* Serial No. 242.

Fernald, A., Taeschner, T., Dunn, J., Papousek, M., de Boysson-Bardies, B., & Fukui, I. (1989). A cross-language study of prosodic modifications in mothers' and fathers' speech to preverbal infants. *Journal of Child Language, 16,* 477–501.

Foster-Cohen, S. (1994). Exploring the boundary between syntax and pragmatics: Relevance and the binding of pronouns. *Journal of Child Language, 21,* 237–255.

Fraser, C., Bellugi, U., & Brown, R. (1963). Control of grammar in imitation, comprehension and production. *Journal of Verbal Learning and Verbal Behavior, 2,* 121–135.

Gerken, L., & Shady, M. E. (1996). The picture selection task. In D. McDaniel, C. McKee, & H. S. Cairns (Eds.), *Methods for assessing children's syntax* (pp. 125–145). Cambridge, MA: MIT Press.

Gleitman, L. (1990). The structural sources of verb meanings. *Language Acquisition, 1,* 3–55.

Gleitman, L. R., & Wanner, E. (1982). Language acquisition: The state of the art. In E. Wanner & L. R. Gleitman (Eds.), *Language acquisition: The state of the art.* Cambridge, MA: Harvard University Press.

Golinkoff, R. M., & Hirsh-Pasek, K. (1995). Reinterpreting children's sentence comprehension: Toward a new framework. In P. Fletcher & B. MacWhinney (Eds.), *The handbook of child language* (pp. 430–461). Oxford: Blackwell.

Goodluck, H. (1996). The act-out task. In D. McDaniel, C. McKee, & H. S. Cairns (Eds.), *Methods for assessing children's syntax* (pp. 147–162). Cambridge, MA: MIT Press.

Gopnik, A., & Choi, S. (1995). Names, relational words, and cognitive development in English and Korean speakers: Nouns are not always learned before words. In M. Tomasello & W. Merriman (Eds.), *Beyond names for things: Young children's acquisition of verbs.* Hillsdale, NJ: Erlbaum.

Grodzinsky, Y., & Reinhart, T. (1993). The innateness of binding and coreference: A reply to Grimshaw and Rosen. *Linguistic Inquiry, 24,* 69–101.

Hakuta, K., de Villiers, J. G., & Tager-Flusberg, H. (1982). Sentence coordination in Japanese and English. *Journal of Child Language, 9,* 193–207.

Hamburger, H., & Crain, S. (1982). Relative acquisition. In S. A. Kuczaj (Ed.), *Language development. Vol. 1. Syntax and semantics.* Hillsdale, NJ: Erlbaum.

Hickey, T. (1991). Mean length of utterance and the acquisition of Irish. *Journal of Child Language, 18,* 553–569.

Hirsh-Pasek, K., & Golinkoff, R. M. (1993). Skeletal supports for grammatical learning: What the infant brings to the language learning task. In C. K. Rovee-Collier (Ed.), *Advances in Infancy Research,* Vol. 10. Norwood, NJ: Ablex.

Hirsh-Pasek, K., & Golinkoff, R. M. (1996). *The origins of grammar: Evidence from early language comprehension.* Cambridge, MA: MIT Press.

Horgan, D. (1978). The development of the full passive. *Journal of Child Language, 5,* 65–80.

Hsu, J. R., Cairns, H. S., Eisenberg, S., & Schlisselberg, G. (1991). When do children avoid backwards coreference? *Journal of Child Language, 18,* 339–353.

Hung, F-S., & Peters, A. M. (1997). The role of prosody in the acquisition of grammatical morphemes: Evidence from two Chinese languages. *Journal of Child Language, 24,* 627–650.

Huttenlocher, J. (1974). The origins of language comprehension. In R. L. Solso (Ed.), *Theories of cognitive psychology: The Loyola symposium.* Potomac, MD: Lawrence Erlbaum Associates.

Hyams, N. M. (1986a). *Language acquisition and the theory of paramters.* Dordrecht: D. Reidel.

Hyams, N. M. (1986b). *Core and peripheral grammar and the acquisition of inflections.* Paper presented at the Eleventh Annual Boston University Conference on Language Development, Boston, NM.

Hyams, N. M. (1989). The null-subject parameter in language acquisition. In O. Jaeggli & K. Safir (Eds.), *The null-subject parameter.* Dordrecht: Kluwer.

Imai, M., & Gentner, D. (1997). A cross-linguistic study of early word meaning: Universal ontology and linguistic influence. *Cognition, 62,* 169–200.

Ingham, R. (1992). The optional subject phenomenon in young children's English: A case study. *Journal of Child Language, 19,* 133–151.

Ingram, D., & Tyack, D. (1979). Inversion of subject NP and auxiliary in children's questions. *Journal of Psycholinguistic Research, 8,* 333–341.

Jackendoff, R. S. (1972). *Semantic interpretation in generative grammar.* Cambridge, MA: MIT Press.

Jeremy, R. J. (1978). Use of coordinate sentences with the conjunction "and" for describing temporal and locative relations between events. *Journal of Psycholinguistic Research, 7,* 135–150.

Jisa, H., & Kern, S. (1998). Relative clauses in French children's narrative texts. *Journal of Child Language, 25,* 623–652.

Johnston, J., & Slobin, D. (1979). The development of locative expressions in English, Italian, Serbo-Croatian, and Turkish. *Journal of Child Language, 6,* 531–547.

Jusczyk, P. W. (1997). *The discovery of spoken language.* Cambridge, MA: MIT Press.

Klima, E., & Bellugi, U. (1966). Syntactic regularities in the speech of children. In J. Lyons & R. Wales (Eds.), *Psycholinguistic papers.* Edinburgh: Edinburgh University Press.

Labov, W., & Labov, T. (1978). Learning the syntax of questions. In R. N. Campbell & P. T. Smith (Eds.), *Recent advances in the psychology of language: Language development and mother-child interaction.* London: Plenum Press.

Leonard, L. (1983, April). *Production before comprehension: Some methodological issues.* Paper presented at the Biennial Meeting of the Society for Research in Child Development, Toronto.

Levy, Y. (1983, October). *Berko's wug technique revisited.* Paper presented at the Eighth Annual Boston University Conference on Language Development, Boston, MA.

Levy, Y (1988). On the early learning of formal grammatical systems: Evidence from studies of the acquisition of gender and countability. *Journal of Child Language, 15,* 179–187.

Levy, Y. (1997). Autonomous linguistic systems in the language of young children. *Journal of Child Language, 24,* 651–671.

Limber, J. (1973). The genesis of complex sentences. In T. E. Moore (Ed.), *Cognitive development and the acquisition of language.* New York: Academic Press.

Maratsos, M. P. (1998). The acquisition of grammar. In W. Damon. (Series Ed.), *Handbook of child psychology* (5th ed.): Vol. 2, D. Kuhn & R. Siegler (Volume Eds.), *Cognition, perception and language.* New York: Wiley.

Marcus, G., Pinker, S., Ullman, M., Hollander, M., Rosen, J., & Xu, F. (1992). Overregularization in language acquisition. *Monographs of the Society for Research in Child Development, 57,* Serial No. 228.

McNeill, D. (1970). *The acquisition of language: The study of developmental psycholinguistics.* New York: Harper & Row.

McNeill, D., & McNeill, N. B. (1968). What does a child mean when he says "no"? In E. M. Zales (Ed.), *Language and language behavior.* New York: Appleton-Century-Crofts.

Meisel, J. (1995). Parameters in acquisition. In P. Fletcher & B. MacWhinney (Eds.), *The handbook of child language* (pp. 10–35). Oxford: Blackwell.

Menyuk, P. (1971). *The acquisition and development of language.* Englewood Cliffs, NJ: Prentice-Hall.

Mervis, C., & Johnson, K. (1987, October). *Acquisition of the plural morpheme: A case study.* Paper presented at the Twelfth Annual Boston University Conference on Language Development, Boston, MA.

Miller, J. F., & Chapman, R. S. (1981). The relations between age and mean length of utterance. *Journal of Speech and Hearing Research, 24,* 154–161.

Miller, W. R., & Ervin, S. (1964). The development of grammar in child language. In U. Bellugi & R. Brown (Eds.), *The acquisition of language. Monographs of the Society for Research in Child Development, 29* (Serial No. 92), 9–34.

Moerk, E. (1980). Relationships between parental input frequencies and children's language acquisition: A reanalysis of Brown's data. *Journal of Child Language, 7,* 105–118.

Morgan, J. L. (1986). *From simple input to complex grammar.* Cambridge, MA: MIT Press.

Naigles, L. (1990). Children use syntax to learn verb meanings. *Journal of Child Language, 17,* 357–374.

O'Grady, W., Peters, A. M., & Masterson, D. (1989). The transition from optional to required subjects. *Journal of Child Language, 16,* 513–529.

Perez-Leroux, A. T. (1998). The acquisition of mood selection in Spanish relative clauses. *Journal of Child Language, 25,* 585–604.

Pine, J. (1999, July). *Tense optionality and children's use of verb morphology: Testing the optional infinitive hypothesis.* Paper presented at the International Association for the Study of Child Language, San Sebastien, Spain.

Pine, J., & Lieven, E. (1997). Slot-frame patterns and the development of the determiner category. *Applied Psycholinguistics, 18,* 123–138.

Pine, J. M., Lieven, E. V. M., & Rowland, C. F. (1998). Comparing different models of the development of the English verb category. *Linguistics, 36(4), 807–830.*

Pinker, S. (1981). On the acquisition of grammatical morphemes. *Journal of Child Language, 8,* 477–484.

Pinker, S. (1984). *Language learnability and language development.* Cambridge, MA: Harvard University Press.

Pinker S. (1987). Constraint satisfaction networks as implementations of nativist theories of language acquisition. In B. MacWhinney (Ed.), *Mechanisms of language learning.* Hillsdale, NJ: Erlbaum.

Pinker, S. (1991). Rules of language. *Science, 253,* 530–535.

Pinker, S., & Prince, A. (1992). Regular and irregular morphology and the psychological status of rules of grammar. In *Proceedings of the 17th Annual Meeting of the Berkeley Linguistics Society.* Berkeley, CA: Berkeley Linguistics Society.

Pizzuto, E., & Caselli, M. C. (1992). The acquisition of Italian morphology: Implications for models of language development. *Journal of Child Language, 19,* 491–557.

Plunkett, K. (1995). Connectionist approaches to language acquisition. In P. Fletcher & B. MacWhinney (Eds.), *The handbook of child language* (pp. 36–72). Oxford: Blackwell.

Plunkett, K., & Marchman, V. (1991). U-shaped learning and frequency effects in a multi-layered perception: Implications for child language acquisition. *Cognition, 38,* 43–102.

Plunkett, K., & Marchman, V. (1993). From rote learning to system building: Acquiring verb morphology in children and connectionist nets. *Cognition, 48,* 21–69.

Pye, C. (1988). *Precocious passives (and antipassives) in Quiche Mayan.* Paper presented at the Child Language Research Forum, Stanford, CA.

Radford, A. (1990). *Syntactic theory and the acquisition of English syntax.* Oxford: Blackwell.

Radford, A. (1994). The syntax of questions in child English. *Journal of Child Language, 21,* 211–236.

Roberts, K. (1983). Comprehension and production of word order in stage I. *Child Development, 54,* 443–449.

Rowland, C. F., & Pine, J. (2000). Subject-auxiliary inversion errors and *wh*-question acquisition: 'What children do know?' *Journal of Child Language,* in press.

Rumelhart, D., & McClelland, J. (1986). On learning the past tense of English verbs. In J. McClelland, D. Rumelhart, and the PDP Research Group (Eds.), *Parallel distributed processing: Explorations in the microstructure of cognition,* Vol. 2, *Psychological and biological models* (pp. 216–271). Cambridge, MA: Bradford Books/MIT Press.

Sachs, J., & Truswell, L. (1978). Comprehension of two-word instructions by children in the one-word stage. *Journal of Child Language, 5,* 17–24.

Scarborough, H. (1985, April). *Measuring syntactic development. The index of production syntax.* Paper presented at the Biennial Meeting of the Society for Research in Child Development, Detroit, MI.

Scarborough, H. (1989). Index of productive syntax. *Applied Psycholinguistics, 11,* 1–22.

Shady, M., & Gerken, L. (1999). Grammatical and caregiver cues in early sentence comprehension. Journal of Child Language, 26, 163–175.

Shi, R., Morgan, J., & Allopena, P. (1998). Phonological and acoustic bases for earliest grammatical category assignment: A cross-linguistic perspective. *Journal of Child Language, 25,* 169–201.

Slobin, D. I. (1966). The acquisition of Russian as a native language. In F. Smith & G. A. Miller (Eds.), *The genesis of language.* Cambridge, MA: MIT Press.

Slobin, D. I. (1973). Cognitive prerequisites for the development of grammar. In C. A. Ferguson & D. I. Slobin (Eds.), *Studies of child language development.* New York: Holt, Rinehart & Winston.

Slobin, D. I. (Ed.). (1985). *The cross-linguistic study of language acquisition: Vol. 1. The data.* Hillsdale, NJ: Erlbaum.

Stromswold, K. (1995). The acquisition of subject and object *wh*-questions. *Language Acquisition, 4,* 5–48.

Stromswold, K. (1996). Analyzing children's spontaneous speech. In D. McDaniel, C. McKee, & H. S. Cairns (Eds.), *Methods for assessing children's syntax* (pp. 23–53). Cambridge, MA: MIT Press.

Suzman, S. (1987). Passives and prototypes in Zulu children's speech. *African Studies, 46,* 241–254.

Tager-Flusberg, H. (1982). The development of relative clauses in child speech. *Papers and Reports on Child Language Development, 21,* 104–111.

Tamis-Lemonda, C. S., Bornstein, M. H., Kahana-Kalman, R., Baumwell, L., & Cyphers, L. (1998). Predicting variation in the timing of language milestones in the second year: An events history approach. *Journal of Child Language, 25,* 675–700.

Tardiff, T. (1996). Nouns are not always learned before verbs: Evidence from Mandarin speakers' early vocabularies. *Developmental Psychology, 32,* 492–504.

Tavakolian, S. L. (1981). The conjoined-clause analysis of relative clauses. In S. L. Tavakolian (Ed.), *Language acquisition and linguistic theory.* Cambridge, MA: MIT Press.

Thornton, R. (1996). Elicited production. In D. McDaniel, C. McKee, & H. S. Cairns, (Eds.), *Methods for assessing children's syntax* (pp. 77–102). Cambridge, MA: MIT Press.

Tomasello, M., & Brooks, P. J. (1999). Early syntactic development: A construction grammar approach. In M. Barrett (Ed.), *The development of language* (pp. 161–190). Hove, Sussex: Psychology Press.

Tomasello, M., Akhtar, N., Dodson, K., & Rekau, L. (1997). Differential productivity in young children's use of nouns and verbs. *Journal of Child Language, 24,* 373–387.

Tyack, D., & Ingram, D. (1977). Children's production and comprehension of questions. *Journal of Child Language, 4,* 211–224.

Vaidyanathan, R. (1991). Development of forms and functions of negation in the early stages of language acquisition: A study of Tamil. *Journal of Child Language, 18,* 51–66.

Valian, V. (1990). Null subjects: A problem for parameter-setting models of language acquisition. *Cognition, 35,* 105–122.

Valian, V. V. (1992). Categories of first syntax: Be, being, and nothingness. In J. Meisel (Ed)., *The acquisition of verb placement: Functional categories and V-2 phenomena.* Dordrecht: Kluwer.

Wason, P. C. (1965). The contexts of plausible denial. *Journal of Verbal Learning and Verbal Behavior, 4,* 7–11.

Weissenborn, J., Roeper, T., & de Villiers, J. G. (1991). The acquisition of *wh*-movement in French and German. In T. Maxfield & B. Plunkett (Eds.), *The acquisition of wh.* University of Massachusetts Occasional Papers in Linguistics. Amherst, MA: University of Massachusetts.

Winzemer, J. A. (1980, October). *A lexical expectation model for children's comprehension of wh-questions.* Paper presented at the Fifth Annual Boston University Conference on Language Development.

Wootten, J., Merkin, S., Hood, L., & Bloom, L. (1979, March). *Wh-questions: Linguistic evidence to explain the sequence of acquisition.* Paper presented at the biennial meeting of the Society for Research in Child Development, San Francisco.

Chapter 6

Language in Social Contexts: Communicative Competence in the Preschool Years

Judith Becker Bryant
University of South Florida

This chapter explores the concept of communicative competence. Consider the following interaction between two four-year-olds. Child A is approaching a large toy car on which Child B has been sitting.

Child A: "Pretend this was my car."
Child B: "No!"
Child A: "Pretend this was our car."
Child B: (reluctantly) "All right."
Child A: "Can I drive your car?"
Child B: "Yes, okay." (smiles and moves away from the car)
Child A: (turns wheel and makes driving noises) (Garvey, 1975, p. 42)

This example illustrates the fact that, when children are learning language, it is important for them to learn more than just phonology, semantics, and syntax. As is probably apparent, being a skilled language user means knowing how to use one's language appropriately and strategically in social situations. Children need to learn **communicative competence** (Hymes, 1967). They must learn how to make language work in interactions with their families, peers, teachers, and others.

Now imagine a three-year-old boy saying "You're a real turkey" to someone. This boy could pronounce the words in this good sentence perfectly, but the sentence certainly would not be appropriate if he said it to his elderly Aunt Gertrude. Whether language is appropriate depends on how it is used in particular contexts. As Hymes

213

put it, appropriateness is a function of the interaction of language and social setting. This is one of the main themes explored in this chapter.

Many skills are involved in communicative competence because we use language for so many purposes. Children need to learn to ask questions, make requests, give orders, express agreement or disagreement, apologize, refuse, joke, praise, and tell stories. They must learn **routines** and polite terms such as "trick or treat," "please" and

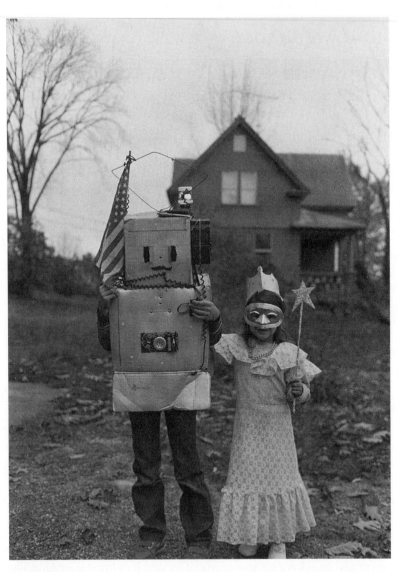

Routines such as "trick or treat" are essential aspects of children's growing communicative competence.

"thank you," "hello" and "goodbye," "excuse me," and ways to address others. They must learn to initiate, maintain, and conclude conversations; know when to speak or be quiet and how to take turns; to provide and respond effectively to feedback; and to stay on topic. They must know and use the appropriate volume and tone of voice. They must learn what styles of speech to use; when to use jargon or particular dialects and languages; and when and whether to talk about certain subjects. With all of these skills, children must learn to be sensitive to their audience and to the situations in which they are communicating.

We can think about audience and situation (i.e., communicative context) as involving many levels (Erickson & Shultz, 1981). There is the immediate context that includes prior conversation, task and setting, relationship between speaker and listener, and listener characteristics. There are also broader contexts such as the culture(s) in which children develop and communicate. To be competent and effective, speakers must learn to take all of these contexts into account.

In this chapter, we refer to the appropriate use of language in social situations using the broad term "communicative competence." Others refer to the same and similar behaviors with other terms such as "pragmatics," "discourse," and "sociolinguistics."

Clearly, the acquisition of communicative competence is complex because it involves so many different skills and requires children to take into account so many contexts. Yet, remarkably, even preschoolers demonstrate some degree of competence, as you will see.

This chapter begins with a section on theories and a section on the development of language in social contexts. Then there is a discussion of why acquisition is difficult for young children. Following this is evidence concerning how children acquire communicative competence. The chapter concludes with a section on why it is important for children to acquire communicative competence.

Theoretical Approaches to the Study of Communicative Competence

Broad theories about language acquisition in all of its aspects will be presented in Chapter 7. Many current theoretical insights specifically related to communicative competence arose from philosophers' ideas about language and from scientists' claims about the nature of children's minds. Two major theories that underlie work in communicative competence are speech act theory and cognitive developmental theory.

Speech Act Theory

Philosopher John Austin (1975) argued that some sentences do not just describe or report information. Rather, when uttered in the appropriate circumstances by the appropriate individuals, they help speakers accomplish things in the world. For example, when the designated person says, "I name this ship 'The Titanic'" while smashing a bottle against the ship's prow, that person is actually naming the ship. Not surprisingly, Austin called such sentences "performatives" or **speech acts.** Speech acts include, for example, orders, requests, warnings, verdicts, promises, and apologies. They are the linguistic realizations of infants' communicative functions that are described in Chapter 2.

Austin also suggested that speech acts have three components:

- the **locutionary act** or the act of saying a sentence that makes sense and refers to something
- the **illocutionary act** or the speaker's purpose in saying that sentence
- the **perlocutionary act** or the effect of that sentence on a listener

For example, someone in a stuffy room might say "It's hot in here" (a locutionary act). By this, the speaker might intend to make a request for a listener to open a window (an illocutionary act). Listeners need to attend to all aspects of the utterance and context or they may misunderstand. For instance, a listener might understand the speaker to be making a simple statement of fact (the perlocutionary act) and agree. Alternatively, someone in a cold room might say "It's hot in here," intending to be ironic, and the listener might open a window, concluding that the speaker is feverish and is making an assertion. An even more obvious example is the use of sarcasm, as when someone says "good move" (a locutionary act) in response to another person's clumsiness. In this example, the speaker intends to be critical (the illocutionary act) and the listener might hear this phrase as praise and feel good (the perlocutionary act). In other words, Austin was arguing that the form of the sentence itself might be different from the function (the intent or effect) of that sentence in specific situations. One needs context in order to determine what the function of a given sentence form might be.

Note that speech act theory does not deal specifically with children or with language acquisition. Nonetheless, it has provided researchers with ideas about which aspects of children's communication to study (i.e., which specific speech acts), the types of at least implicit knowledge children should acquire about communication, and the other competencies (e.g., the ability to draw inferences) that may underlie communicative competence.

Cognitive Developmental Theory

Also influential in the study of the development of communicative competence is Jean Piaget's cognitive developmental theory, which is also discussed in Chapter 7. Piaget, a Swiss biologist who became interested in psychology, described the notion of **egocentrism.** Examples of egocentric behavior are when a child waves at the telephone rather than saying "hello" to Grandma at the other end of the line, or talks to his parents at home about "the book" his teacher read at school without explaining which book it was. In Piaget's view, egocentrism is the inability to take another person's point of view, the inability to recognize that others have different knowledge, feelings, thoughts, and perceptions or to know what the different knowledge, feelings, thoughts, and perceptions might be.

In his 1926 book *The Language and Thought of the Child* (1926/1974; Ginsburg & Opper, 1988), Piaget argued that young children think and act more egocentrically than adults. Piaget came to this conclusion after observing the language of two six-year-old boys in everyday activities in their schools. He and his colleagues sorted the boys' sentences into three categories of egocentric speech (Piaget, 1926/1974):

1. **Echolalia:** When a child repeats words and syllables "for the pleasure of talking, with no thought of talking to anyone, nor even at times of saying words that will make sense" (p. 32). For example, one boy says to another, "Look, Ez, your pants are showing." From another part of the classroom, a different boy echoes, "Look, my pants are showing, and my shirt, too" (p. 35).

2. **Simple Monologue:** When a child "talks to himself as though he were thinking aloud" and without addressing someone else (p. 32). For example, a child may draw alone at a table and say, "I want to do that drawing, there.... I want to draw something, I do. I shall need a big piece of paper to do that" (p. 37).

3. **Collective Monologue:** When a child "talks aloud to himself in front of" someone else (p. 40), but "the point of view of the other person is never taken into account; his presence serves only as a stimulus" (p. 33). For example, a child twice asks someone "What did you say?" but never listens for an answer (p. 41).

Piaget also counted a group of sentences that involved more socialized, nonegocentric speech. These sentences included information adapted to the listener's point of view as well as requests and threats. Egocentric speech comprised nearly half of the spontaneous language of the two boys.

Piaget attempted to replicate his findings by observing in their schools twenty other boys and girls between the ages of four and seven years. The average amount of egocentric speech across these children was, again, just less than half. There also appeared to be stages in the development of socialized speech, with the amount of egocentric speech decreasing with age. From these findings, Piaget placed "the beginnings of socialization of thought somewhere between seven and eight" (p. 81).

To test his ideas further, Piaget also conducted more formal experiments in which he asked children between the ages of six and eight years to retell stories, relay messages, and explain to a same-aged peer how a faucet or syringe works. Once again, children's language was relatively egocentric. For example, children called story characters "she" or "it" without explaining to whom they were referring, left out important information, and did not present events in the correct order, as if they assumed that their listeners already understood what they were talking about. From these data, Piaget concluded that preschoolers are egocentric and unable to take their listeners' perspectives, that "the effort to understand other people and to communicate one's thought objectively does not appear in children before the age of about seven or seven and one-half" (p. 139).

It should be clear that both speech act theory and Piaget's cognitive developmental theory stress the relevance of context for using and understanding language. For the speech act theorists, context meant the participants as well as the task or setting and prior conversation. For Piaget, context meant the immediate physical context as well as characteristics of the listener (what the listener knows, etc.). As we will see, subsequent researchers have investigated preschoolers in many contexts to see which contextual factors affect the children's language. That is, they assessed specific claims and aspects of these theories.

Language in Social Contexts

Communicative competence entails the appropriate use of language in social contexts. It is precisely because communicative behaviors are so contextually sensitive that it is difficult to describe clear developmental progressions for each of them. Preschoolers usually perform differently in laboratory experiments than in everyday interaction and converse differently with strangers than with those who are more familiar, making it hard to define and identify level of competence. This section therefore focuses on several domains that provide relatively clear information about development in the preschool years: egocentric language, requests, and language varieties.

Early Work on Egocentric Language

In some of the earliest efforts to assess young children's communicative competence, researchers asked whether preschoolers communicate egocentrically. Using research procedures modeled after Piaget's, these researchers demonstrated that young children have the capacity to take the perspective of the listener in certain circumstances. For example, Michael Maratsos (1973) asked three- to five-year-olds to tell an experimenter which of several toy animals to put in a toy car before it rolled down a hill. The experimenter either had her eyes open or closed. Children were significantly more explicit verbally and pointed less for the experimenter when her eyes were closed than when her eyes were open. In other words, the children took the experimenter's sightedness into account when communicating.

In a similar study of **referential communication,** Sam Glucksberg and Robert Krauss (1967; Glucksberg, Krauss, & Weisberg, 1966) had young children describe a set of blocks so that another child on the opposite side of a screen could stack them in the same order. When the blocks had pictures of familiar animals on them, preschoolers could play the game perfectly. By contrast, when the blocks had unusual, abstract designs on them, Kindergartners produced ineffective messages such as "It's like a hat" and "Daddy's shirt" and sometimes simply traced the design with their fingers.

Carole Menig-Peterson (1975) had three- and four-year-olds participate in eight different tasks (e.g., helping to clean up a spilled drink) during two play sessions. One week after each session, they talked about their experiences with someone who had been present and someone who had not. The children were able to provide more information for the listener unfamiliar with the tasks than they did for the familiar listener.

Taking a different approach to the question of egocentrism, Marilyn Shatz and Rochel Gelman (1973) investigated whether four-year-olds would speak differently depending on who their listeners were. The preschoolers were asked to tell both an adult and a two-year-old about a toy. Speech to the two-year-olds tended to be shorter and simpler than that to adults, and it contained more phrases to get and hold attention (e.g., *hey, look*). Interestingly, these same four-year-olds tended to perform poorly on a referential communication task and a physical perspective-taking task.

So *are* preschoolers egocentric in their attempts to communicate? The answer depends on context, in these cases the type of task. When preschoolers are familiar with a fairly simple task and are motivated to do it, their language does not appear to be completely egocentric. Although it may seem that this conclusion is inconsistent with Piaget's theory, it really is not. Piaget observed that preschoolers sometimes use egocentric language and sometimes use more social language. They are not inherently egocentric. Rather, they may *behave* egocentrically in certain situations and are more likely to behave egocentrically than older children and adults, especially when the cognitive, linguistic, and social demands on them are great.

Requests

Requests are interesting parts of communicative competence for at least two reasons. First, requests exemplify the distinctions Austin made among the three components of speech acts: locutionary, illocutionary, and perlocutionary acts. Listeners must understand that very indirect, vague locutionary acts (e.g., "I'm bored," "Do you remember that book I lent you?") and very direct, explicit locutionary acts (e.g., "Entertain me," "Give me that book") may have the same illocutionary purpose and perlocutionary effect. Adults are thought to infer the meaning of **indirect requests** by considering both their form and the context of their use. Researchers are interested in whether young children have this understanding and therefore investigate children's comprehension of indirect requests.

Second, effective speakers take context into account by varying the requests they use in different situations. Speakers have many forms of requests at their disposal, not only in terms of their direct and indirect structure, but in terms of whether they contain **semantic aggravators** (words or phrases that intensify the request; e.g., "or else," "right now") or **semantic mitigators** (words or phrases that soften the request; e.g., "please," reasons). Researchers are thus interested in how children produce requests and whether they recognize the relationship between the forms and functions of requests (see Becker, 1982, 1984).

Preschoolers' Comprehension of Indirect Requests

Both observational and experimental research indicates that preschoolers respond to indirect requests as requests for action. Two-year-olds respond as appropriately to requests their mothers phrase as questions as to those phrased directly (Shatz, 1978), and three- and four-year olds respond with appropriate actions when, for instance, telephone callers ask "Is your Daddy there?" and when someone hints "It's noisy in here" (Ervin-Tripp, 1974, 1977).

Other evidence that preschoolers understand indirect requests to be requests for action is found in the way children normally refuse such requests. Catherine Garvey (1975) observed thirty-six preschool dyads. When children did not want to comply with indirect requests, they often justified and explained in terms of their inability to perform the requested act (e.g., "I can't"), lack of willingness (e.g., "I don't want to"), lack of obligation to comply (e.g., "I don't have to"), or their inappropriateness as the person being asked to comply (e.g., "No, you"). Their comments reveal not only that they viewed indirect requests as requests, but that they understood the conditions under which they could legitimately make requests and the conditions under which they should respond.

Experiments also show that preschoolers understand the intent of indirect requests. Leonard and his colleagues (Leonard, Wilcox, Fulmer, & Davis, 1978) assessed children's comprehension of embedded imperatives such as "Can you X?" and "Will you X?" Children watched videotapes of everyday interactions in which an adult used an embedded imperative to make a request of another adult. Children judged whether the listener's subsequent behavior was in compliance with the request. Even four- and five-year-olds performed at better than chance on these requests, even when the requests were that the listener stop or change a behavior. Ervin-Tripp, Strage, Lampert, and Bell (1987) obtained similar results.

It may be that indirect requests like hints are not very opaque or difficult for young children to understand. They may not require logical reasoning or the conscious consideration of form and context because some indirect requests are so common in everyday speech (Gordon & Ervin-Tripp, 1984). Preschoolers may routinely hear requests such as "Lunch time" (meaning "clean up") so that their intent has become obvious and the response, automatic.

Preschoolers' Production of Requests

Many contextual factors affect the forms of requests adults use in different situations. They include the roles of the two people conversing, whether the setting is personal or transactional, whether the requested action can normally be expected of the listener, and the relative status or power of these two people (Ervin-Tripp, 1976). Most of the research on children has focused on status.

In general, like adults, children tend to address direct requests with semantic aggravators to listeners of lower status and indirect requests with semantic mitigators to listeners of higher status. For example, preschoolers are more likely to use an imperative (e.g., "Gimme an X") with a peer and a more indirect request (e.g., "May I have an X?" "Do you have an X?") with an adult (Ervin-Tripp, 1974, 1977; Gelman & Shatz, 1977; Gordon & Ervin-Tripp, 1984; James, 1978; McTear, 1980; Sachs & Devin, 1976; Shatz & Gelman, 1973). During role play, they have dominant puppets enact more direct requests than submissive puppets do (Andersen, 1986, 1990; Corsaro, 1979). They even make more subtle differentiations, using requests that are more indirect with more dominant, bigger peers than with less powerful peers (Ervin-Tripp, 1974; Wood & Gardner, 1980).

Preschoolers are, at least to some degree, aware of the association between request forms and the relative status of speakers and listeners and can recognize the social messages that requests convey. Preschool-aged children reported that direct requests with semantic aggravators were "bossier" than less direct requests with semantic mitigators, which were seen as "nicer" (Becker, 1986). When asked to make bossy and nice requests, these children produced bossy requests that were more direct and aggravated than their nice requests. In other words, a peer who requests the way a higher status person requests is bossy, whereas one who requests the way a lower status person requests is nice. Requests themselves are not inherently bossy or nice. Rather, it is the use of the forms in particular contexts by particular people that imbues them with social nuances.

By elementary school, children are capable of using their requests to comment on and manipulate social relationships. Children as young as seven years have been observed to set **imperative traps** in which they successfully address direct requests to older children. Claudia Mitchell-Kernan and Keith Kernan (1977) described one such girl who said to an eleven-year-old, "Bring your li'l self here." To a third party who asked "Who you think you are?" the girl replied, "I think I'm somebody big" (p. 204). In contrast, a child who forces a peer to produce a "courtesy phrase" (an unusually indirect request with semantic softeners such as "Pretty please with sugar on it could you stop punching me?") is forcing that child to act submissively. The social power of imperative traps and courtesy phrases clearly shows that children are aware of the connection between language form and language function in those contexts.

In summary, preschoolers are quite adept at comprehending and producing different request forms. They respond appropriately to indirect requests and understand conditions of their use. They also vary the forms of their requests systematically when speaking with individuals who are more or less powerful than they are.

Choices Among Language Varieties

Another aspect of communicative competence involves the choices speakers make among language varieties. For example, one would speak differently while giving a formal presentation at school than when playing in one's neighborhood; when talking to chess buddies about strategy than when talking with younger siblings about television shows; when talking with one's elderly Cuban grandparents than with younger European American neighbors. These language varieties include **registers, dialects,** and languages. Registers (sometimes called speech "codes" or "styles") are usually thought of as forms of language that vary according to participants, settings, and topics. Dialects are usually thought of as mutually intelligible forms of language associated with a particular region or defined group of people. And languages are forms that are typically not intelligible across groups. The distinctions among these three forms are not always great; they are often based on social and political, rather than linguistic, considerations (Linguistic Society of America, 1999). The Linguistic Society of America notes, for example, that different varieties of Chinese are considered dialects even though speakers of these different forms cannot understand each other and that Swedish and Norwegian are separate languages, but users of each understand the other.

No one language variety is inherently more appropriate than another (though listeners have many stereotypes and prejudices concerning them). As with other aspects of communicative competence, whether a given variety is appropriate and effective depends on the context in which it is used. Two examples of language varieties are those associated with ethnicity and gender. Keep in mind that these varieties are only *associated* with ethnicity and gender; there are tremendous differences across group members.

Language and Ethnicity: African American Vernacular English

Interest in and concern about children's dialects came to the fore in 1996 when the Oakland (California) School Board made a controversial decision. It declared that "Ebonics," a variety of English spoken by many African Americans, should be recognized and taken into account in teaching "Standard English" (SE).

"Ebonics," most commonly referred to as **African American Vernacular English** (AAVE; Mufwene & Rickford, 1998), is characterized in adult usage by its phonological, syntactic (see Table 6.1), and pragmatic features. Phonological features that best distinguish it from most other varieties of English include simplification processes such as final consonant cluster reduction and consonant reversals (Bailey & Thomas, 1998). For example, the word "cold" is reduced to "cole" and "ask" changes to "aks." Syntactic features include multiple negation as in "He ain't got no car" and subject-verb disagreement as in "What do this say?" (Martin & Wolfram, 1998). There are also pragmatic features such as the use of **signifying** (also referred to as "sounding"

	SE	AAVE
Zable 6.1 **Sample Differences Between Standard English and African American Vernacular English**		

Phonology

	SE	AAVE
consonant deletions		
final consonant cluster reduction	test	tes
unstressed syllable deletion	government	gov'ment
final consonant deletion	hive	hi
consonant substitutions		
final stop devoicing	bad	bat
/f/ and /v/ for medial and final /th/	mouth	mouf
/d/ for initial /th/	these	dese
consonant reversals		
final /s/ + stop	ask	aks

Syntax

	SE	AAVE
multiple negation	"doesn't have"	"ain't got no"
noninverted question	"Who is that?"	"Who that is?"
deletion of auxiliary	"How do you do this?"	"How you do this?"
subject-verb disagreement	"this says"	"this say"
invariant "be"	"She usually drives"	"She be driving"
regularized possessive	"He walks by himself"	"He walks by hisself"

(Compiled from Bailey & Thomas, 1998, and Martin & Wolfram, 1998)

and "playing the dozens"; Morgan, 1998). Signifying is a type of sarcastic or witty language play that allows users to make indirect comments upon socially significant topics. For example, one can comment upon appearance by saying, "You're so ugly, you went into a haunted house and came out with a job application" (Morgan, 1998, p. 268). Another pragmatic characteristic of AAVE is the use of topic-associating (rather than topic-focused) narratives, which you will read more about in Chapter 10.

According to the Linguistic Society of America, this language variety has systematic and expressive grammatical and pronunciation patterns. The Society's 1997 resolution states, "Characterizations of Ebonics as 'slang,' 'mutant,' 'lazy,' 'defective,' 'ungrammatical,' or 'broken English' are incorrect and demeaning" (Linguistic Society of America, 1999).

Like any other form of English, children's production of AAVE differs from that of adults. Unfortunately, little research has been devoted to the development of this

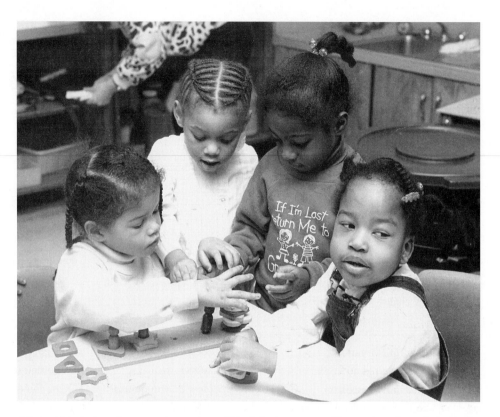

Many African Americans speak a variety of English characterized by its phonological, syntactic, and pragmatic features.

form (Washington, 1996; Wyatt, 1995). Preschoolers have been observed in pragmatic performances such as signifying (Wyatt, 1995). Many other characteristics that distinguish AAVE from SE do not emerge until after the preschool years (Battle, 1996; Terrell, Battle, & Grantham, 1998). Some of the earliest characteristics to appear are those involving the verb phrase, deletion of the auxiliary, and negation (Battle, 1996; Washington & Craig, 1994). In contrast, forms involving the habitual, invariant "be" and virtually all of the phonological features emerge much later (Battle, 1996; Terrell, Battle, & Grantham, 1998).

In addition to age, factors such as socioeconomic status and context affect how often children use AAVE and which features they produce (Battle, 1996). AAVE is more commonly used among working-class and low-income African Americans (Washington, 1996) and in informal situations (Battle, 1996). One five-year-old African American girl (Wyatt & Seymour, 1990) used AAVE features 10 percent of the time while describing pictures and photos, but 43 percent of the time when discussing the characteristics, feelings, actions, and comments of other children. She omitted these features completely when addressing her Caucasian classroom teacher and used them approximately 40 percent of the time when speaking to African American peers. Some elementary-school-age African American children use AAVE at home and in other informal settings and switch to SE in more formal, academic settings, a tendency that is more pronounced in adolescence as children become more aware of the social significance of SE (Battle, 1996).

Why would speakers vary their speech so much across settings? According to William Hall (1976), their behavior is due to their perceptions of the relative risks as opposed to the gains or benefits to be derived from speaking different varieties. In some settings, using a certain form enables speakers to establish and maintain social bonds and to display cultural pride. In other settings, speakers may focus on the social consequences of language variety for teachers' attitudes. They may recognize that using a certain variety has implications for educational and occupational access and success.

Language and Gender

Some research has suggested that there are feminine and masculine speech styles. For example, women are said to be more likely to use standard phonetic forms than are men (e.g., pronouncing the final "-ing" in words), use polite forms such as tag questions or requests, react rather than initiate in conversations, and use particular lexical items (e.g., intensifiers, meaningless particles, politeness markers, rare color terms, expressive adjectives, and euphemisms) (Andersen, 1990, p. 41). There is a great deal of controversy about whether, in fact, there really are such gender differences and whether these characteristics are more stereotypes or a function of role rather than of gender *per se*.

Even though they do not appear to use many of these language features, young children associate them differentially with men and women. In a study by Edelsky (1977), first graders tended to agree that women are more likely than men to use the word "adorable," and almost all agreed that men are more likely than women to say "damn it." Consensus about other features increased with age, and stereotypes became more like those of adults.

Overall, the language boys and girls produce is more similar than different. The most consistent difference with respect to communicative competence is that young girls tend to use more collaborative, supportive, and mitigated speech styles whereas young boys tend to use more controlling and unmitigated speech styles in interaction with peers (Austin, Salehi, & Leffler, 1987; Cook, Fritz, McCornack, & Visperas, 1985; DeHart, 1996; Leaper, 1991; Miller, Danaher, & Forbes, 1986; Sachs, 1987). For example, girls are more likely to ask something like "Will you be the doctor for a few minutes?" and "She needs the little pill, right?" In contrast, boys are more likely to produce such sentences as, "Come on, be a doctor" and "Gimme your arm" (Sachs, 1987).

Amy Sheldon has conducted detailed, qualitative analyses of preschoolers' disputes. In one study (1990), she observed triads of same-gender children during dramatic play in the housekeeping area of their preschool. Focusing on disputes two triads had over a toy pickle, she found more negotiation among the girls:

> *Sue:*   "No, Lisa wants pickle."
> *Mary:*   "She gots…"
> *Sue:*   "You want pickle, Lisa?"
> *Lisa:*   "Mmmhm."
> *Sue:*   "Lisa says she wants pickle."
> *Mary:*   "I'll cut it in half."
> *Lisa:*   "No, that's not fair!"
> *Sue:*   (looks for other food) "And the oranges."
> *Mary:*   "I need, I need to cut it in half, one for dessert and one for you." (p. 17)

Ultimately the dispute was resolved and play continued. A dispute among three boys was quite different as two of them struggled for control:

> *Nick:*   "No, I have to cut that!" (tries to take pickle)
> *Kevin:*   "No, I cut it."
> *Nick:*   "No! No, no, *no*! You're the children!"
> *Kevin:*   "No, I'm not!"
> *Nick:*   "Kevin, but the, oh, I *have* to cut it! I want to cut it! It's mine!"
> *Nick:*   (whining to Joe) "Kevin is not letting me cut the pickle."
> *Joe:*   "Oh, I know! I can pull it away from him and give it back to you. That's an idea!"
> *Kevin:*   "Joe!"
> *Nick:*   "I can pull it, take it away from you and put it in the oven."
> *Kevin:*   "Don't, Joe, don't, don't, don't, don't!"
> *Nick:*   "You have to make a pickle salad! I'll put it in the pot."
> *Kevin:*   "Don't." (pp. 22–23)

This dispute escalated and continued through many rounds of opposition.

There are many differences across children in the extent to which they use these gender-related speech styles. Moreover, their tendency to use these styles varies contextually. Preschoolers are more likely to use them with peers of the same gender than with peers of the other gender (Killen & Naigles, 1995; Leaper, 1991; Miller et al., 1986) and more with peers than with siblings (DeHart, 1996). Gender differences also become more pronounced with age, as you will see in Chapter 10.

Language in Role Play

Another indication that children understand the connection between different language forms and context is the way they role play. That is, by speaking differently when enacting the roles, they reveal their knowledge of language registers. Elaine Andersen (1986, 1990) asked eighteen four- five- and six-to-eight-year-olds to use puppets to enact a family situation with mother, father, and young child puppets; a classroom situation with a teacher and two child puppets; and a doctor situation with a patient puppet and male and female puppets in medical attire. Children marked the different roles phonologically (mostly through pitch differences, but also through intonation, volume, rate, and voice quality), lexically (e.g., some use of technical medical terminology), and syntactically. In the family situation, for example, children used deep, loud voices as fathers, higher pitch for mothers, and even higher pitch and often nasalization or whining for children. When pretending to have the child address the father, they used more indirect requests such as "Would you button me?" than they did when pretending to address the mother. To her, they were more likely to use direct requests such as "Gimme Daddy's flashlight" (1990, p. 134). When pretending to be fathers, children often used speech that was straightforward, unqualified, and forceful, and for mothers they used speech that was more polite, qualified, and indirect (e.g., using many hints such as "Baby's sleepy;" 1986, p. 159). With age, children were able to use more linguistic devices to mark the different roles. Initially, they relied on phonological features, then added differentiated vocabulary and topics, and finally utilized syntax. Older children were also better able to maintain these contrasts throughout their role play.

Preschoolers can spontaneously correct their speech as they enact roles (Andersen, 1990) and have even been overheard to make comments upon role-related language. A three-year-old girl playing the role of baby, for example, told a boy playing a parent, "Say, 'Go to sleep now.'... Say, 'Go to sleep. Put your head down'" (Garvey, 1990, pp. 83–84).

As you have seen, preschoolers have many language varieties at their disposal, including dialects and registers. Many African American preschoolers are beginning to acquire the features of African American Vernacular English and to use them differently in different settings. Girls and boys are developing somewhat different styles, with girls communicating more collaboratively with peers than boys do. During play, young children demonstrate basic knowledge of the registers associated with different roles. Preschoolers clearly have a command of some of the culturally determined components of communication.

Areas of Preschoolers' Communicative Incompetence

Thus far preschoolers have been portrayed as having a great deal of communicative competence. Lest you think that there is little for children to achieve after the age of five, it is important to realize that there are also ways in which preschoolers' competencies have yet to develop (see Chapter 10 and Romaine, 1984). Recall Piaget's observation that egocentric speech comprised nearly 50 percent of preschoolers' speech and that his experiments showed that they convey confusing, incomplete messages. According to Ninio and Snow (1996), "It is easy to characterize children as precocious or as hopelessly unskilled depending on what aspect of conversation one focuses on" (p. 150). There are a number of communicative skills preschoolers typically lack, including sophisticated use of deictic terms as well as conversational skills.

Deictic Terms

Deictic terms are those that point to components of a situation without actually naming them. (The word "deixis" comes from the Greek word "deiktikos" meaning "capable of showing.") Deictic terms indicate people (e.g., "I" and "you"), objects (e.g., "this" and "that"), motions (e.g., "come" and "go"), time (e.g., "before" and "after"), and locations (e.g., "here" and "there"). "I" and "you" do not refer to particular people. Instead, their referents depend on context, specifically, who is speaking and who is listening. Similarly, "here" and "there" are not always the same place. "Here" refers to locations close to the speaker, and "there" refers to locations that are further away. These are abstract words and their meanings vary across contexts, so they are relatively difficult for children to learn.

Full comprehension of deictic terms comes relatively late (Garvey, 1984; Tanz, 1980). Pronouns such as "I" and "you" are acquired earliest (usually before the age of two), followed by terms for location and objects. Verbs of motion may not be learned until elementary school. Chapter 4 presents details about several studies of deictic terms.

Conversational Skills

By the end of preschool, children are remarkably good conversationalists, but their ability to conduct a coherent, sustained conversation improves with age. There are several areas in which they have some difficulties:

- For one thing, preschoolers are less capable than older children of maintaining a conversation. The don't find it easy to develop a topic (Ninio & Snow, 1996). They also have difficulty giving and responding to feedback in conversations. For example, preschoolers are inconsistent and often inept at asking for clarification when others' communication is unclear and at repairing their own speech, especially when their listener's feedback is not explicit (Patterson & Kister, 1981; Robinson, 1981). It is not until nearly adolescence that children are able to insert "uh-huhs" and head nods at appropriate moments to indicate continuing attention and satisfactory comprehension (Garvey, 1984).

- Preschoolers also lack the precise timing of conversational turns that adults exhibit, although they rarely overlap turns. They tend to rely on obvious cues that a speaker is done, rather than anticipating upcoming conversational boundaries, which often results in long pauses between turns (Garvey, 1984). Turn-taking is particularly difficult when there are more than two speakers (Ervin-Tripp, 1979).

- Conversations over the telephone also pose problems for preschoolers even though they have many experiences using telephones. Amye Warren and Carol Tate (1992) taped twenty children between the ages of two and six years as they talked on the telephone with familiar adults. These conversations were hard for children to maintain. Even the oldest ones gave inappropriate responses and occasionally gestured. The latter was the case with a boy of four years, ten months who answered his grandfather's questions about his age by repeatedly holding up four fingers and saying, "Dis many" (p. 259).

The Difficulty of Acquiring Communicative Competence

The foregoing discussion shows that children must adapt their language to different contexts. They must learn, for example, that they may yell when they are playing outdoors, but must use quieter voices inside and perhaps not even talk at all in settings such as movie theaters and churches. Similarly, they must learn that they may discuss toileting matters and details of recent illnesses with family members and physicians, but not with strangers, and that members of their soccer team may understand soccer jargon and expressions, but that they must use other phrases with nonplayers. Not only must children acquire a repertoire of communicative behaviors, they must be able to recognize characteristics of different contexts and then use the behaviors that are expected, appropriate, and effective. This is clearly a difficult task for them.

In contrast with the morphological and syntactic rules described in Chapter 5, there are usually not strict rules for communicative competence (Becker, 1990). Rather, in specific contexts, using or omitting a particular communicative behavior is seen as relatively appropriate or inappropriate. For example, children do not always have to say "please" in order to be polite and appropriate. There are other ways to make polite requests, such as saying "May I have a cookie?" The lack of hard and fast rules probably makes it difficult for children to learn whether and when to exhibit different behaviors.

Another factor that makes acquisition of communicative competence difficult is that many polite forms have no clear referents. That is, it is not obvious what a form such as "please" means. Furthermore, some forms such as "thank you" that seem to have a meaning (in this case, being thankful) are often supposed to be used in situations when their meaning is contradicted (such as when it is appropriate to thank elderly Aunt Gertrude for the hideous socks she sent for one's birthday) (Berko Gleason, Perlmann, & Greif, 1984). Therefore, the learning process is probably different from that described for other words in Chapter 4.

Another complicating factor is that the conventions for competent communication in one setting (e.g., home) are often different from those in other settings (e.g., school). To the extent that these conventions are different, children may have trouble learning and adjusting to those of school. The implications of this mismatch between home and school are dramatically illustrated by children whose cultures are different from those of teachers and the classroom.

In a classic study, Susan Philips (1970) observed Native American children on the Warm Springs Indian Reservation in Oregon. These children had acquired culturally appropriate ways of communicating as they learned traditional skills in their community. In first-grade classrooms, they rarely volunteered to speak and were reluctant to answer teachers' questions. When they did speak, they did so very softly. Teachers tended to view these children as shy and, at times, uncooperative. Teachers had difficulty assessing their knowledge. When they adjusted their teaching styles to make them more compatible with the students' cultural tendencies, the teachers failed to provide the children with experiences necessary to develop the communicative skills needed for further school success. These results are not unique to Native Americans. Australian Aboriginal children (Malcolm, 1979, 1982) and others may encounter similar difficulties (Battle, 1996; Boggs, 1985; Crago & Cole, 1991; Crago & Eriks-Brophy, 1994; Harris, 1998; Iglesias, 1985; Schieffelin & Eisenberg, 1984; Tharp, 1989).

Influences on the Acquisition of Communicative Competence

Acquiring communicative competence is difficult, but children have some help. There are a number of ways that families and schools contribute to the acquisition process. Furthermore, children's knowledge and their efforts to learn about communication also facilitate their communicative development.

Family Influences on the Acquisition of Communicative Competence

In general, it can be said that caregivers "socialize" language. They use language to help their children become competent members of their societies and cultures, competence reflected in part in the children's language usage (Ely & Berko Gleason, 1995; Schieffelin & Ochs, 1996). This section will focus primarily on literature describing middle-class, American families because that is the population on which most of the research has been done. (See Battle & Anderson, 1998; Blum-Kulka, 1990, 1997; Rabain-Jamin, 1998; Schieffelin & Ochs, 1986, for information about the socialization of communicative competence in other cultures.) Given that societies and cultures vary greatly, though, you must recognize that characteristics of caregiver–child interactions as well as the language behaviors socialized vary across cultures (Crago, 1994; Crago & Cole, 1991; Schieffelin & Ochs, 1986).

Virtually from birth, infants begin to receive information about some of the communicative behaviors that will help them meet their social needs. You have probably seen many parents wave the hands of their little, preverbal infants and say such things for them as "Say 'hi' to Mrs. Stanley" or "Bye bye, Grandpa."

Much of the structure of conversations may be learned in early interactions between infants and caregivers, as Jacqueline Sachs indicated in Chapter 2. Actions and talk (e.g., the use of "hello," "please," and "thank you") are highly organized and predictable during social games or routines such as "peek-a-boo" and in give and take with objects (Bruner, 1974/75, 1975). Such games provide clear and consistent information about a small number of socially significant phrases. In these interactions, infants also learn about taking turns, the responsibilities of both participants to keep the interaction going, how to focus on a theme or topic, and how to make the interaction cohere. Caregivers find ways to pull their infants into the interaction, to help infants respond and participate, much as if they were having a conversation (Ninio & Snow, 1996; Snow, 1977).

Once children exhibit some basic communicative competence, begin to participate more actively in interactions, and can anticipate sequences of behavior in the routines, caregivers adapt their interactions (Becker, 1990). A number of interesting studies have been conducted on how they do this during the preschool years.

In a simple and clever study, Jean Berko Gleason and Sandra Weintraub (1976) tape-recorded what happened at two homes as trick-or-treaters arrived on Halloween evening. They also followed two mothers and their children as they went door-to-door trick-or-treating. Berko Gleason and Weintraub observed that many parents insisted that their children say "trick or treat" and "thank you," often using the prompt "say." Their teaching is illustrated in the following example:

> *Girl's mother:*   (Approaching a house) "Don't forget to say 'thank you.' (Children go to door and return to sidewalk.) "Did you say 'thank you,' Sue, did you say 'thank you'?"
> *Sue:*   "Ya."
> *Mother:*   "Good."
> *Boy's mother:*   "Ricky, did *you* say 'thank you'?"
> *Girl's mother:*   "Did you say 'trick or treat,' Sue?"
> *Boy's mother:*   (Approaching another house) "Will you remember to say 'trick or treat' and 'thank you'?"
> *Girl's mother:*   (Children have walked to door. She calls to them from the sidewalk.) "Don't forget to say 'thank you'!" (Berko Gleason & Weintraub, 1976, p. 134)

Berko Gleason and other colleagues (Berko Gleason et al., 1984; Greif & Berko Gleason, 1980; Snow, Perlmann, Berko Gleason, & Hooshyar, 1990) as well as other researchers (Eisenberg, 1982; Pellegrini, Brody, & Stoneman, 1987) have made similar observations.

In order to replicate and extend these findings I conducted a one-year longitudinal study of five families (Becker, 1994). Parents audiotaped everyday interactions between themselves and their preschoolers in their homes. In our analyses of the transcribed tapes we found that parents commented about a wide variety of communicative behaviors. They provided input about what children were expected to say ("please," "thank you," polite requests, "goodbye," routines such as "trick or treat," address terms, slang, appropriate subject matter, and apologies), how children were expected to speak (using the appropriate volume, tone of voice, and clarity), when children should speak (knowing when to speak, responding verbally), and how to stay on topic.

Parents also used a variety of strategies in their comments about and reactions to their preschoolers' communicative behaviors. They prompted in several different ways, modeled, and reinforced, and occasionally posed hypothetical situations, evaluated behavior after the fact, addressed children's comments about communication, and evaluated others' communicative behavior (see Table 6.2).

One of the provocative aspects of these findings is that most of the parents' input was indirect. Specifically, parents' indirect comments on errors and omissions comprised an average of 61 percent of the total input (49–91% across the families). Indirectness seems a risky way to teach communicative competence because children might not understand what they are supposed to do. The finding that so much parental input is indirect is counterintuitive because parents believe that displaying competence is important and a reflection of their own socialization competence (Becker & Hall, 1989; Bryant, 1999). One would think that parents would be explicit in order to maximize the chances of their children performing correctly. Although these are not experimental findings and therefore causal conclusions cannot be drawn, it is likely that indirectness challenges children more cognitively and provides more information about communicative conventions than does direct, explicit input (Becker, 1988). In fact, mothers of preschoolers believe that indirect responses place cognitive burdens on children by helping them "to think rather than just parrot" and "figure it out on [their] own" (Bryant, 1999, p. 134).

Parents are not the only family members who socialize communicative competence. Siblings in several cultures have been observed to prompt appropriate behavior (Berko Gleason, Hay, & Cain, 1989; Demuth, 1986; Wilhite, 1983). For example, a five-year-old girl apparently imitated her parents by instructing her younger sister, "Don't talk while you're eating" (Berko Gleason et al., 1989).

A number of researchers have suggested that, although different family members may contribute to the acquisition of communicative competence, each does so in a different and potentially important way. That is, family members who know the child less intimately (e.g., fathers who are secondary caregivers) or who lack the capacity and motivation to tune in to the child's needs (e.g., older siblings) may pressure the child to communicate more clearly and appropriately than would family members who know the child most intimately (e.g., mothers who are primary caregivers) (Barton & Tomasello, 1994; Berko Gleason, 1975; Brown, 1973; Mannle & Tomasello, 1987; Rondal, 1980). Thus, fathers and siblings may serve as "bridges" to the outside world, "leading the child to change her or his language in order to be understood" (Berko Gleason, 1975, p. 293). Fathers and siblings, in this view, challenge children to adapt and broaden their communicative skills and thus prepare them to talk with strangers and about unfamiliar topics.

$\mathcal{T}able\ 6.2$	**Categories of Parental Input Regarding Preschoolers' Communicative Behaviors**

Prompts

direct comment on omission
  explicitly point out the omitted behavior or that the child must produce this behavior; e.g., "Say 'excuse me' when you cough"

indirect comment on omission
  allude to the omission; e.g., "What's the magic word?"

direct comment on error
  explicitly point out the child's error or that the child must correct behavior; e.g., "Don't talk with your mouth full"

indirect comment on error
  allude to the error; e.g., "What did you say?"

anticipatory suggestion
  suggest a behavior prior to an omission or error; e.g., "Don't forget to say 'night-night' to Daddy"

Modeling

modeling
  provide the appropriate behavior before the child has the opportunity to produce it; e.g., "Excuse me" as the child coughs

teaching sibling
  modeling for the preschooler by commenting on younger sibling's behavior; e.g., Mother: "What do you say?" Infant: "Thank you." Mother: "You're welcome. Very good!"

parents demonstrate
  parents demonstrate prompts and behaviors as instruction; e.g., Father: "Go get my milk." Mother: "Well, what do you say?" Father: "Please."

Reinforcement

verbal reinforcement following preschoolers' appropriate usage; e.g., "I like the way you say [X]."

Other Forms of Input

hypothetical situation
  pose a hypothetical situation for didactic purposes; e.g., "What would you say if that ape came up to you and said 'hi'?"

retroactive evaluation
  comment on child's appropriateness well after the fact; e.g., "She said her prayers [earlier at lunch] all by herself! Word for word, too. I'm really happy about that."

address child's comment
  respond to child's question, statement, or prompt about communicative competence; e.g., Child: "It's a bad word, 'ugly.'" Mother: "It's not a bad word, you just use it wrong."

evaluate another
  seek child's evaluation of another person's behavior; e.g., "Right, Jane?"

(Becker, 1994, pp. 136–137)

There is some evidence to support the bridge hypothesis. Relative to mothers, fathers of infants have been observed to have more breakdowns in communication, spend less time focused on the same object or action, be less successful at tuning in to their children's current focus of attention, make more off-topic replies, and request clarification more often (Mannle & Tomasello, 1987; Tomasello, Conti-Ramsden, & Ewert, 1990). Fathers of preschoolers also use more imperatives with their children than do mothers (Berko Gleason, 1975; Gleason, 1975; Malone & Guy, 1982). A recent meta-analysis (a statistical review of many studies) demonstrated that, across studies, mothers are more supportive (e.g., they praise, acknowledge), more negative (e.g., they are critical, disagree), and less directive in their speech than fathers (Leaper, Anderson, & Sanders, 1998). In general, fathers appear to be less tuned in to children than mothers are.

Note that less supportive conversational interaction is not necessarily a good thing: Parents who fail to give their preschoolers time to respond to requests tend to have children with poor turn-taking skills (Black & Logan, 1995).

Not surprisingly, older siblings are even less tuned in and conversationally responsive than fathers. Erika Hoff-Ginsberg (now Erika Hoff) and Wendy Krueger (1991) observed toddlers interacting with preschool-aged siblings, seven-to-eight-year-

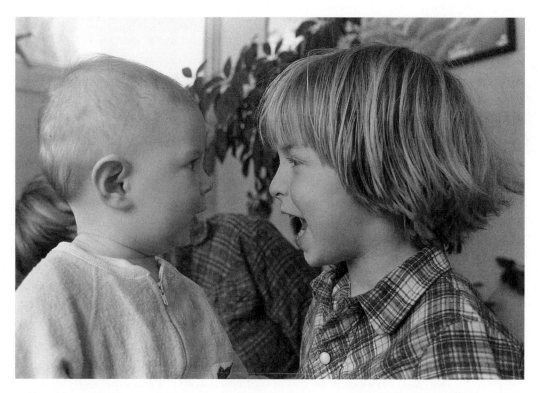

Older siblings contribute to communicative competence in several ways. Like their parents, they sometimes prompt younger siblings to use appropriate behavior.

old siblings, and their mothers. The older siblings were conversationally more like their mothers than were the preschoolers, but neither group of siblings adapted their speech adequately to their younger siblings' age. They did not adjust their rate of directives, conversation-eliciting utterances, recasts of the toddlers' utterances, or tendency to continue the toddlers' topic. Similarly, Michael Tomasello and Sara Mannle (1985) found that preschool-aged siblings of infants used more directives, asked fewer questions, recast and continued topics less frequently, were less capable of sharing attentional focus and interacting jointly than were their mothers, and, most unsupportively, acknowledged fewer utterances. Mannle, Barton, and Tomasello (1991) observed those differences even when infants did not differ in their conversational behavior with their mothers and siblings. In general, siblings are more directive, less responsive, and less adept than their mothers at using techniques for maintaining conversations with younger siblings and at taking into account the siblings' conversational immaturity.

Siblings can affect communicative competence in additional ways. Some researchers argue that younger siblings are motivated to participate in conversations between their mothers and older siblings. Therefore, they learn how to enter conversations effectively (Barton & Tomasello, 1991; Dunn & Shatz, 1989) as well as to maintain a topic and take turns in such complex, triadic conversations (Barton & Tomasello, 1994; Hoff-Ginsberg & Krueger, 1991; Woollett, 1986). Younger siblings also have the opportunity to observe conversations between their mothers and older siblings and are thereby exposed to a variety of communicative styles (Woollett, 1986).

If siblings affect the acquisition of communicative competence, one would expect first-born children to differ from later-born children in their communicative skills. Hoff-Ginsberg (1998) investigated this possibility with one-and-one-half- to two-and-one-half-year-olds. Although, as previous research has shown, the first-born children exhibited more advanced lexical and grammatical development, the later-born children had more advanced conversational skills in interactions with their mothers.

There are several limitations in this literature that should be noted:

- First, causal conclusions cannot be drawn because the research is descriptive and correlational. Neither experimental studies nor interventions have been done on the influences of families on the acquisition of communicative competence.

- Second, there are many variations across families with similar configurations (Mannle & Tomasello, 1987). Not all mothers behave the same way, nor do all fathers or all siblings. For example, Davidson and Snow (1996) failed to find that middle-class, highly educated fathers of kindergartners used more challenging language than mothers. We must also exercise caution in generalizing results of studies of relatively few families.

- Third, context influences parental behavior to a greater extent than parental gender does (Lewis, 1997). The setting, the task, and other situational characteristics strongly affect how parents interact with their preschoolers.

School's Influence on the Acquisition of Communicative Competence

Teachers who provide opportunities and encourage children to talk for a wide variety of purposes, in different situations, and with different audiences also help children learn to communicate effectively (Chall & Curtis, 1991). More specifically, children need a variety of experiences communicating in order to learn the functions of language, different forms of discourse, and the conventions for using language appropriately. Valuable experiences include informal conversations between children and teachers and among children (not to mention with the principal, other teachers, parents, and members of the community), games, small group projects, storytelling, role playing, and the integration of communication training across the curriculum (Chall & Curtis, 1991). Researchers have concluded that children should not just be talked *to,* but should be able to develop communicative competence in relevant, interesting, everyday situations. Having access to a variety of materials, interacting in small areas or centers within the classroom, and having longer periods for interaction also appear to promote communicative competence in the preschool years (Cole, 1995).

Furthermore, teachers explicitly teach some rules governing communicative behavior specific to the classroom (Fivush, 1983). Effective teachers announce both restrictive rules (e.g., no screaming) and prescriptive rules (e.g., pay attention, follow routines) from the beginning of the school year and attempt to correct children's violations of these rules. In contrast, there are other rules that children must infer from the ongoing interaction. Fivush observed that teachers do not explicitly teach children about turn-taking and that only teachers can initiate topics.

School also affords children the opportunity to interact with peers. Peers probably affect communicative competence in a variety of ways. They may be similar to siblings as relatively uncooperative conversational partners, and thus contribute to the pressure preschoolers feel to communicate more clearly and effectively (Mannle & Tomasello, 1987). Peers also participate in forms of communication that are different from those of adult-child speech (Ely & Berko Gleason, 1975; Gleason, 1995). Their special kinds of humor and disagreements, the topics about which they talk, and their explicit socialization about language provide communicative experiences that no doubt complement those experienced with adults. (See Chapter 10 for further discussion of interaction with peers.)

Preschoolers' Cognitions and Efforts to Achieve Communicative Competence

Families and schools influence acquisition in part because they support and build on children's cognitive abilities and social predispositions (Snow, 1999).

Knowledge and Cognitive Abilities

Communicative competence requires a great deal of knowledge. Speakers must have a repertoire of terms and routines as well as language varieties. They must know something about situations and about relationships. Particular cognitive skills are thought to underlie specific communicative skills (e.g., spatial perspective taking as a prerequisite for the acquisition of deictic uses of "I" and "you"; Loveland, 1984). More general skills that also appear to influence communicative competence are knowledge of scripts and the ability to test hypotheses about communication.

Scripts

When children possess abstract knowledge about familiar, everyday events they are better able to communicate (Goodman, Duchan, & Sonnenmeier, 1994). This knowledge about an event is referred to as a **script.** Scripts are the way we represent familiar events in our memories. These representations contain information about sequences of actions, the usual functions of objects, roles of the people involved, and the kind of language used during the events—what one sees, does, and says in what order. For example, a script about going to the zoo might contain information about asking the ticket seller for a ticket, presenting it to the ticket taker, seeing exhibits in a particular order, feeding animals in the petting zoo, visiting the gift shop, and then leaving. The more familiar an event, the more likely children are to have a script for it and the more easily they can draw on the script structure and content to communicate in that situation or a reenactment of it.

Hypothesis Testing

It is important to remember that children are not passive acquirers of communicative competence (or much else, for that matter) (Becker, 1990). They naturally notice regularities across their experiences and organize those experiences. They associate communicative behaviors, conventions, and meanings with specific situational and contextual conditions and thereby "develop a sense of what is preferred and expected" (Schieffelin & Ochs, 1996, p. 258). They form hypotheses about communicative conventions and then test these hypotheses through trial and error and by asking questions and commenting upon communicative behavior.

Just as they overextend vocabulary and overregularize grammatical rules, young children sometimes misapply communicative conventions. It is common for infants to use "thank you" both when receiving and giving objects (Bruner, 1974/75; Gopnik & Meltzoff, 1986) and to interchange "hello" and "goodbye" (Gopnik & Meltzoff, 1986). An unusual example of a misapplied behavior is the one-year-old girl who said "phew" when her mother came into her room in the morning (Ferrier, 1978). She had obviously heard her mother use this term upon entering the bedroom and smelling a dirty diaper and had apparently understood it to be a greeting. Such overextensions suggest that infants are going beyond the evidence their environments have provided and are formulating generalizations about behaviors.

When they are older, children may seek verification for their hypotheses. For example, one of the preschool girls in my research had been taught to say "yes, Daddy" and "yes, Mommy." One day she said to her father, "Daddy. I just made up another one: 'No, Daddy. No, Mommy.' Is that right?" (Becker, 1990).

It is apparent that preschoolers know that there are specific aspects of communicative conventions to be learned, including what words to say and when, how, and why one should say them. Their active, conscious efforts to obtain this information are illustrated in the following excerpt from a conversation about events that will occur in the future on Christmas. Keep in mind that the preschooler in this example had had limited experience with Christmas and had relatively recently celebrated Halloween.

> *Girl:* "Maybe somebody, we are gonna coming in say 'trick or treat'?"
> *Mother:* (laughs) "No. They're not going to say 'trick or treat' on Christmas."
> *Girl:* "....What say then?"
> *Mother:* "Say 'Merry Christmas.'"
> *Girl:* "'Merry Christmas'?"
> *Mother:* "At Christmas time you say...And wish everybody a Merry Christmas. That means you hope they have a good time on Christmas day."
> *Girl:* "When they're sleeping, huh?"
> *Mother:* "No, when they're awake." (Becker, 1994, p. 141).

The daughter first attempts to ascertain what the appropriate verbal routine is for this occasion and then wonders what the phrase might mean. Finally, she inquires about the appropriate time at which one would use the phrase.

To summarize, families and schools afford a variety of opportunities for children to learn about the language considered appropriate in different contexts. Mothers, fathers, siblings, teachers, and peers appear to contribute differently to the acquisition of communicative competence by providing different types of information, feedback, and pressure. Children bring to these interactions their knowledge and their efforts to learn about communication. There are many influences on the acquisition of communicative competence and no doubt many possible paths to its achievement, a view consistent with the social interaction approach to language acquisition you will read about in Chapter 7.

The Significance of Communicative Competence

There are several reasons communicative competence is important to children's lives. Communicative competence predicts later literacy skills, is necessary for understanding and functioning in the classroom, and is associated with being liked more by peers and adults:

- First, some components of communicative competence in the preschool years are predictive of (and may in fact prepare children for) later literacy skills (Gillam, McFadden, & van Kleeck, 1995; Reeder, Shapiro, Watson, & Goelman, 1996; Wallat, 1991). For example, oral narrative skills may provide a bridge to literacy because they promote the enjoyment of stories and help children learn about the conceptual organization and linguistic conventions of stories (Gillam et al., 1995; Goelman, 1996; Snow, 1994). Kenneth Reeder and his colleagues have found a relationship between pragmatic awareness and early writing ability (Reeder & Shapiro, 1997). They argue that having the metalinguistic skills to attribute intentions and motives to speakers, to differentiate what is said from what is meant, may help children develop the ability to understand written language that provides no clues from social interactions (Goelman, 1996; Reeder & Shapiro, 1996).

- A second way in which communicative competence is important is that some degree of such competence is necessary for children to understand and function in preschool and kindergarten classrooms (Creaghead & Tattershall, 1985; Pinnell & Jaggar, 1991). Children must learn when and how to speak and respond to teachers and peers, to display their knowledge and obtain information appropriately, to comprehend nonliteral language (such as knowing that when teachers say "lunch time" they usually intend that children clean up their toys and wash their hands), and to communicate appropriately in different school settings (e.g., playground, lunch, rest time). Communicative competence (or the lack thereof) affects teachers' judgments of children's abilities and motivations (Becker, Place, Tenzer, & Frueh, 1991; Fivush, 1983; Heath, 1983; Mehan, 1979; Rice, 1993b) as well as children's opportunities for learning through interactions with peers and teachers (Chall & Curtis, 1991; Donahue, 1985; Rice, 1993b; Silliman & Wilkinson, 1991). (Note, by the way, that speech and language clinicians also make judgments based on children's communicative competence; American Speech-Language-Hearing Association Joint Subcommittee of the Executive Board on English Language Proficiency, 1998; Battle, 1998.)

- A third way in which communicative competence is important is that competent children are better liked than those who are less skilled. The editor of this textbook, Jean Berko Gleason (Berko Gleason et al., 1989), wrote about driving in a carpool when her children were young. One boy never said "thank you" or "good bye" when she dropped him off at his house. "Many years later," said Berko Gleason, "it is impossible to think of him with anything but distaste." As we all know, people who are rude, who demand and interrupt, are not very pleasant to be around. Wrote Dell Hymes, the apparent originator of the term "communicative competence," "A child capable of any and all grammatical utterances, but not knowing which to use, not knowing even when to talk and when to stop, would be a cultural monstrosity" (1967, p. 16).

There is empirical evidence for Berko Gleason's and Hymes' impressions about the relationship between communicative competence and liking. Many researchers have shown that children who are skilled at gaining entry to ongoing social interactions are more popular than children who are less skilled (Dodge, Schlundt, Schocken, & Delugach, 1983; Putallaz & Gottman, 1981). That is, it is advantageous to be able to employ such verbal strategies as greeting, suggesting, requesting to join in, and making substantive contributions to the interaction (Craig & Washington, 1993). Nancy Hazen and Betty Black (1989) have shown that three-and-one-half- to five-and-one-half-year-olds who are well-liked by their peers (as contrasted with those who are disliked) are better able to initiate and maintain coherent conversations. These children clearly direct their communication to specific peers, respond appropriately when others try to communicate with them, and can attend to two playmates rather than just focusing on one of them. Furthermore, when interacting with unfamiliar children, popular preschoolers are also more responsive and better able to carry on a coherent conversation than are unpopular children (Black & Hazen, 1990). Other researchers have obtained similar findings (Black & Logan, 1995; Gertner, Rice, & Hadley, 1994; Rice, 1993a). Mabel Rice and her colleagues have even suggested that something as simple as being able to address peers by name rather than as "hey, you" has implications for popularity.

The nature of the causal relationship between communicative competence and popularity is complex (Black & Logan, 1995; Weinert, 1993; Windsor, 1995). Black and Hazen (1990) argued that some communication skills (such as the ability to make relevant comments and respond positively and contingently to peers) contribute to young children's initial popularity. Then, further differences in communication skills emerge after children's reputations as being popular or unpopular are established. That is, unpopular children may avoid communicating with peers in order to avoid rejection. Their poor communication skills serve to maintain their lower status and may preclude their involvement in positive interactions that would help them learn better skills and develop better self-concepts.

In elementary school, skills such as being able to adjust messages to meet listeners' needs, ask appropriate questions, initiate and maintain conversations, communicate intentions clearly, address all participants when joining a group, make more positive than negative comments, and persuade and verbally comfort are all related to popularity with peers (Brinton & Fujiki, 1995; Burleson, Delia, & Applegate, 1992; Gallagher, 1991; Windsor, 1995). The effect of communicative competence on popularity is further supported by experimental work Karen Place and I conducted (Place & Becker, 1991) in which elementary-aged girls reported liking an unfamiliar girl who displayed communicative competence better than they liked unfamiliar girls who made rude requests, interrupted, or strayed off topic.

How well children get along with others is not a trivial matter. The quality of peer relationships has implications for future psychological well-being. Difficulty with peers puts children at risk for subsequent academic problems and psychological maladjustment (Rubin, Bukowski, & Parker, 1998).

This chapter opened with an example of preschoolers' conversation that illustrated the importance of communicative competence. Let's close with another. In this example, friends David and Josh, both four years old, are walking around pretending to be robots:

> *David:*   "I'm a missile robot who can shoot missiles out of my fingers. I can shoot them out of everywhere—even out of my legs. I'm a missile robot."
> *Josh (tauntingly):*   "No, you're a fart robot."
> *David (protestingly):*   "No, I'm a missile robot."
> *Josh:*   "No, you're a fart robot."
> *David (hurt, almost in tears):*   "No, Josh!"
> *Josh (recognizing that David is upset):*   "And I'm a poo-poo robot."
> *David (in good spirits again):*   "I'm a pee-pee robot." (Rubin, 1980, p. 55)

David's competent use of language shows us again just how powerful preschoolers' language may be in social contexts.

Summary

Communicative competence is the ability to use language appropriately and strategically in social contexts. That is, it involves knowing what, where, how, and to whom one should communicate. Communicative behaviors include routines, polite terms, conversational skills, and language varieties such as dialects and registers. It is important that children acquire communicative competence because it predicts later literacy skills, helps children succeed in school, and is associated with popularity among peers.

There are two major theoretical approaches to the study of communicative competence, speech act theory and cognitive developmental theory. Austin's speech act theory breaks communication into three components (locutionary, illocutionary, and perlocutionary acts) in order to illustrate how the interaction between the form of a sentence and context relates to a speaker's intentions and a listener's understanding. This theory also identifies a set of speech acts or communicative behaviors. Piaget's cognitive developmental theory describes preschoolers as being relatively unskilled at taking their listeners' perspectives into account when communicating.

Research indicates that preschoolers are able to use a wide range of communicative behaviors and adjust their communication for different listeners and in different situations. They comprehend indirect requests in which form does not obviously match function and produce different request forms for listeners of different statuses, suggesting that they have some understanding of the relationship between form and power. Preschoolers are also acquiring language varieties associated with ethnicity, gender, and social roles. However, they still have some difficulty with deictic terms, whose meanings vary across situations of use, and with conducting long conversations.

The task of acquiring communicative competence is difficult, and families and schools appear to play a role in this process. Mothers, fathers, and siblings provide instruction about communicative behaviors, each pressuring preschoolers in complementary ways to communicate appropriately. Teachers and peers also offer opportunities for communicative development. Preschoolers' experiences as well as their knowledge of scripts and their natural tendency to form hypotheses about communication drive the acquisition process.

Key Words

African American Vernacular English (AAVE)	locutionary act
	perlocutionary act
collective monologue	referential communication
communicative competence	register
deictic term	routine
dialect	script
echolalia	semantic aggravator
egocentrism	semantic mitigator
illocutionary act	signifying
imperative trap	simple monologue
indirect request	speech act

Suggested Projects

1. Consider the ways that the meaning of a particular utterance varies according to context. (Remember the example in the chapter of "It's hot in here" being a request for the listener to open a window or an ironic statement about a cold room?) That is, a particular locutionary act can be associated with a variety of illocutionary acts depending on the contexts in which it is produced. Write one such sentence and describe different contexts (e.g., in terms of settings or participants) in which it could be produced. Also, explain how listeners consider the contexts and the sentence in determining the sentence's meanings.

   Now think about how a particular meaning (e.g., agreement) may be expressed differently in different contexts (e.g., "Yeah" to a friend; "Aye, aye, sir" to a Navy superior; "Okee dokee" to an old-fashioned uncle). If a speaker used one of these expressions in an unexpected context, more meaning would be conveyed than just agreement. For example, if a student responds to a simple request from a professor by saying "Aye aye, sir," the student would not simply be agreeing to the professor's request! Consider the following situation: When I come in to the office in the morning, my secretary usually says, "Good morning, Dr. Bryant." How might she greet me differently to convey that she is angry with me? How might she greet me in another way if she wanted to convey embarrassment because she inadvertently erased something of mine from a computer disk? Explain both your answers and explain how I would figure out what my secretary meant.

2. Observe children between the ages of three and five years in their preschool or day care center. Compare and contrast their language with teachers vs. peers and in different activities (e.g., lunch, role play, story time). Note, for example, children's topics, requests, volume and tone of voice, and turn-taking in these different contexts.

3. Review transcripts of children's conversations available through the Child Language Data Exchange System (CHILDES) that was described in Chapter 1. Using your computer's web browser, access the CHILDES database at http:// childes.psy.cmu.edu. Scroll to and click "The database and the database manual." Go to the section for Macintosh or Windows, depending on what kind of system you have. Then scroll to and click "English corpora." Scroll to "MacWhinn.zip" and click to open. The file can be opened from the server location or downloaded to your computer. (Note that you must have software installed on your computer to unzip the file. If you do not already have this software, follow the instructions for downloading it that are provided by CHILDES.) This file contains transcripts involving Ross (29 files that span ages 5<< to 8 years) and his brother Mark (files from 2 << to 5 years, 4 months). Open for viewing the earliest (boys61) and latest (boys94) files to find transcripts of the two boys talking with their father during various activities (e.g., making a peanut butter and jelly sandwich and assembling a toy robot). Note the specific ways in which the boys' communicative competencies have changed over time.

4. Go into the CHILDES English database again. This time, click on the "Gleason.zip" file in which you will find transcripts for 24 children (aged 2–5 years) who were observed while playing with their parents in the laboratory and while having dinner at home with their families. Review transcripts from both the laboratory and the home. Note the specific ways in which the children communicate differently in these different contexts.

5. Interview adolescents or adults who speak more than one dialect or language. Ask them about the situations in which they use one of these language varieties as opposed to another. Get their impressions of why they switch and how they and others would react if they did not switch.

6. Prepare a handout about communicative competence for parents and teachers of preschoolers. Explain what communicative competence is, how teachers and parents can help in its development, and why it is important for children to acquire. Try to use everyday language in your explanations. Give the handout to several teachers and parents and get their feedback about it.

Suggested Readings

Becker, J. (1994). Pragmatic socialization: Parental input to preschoolers. *Discourse Processes, 17,* 131–148.

Berko Gleason, J., & Weintraub, S. (1976). The acquisition of routines in child language. *Language in Society, 5,* 129–136.

Black, B., & Logan, A. (1995). Links between communication patterns in mother–child, father–child, and child–peer interactions and children's social status. *Child Development, 66,* 255–271.

Ervin-Tripp, S., & Mitchell-Kernan, C. (1977) (Eds.). *Child discourse.* New York: Academic Press.

Garvey, C. (1984). *Children's talk.* Cambridge, MA: Harvard University Press.

Hoff-Ginsberg, E. (1998). The relation of birth order and socioeconomic status to children's language experience and language development. *Applied Psycholinguistics, 19,* 603–629.

Linguistic Society of America. (1999). LSA resolution on the Oakland "Ebonics" issue [Online]. Available: http://www.lsadc.org/ebonics.html.

Mufwene, S., Rickford, J., Bailey, G., & Baugh, J. (1998) (Eds.), *African-American English: Structure, history, and use.* London: Routledge.

Philips, S. (1970). Acquisition of rules for appropriate speech usage. In J. Alatis (Ed.), *Report of the 21st Annual Round Table Meeting on Linguistics and Language Studies: Bilingualism and language contact: Anthropological, linguistic, psychological, and sociological aspects* (pp. 77–101). Washington, DC: Georgetown University Press.

Piaget, J. (1926/1974). (Trans. M. Gabain). *The language and thought of the child.* New York: New American Library.

Sheldon, A. (1990). Pickle fights: Gendered talk in preschool disputes. *Discourse Processes, 13,* 5–31.

References

American Speech-Language-Hearing Association Joint Subcommittee of the Executive Board on English Language Proficiency. (1998). Students and professionals who speak English with accents and nonstandard dialects: Issues and recommendations. Position statement and technical report. *Asha, 40* (suppl. 18), 28–31.

Andersen, E. (1986). The acquisition of register variation by Anglo-American children. In B. Schieffelin & E. Ochs (Eds.), *Language socialization across cultures* (pp. 153–161). New York: Cambridge University Press.

Andersen, E. (1990). *Speaking with style: The sociolinguistic skills of children.* New York: Routledge.

Austin, A., Salehi, M., & Leffler, A. (1987). Gender and developmental differences in children's conversations. *Sex Roles, 16,* 497–510.

Austin, J. L. (1975). *How to do things with words.* Cambridge, MA: Harvard University Press.

Bailey, G., & Thomas, E. (1998). Some aspects of African-American Vernacular English phonology. In S. Mufwene, J. Rickford, G. Bailey, & J. Baugh (Eds.), *African-American English: Structure, history, and use* (pp. 85–109). London: Routledge.

Barton, M., & Tomasello, M. (1991). Joint attention and conversation in mother–infant–sibling triads. *Child Development, 62,* 517–529.

Barton, M., & Tomasello, M. (1994). The rest of the family: The role of fathers and siblings in early language development. In C. Gallaway & B. Richards (Eds.), *Input and interaction in language acquisition* (pp. 109–134). New York: Cambridge University Press.

Battle, D. (1996). Language learning and use by African American children. *Topics in Language Disorders, 16,* 22–37.

Battle, D. (1998). (Ed.), *Communication disorders in multicultural populations.* Boston: Butterworth-Heinemann.

Battle, D., & Anderson, N. (1998). Culturally diverse families and the development of language. In D. Battle (Ed.), *Communication disorders in multicultural populations* (pp. 213–245). Boston: Butterworth-Heinemann.

Becker, J. (1982). Children's strategic use of requests to mark and manipulate social status. In S. Kuczaj (Ed.), *Language development: Language, thought, and culture* (pp. 1–35). Hillsdale, NJ: Lawrence Erlbaum Associates.

Becker, J. (1984). Implications of ethology for the study of pragmatic development. In S. Kuczaj (Ed.), *Discourse development* (pp. 1–17). New York: Springer-Verlag.

Becker, J. (1986). Bossy and nice requests: Children's production and interpretation. *Merrill-Palmer Quarterly, 32,* 393–413.

Becker, J. (1988). The success of parents' indirect techniques for teaching their preschoolers pragmatic skills. *First Language, 8,* 173–181.

Becker, J. (1990). Processes in the acquisition of pragmatic competence. In G. Conti-Ramsden & C. Snow (Eds.), *Children's language* (Vol. 2, pp. 7–24). Hillsdale, NJ: Lawrence Erlbaum Associates.

Becker, J. (1994). Pragmatic socialization: Parental input to preschoolers. *Discourse Processes, 17 ,* 131–148

Becker, J., & Hall, M. (1989). Adult beliefs about pragmatic development. *Journal of Applied Developmental Psychology, 10,* 1–17.

Becker, J., Place, K., Tenzer, S., & Frueh, C. (1991). Teachers' impressions of children varying in pragmatic skills. *Journal of Applied Developmental Psychology, 12,* 397–412.

Berko Gleason, J. (1975). Fathers and other strangers: Men's speech to young children. In D. Dato (Ed.), *Developmental psycholinguistics: Theory and applications. Georgetown University Roundtable on Language and Linguistics* (pp. 289–297). Washington, DC: Georgetown University Press.

Berko Gleason, J., Hay, D., & Cain, L. (1989). Social and affective determinants of language acquisition. In M. Rice & R. Schiefelbusch (Eds.), *The teachability of language* (pp. 171–186). Baltimore: Paul H. Brookes.

Berko Gleason, J., Perlmann, R., & Greif, E. (1984). What's the magic word: Learning language through politeness routines. *Discourse Processes, 7,* 493–502.

Berko Gleason, J., & Weintraub, S. (1976). The acquisition of routines in child language. *Language in Society, 5,* 129–136.

Black, B., & Hazen, N. (1990). Social status and patterns of communication in acquainted and unacquainted preschool children. *Developmental Psychology, 26,* 379–387.

Black, B., & Logan, A. (1995). Links between communication patterns in mother–child, father–child, and child–peer interactions and children's social status. *Child Development, 66,* 255–271.

Blum-Kulka, S. (1990). You don't touch lettuce with your fingers: Parental politeness in family discourse. *Journal of Pragmatics, 14,* 259–288.

Blum-Kulka, S. (1997). *Dinner talk: Cultural patterns of sociability and socialization in family discourse.* Mahwah, NJ: Lawrence Erlbaum Associates.

Boggs, S. (1985). *Speaking, relating, and learning: A study of Hawaiian children at home and at school.* Norwood, NJ: Ablex.

Brinton, B., & Fujiki, M. (1995). Conversational intervention with children with specific language impairment. In M. Fey, J. Windsor, & S. Warren (Eds.), *Language intervention: Preschool through the elementary years* (Vol. 5, Communication and Language Intervention Series, pp. 183–212). Baltimore, MD: Paul H. Brookes.

Brown, R. (1973). *A first language: The early stages.* Cambridge, MA: Harvard University Press.

Bruner, J. (1974/75). From communication to language: A psychological perspective. *Cognition, 3 ,* 255–287.

Bruner, J. (1975). The ontogenesis of speech acts. *Journal of Child Language, 2,* 1–19.

Bryant, J. B. (1999). Perspectives on pragmatic socialization. In A. Greenhill (Ed.), *Proceedings of the 23rd Annual Boston University Conference on Language Development* (Vol. 1, pp. 132–137). Somerville, MA: Cascadilla Press.

Burleson, B., Delia, J., & Applegate, J. (1992). Effects of maternal communication and children's social-cognitive and communication skills on children's acceptance by the peer group. *Family Relations, 41,* 264–272.

Chall, J., & Curtis, M. (1991). Responding to individual differences among language learners: Children at risk. In J. Flood, J. Jensen, D. Lapp, & J. Squire (Eds.), *Handbook of research on teaching the English language arts* (pp. 349–720). New York: MacMillan.

Cole, K. (1995). Curriculum models and language facilitation in the preschool years. In M. Fey, J. Windsor, & S. Warren (Eds.), *Language intervention: Preschool through the elementary years* (Vol. 5, Communication and Language Intervention Series, pp. 39–60). Baltimore, MD: Paul H. Brookes.

Cook, A., Fritz, J., McCornack, B., & Visperas, C. (1985). Early gender differences in the functional usage of language. *Sex Roles, 12,* 909–915.

Corsaro, W. (1979). Young children's conception of status and role. *Sociology of Education, 52,* 46–59.

Crago, M. (1994). Ethnography and language socialization: A cross-cultural perspective. In K. Butler (Ed.), *Cross-cultural perspectives in language assessment and intervention* (pp. 3–14). Gaithersburg, MD: Aspen. (Reprinted from *Topics in Language Disorders,* 1992, *12 (3),* 28–39.)

Crago, M., & Cole, E. (1991). Using ethnography to bring children's communicative and cultural worlds into focus. In T. Gallagher (Ed.), *Pragmatics of language: Clinical practice issues* (pp. 99–131). San Diego, CA: Singular Publishing Group.

Crago, M., & Eriks-Brophy, A. (1994). Culture, conversation, and interaction: Implications for intervention. In J. Duchan & R. Sonnenmeier (Eds.), *Pragmatics: From theory to practice* (pp. 43–58). Englewood Cliffs, NJ: Prentice Hall.

Craig, H., & Washington, J. (1993). Access behaviors of children with specific language impairment. *Journal of Speech and Hearing Research, 36,* 322–337.

Creaghead, N., & Tattershall, S. (1985). Observation and assessment of classroom pragmatic skills. In C. Simon (Ed.), *Communication skills and classroom success* (pp. 105–127). San Diego, CA: College-Hill Press.

Davidson, R., & Snow, C. (1996). Five-year-olds' interactions with fathers versus mothers. *First Language, 16,* 223–242.

DeHart, G. (1996). Gender and mitigation in 4-year-olds' pretend play talk with siblings. *Research on Language and Social Interaction, 29,* 81–96.

Demuth, K. (1986). Prompting routines in the language socialization of Basotho children. In B. Schieffelin & E. Ochs (Eds.), *Language socialization across cultures* (pp. 51–79). New York: Cambridge University Press.

Dodge, K., Schlundt, D., Schocken, I., & Delugach, J. (1983). Social competence and children's sociometric status: The role of peer group entry strategies. *Monographs of the Society for Research in Child Development, 5* (Serial No. 213).

Donahue, M. (1985). Communicative style in learning disabled students: Some implications for classroom discourse. In D. Ripich & F. Spinelli (Eds.), *School discourse problems* (pp. 97–124). San Diego, CA: College-Hill Press.

Dunn, J., & Shatz, M. (1989). Becoming a conversationalist despite (or because of) having an older sibling. *Child Development, 60,* 399–410.

Edelsky, C. (1977). Acquisition of an aspect of communicative competence: Learning what it means to talk like a lady. In S. Ervin-Tripp & C. Mitchell-Kernan (Eds.), *Child discourse* (pp. 225–243). New York: Academic Press.

Eisenberg, A. (1982). Understanding components of a situation: Spontaneous use of politeness routines by Mexicano two-year-olds. *Papers and Reports on Child Language Development, 21,* 46–54.

Ely, R., & Berko Gleason, J. (1995). Socialization across cultures. In P. Fletcher & B. MacWhinney (Eds.), *The handbook of child language* (pp. 251–276). Cambridge, MA: Blackwell.

Erickson, F., & Shultz, J. (1981). When is a context? Some issues and methods in the analysis of social competence. In J. Green & C. Wallat (Eds.), *Ethnography and language in educational settings* (pp. 147–160). Norwood, NJ: Ablex.

Ervin-Tripp, S. (1974). The comprehension and production of requests by children. *Papers and Reports on Child Language Development, 8,* 188–196.

Ervin-Tripp, S. (1976). Is Sybil there? The structure of some American English directives. *Language in Society, 5,* 25–66.

Ervin-Tripp, S. (1977). Wait for me, roller skate! In S. Ervin-Tripp & C. Mitchell-Kernan (Eds.), *Child discourse* (pp. 165–188). New York: Academic Press.

Ervin-Tripp, S. (1979). Children's verbal turn-taking. In E. Ochs & B. Schieffelin (Ed.), *Developmental pragmatics* (pp. 391–413). New York: Academic.

Ervin-Tripp, S., Strage, A., Lampert, M., & Bell, N. (1987). Understanding requests. *Linguistics, 25,* 107–143.

Ferrier, L. (1978). Some observations of error in context. In N. Waterson & C. Snow (Eds.), *The development of communication* (pp. 301–309). New York: Wiley.

Fivush, R. (1983). Negotiating classroom interaction. *The Quarterly Newsletter of the Laboratory of Comparative Human Cognition, 5,* 83–87.

Gallagher, T. (1991). Language and social skills: Implications for assessment and intervention with school-age children. In T. Gallagher (Ed.), *Pragmatics of language: Clinical practice issues* (pp. 11–41). San Diego, CA: Singular Publishing Group.

Garvey, C. (1975). Requests and responses in children's speech. *Journal of Child Language, 2,* 41–63.

Garvey, C. (1984). *Children's talk.* Cambridge, MA: Harvard University Press.

Garvey, C. (1990). *Play* (2nd ed.). Cambridge, MA: Harvard University Press.

Gelman, R., & Shatz, M. (1977). Appropriate speech adjustments: The operation of conversational constraints on talk to two-year-olds. In M. Lewis & L. Rosenblum (Eds.), *Interaction, conversation, and the development of language* (pp. 27–61). New York: Wiley.

Gertner, B., Rice, M., & Hadley, P. (1994). Influence of communicative competence on peer preferences in a preschool classroom. *Journal of Speech and Hearing Research, 37,* 913–923.

Gillam, R., McFadden, T., & van Kleeck, A. (1995). Improving narrative abilities: Whole language and language skills approaches. In M. Fey, J. Windsor, & S. Warren (Eds.), *Language intervention: Preschool through the elementary years* (Vol. 5, Communication and Language Intervention Series; pp. 145–182). Baltimore, MD: Paul H. Brookes.

Ginsburg, H., & Opper, S. (1988). *Piaget's theory of intellectual development* (3rd Ed.). Englewood Cliffs, NJ: Prentice Hall.

Glucksberg, S., & Krauss, R. (1967). What do people say after they have learned how to talk? Studies of the development of referential communication. *Merrill-Palmer Quarterly, 13,* 309–316.

Glucksberg, S., Krauss, R., & Weisberg, R. (1966). Referential communication in nursery school children: Method and some preliminary findings. *Journal of Experimental Child Psychology, 3,* 333–342.

Goelman, H. (1996). Literate apprenticeships and oral discourse. In K. Reeder, J. Shapiro, R. Watson, & H. Goelman (Eds.), *Literate apprenticeships: The emergence of language and literacy in the preschool years* (pp. 101–118). Norwood, NJ: Ablex.

Goodman, G., Duchan, J., & Sonnenmeier, R. (1994). Children's development of scriptal knowledge. In J. Duchan & R. Sonnenmeier (Eds.), *Pragmatics: From theory to practice* (pp. 120–133). Englewood Cliffs, NJ: Prentice Hall.

Gopnik, A., & Meltzoff, A. (1986). Words, plans, things, and locations: Interactions between semantic and cognitive development in the one-word stage. In S. Kuczaj & M. Barrett (Eds.), *The development of word meaning* (pp. 199–223). New York: Springer-Verlag.

Gordon, D., & Ervin-Tripp, S. (1984). The structure of children's requests. In R. Schiefelbusch & J. Pickar (Eds.), *The acquisition of communicative competence* (Vol. VIII: Language Intervention Series; pp. 295–321). Baltimore, MD: University Park Press.

Greif, E., & Berko Gleason, J. (1980). Hi, thanks, and goodbye: More routine information. *Language in Society, 9,* 159–166.

Hall, W. (1976). Black and white children's responses to Black English Vernacular and Standard English sentences: Evidence for code-switching. In D. Harrison & T. Trabasso (Eds.), *Black English: A seminar* (pp. 201–208). Hillsdale, NJ: Erlbaum.

Harris, G. (1998). American Indian cultures: A lesson in diversity. In D. Battle (Ed.), *Communication disorders in multicultural populations* (pp. 117–156). Boston, MA: Butterworth-Heinemann.

Hazen, N., & Black, B. (1989). Preschool peer communication skills: The role of social status and interaction context. *Child Development, 60,* 867–876.

Heath, S. (1983). *Ways with words.* Cambridge: Cambridge University Press.

Hoff-Ginsberg, E. (1998). The relation of birth order and socioeconomic status to children's language experience and language development. *Applied Psycholinguistics, 19,* 603–629.

Hoff-Ginsberg, E., & Krueger, W. (1991). Older siblings as conversational partners. *Merrill-Palmer Quarterly, 37,* 465–482.

Hymes, D. (1967). Models of the interaction of language and social setting. *Journal of Social Issues, 23 (2),* 8–28.

Iglesias, A. (1985). Cultural conflict in the classroom: The communicationally different child. In D. Ripich & F. Spinelli (Eds.), *School discourse problems* (pp. 79–96). San Diego, CA: College-Hill Press.

James, S. (1978). Effect of listener age and situation on the politeness of children's directives. *Journal of Psycholinguistic Research, 7,* 307–317.

Killen, M., & Naigles, L. (1995). Preschool children pay attention to their addressees: Effects of gender composition on peer disputes. *Discourse Processes, 19,* 329–346.

Leaper, C. (1991). Influence and involvement in children's discourse: Age, gender, and partner effects. *Child Development, 62,* 797–811.

Leaper, C., Anderson, K., & Sanders, P. (1998). Moderators of gender effects on parents' talk to their children: A meta-analysis. *Developmental Psychology, 34,* 3–27.

Leonard, L., Wilcox, J., Fulmer, K., & Davis, A. (1978). Understanding indirect requests: An investigation of children's comprehension of pragmatic meanings. *Journal of Speech and Hearing Research, 21,* 528–537.

Lewis, C. (1997). Fathers and preschoolers. In M. Lamb (Ed.), *The role of fathers in child development* (pp. 121–142). New York: John Wiley and Sons.

Linguistic Society of America (1999). LSA resolution on the Oakland "Ebonics" issue [Online]. Available: http://www.lsadc.org/ebonics.html.

Loveland, K. (1984). Learning about points of view: Spatial perspective and the acquisition of "I/you." *Journal of Child Language, 11,* 535–556.

Malcolm, I. (1979). The West Australian Aboriginal child and classroom interaction: A sociolinguistic approach. *Journal of Pragmatics, 3,* 305–320.

Malcolm, I. (1982). Speech events in the Aboriginal classroom. *International Journal of the Sociology of Language, 36,* 115–134.

Malone, M. J., & Guy, R. (1982). A comparison of mothers' and fathers' speech to their three-year-old sons. *Journal of Psycholinguistic Research, 11,* 599–608.

Mannle, S., Barton, M., & Tomasello, M. (1991). Two-year-olds' conversations with their mothers and preschool-aged siblings. *First Language, 12,* 57–71.

Mannle, S., & Tomasello, M. (1987). Fathers, siblings, and the bridge hypothesis. In K. E. Nelson & A. van Kleeck (Eds.), *Children's language* (Vol. 6) (pp. 23–41). Hillsdale, NJ: Lawrence Erlbaum Associates.

Maratsos, M. (1973). Non-egocentric communication abilities in preschool children. *Child Development, 44,* 696–700.

Martin, S., & Wolfram, W. (1998). The sentence in African-American Vernacular English. In S. Mufwene, J. Rickford, G. Bailey, & J. Baugh (Eds.), *African-American English: Structure, history, and use* (pp. 11–36). London: Routledge.

McTear, M. (1980). Getting it done: The development of children's abilities to negotiate request sequences in peer interaction. *Belfast Working Papers in Language and Linguistics, 4,* 1–29.

Mehan, H. (1979). *Learning lessons: Social organization in the classroom.* Cambridge, MA: Harvard University Press.

Menig-Peterson, C. (1975). The modification of communicative behavior in preschool-aged children as a function of the listener's perspective. *Child Development, 46,* 1015–1018.

Miller, P., Danaher, D., & Forbes, D. (1986). Sex-related strategies for coping with interpersonal conflict in children aged five and seven. *Developmental Psychology, 22,* 543–548.

Mitchell-Kernan, C., & Kernan, K. (1977). Pragmatics of directive choice among children. In S. Ervin-Tripp & C. Mitchell-Kernan (Eds.), *Child discourse* (pp. 189–208). New York: Academic Press.

Morgan, M. (1998). More than a mood or an attitude: Discourse and verbal genres in African-American culture. In S. Mufwene, J. Rickford, G. Bailey, & J. Baugh (Eds.), *African-American English: Structure, history, and use* (pp. 251–281). London: Routledge.

Mufwene, S., & Rickford, J. (1998). Introduction. In S. Mufwene, J. Rickford, G. Bailey, & J. Baugh (Eds.), *African-American English: Structure, history, and use* (pp. 1–7). London: Routledge.

Ninio, A., & Snow, C. (1996). *Pragmatic development.* Boulder, CO: Westview Press.

Patterson, C., & Kister, M. (1981). The development of listener skills for referential communication. In W. P. Dickson (Ed.), *Children's oral communication skills* (pp. 143–166). New York: Academic.

Pellegrini, A., Brody, G., & Stoneman, Z. (1987). Children's conversational competence with their parents. *Discourse Processes, 10,* 93–106.

Philips, S. (1970). Acquisition of rules for appropriate speech usage. In J. Alatis (Ed.), *Report of the 21st Annual Round Table Meeting on Linguistics and Language Studies: Bilingualism and language contact: Anthropological, linguistic, psychological, and sociological aspects* (pp. 77–101). Washington, DC: Georgetown University Press.

Piaget, J. (1926/1974) (Trans. M. Gabain). *The language and thought of the child.* New York, New York: New American Library.

Pinnell, G., & Jaggar, A. (1991). Oral language: Speaking and listening in the classroom. In J. Flood, J. Jensen, D. Lapp, & J. Squire (Eds.), *Handbook of research on teaching the English language arts* (pp. 691–720). New York: MacMillan.

Place, K., & Becker, J. (1991). The influence of pragmatic competence on the likeability of grade-school children. *Discourse Processes, 14,* 227–241.

Putallaz, M., & Gottman, J. (1981). An interactional model of children's entry strategies into peer groups. *Child Development, 52,* 986–994.

Rabain-Jamin, J. (1998). Polyadic language socialization strategy: The case of toddlers in Senegal. *Discourse Processes, 26,* 43–65.

Reeder, K., & Shapiro, J. (1996). A portrait of the literate apprentice. In K. Reeder, J. Shapiro, R. Watson, & H. Goelman (Eds.) (1996). *Literate apprenticeships: The emergence of language and literacy in the preschool years* (pp. 119–133). Norwood, NJ: Ablex.

Reeder, K., & Shapiro, J. (1997). Children's attributions of pragmatic intentions and early literacy. *Language Awareness, 6,* 17–31.

Reeder, K., Shapiro, J., Watson, R., & Goelman, H. (Eds.) (1996). *Literate apprenticeships: The emergence of language and literacy in the preschool years.* Norwood, NJ: Ablex.

Rice, M. (1993a). "Don't talk to him; he's weird": A social consequences account of language and social interaction. In A. Kaiser & D. Gray (Eds.), *Enhancing children's communication: Research foundations for intervention* (pp. 139–158). Baltimore: Paul H. Brookes.

Rice, M. (1993b). Social consequences of specific language impairment. In H. Grimm & H. Skowronek (Eds.), *Language acquisition problems and reading disorders: Aspects of diagnosis and intervention* (pp. 111–128). New York: Walter de Gruyter.

Robinson, E. J. (1981). The child's understanding of inadequate messages and communication failure: A problem of ignorance or egocentrism? In W. P. Dickson (Ed.), *Children's oral communication skills* (pp. 167–188). New York: Academic.

Romaine, S. (1984). *The language of children and adolescents.* New York: Basil Blackwell.

Rondal, J. (1980). Fathers' and mothers' speech in early language development. *Journal of Child Language, 7,* 353–369.

Rubin, K., Bukowski, W., & Parker, J. (1998). Peer interactions, relationships, and groups. In W. Damon (Series Ed.) & N. Eisenberg (Vol. Ed.), *Handbook of child psychology: Vol. 3. Social, emotional, and personality development* (5th ed., pp. 619–700). New York: Wiley.

Rubin, Z. (1980). *Children's friendships.* Cambridge, MA: Harvard University Press.

Sachs, J. (1987). Preschool boys' and girls' language use in pretend play. In S. Philips, S. Steele, & C. Tanz (Ed.), *Language, gender, and sex in comparative perspectives* (pp. 178–188). Cambridge: Cambridge University Press.

Sachs, J., & Devin, J. (1976). Young children's use of age-appropriate speech styles in social interaction and role playing. *Journal of Child Language, 3,* 81–98.

Schieffelin, B., & Eisenberg, A. (1984). Cultural variation in children's conversations. In R. Schiefelbusch & J. Pickar (Ed.), *The acquisition of communicative competence* (pp. 377–420). Baltimore, MD: University Park Press.

Schieffelin, B., & Ochs, E. (1986). (Eds.). *Language socialization across cultures.* New York: Cambridge University Press.

Schieffelin, B., & Ochs, E. (1996). The microgenesis of competence: Methodology in language socialization. In D. Slobin, J. Gerhardt, A. Kyratzis, & J. Guo (Eds.), *Social interaction, social context, and language: Essays in honor of Susan Ervin-Tripp* (pp. 251–263). Mahwah, NJ: Erlbaum.

Shatz, M. (1978). Children's comprehension of their mothers' question directives. *Journal of Child Language, 5,* 39–46.

Shatz, M., & Gelman, R. (1973). The development of communication skills: Modifications in the speech of young children as a function of listener. *Monographs of the Society for Research in Child Development, 38* (5, Serial No. 152).

Sheldon, A. (1990). Pickle fights: Gendered talk in preschool disputes. *Discourse Processes, 13,* 5–31.

Silliman, E., & Wilkinson, L. (1991). *Communicating for learning: Classroom observation and collaboration.* Gaithersburg, MD: Aspen.

Snow, C. (1977). The development of conversation between mothers and babies. *Journal of Child Language, 4,* 1–22.

Snow, C. (1994). What is so hard about learning to read? A pragmatic analysis. In J. Duchan, L. Hewitt, & R. Sonnenmeier (Eds.), *Pragmatics: From theory to practice* (pp. 164–184). Englewood Cliffs, NJ: Prentice Hall.

Snow, C. (1999). Social perspectives on the emergence of language. In B. MacWhinney (Ed.), *The emergence of language* (pp. 257–276). Mahwah, NJ: Erlbaum.

Snow, C., Perlmann, R., Berko Gleason, J., & Hooshyar, N. (1990). Developmental perspectives on politeness: Sources of children's knowledge. *Journal of Pragmatics, 14,* 289–305.

Tanz, C. (1980). *Studies in the acquisition of deictic terms.* New York: Cambridge University Press.

Terrell, S., Battle, D., & Grantham, R. (1998). African American cultures. In D. Battle (Ed.), *Communication disorders in multicultural populations* (pp. 31–71). Boston, MA: Butterworth-Heinemann.

Tharp, R. (1989). Psychocultural variables and constants: Effects on teaching and learning in schools. *American Psychologist, 44,* 349–359.

Tomasello, M., Conti-Ramsden, G., & Ewert, B. (1990). Young children's conversations with their mothers and fathers: Differences in breakdown and repair. *Journal of Child Language, 17,* 115–130.

Tomasello, M., & Mannle, S. (1985). Pragmatics of sibling speech to one-year-olds. *Child Development, 56,* 911–917.

Wallat, C. (1991). Child-adult interaction in home and community: Contributions to understanding literacy. In S. Silvern (Ed.), *Advances in reading/language research: Literacy through family, community, and school interaction* (Vol. 5, Series Ed. B. Hutson; pp. 1–36). Greenwich, CT: JAI Press.

Warren, A., & Tate, C. (1992). Egocentrism in children's telephone conversations. In R. Diaz & L. Berk (Eds.), *Private speech: From social interaction to self-regulation* (pp. 245–264). Hillsdale, NJ: Erlbaum.

Washington, J. (1996). Issues in assessing the language abilities of African American children. In A. Kamhi, K. Pollock, & J. Harris (Eds.), *Communication development and disorders in African American children: Research, assessment, and intervention* (pp. 35–54). Baltimore, MD: Paul H. Brooks.

Washington, J., & Craig, H. (1994). Dialectal forms during discourse of poor, urban, African American preschoolers. *Journal of Speech and Hearing Research, 37,* 816–823.

Weinert, S. (1993). Commentary on Rice: What do we know about the sequelae of socioemotional and cognitive consequences of specific language impairment? In H. Grimm & H. Skowronek (Eds.), *Language acquisition problems and reading disorders: Aspects of diagnosis and intervention* (pp. 129–137). New York: Walter de Gruyter.

Wilhite, M. (1983). Children's acquisition of language routines: The end-of-meal routine in Cakchiquel. *Language in Society, 12,* 47–64.

Windsor, J. (1995). Language impairment and social competence. In M. Fey, J. Windsor, & S. Warren (Eds.), *Language intervention: Preschool through the elementary years* (Vol. 5, Communication and Language Intervention Series; pp. 213–238). Baltimore, MD: Paul H. Brookes.

Wood, B., & Gardner, R. (1980). How children "get their way": Directives in communication. *Communication Education, 29,* 264–272.

Woollett, A. (1986). The influence of older siblings on the language environment of young children. *British Journal of Developmental Psychology, 4,* 235–245.

Wyatt, T. (1995). Language development in African American English child speech. *Linguistics and Education, 7,* 7–22.

Wyatt, T., & Seymour, H. (1990). The implications of code-switching in Black English speakers. *Equity & Excellence, 24,* 17–18.

Chapter 7

Theoretical Approaches to Language Acquisition

John N. Bohannon III
Butler University

John D. Bonvillian
University of Virginia

Developmental psycholinguists have been accumulating facts about language acquisition for almost forty years. Unfortunately, theory construction has lagged behind data collection. In fact, some researchers have described the process of language acquisition as seeming "magic" (Bloom, 1983) or "mysterious" (Gleitman & Wanner, 1982). Perhaps constructing a general theory of language development is hindered by the broad scope of "language" behavior. The breadth of this book illustrates this complexity. "Language" includes phonology, semantics, syntax, and pragmatics. There are few explanatory developmental principles common to all these domains. A true theory of how language develops should organize the facts from these varied sources, generate testable hypotheses, and provide an explanation of the acquisition process. It appears that none of the existing "theories" qualifies according to these requirements.

Another reason many have despaired of organizing the current mass of data is that some of the facts appear to be contradictory or even irrelevant to particular research issues. Researchers, therefore, have typically focused upon narrowly circumscribed problems within each area (phonology, semantics, etc.). This has allowed limited explanations specific to the problem without reference to broader issues. Other researchers have devised models of the language acquisition process (e.g., MacWhinney, 1987, 1989; Pinker, 1994; Wexler & Culicover, 1980). A model differs from a theory in that it is an analogy based upon some known mechanism. A model describes a process by simulation, invoking similarities between some already understood process and the phenomenon under investigation. For example, computers are often used to model the human memory system.

Chomsky (1957, 1965) proposed that descriptions, models, and theories are all part of an overall taxonomy of theoretical adequacy.

Descriptive adequacy, Chomsky's first level, requires cataloging all behaviors relevant to language and distinguishing them from nonlanguage behaviors. Language acquisition research has made progress towards this descriptive goal. On the other hand, children's language is creative and, potentially, infinitely variable. Therefore, an exhaustive list of all possible language productions, even from children, might be impossible to complete. Even if an exhaustive list existed, it would lack explanatory power, conveying little understanding of the mechanisms that produced the behavior.

Model adequacy, the second level, is achieved when some finite number of unifying principles are identified that account for the appearance of the various language behaviors. These principles predict the known facts of development, but are not necessarily the principles by which language-learning children actually operate. This second level is, in fact, theoretical modeling such as learnability approaches. Most grammars written from transcripts of children's speech are attempts to determine the rules that account for the observed data. However, few researchers would insist that their grammars are the actual rules children use when speaking or understanding speech.

Theoretical adequacy, the last and most ambitious level, is achieved when a finite set of principles is discovered that not only accounts for all the language behaviors observed, but also is the actual set of mechanisms used by language-learning children; the principles have psychological reality for the speakers.

A theory of language acquisition must explain not only why children say what they do, but also why they eventually speak like adults. This developmental perspective obviously presents researchers with additional concerns. Derwing (1973) argued that any theory of adult language would be inadequate if it did not include the developmental implications of the theory. In contrast, Gleitman and Wanner (1982) argued that any theory of child language would be similarly impaired unless it took mature language behavior as its ultimate goal. The trouble with the current state of affairs is that few can agree on what either adults or children are doing when they speak and understand (Gleitman & Wanner, 1982; Ritchie & Bhatia, 1999).

Distinguishing Features of Theoretical Approaches

Despite the bleak picture presented above, language acquisition research and speculation goes on undiminished. These speculations may be grouped into several general theoretical approaches to the problem. The rest of this chapter will attempt to outline these competing approaches and compare them on some critical features relevant to their explanations of both steady-state language behavior and language development. These features include emphasis on: (1) **structuralism** or **functionalism,** (2) **competence** or **performance,** and (3) **nativism** or **empiricism.**

In addition, the methods and relevant data for each approach will be considered. It is important to note that the distinctions to be described are, in a sense, artificially bipolar dimensions. As will be apparent, some of the extreme positions are complementary rather than truly opposite (see Zimmerman & Whitehurst, 1979, or Segal, 1977, for a discussion of structuralism versus functionalism). However, these features should facilitate recognition of critical similarities and differences between various approaches, thus providing a clearer picture.

Structuralism Versus Functionalism

A *structural* description of behavior attempts to discover *invariant* processes or mechanisms underlying observable data. Chomsky's rules of grammar and Watson's stimulus-response bonds are examples of structures that are used to explain observable behavior. *Functional* accounts of behavior seek to establish predictive *relationships* between environmental or situational variables and language. The aim of a functional account of language is the prediction and control of verbal behavior in different contexts and individuals.

The structural-functional distinction may be illustrated by the following example. If a child said, "I want milk," structuralists would analyze the form of the utterance, finding it to be composed of a subject (*I*), a main verb (*want*), and an object (*milk*). They might then take this sentence as evidence that the child knows the English word-order rule governing active, declarative sentences (i.e., subject-verb-object). Knowledge of this rule should enable the child to create an unlimited number of similar sentences from it. Functionalists would examine the situation in which the utterance "I want milk" occurred. They might determine that this particular utterance, if said in the presence of the mother, frequently yields a glass of milk. The utterance is jointly determined by the context (presence of mother) and its result (receiving a glass of milk). Notice that in this case, structuralists and functionalists are describing different aspects of language behavior, the former accounting for syntax and the latter explaining the pragmatic, social use of language. These perspectives are complementary, and both are necessary to fully explain the child's language behavior.

Competence Versus Performance

Competence refers to the individual's knowledge of language, or the underlying rules that may be deduced from language behavior. *Performance* refers to actual language use. In other words, competence and performance refer to the individual's abstract linguistic knowledge and to the use of this knowledge. For example, mature speakers of English might slip and say, "She will be home yesterday," although they know that such an utterance is ill formed. Mistakes of this type are typically attributed to performance problems such as lapses of attention or memory, rather than to a basic ignorance of the rules of English grammar. The concept of competence is important to linguists; for instance, one must be very careful that the utterances used for determining grammatical rules are not cluttered with performance mistakes. For this reason, many researchers use judgments of grammaticality rather than language use to infer a speaker's linguistic competence (e.g. de Villiers & de Villiers, 1972; Gleitman, Gleitman, & Shipley, 1972). In addition, note that only structuralists are typically concerned with competence, since functionalists are more concerned with particular instances of language use (performance).

Nativism Versus Empiricism

The third dimension along which theories differ concerns the emphasis placed upon either the child or the environment in the process of language acquisition. This is another example of the old nature–nurture issue. On the one side, nativists insist that language is too complex and is acquired too rapidly to have been learned through any known methods (e.g., **imitation**), so some critical aspects of the language system must be innate. By contrast, empiricists place most of the responsibility for language acquisition upon environmental agents. Proponents of this view feel that language is not essentially different from any other behavior. Therefore, it is learned like any other behavior and subject to all the laws and principles of learning derived from the study of simpler behaviors and simpler organisms.

Language researchers typically do not adhere strictly to either extreme position on the nativist-empiricist continuum. Few will disagree that language acquisition is determined both by children's innate capacities and their linguistic experiences. The course of early development is too invariant across many languages and contexts not to have some innate component. Similarly, children with no linguistic experience, such as normal children of deaf parents (Sachs & Johnson, 1976), do not learn to speak. Despite the necessity of both factors, rarely are they given equal explanatory credit.

Evaluating Research Methods

The major approaches to language acquisition may also be compared with respect to the methods frequently used and the data that each theory attempts to explain. The theoretical inclinations of researchers usually determine the data and methods they consider relevant. Unfortunately, this sometimes leads to a complete separation of research efforts, with one group pursuing longitudinal observations of the changing grammars of a small number of children, and others performing experiments on sizable groups of children to change the frequency of occurrence of particular verbal behaviors. The developmental perspective and the subjects chosen for study also depend on the researchers' theoretical views. For example, those who hold that language is uniquely human, largely maturational, and composed of syntactic structures would observe maturing grammars in human children. Studies of adults or nonhuman subjects would be considered irrelevant, and experimentation fruitless. By contrast, those who believe that language differs little from other motor activities and is learned in much the same way might try to reinforce communicative behavior in chimpanzees.

Is any agreement possible when the theoretical approaches differ so drastically? In any scientific endeavor, diversification of research methods and strategies should ultimately lead to **convergent validity.** That is, the more one examines a problem from different angles, the more likely it is that a solution will be discovered. Moreover, the broad range of language behavior needing explanation (phonology, semantics, etc.) may require just as much diversity to answer all the resulting questions. These points justify the hope that some unifying principles will be discovered, despite the splintered nature of current language development research.

In the sections to follow, some of the competing approaches offering explanations of language acquisition will be outlined. They are organized into three main groups, the behavioral, linguistic, and interactionist. The interactionist position is further subdivided into the cognitive interactionist approach and the social interactionist approach. Each area will be outlined according to the distinctions previously delineated (e.g., structural-functional). Finally, a brief evaluation of all the approaches will be presented, in order to highlight the strengths and weaknesses of each.

Behavioral Approaches

General Assumptions

There are many different hypotheses concerning language acquisition that come under the general heading of behaviorism. In spite of their differences, all share a common focus on the observable and measurable aspects of language behavior. Whenever possible, behaviorists avoid mentalistic explanations of language behavior that rely on such constructs as intentions or "implicit knowledge" of grammatical rules. Because these mental processes are not easily defined nor accessible for measurement, behaviorists search for observable environmental conditions (stimuli) that co-occur and predict specific verbal behaviors (responses). Behaviorists do not deny the existence of internal mechanisms. They recognize that overt behavior has an internal physiological base, and that research into these physiological processes is necessary for a better understanding of behavior (for example, the relationship between language dysfunction and specific brain structures; see Menn & Obler, 1990). What behaviorists reject are internal structures or processes with no specific physical correlate, such as grammars (Zimmerman & Whitehurst, 1979).

Clearly, behaviorists emphasize performance over competence. In fact, few behaviorists acknowledge the existence of competence or any knowledge that is separate from observable behavior. Eschewing the structure of language, behaviorists focus on the functions of language, the stimuli that evoke verbal behavior, and the consequences of language performance. Skinner (1957) argued that behavioral psycholinguists should search for functional language units as they naturally occur, and then discover the functional relationships that predict their occurrence. He viewed linguistic approaches as irrelevant to this task.

Behaviorists also focus on learning because they regard language as a skill, not essentially different from any other behavior. For example, Watson (1924) stated that "Language as we ordinarily understand it, in spite of its complexities, is in the beginning a very simple type of behavior. It is really a manipulative habit." Skinner (1957) argued that language is a special case of behavior only because it is behavior that is reinforced exclusively by other organisms. Apart from the effect that language has on someone else, verbal behavior does not produce any reinforcement in and of itself.

The emphasis on learning places behaviorists toward the empirical end of the nativism–empiricism continuum. Although they admit that humans have specialized physiological structures (e.g., fine motor control of the lips, tongue, larynx, etc.) that allow them to speak, speaking is assumed to be learned through the same principles that rats learn to run mazes. Speaking (and understanding speech) must be brought under the control of stimuli in the environment by imitation, reinforcement, and successive approximations of mature performance (known as shaping). The child is typically viewed as a passive recipient of environmental pressures, much as a malleable piece of clay is molded into new shapes. Behaviorists rarely acknowledge that children, in turn, may affect their environment. In fact, Skinner (1957) states that the speakers should be considered as merely "interested bystanders," having no active role in the process of their own language behavior or development.

Behavioristic Language Learning

One of the simplest ways of explaining changes in behavior is through the connection or association of stimuli in the environment and certain responses of the organism. The process of forming such associations is known as **classical conditioning** (see Chapter 4). The associations formed between external verbal stimuli and internal responses are often cited as the source of word meanings (Staats, 1971). For example, a child may learn the word milk in the following manner: Milk fed to a hungry infant causes physiological responses in the infant. The milk itself is the unconditioned stimulus (UCS) and the physiological response is the unconditioned response (UCR). When the infant's mother says the word milk prior to or during feeding, this word (the conditioned stimulus, or CS) becomes associated with the primary stimulus of the milk and gradually the word acquires the power to elicit a conditioned response (CR) in the child that is similar to the response to the milk itself.

Once a CS (a word) has come to elicit a CR, it can then be used as a UCS to modify the response to another CS. For example, if a new CS, such as the word bottle, frequently occurs with the word milk, the new word may come to elicit a CR similar to the response to milk. The associations formed between several stimuli (CSs) and a single response lead to the formation of associations between the stimuli themselves. Thus, not only may arbitrary verbal CSs be associated with specific internal meanings (CRs), but the words themselves may be connected by stimulus–stimulus associations. In this way, classical conditioning is used to account for the interrelationship of words and word meanings.

Whereas behaviorists use the principles of classical conditioning to account for the child's development of receptive vocabulary, additional learning principles must be invoked to explain productive speech. **Operant conditioning** is the form of learning most often used to fill this role (Moerk, 1983; Mowrer, 1960; Osgood, 1953; Staats, 1971). Operant conditioning concerns changes in voluntary, nonreflexive behavior that arise due to environmental consequences contingent upon that behavior. Simply put, behaviors that most frequently result in rewards tend to be repeated, whereas behaviors that are ignored or result in punishment tend to vanish. All behavioristic accounts of language acquisition assume that children's productive speech is shaped by by environmental agents (e.g., parents). Behaviorists assume that children's speech that more closely approximates adult speech is rewarded, whereas meaningless or inappropriate speech is ignored or punished. Gradually, the response unit will change from simple sounds to whole words as the parents change their reinforcement practices, eventually restricting rewards to only those utterances that are meaningful and adultlike.

Behaviorists assume that throughout development, children's caretakers industriously train children to perform verbal behaviors, usually after the parent has provided an example: "Say bye-bye. Bye-bye." In this way, the adult provides the child with both mature speech exemplars and training in imitation, another form of learning. When children successfully imitate what the adult just pronounced, the children are rewarded. In addition, the word dog is provided in the presence of dogs, boy in the presence of boys, and so on. Thus, the acquisition of both receptive and productive vocabulary begins to accelerate as all the types of learning—classical, operant, and imitative—converge to direct and control the child's language behavior. Behaviorists assume that the course of language development is largely determined by the course of training, not maturation.

Children's word combinations are assumed to be acquired in much the same ways as single words. Parents teach simple word combinations through **shaping** and imitation training, rewarding successive approximations to adultlike word strings. Some behaviorists explain these word combinations as response chains, with the first word and current context serving as a stimulus for the second word, which with the context serves as a stimulus for the next word, and so forth. These word chains are also known as *Markov models of sentences* (Mowrer, 1960). Some theorists (Osgood, 1953, 1963) include internal stimuli within the system that may alter the chain by eliciting different overt responses, but they are, in essence, still Markov models. Clearly, the child need not have heard every possible chain or string of words in order to produce and understand them. It is only necessary for the child to have associations between pairs of words, between individual words and the environmental context, and between words and possible internal mediating stimuli.

Behavioral interpretations assume increasing complexity in the response unit. Just as sounds were shaped into words in infancy, such that words become the functional response unit, combinations of words come to serve as new, larger response units. Whitehurst (1982) argues that some word patterns (e.g., the boy's shoe, the boy's bike, the boy's dog) become grammatical frames (the boy's X), where insertion of novel lexical items with similar properties is allowed (the boy's toothbrush). It should be noted, however, that most behaviorists do not view such grammatical frames as true grammatical rules, since children are not explicitly aware of them.

The basic processes of learning (i.e., classical and operant conditioning) are assumed to direct and control the increasing complexity of children's verbal behavior. These processes continue to function into adulthood, but the rapid rate of learning during childhood requires additional learning principles, and behaviorists rely on imitation as one especially important factor in language learning. Imitation allows a shortcut to mature behavior without the laborious shaping of each and every verbal response. Imitation may be an exact copy of observed behavior, but it is not limited to exact copies (Bandura & Walters, 1963). Through imitation children may perform behaviors that only partially resemble the modeled behavior. Whitehurst and Vasta (1975) suggest that children can acquire grammatical frames through imitation, substituting their own words appropriate to the new context in which the utterance occurs. Imitation is not limited to behaviors that immediately follow modeled behavior; imitations may occur after a considerable delay. When children successfully imitate new words and forms, behaviorists assume that reinforcement occurs, either from adults or from the children themselves. The fact that the very process of imitating becomes reinforcing in itself suggests that children will use imitation more frequently over time. Thus, imitation serves as a relatively flexible and frequently used learning strategy that enables rapid learning of complex language behaviors.

In summary, behaviorists focus on learning principles. Language development is considered to be a problem of linking various stimuli in the environment to internal responses, and these internal responses to overt verbal behavior. Language development is viewed as a progression from random verbalizations to mature communication through the application of classical and operant conditioning and imitation. The time it takes children to acquire language is seen as a limitation of the training techniques of the parents rather than maturation of the child.

Evaluation of the Behavioral Approach

Supporting Evidence

Many accounts of word meaning have shown that networks of interstimulus and stimulus–response associations of varying qualities and strength may be involved in semantics (Smith, 1978). The questions remain, though, how are these associations learned initially, and are word meanings actually acquired through these associations? Behaviorists suggest that classical conditioning is primarily responsible. Staats, Staats, and Crawford (1962) asked adult subjects to learn a list of words, during which they received intermittent electric shocks. The words that preceded the shocks eventually came to be rated as unpleasant and generated emotional reactions similar to the shock itself. Staats (1971) argued that similar conditioning processes during the course of development are responsible for the differential reactions to words, such as *horror, ugly,* and *disaster* versus *graceful, gift,* and *pretty.* Moreover, word stimuli may modify each other through occasional pairing. Staats and Staats (1957) paired nonsense syllables (GIW, WUH, etc.) with either pleasant or unpleasant words. Those syllables paired with the negative words (*ugly, bitter*) were rated significantly more unpleasant by college-age subjects than those syllables paired with positive words (*beauty, gift*). Thus, classical conditioning may alter the meanings of words.

Probably the most notable successes of the behavioral approach to language learning have taken place with mentally retarded children (Sailor, 1971) and children with autistic disorder (Lovaas, 1977). Through the careful application of such behavior modification techniques as shaping and reinforcement, many children with very limited speech skills have made considerable progress in learning to speak (Lovaas, 1977, 1987). In many instances, the gains by these behaviorally trained children contrasted markedly with records of virtually no progress for children in more traditional therapy programs. Although these findings of language gains in low-functioning children are quite impressive, it should also be recognized that the processes involved in language learning in these children may not be the same for children with normal abilities.

The effects of imitation have also been studied extensively by behaviorists (for a review see Speidel & Nelson, 1984; Whitehurst & Vasta, 1975). These studies usually involve an adult model who uses particular grammatical forms in differing sentential contexts. Unfortunately, the simple provision of novel grammatical exemplars by adult models has not yielded convincing evidence that children will always learn the modeled form (Bandura & Harris, 1966; Liebert, Odum, Hill, & Huff, 1969). Whitehurst and Novak (1973) demonstrated new grammatical forms to children under two conditions. In the first condition, an adult simply modeled the target rule for the child. The second condition involved "imitation training," which encouraged the child to try to reproduce the form. Such imitation training proved much more effective in getting the children to use the targeted linguistic rule in novel sentences.

Behaviorists have often trained adults in miniature artificial languages in attempts to model the processes involved in children's language learning. Palermo and

Eberhart (1968) asked adults to learn a language of nonsense syllables with both regular and irregular forms. Mirroring the patterns of occurrence in English, the experimental language used the irregular forms more frequently than the regular forms. The pattern of adult acquisition of the experimental language paralleled children's progress in learning English, in that the adults began using the frequent irregular forms correctly until they learned the regular rules. After discovering the regular forms, the adults overgeneralized the regular rule to the irregular items. The authors concluded that children's overgeneralizations in language were due to typical learning patterns that result from the frequency of occurrence of the materials to be learned.

Contrary Evidence

The problem with much of the research noted above concerns a very important distinction between changing existing behavior and acquiring new behaviors. Clearly, to increase adults' use of known grammatical structures is quite a different proposition from teaching children new grammatical rules. Thus, getting an adult to use more prepositions through verbal reinforcement tells us little about how children come to use prepositions in the first place. Moreover, the adults in the Palermo and Eberhart (1968) study had extensive experience with the distributional frequencies of regular and irregular verb forms in English, which may have caused the similar patterns of acquisition. In other words, the behaviorists must test their assumptions in experiments on the subjects about whom they theorize, namely children. Further, they must search for evidence of their critical factors such as shaping and reinforcement in children's natural home environments.

If a factor proven to be effective in increasing learning in the lab does not exist in the child's natural environment, then that factor cannot be relied upon to explain language acquisition. Many researchers (Morgan, 1986; Morgan, Bonamo, & Travis, 1995; Pinker, 1984, 1994; Wexler & Culicover, 1980) have argued that children are not carefully shaped and tutored in the home, regardless of the effectiveness of these techniques in the lab. McNeill (1966) cited the following example as reflecting the importance of maturation in the acquisition process:

> *Child:*   Nobody don't like me
> *Mother:*   No. Say, "Nobody likes me."
> *Child:*   Nobody don't like me.
> (Eight repetitions of the above)
> *Mother:*   Now listen carefully. Say, "Nobody likes me."
> *Child:*   Oh! Nobody don't likes me. (p. 69)

The failure of careful tutoring is clear in this instance, but this evidence is only anecdotal. Further studies of naturally occurring conversations between children and parents have drawn similar conclusions from much more data. Several studies (Brown & Hanlon, 1970; Hirsh-Pasek, Treiman, & Schneiderman, 1984; Penner, 1987) found that parents do not verbally reward or praise their children for producing grammatically correct utterances, nor do they punish them for producing ungrammatical statements. Instead, these researchers found that parents were more likely to respond positively with "Right" or "Good" when the content of an utterance was true, whether or not the utterance was syntactically appropriate. Parents were more likely to say "No" or "Wrong" when the semantic content of an utterance was false, even if it had been expressed in grammatically correct form.

The assumption that language is "just another behavior" is also seriously questioned. There is simply too much data to suggest that humans are uniquely constructed to detect language stimuli in the environment and process language information differently from other information. For instance, Condon and Sander (1974) found that newborns move in synchrony with human voices but not with other sounds. Molfese (1977) found that the brains of newborns respond asymmetrically to speech and nonspeech stimuli. He reported greater left hemisphere responses to speech sounds and greater right hemisphere responses to nonspeech sounds. In addition, human language behavior is clearly not sequentially organized into the S-R chains used to explain other behaviors (Ervin-Tripp, 1971). Sequential Markov models cannot account for the hierarchical organization and recursive nature of sentences with multiple embedded clauses (McNeill, 1966). As Miller (1965) pointed out, the total number of possible sentences in language is so great that it would be impossible to learn each one through association with a particular set of environmental stimuli.

In summary, the behavioral approach has belied its original promise of prediction and control of language behavior. Although language performance has been shown to be responsive to shaping in the laboratory, researchers are hard put to (1) find clear instances of successful tutelage in the home and (2) prove that children's language gains are equally susceptible to manipulation via reinforcement. One reason for this failure may be that behaviorists have rarely tested their assumptions in relevant contexts (i.e., with language-learning children in natural settings), thus making generalizations difficult or impossible. In spite of the major failures of the behavioral approach, it should be remembered that language acquisition is a form of behavioral change over time. As such, the study of language acquisition must incorporate some aspects of general learning mechanisms, which the behavioral approach has studied extensively. To neglect the learning approach totally would be tantamount to throwing the baby out with the bathwater.

Linguistic Approaches

General Assumptions

All linguistic approaches assume that language has a structure or grammar that is somewhat independent of language use. This independent rule system specifies the sentences that are "grammatical" or permissible in any particular language. A **grammar** is a finite set of rules, shared by all the speakers of a language; it allows the generation of an infinite set of permissible sentences. The rules of grammar are not unlike the rules that govern mathematics (e.g., associativity, commutativity, etc.), which allow the solution of an infinite number of problems with a finite set of theorems. Chomsky (1957) argued that an adequate grammar must be generative or creative in order to account for the myriad sentences that native speakers of a language can produce and understand. Adult speakers of any language can produce and understand sentences they have never said or heard before, simply by using a single grammatical rule and inserting various lexical items. Chomsky (1957) argued that a true grammar should describe the speaker's knowledge of all permissible utterances (competence) rather than just the utterances typically produced (performance).

As Chapter 5 noted, Chomsky's grammatical theory has undergone continuous revision over the years. One influential version (1982, 1988, 1999) is known as **government and binding theory (GB)**. GB includes phrase structure rules that specify the permissible constituent structures or elements of phrases. For example, S → NP + VP means that a sentence (S) may consist of a noun phrase followed by a verb phrase. There are further rules specifying the elements of the noun phrase, the verb phrase, and so on. GB also includes the lexicon, which specifies the semantic, syntactic, and phonological features of each word, as well as the thematic role the item plays in the sentence (see Chapter 5). Lexical insertion rules essentially describe the restrictions on placement of lexical items into particular phrase elements. Lexical items from the appropriate syntactic category and with the appropriate features are placed into the nodes of a phrase structure "tree" diagram, resulting in a d-structure. These d-structures may be further modified. Transformational rules, such as [move a], meaning move any part of the sentence to a new position, applied to the d-structure produce various syntactic surface forms while retaining the meaning or intent of the original. For example, the passive form of [move a] may be applied to the string *She hit me* to produce *I was hit by her.* The sentences that result after all transformational rules have been applied are called s-structures. The s-structure is the form that most closely resembles the actual utterance of a sentence. A single deep structure may be transformed into many different s-structures. Conversely, a single overt s-structure, such as *She was killed by the river,* may be produced from two different d-structures (i.e., *The river killed her,* or *Someone killed her near the river*). Thus, one of the most important tasks confronting the language-learning child is how to derive meaning from the ambiguous surface structure exemplars provided in the language environment (Gleitman & Wanner, 1982; Pinker, 1984, 1994).

Those investigators following a linguistic approach argue that language is innate in humans. In recent decades, this position has been the source of fierce controversy among child language researchers. Helping to fuel the debate is the problem that investigators differ in what they mean when they say a behavior is innate. For some, behavior is considered innate when its course of development is significantly constrained, given expected inputs from the environment (Elman, 1999). Chomsky

(1988) and many others, however, argue for a stronger nativist position. Chomsky advances the view that there is a genetically determined, biological endowment for language, and that a special capacity has evolved for grammar. This view has been interpreted as indicating that "children must therefore have built into their brain a universal grammar, a plan shared by the grammars of all natural languages" (Kandel, Schwartz, & Jessell, 1995, p. 639).

What is meant by this term Universal Grammar (UG)? According to Chomsky (1982, 1988), UG is part of the biological endowment of all human beings and consists of the principles and restrictions that hold for the structure of all human languages. UG is based on the assumption that the same symbol-processing capacities underlie all the world's languages. UG also refers to the capacity inherent in the brains of all children to master the grammar of their parents' language. Because there is substantial variation in the form that the world's languages may take, Chomsky proposed that UG is supplemented by a number of language-particular **parameters.** These parameters allow for a specific and limited set of options in language form and they operate within the restrictions of UG. Once a specific parameter is set for a language, it can have a substantial effect on the superficial appearance of that language.

These assumptions about the nature of language and the learning situation confronting children have profound implications. First, there is a "formal chasm between the input and output of language learning" (Pinker, 1987). In general, this means that what the child hears in speech is only indirectly related to the formal grammatical rules that are assumed to be the end product of language learning. If language learning consists of children forming a succession of hypotheses about grammatical rules, there is simply too much ambiguity in the language children hear for language to be learned. Second (and contrary to the behaviorists), linguists assume that children are never told which sentences are correct and incorrect, either in the speech they hear or through correction of their own productive errors (Morgan et al., 1995; Pinker, 1994; and many others).

LAD and Development

The innate language component has been defined as a **language acquisition device,** or LAD (Chomsky, 1982, 1999; Lenneberg, 1967), that bestows upon the child a host of information about grammatical classes, d-structure, and possible transformations. The LAD operates on the raw linguistic data to which children are exposed to produce the particular abstract grammar of the children's native tongue. The LAD is assumed to be a physiological part of the brain that is a specialized language processor. Just as wings allow birds to fly, the LAD allows children enough innate knowledge of language to speak (Pinker, 1994). The innate knowledge must consist of aspects of language that are universal to all languages. Since children initially have the capacity to learn any language, the properties of the LAD cannot be specific to any one tongue, such as English. The exact nature of the LAD and its attendant mechanisms is a matter of great debate (see Morgan, 1990; Ritchie & Bhatia, 1999).

In an early formulation, McNeill (1970) argued that children are innately endowed with "strong linguistic universals" such as the concepts of "sentence" and grammatical classes and some aspects of phonology, all of which were necessary for the proper development of a grammar. More recently, others have confined the innate linguistic capacities to some inherent constraints and biases to treat the language environment in special ways (Wexler, 1999). Children are regarded as "little cryptographers," who must employ their inherent knowledge of languages to decipher their mother tongue. As children are exposed to their native language, a series of linguistic parameters are set. For example, a child hearing English would over time be "set" to use word order to signal relations between words, whereas someone hearing Italian might be "set" to use verb inflections. Slobin (1979) describes the natural linguistic tendencies as "operating principles" that facilitate the acquisition of grammar. For example, Slobin argues that children "pay attention to the ends of words," which insures that they will note grammatical morphemes that cause changes in word meaning, such as the addition of the morpheme -s to denote plurality. Another proposed operating principle is that "there are linguistic elements that encode relations between words." This principle argues that children know that separate words, when strung together, not only relate to the environment but also to each other. These two important operating principles, when taken together, should aid the child in decoding the relations between spoken strings of words and their d-structure meanings.

Obviously, the linguistic approach is biased towards the structural and nativist ends of the continuum. Linguists search for commonalities across children, cultures, and languages to discover the inherent organization that can be deduced from features that are universal to all languages. As Pinker (1994) put it, "Differences between individuals are so boring!" It should be noted here that the linguistic approach recognizes the need for experience with the language environment. However, this approach insists that the environment merely triggers the maturation of a physiologically based language system (LAD), or sets certain parameters, but does not shape or train verbal behavior. In addition, the linguistic approach favors competence over performance, although both concepts are considered acceptable topics of research. Competence is emphasized because it consistently reflects the formal organization of grammar, whereas children's performance is too susceptible to errors irrelevant to the structure of language.

The child's task of acquiring a language, within this view, is made considerably simpler when certain critical aspects of the task are assumed to be present at birth within the LAD. Newborns immediately begin to detect the sounds in the environment that are linguistically significant. As their ability to control the articulatory mechanisms matures, they begin to produce only those sounds that have been present in their linguistic environment. This process may be facilitated by some innate imitative tendencies, through which the child automatically reproduces facial motor movements (lip and tongue configurations that correlate with different sounds) seen in adults (Field, Woodson, Greenberg, & Cohen, 1982). As the skills of phonetic production mature, children are simultaneously forming primitive, unlabeled concepts

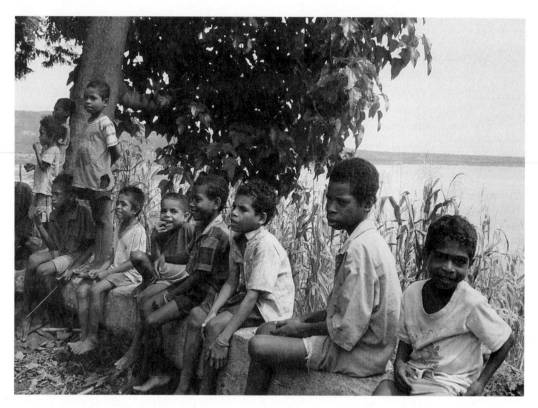

According to linguistic theory, children like these Indonesian Islanders develop language in just the same way that children in New York or Paris do: through the action of their innate Language Acquisition Device.

for referents in their environment, such as milk (Bloom, 1999; Nelson, 1981). At some point, the child may hear an adult say, "Do you want some milk?" and conclude that milk is the label that refers to the primitive concept of milk, even though this word was not taught specifically. The reason that the word milk was chosen by the child to represent the concept, rather than the other words in the string, is that the child possesses mechanisms for categorizing words into appropriate grammatical classes. In other words, children can, almost automatically, differentiate nouns from verbs by their differing patterns of usage in adult speech.

Many have speculated that children are particularly sensitive to commonalities in usage and meaning (Pinker, 1991, 1994). For example, nouns usually refer to things, verbs to actions or relations. Moreover, these classes of words (things versus acts) tend to occur in predictable combinations with other words. Thus, the word *snurt* used in the medial position in the sentence "He snurt himself" conveys considerable information about the permissible uses of the word in other sentences such as "Can I snurt the bread?" or "I snurted until my brains fell out." These critical combinatorial cues may also derive from examples of how the word combines with grammatical morphemes, such as -ed, usually meaning that the root is a verb (Gleitman & Gillette, 1999; Landau & Gleitman, 1985). This may be an example of one mechanism responsible for Slobin's (1979) second operating principle that searches for linguistic elements that encode changes in meaning.

Children move rapidly from the acquisition of their first word to the realization that "everything has a name" (Bates, Bretherton, & Snyder, 1988), which leads to great increases in vocabulary size. In spite of the fact that children now know many words, they use only one word per utterance during this stage. Although each word occurs in isolation, the linguistic approach assumes that each word is governed by grammatical relations or rules. That is, each word constitutes a sentence, and is assumed to be a direct expression of children's intentions or d-structure. The child does not string more words together in this stage only because of performance limitations, such as memory or attentional factors. The child's notion of a hierarchically organized sentence structure is further differentiated over time into noun phrases, verb phrases, and so on. Thus, children move from the one-word stage to two words at a time to multiword utterances by testing their own evolving grammars against the data provided by the environment. Some have called this process hypothesis testing to highlight the child's active role in the acquisition of syntactic rules (see Lust, 1999; Pinker, 1991).

Evaluation of the Linguistic Approach

Supporting Evidence

Research supporting the linguistic approach has followed several lines. The first attempted to support the concept of grammatical rules as links between what is meant and what is said. Such evidence would support Chomsky's (1957, 1965, 1982) distinction between d-structure and the overt s-structure. Besides the intuition that underlying structures are necessary to account for ambiguous sentences, some empirical data have been sought to confirm the existence of grammatical structures.

Several classic studies (Clifton & Odum, 1966; Savin & Perchonock, 1965) demonstrated that simple sentences more closely approximating base structures were processed more quickly and were easier to recognize than more complex, transformed sentences. For example, in early versions of Chomsky's grammar, the passive sentence was considered to be more complex than the active, because it involved at least one transformation. Thus, a passive sentence should be psychologically more complex and take longer to process for comprehension, which was confirmed (e.g., Gough, 1966; Slobin, 1966). Sachs (1967) found that regardless of the surface form of a sentence, only the baselike meaning of the sentence was remembered, suggesting that subjects somehow transform surface structures back into deep structure in order to comprehend sentences. Lastly, in two studies, if subjects heard a "click" while processing a sentence, they perceived the sound as having occurred at the nearest constituent boundary, regardless of when it actually occurred (Garrett, Bever, & Fodor, 1966). Thus, even the perception of sentences is determined by syntactic parsing. Taken together, the research suggests that comprehending a sentence consists of actively processing the hierarchical sentence structure to determine the major syntactic units and deriving the transformations of those structures to attain the base structure meaning (Bock, 1982; Chomsky, 1982).

Evidence of the emergence of linguistic rules was also sought in children's spontaneous speech, primarily using longitudinal, in-depth observations of small numbers of children. (For a review of these early studies, see Brown, 1973; Roeper, 1988.) Many studies focused on the phenomenon of overregularization, defined as the inappropriate application of a grammatical rule. For example, a child might say, "I taked a cookie." This utterance may be taken as evidence that the child knows the rule for the formation of past tense for regular verbs (add *-ed* to the root) and has overapplied this rule to irregular forms (see Pinker, 1991). Brown and Bellugi (1964) concluded that children must be inducing the latent structure of language since they could never have heard these errors in adult speech. Moreover, many studies have found evidence of similar rule use in children from a wide range of languages and cultures, including Finnish (Bowerman, 1973), Turkish (Slobin, 1982), Russian (Slobin, 1966), and Japanese (Hakuta, 1977). The orderly patterns of rule appearance in these varied contexts and cultures resembled the simple maturation of motoric development (Lenneberg, 1967).

The cross-cultural or cross-linguistic perspective has also proven to be a rich source of data concerning the biological basis of language (Slobin, 1986). Because the LAD is assumed to function in all children, it must allow the acquisition of any language (Pinker, 1994), so similar patterns of development across several languages are taken as evidence of the LAD's operation. Slobin (1982) found that young children use subject-object word order, regardless of the order used by mature speakers of their native language, thus it may be a universal. McNeill (1966) argued that the LAD also allows children to presuppose the existence of grammatical classes, such as nouns, verbs, and so on, because these classes are common to all languages and are acquired relatively early in development.

The surprising abilities of infants to perceive relevant acoustic dimensions may also bolster the maturational view of language development. Many studies (for a review, see Molfese, Molfese, & Carrell, 1982) document categorical perception of consonants and vowels within months of birth. Molfese (1989) even found that infants' brains responded asymmetrically to language versus nonlanguage sounds. Thus, children seem to be especially sensitive to human language and quickly achieve adultlike sound discrimination abilities. Moreover, the early patterns of babbling in infancy are comparable across many languages and situations (Levitt & Uttman, 1992).

Some of the most compelling evidence that human beings are endowed with a capacity to generate symbols and to organize their communicative expressions systematically has come from a longitudinal investigation of ten deaf children of hearing parents who elected not to sign with their children. Rather, these parents worked diligently to develop spoken language skills in their children. These efforts, however, proved unsuccessful. The children, as a result, were reared in a loving environment that did not provide them with a useful language model. How children would respond to such a situation has been the focus of Goldin-Meadow and her associates' research for a number of years.

Early in their development, all ten of the children were observed producing several different types of gestures (Goldin-Meadow & Feldman, 1977; Goldin-Meadow & Mylander, 1984, 1990). One group, deictic gestures, was used by the children to indicate specific objects, persons, and locations in their immediate environment. In most instances, these gestures consisted of points. The second group, characterizing gestures, were stylized pantomimes. These mimetic gestures clearly resembled the actions or objects to which the children were referring. The third group of gestures, known as markers, were quite similar to gestures used by most members of American society. Examples of markers included nodding the head for an affirmation or extending a finger to signify "wait." By combining their gestures, these children were able to convey a wide range of semantic relations.

One of the ten original children, David, has been the focus of continuing investigation. Systematic analyses of David's gestural production have shown that David's gestural communication has become more language-like as he got older. David learned to refer to absent objects (Butcher, Mylander, & Goldin-Meadow, 1991) and to form his characterizing gestures slightly differently depending upon whether the gestures served a noun or verb role (Goldin-Meadow, Butcher, Mylander, & Dodge, 1994). Finally, many of David's gestures began to resemble structurally signs from sign languages used by deaf persons. That is, many of David's signs were made in the same locations and involved the same movements as signs from sign languages (Singleton, Morford, & Goldin-Meadow, 1993). Thus, David, with very little if any useful input, appears to have created a communication system with a number of properties in common with languages.

Further support for the nativist position comes from two additional sources. First, the available data on those immersed in a second language suggests that there may be a sensitive or critical period, after which acquisition becomes difficult (Johnson & Newport, 1989). Also, studies of Genie, who was almost totally deprived of any linguistic input until age thirteen, show that she did not acquire syntax after years of intensive training, even though her semantic (and cognitive) development advanced more normally (Curtiss, 1981). Second, those concerned with the species-specificity of language have determined that only humans have the ability to create and understand potentially infinite combinations of linguistic symbols (Terrace & Bever, 1976). The communication systems of other animals are thought to be stimulus bound and not generative or creative (Umiker-Sebeok & Sebeok, 1980).

In the early 1990s, Gopnik (1990; Gopnik & Crago, 1991) reported a family in England with a grammatical deficit called **feature-blind dysphasia** that appeared to follow Mendelian dominant inheritance patterns. Specifically, Gopnik (1990) reported that afflicted family members had particular trouble with grammatical morphemes such as -ed to denote past tense. It appeared that normal syntactic generalization was not available to these individuals, and they had to learn each verb and its past tense form individually. Using of this evidence of a genetic basis for the acquisition of the regular morphemes, Pinker (1991) argued for a dissociation between regular and irregular forms. He suggested that genetic specification for innate grammar had been unequivocally supported, although he doubted if a single gene controlled regular grammatical morpheme use.

Some linguists have tried to test the formal learnability of certain grammars, much as mathematicians test the adequacy of a set of axioms in proving a theorem. Learnability theorists (Pinker, 1984; Wexler & Culicover, 1980) reasoned that if languages are acquired by learning syntactic rules, then those rules must be discoverable from the raw linguistic data provided by the environment. Their basic assumption is that the strings of words that children hear are all positive exemplars of permissible constructions, and that children are given no **negative evidence,** that is, information about unacceptable strings. This type of learning situation is called **text presentation** (Gold, 1967). Without any information about their errors, children could never learn the correct rules, so some rules must be innate, or some alternatives must be ruled out a priori. One recent paper (Morgan et al., 1995) investigated the possible effects of one kind of negative evidence on children's emerging language. Using Brown's Adam, Eve, and Sarah data, Morgan and colleagues (1995) applied sophisticated synchronous and time series regression techniques to detect the effects of error correction on children's emerging grammar. They reported significant negative correlations between the amount of parental corrections and the proportion of syntactically correct children's forms. These authors concluded that parental recasts did not facilitate language learning and actually impeded it. The general conclusion, given the assumption of text presentation, is that grammar is unlearnable through any known principles and must be largely innately programmed (see Wexler, 1999).

Contrary Evidence

Ironically, the same assumptions thought to be the strong points of the linguistic approach in the 1960s became targets of serious criticism. Some linguists adhered too closely to the concept of competence, discarding much of the actual data from adults and children as irrelevant to linguistic theory (e.g., Bever, 1982). Many agree that because linguistic grammars do not correspond well to processes observed in language performance (Palermo, 1978), these grammars are untestable as psychological theories (see Morgan, 1990). A similar problem exists with formal tests of the "learnability" of generative grammars (i.e., Chomsky, 1957). After Wexler (1982; Wexler & Culicover, 1980) showed that an early grammar was "unlearnable," Chomsky (1982) replaced it with the current GB system. Rather than concluding that grammar is by nature unlearnable, it is just as reasonable to assume that the grammar tested was a false description of language, as Chomsky himself later suggested. Moreover, concluding that grammar is not learned through any known principles is not equivalent to concluding that it is innate. Pinker (1984, 1994) calls this the **poverty of imagination** postulate, meaning that just because someone cannot imagine how a particular behavior might have been learned, it does not necessarily follow that it was not learned (i.e., is innate).

Probably the most vulnerable aspect of the linguistic approach concerns the assumptions related to text presentation, or the lack of negative evidence (Gold, 1967; Pinker, 1994). This *no negative evidence* postulate is so central to learnability theory that it may be the "smoking gun" (Moerk, 1991b; Pinker, 1984, 1994). If children are provided any information at all about the acceptability of sentences in their language, then the elaborate arguments of learnability do not hold (see Bohannon, MacWhinney, & Snow, 1990; Valian, 1999). Several reports have clearly questioned the negative evidence issue. One study (Bohannon & Stanowicz, 1988) examined both parents and nonparents conversing with children. They found that over 90 percent of adults' exact imitations of their children's speech followed children's well-formed utterances, whereas over 70 percent of adults' **recast** or expanded imitations followed children's language errors. In this study, both parents and nonparents rarely reproduced a child's language error. Children's language errors were *changed* into correct alternative forms and presented immediately following the child's error. Farrar (1992) also reported that children are more likely to imitate their parents' recasts and expansions than any other utterances. Finally, two recent studies by Saxton and his associates (Saxton, Gallaway, & Backley, 1999; Saxton, Kulcsar, Marshall, & Rupra, 1998) have examined the role that corrective adult input plays in children's grammatical development. The investigators found relatively long-term improvements in the grammaticality of children's speech when adults provided them with corrective recasts, and that improvements were particularly striking when the children were provided instances of negative evidence. Thus, children seem to be sensitive to the adult responses that follow their errors. In summary, the most basic assumption of the linguistic approach seems to be erroneous. Adults do respond differentially to well-formed versus ill-formed child utterances, and children, in turn, respond to the adults' feedback.

Some of the other evidence supporting the linguistic approach has also turned out to be problematic. Although the ability of very young infants to perceive human speech sounds categorically (Eimas, Siqueland, Jusczyk, & Vigorito, 1971) often has been interpreted as strong evidence of innate language capacities in humans, much less attention has been paid to findings that other animals have been shown to perceive these sounds similarly. Needless to say, investigators have not advanced the view that these animals are demonstrating innate language-processing abilities. A better interpretation of these findings of categorical speech perception probably would be that human communication evolved to use more perceptually salient sounds (Kuhl, 1993), rather than claiming that humans evolved special language-processing skills.

Similarly, Gopnik's (1990) report on the specific "grammar gene" may have been premature. A full report of the original investigators has shown that the inherited dominant-gene disability was not limited to grammar but impaired most aspects of the language of this family. The report by Morgan and colleagues (1995) on the inhibitory effects of recasts also has turned out to have equivocal results: Bohannon,

Padgett, Nelson, and Mark (1996) employed a formal modeling procedure to test the statistical procedures used by Morgan and colleagues. They found that the analyses used by these authors could not discriminate between the data generated by models where (1) recasts totally determined grammatical learning, (2) recasts supplemented other learning, (3) recasts inhibited learning, or (4) recasts had nothing to do with grammatical learning whatsoever.

Some of the other assumptions of the linguistic approach are also open to criticism. Language does not develop as rapidly as had been supposed (McNeill, 1966); in fact, the acquisition of complex structures and the subtleties of syntax continues well past age four and possibly through adulthood (Chomsky, 1969; Menyuk, 1977). Furthermore, no neurological basis for rapid early development and slower or nonexistent later development (i.e., for a critical period) has been clearly identified. Studies indicate that language lateralization occurs fairly early, and not during adolescence (Molfese et al., 1982), and that languages can be learned after adolescence (e.g., Krashen, 1975). Lastly, the assertion that human language is due to a species-specific LAD (Pinker, 1994) is controversial. As noted in Chapter 1, chimpanzees and gorillas have learned a variety of communication systems. Depending upon one's definition of language, then, there is research to support either a species-specific argument or the position that human language is merely one end of a continuum of symbolic communication (Bohannon, 1982).

The linguistic approach has generally minimized the effects of differing language environments. Taken to its extreme (e.g., Pinker, 1994; Wexler, 1999), this view suggests that the LAD could construct a grammar from any kind of linguistic textual presentation, no matter how abstract, complex, or error-filled. However, children exposed to language only through the medium of television, for instance, do not learn a language. Sachs, Bard, and Johnson (1981) reported on a young family from Connecticut in which both parents were deaf and both children had normal hearing. The parents elected not to interact with their two sons through the signs they used with one another, but chose instead to stress spoken language acquisition. The parents' spoken language skills, however, were extremely limited and they had no hearing relatives in the state and no hearing family friends. As a result, the boys had very little contact with adult speakers of English, but were exposed to English through frequent television viewing. When the older boy, Jim, began attending a preschool program, it soon became apparent that he had very limited language skills. Although he was nearly four years old, he produced no spontaneous utterances and his responses to questions were only one or two words in length. Moreover, his speech revealed a serious articulation problem and many unintelligible utterances. His comprehension was also poor. An analysis of his spoken utterances showed that many did not conform with English word order; his mean length of utterance was only 2.92, way below normative expectations. He used few grammatical morphemes and was unable to use syntactic devices to combine relations in a sentence. Jim's serious linguistic limitations did not persist for long. After only a few months in nursery school, and with speech language therapy, structures typical of normal child speech emerged. In subsequent years his language moved into the normal range. In this example, at least, mere exposure to a copious sample of language on television did not ensure that the child would acquire language.

Probably the most criticized aspect of the linguistic approach is the tendency to resort to innateness as an explanation, without giving serious consideration to alternative hypotheses. As pointed out earlier, this may be due to a "poverty of imagination." Many researchers (e.g., Gleitman, Newport, & Gleitman, 1984; Goldin-Meadow, 1982; Landau & Gleitman, 1985; Shatz, 1982) have accepted the "null hypothesis," offering nativist interpretations whenever any environmental factor appears not to have an effect upon children's language, although there could be many other explanations for such findings (Moerk, 1991a).

Interactionist Approaches

General Assumptions

If the behaviorist and linguistic approaches are radical complements on the ends of each theoretical continuum, then interactionist theory might be considered a moderate compromise. This approach recognizes and often accepts the more powerful arguments from both camps. Interactionists, as the name implies, assume that many factors (e.g., social, linguistic, maturational/biological, cognitive, etc.) affect the course of development, and that these factors are mutually dependent upon, interact with, and modify one another. Not only may cognitive or social factors modify language acquisition, but language acquisition will in turn modify the development of cognitive and social skills (Vygotsky, 1962). Thus, not only are these variables interactive, the causal relationships among them are reciprocal.

There are three basic types of interactive approaches. First, the developmental cognitive theory of Jean Piaget has a number of important implications for the development of language. Second, our growing knowledge of human cognition (perception, problem solving, memory) has encouraged applications of the information processing paradigm to language behavior. We will focus on one of the newer information processing cognitive models, the competition model (Bates & MacWhinney, 1989). Finally, the fact that language acquisition emerges from and develops within social interaction demands that social factors be explored as causal candidates in language development.

Piaget's Cognitive Approach

The cognitive theory of Jean Piaget shares many important features with the traditional linguistic account of language acquisition. Both emphasize internal structures as the ultimate determinants of behavior. They also agree upon the basic nature of language as a symbolic system for the expression of intention or meaning. The distinctions between competence and performance, and between underlying (deep) structure and surface structure, are typically retained by cognitive researchers. In spite of these similarities, there are also some major theoretical differences between the two. Most important is Piaget's assumption that language per se is not a separate faculty, but is rather only one of several abilities that result from cognitive maturation. According to Piaget (1954), language is structured or constrained by reason; basic linguistic developments must be based upon or derived from even more basic, general changes in cognition (Bates & Snyder, 1985). The sequence of cognitive development, then, determines the sequence of language development.

In 1975, Piaget and Chomsky met and debated the issue of nativism in language, with Chomsky asserting that the general mechanisms of cognitive development cannot account for the abstract, complex, and language-specific structures of language. Moreover, he stated (as discussed previously) that the linguistic environment is also unable to account for the structures that appear in children's language. Therefore, language, or at least aspects of linguistic rules and structure, must be innate. Piaget, on the other hand, insisted that the complex structures of language might be neither innate nor learned. Instead, these structures emerge as a result of the continuing interaction between the child's current level of cognitive functioning and his or her current linguistic, and nonlinguistic, environment. This interactive approach is known as *constructivism* as opposed to strict nativism or empiricism. Bates and Snyder (1985) explain that the resulting structure in language may not resemble either the structure of external reality or the structure of the simple, innate cognitive schemas with which the child began exploring his environment. Instead, the structure is:

> ...an inevitable emergent solution to a series of interactions. Because that structure is inevitable, it does not have to be innate. There is no reason for nature to waste perfectly good genes on an outcome that is going to happen anyway. Applied to language, this approach suggests that the semantic and grammatical structures of language are the inevitable set of solutions to the problem of mapping certain nonlinguistic, cognitive meanings and social intentions onto the highly constrained linguistic channel, and vice-versa. (Bates & Snyder, 1985)

Another related point of contention between traditional linguistic and cognitive interactionist approaches is the data that each regards as relevant to the explanation of child language acquisition. Whereas both approaches preserve a distinction between competence and performance, typically linguists insist that only competence is important to theories of grammar and that performance factors are simply annoying complications. To Piagetians, on the other hand, performance "limitations" provide some of the most useful data. The child's cognitive capacities are assumed to be qualitatively, as well as quantitatively, different from those of adults. Thus, the different way in which the child reasons about the world will affect the way in which she approaches the language acquisition task. Children's linguistic performance, including their errors, may reveal not only their knowledge of the structure of language, but also the structure of their knowledge. The cognitive constraints and abilities that determine linguistic performance are assumed to be the same ones that underlie the child's language competence.

To illustrate the relation between cognitive development and language development, we will examine the earliest stage in Piaget's (1954) account of the development of intelligence. In this account, the period of development from birth to approximately eighteen to twenty-four months of age is described as the period of sensorimotor intelligence. According to Piaget (1945/1962, 1936/1963), the child needs to complete, or nearly complete, the sensorimotor period prior to using language. This period of development is depicted as prelinguistic since the child has not yet acquired the mental representational skills that are necessary for symbol usage. Words, because they can represent or stand for objects, events, and properties, constitute the quintessential symbol. In Piaget's account, children in the sensorimotor period understand the world only through direct sensation of it (sensory) and the activities they perform upon it (motor). These children do not yet recognize the separate and continued existence of objects, apart from their own direct experience of them. Objects that are out of sight are also out of mind, ceasing to exist as soon as they are not in the child's immediate perceptual environment.

During the second year of life, children establish the concept of object permanence, understanding that objects have a permanence and an identity apart from their own perception. The acquisition of this concept often is measured by evaluating children's performance on an object-permanence task. If young children search accurately for an object after hidden displacements, then such behavior is interpreted by Piaget as indicating that the children have formed a mental image or representation of the hidden object. Symbolic play in children also is seen by Piaget as utilizing mental representational skills, and thus is related to language development as well.

Sinclair-deZwart (1969) argued that a child in the sensorimotor period has no need for symbols to represent objects in the environment since the objects are either present, hence serving as their own referents, or they are totally absent and nonexistent for the child. Once object permanence is achieved, the child may begin to use symbols to represent objects that are no longer present, and these symbols become the child's first true words. In this view, then, object permanence is a necessary precursor for language.

Similarly, other cognitive developments are assumed to occur before they are reflected in the child's linguistic skills. For example, children's first word combinations have been posited to be dependent upon the child's perception of semantic relations among objects and people in the world (Bowerman, 1982). With the realization that animate beings typically act upon inanimate things, the child then combines the symbols for these concepts in a similar fashion. Thus the child's first grammar is composed of semantic classes, with animate actors (subjects) followed by actions (verbs) and inanimate acted-upons (objects). It is only later in the course of development that the more abstract grammatical classes of noun phrases, verb phrases, and so on, are formed through the reorganization of the more primitive semantic categories. This linguistic reorganization is assumed to reflect an underlying restructuring of cognitive schemas.

In summary, the Piagetian cognitive approach suggests that language is only one expression of a more general set of human cognitive activities. Proper development of the cognitive system is considered a necessary precursor of linguistic expression. The major task facing the cognitive interactionist, then, is to identify the sequence of cognitive maturation and to explain how these cognitive developments are reflected in language acquisition.

Evaluation of the Cognitive Perspective

Supporting Evidence. Piaget's model of language acquisition depicts language as emerging from or intimately tied to advances in children's cognitive development. Researchers who have examined this model have sought evidence that the attainment of certain basic cognitive abilities precedes or co-occurs with the children's expressive language. A number of studies have shown that the achievement of various early language milestones often coincides or correlates with many nonlinguistic attainments, such as symbolic play with objects, imitation of gestures and sounds, and tool use (for reviews, see Bates, Benigni, Bretherton, Camaioni, & Volterra, 1979; Bates & Snyder, 1985; Corrigan, 1978). Bates (1976) found that children's first words typically occurred after the realization that other people may serve as agents. Furthermore, in most children, there is a precipitous increase in vocabulary and volubility—the vocabulary spurt—that takes place in the latter half of the second year (Bloom, Lifter, & Broughton, 1985; Nelson, 1973). This dramatic increase in vocabulary size, moreover, coincides in most children with their attainment of the last stage of sensorimotor development.

Nonlinguistic accomplishments related to other aspects of language acquisition also have been demonstrated. Corrigan (1978) discovered that the appearance of two-word combinations was related to Piaget's final stage of sensorimotor intelligence. Other investigators (e.g., Branigan, 1979; Case, 1980; Fenson & Ramsey, 1980) reported that children begin joining two or more words into a single intonational contour, or two or more gestures into single, planned motor units, around twenty months of age. Further, Bates and her colleagues have found significant correlations between the appearance of multiword speech and multischema gestures. Taken together, these results indicate that the transition from one-word to multiword speech is part of the more general shift toward "chunking" and the planning of higher-order motor schemas (Bates, Beeghly-Smith, Bretherton, & McNew, 1983).

The work of Slobin (1979) and others (e.g., Block & Kessel, 1980) further suggests that the acquisition of a particular productive morpheme (e.g., tense or plural markers) follows the child's understanding of the semantic properties that the morpheme encodes. In other words, children do not grammatically mark relationships in their spontaneous productive speech until they know the concept that the marker denotes. On this basis, Slobin (1982) suggests that new functions are first expressed in old forms and new forms first express old functions. For example, children must first grasp the primitive concept of past before they will talk about past events using old forms (e.g., "The other day" to refer to a displacement in time), and after this they may use the new form (e.g., past tense markers on the main verb). A related argument (Bowerman, 1982; Sinclair-deZwart, 1973) suggests that cognitive-semantic categories of agent, action, and patient more adequately describe early sentences than the abstract syntactic forms of subject, verb, and object. Bates and her colleagues (1983) concluded that children use cognitively based meanings to decipher the grammatical code in their language. Indeed, early grammars based upon cognitive-semantic categories seem to be the strongest asset of the cognitive-interactionist approach (Pinker, 1984).

Contrary Evidence. The cognitive-interactionist approach avoids many of the problems inherent in the extreme nativist position that language in and of itself is not innate, but that perhaps nonlinguistic, cognitive percursors of language are to a large extent. However, there are several other criticisms that may be leveled at the Piagetian cognitive view. Many of the studies relating cognitive and language development implicitly assume that abilities that emerge at the same point in development (e.g., the acquisition of object permanence and the onset of the vocabulary spurt) share underlying cognitive mechanisms. In addition, positive correlations between cognitive and linguistic achievements often are taken as reflections of causal relationships. As Curtiss (1981) and others (Newport, Gleitman, & Gleitman, 1977) have pointed out, age-related correlations and co-developments occur frequently, such as first molar teeth appearing around the time of first words, yet such co-occurrences are rarely assumed to be causally related.

A better method of sorting out these relations is to identify cognitive achievements that always precede particular linguistic attainments. Then, if any child develops the linguistic skill without also displaying the supposedly prerequisite cognitive skill, the hypothesis would be clearly disproven. Unfortunately, as Bates and Snyder (1985) point out, such clear instances are very difficult to find. But there are sufficient instances to seriously call into question Piaget's claim that completion, or near completion, of the sensorimotor period is a prerequisite for language use. Children learning to sign from their deaf parents often demonstrate symbolic sign usage and combine signs long before they attain full object permanence or complete the sensorimotor period (Bonvillian, Orlansky, Novack, & Folven, 1983). Similarly, a small percentage of children are quite precocious in their spoken language development while appearing to develop normally in other ways (Ingram, 1981). In light of these findings, it would appear necessary to revise considerably Piaget's model of language emergence. Perhaps the cognitive skills that children need to master before using language are the abilities to recognize and identify objects and that objects continue to exist when they are no longer in view. The ability to identify objects and to conduct elementary searches for nonpresent objects emerges in children months before children attain the full range of sensorimotor skills.

As noted previously, Sinclair-deZwart (1973) suggested that development of the object concept should precede the child's first true words. As we have observed, this does not appear to be the case in some instances. There is, however, a growing body of evidence that more specific cognitive attainments *do* correlate with particular linguistic milestones (Corrigan, 1978; Gopnik, 1984; Gopnik & Meltzoff, 1987; Halpern & Aviezer, 1976). For example, the development of "disappearance" words (e.g., *allgone*) is related to object permanence acquisition; "success and failure" terms (e.g., *There! Uh-oh*) appear around the same time as means-ends understanding (solving problems through insight rather than trial and error); and certain ways of categorizing or grouping objects, which develop around 18 months of age, coincide with the vocabulary spurt in children. Gopnik and Meltzoff (1987) as advocates of the "specificity hypothesis" avoid some of the pitfalls present in assessing causal connections between cognition and language by asserting that children learn *specific* words related to the very specific cognitive problems that interest them at a given time. They do not attempt to answer the chicken or egg question—"Which came first?—but focus on the fact that certain cognitive and linguistic events do coincide.

Finally, the work of Curtiss and her colleagues (Curtiss, 1981; Curtiss, Yamada, & Fromkin, 1979) has identified situations in which language and cognitive skills may be separable. Children with Turner's syndrome score quite poorly on cognitive tasks yet exhibit normal language skills. The case study of Genie suggests that semantic and cognitive development are parallel (both were proceeding normally with training), but syntax and morphology are quite different (these were delayed). In other cases, syntax and morphology are normal or even advanced whereas semantic development lags, apparently due to cognitive disabilities. Thus, Curtiss (1981) argues that the acquisition of syntax and morphology must be somewhat independent of other cognitive developments. More recently, Bates (1993) and others (e.g., Newport, 1986) have suggested that during infancy and early childhood cognitive and linguistic development proceed more or less in tandem, but then they begin to take different paths. Although these case studies of atypical language development cannot provide compelling counterevidence, they should caution us against making sweeping statements about the cognitive bases of language acquisition.

In summary, the broad assertion by Piaget that cognitive development determines language development has been seriously questioned by a number of researchers. Moreover, despite an abundance of correlational evidence in this area, methodological problems prevent a clear causal interpretation of much of the data. However, the studies so far indicate that continued research atimed at specific relations between cognition and language should prove more rewarding.

Information Processing Approach

One of the most recent cognitive approaches to language learning is derived from the information processing paradigm. This paradigm is common in experiments on human memory, perception, and problem solving. In essence, the human information processing system is a mechanism that encodes stimuli from the environment, interprets those stimuli, stores in memory stimulus representations and results of operations on them, and allows information retrieval. As we noted previously, one way of approaching language acquisition is to begin with mature language use and then consider how such a system might develop (Gleitman & Wanner, 1982). There is considerable evidence about the nature of adult language processing and memory (Bock, 1982), and this approach views children, however naive and primitive they may be, as qualitatively similar to adults. Simply put, children are information processors in transition from novice to skilled status.

Although there are several recent information processing approaches to language, we will focus on one of these, known as the **competition model** (Bates & MacWhinney, 1989; MacWhinney, 1989). This model emphasizes both structure and function in learning language, but in a novel way. Specifically, the functions involved are communicative functions, such as establishing topicality, requesting, and identifying a location. The structures are language mechanisms that produce strings of spoken words that encode those communicative functions. As Bates and MacWhinney (1987) argue, the structure emerges from the communicative function that the structure serves. "The idea that grammars routinely...spawn forms that play no role in facilitating communication is foreign to...the position" (p. 160). Information processing models such as the competition model are meant to address language performance rather than competence, but it is their position that the structures that produce language performance at any time, even during development, are the same structures that allow linguists to make grammatical judgments (competence). Thus, although this approach explicitly models language performance, it may also account for the nature of linguistic competence.

Before elaborating the details of the competition model, it will be necessary to distinguish between two basic types of information processing. In **serial processing,** operations are performed one at a time, sequentially, whereas in parallel processing multiple operations may occur simultaneously. The linguistic approach discussed previously relies largely on serial processing, in that d-structures are formulated first, prior to application of transformations (e.g., passives, questions, etc.), which are also performed in serial order. Moreover, current conceptions of the linguistic approach suggest that innate linguistic parameters such as word order are set sequentially through exposure.

More recent cognitive approaches assume that parallel processing underlies language. In parallel processing, networks of processors are connected such that several operations or decisions may proceed concurrently. These networks have come to be called **parallel distributed processors,** or **PDPs** (McClelland & Rummelhart, 1981). An example of a PDP network is shown in Figure 7.1. PDP models consist of a series of processing units called *activation nodes.* These are meant to resemble or model individual neurons or assemblies of neurons in the brain. Each node is connected to other nodes by pathways that vary in the strengths of their connections. (Hence, these models are sometimes called *connectionist models.*) The pathways are meant to model the dendrites and axons that connect neurons in the brain. Activation nodes, like neurons, are decision mechanisms. They receive input from other nodes across pathways of varying strength,

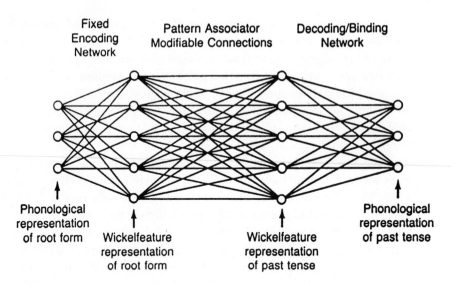

Figure 7.1

The basic structure of the model.   (From *"Learning the Past Tense of English Verbs: Implicit Rules or Parallel Distributed Processing"* [p. 201] by D. Rummelhart and J. McClelland, 1987, in B. MacWhinney (Ed.), *Mechanisms of Language Acquisition,* Hillsdale, NJ: Erlbaum. Reprinted by permission.)

weigh the input, then "decide" whether to "fire" and send information to subsequent levels. For example, a series of phonetic features that make up the word *bat* would be fed to the earliest input level of the network (far left in Figure 7.1). The resulting pattern of activation (decisions of each node) is passed to the initial level of a pattern associator network. The initial word features are further modified, then passed to the second level of the pattern associator. The output connections, known as a decoding network, take these modified word features and generate another pattern of activation that represents the output pattern of sound sequences (see far right portion of Figure 7.1). The place where all learning occurs is in the middle set of nodes called the pattern associator.

The way the system "learns" new patterns, such as the formation of plurals, is through changing the way input patterns are transferred from the encoding to the output level. Depending upon whether the output pattern generated by the system successfully matches a criterion, the relative strengths of the connections between the associator nodes are adjusted. For example, the system might try to generate the plural of *house.* The phonetic representation of house is fed into the associator network as a pattern of activation strengths. The associator network sends another pattern of activation to the decoding network. The criterion plural, houses, is then compared to the output. If the system, in fact, generated the match, *houses,* then the connections in the pattern associator responsible for that guess are left alone. If, on the other hand, the system generates a mismatch (e.g., when presented the word *mouse,* it generates the response *mouses,* which does not match the criterion plural *mice*), this would result in a backwards adjustment of the connections in the pattern associator. If an output node should have been activated but was not, the connections are strengthened by some small incremental amount. If the output node was activated but should not have been, then the strength of the prior connections is decreased by the same, small amount. With sufficient presentations of root word forms, such as *mouse, house, horse, moose,* and so on, and their corresponding correct plural forms, the system will eventually converge, through these incremental adjustments, on the correct plural representation for each root item. Note that the system would also proceed through an error stage, since similar-sounding words would lead to overgeneralization errors. In the example above, a PDP network after being presented with *house* and *houses,* is likely to respond with *mouses* when presented with *mouse,* because the activation patterns are similar.

Using PDP models as a base, Bates and MacWhinney (1989) have proposed their derivative *competition model.* They argue that PDP networks may be thought of as allowing all known syntactic forms, words, and phonetic patterns to compete simultaneously to represent any particular meaning and communicative function. For example, *mice* and *mouses* are both present as possible activation patterns. Which of these is ultimately used depends upon the current levels of activation of each. Over the course of development, the patterns that most successfully match the various criteria are more likely to occur again (are strengthened), and errorful, primitive patterns will eventually disappear. This critical matching function takes place when children's responses are matched against the criteria of adult speech the children hear. Thus, PDP models in general, and the competition model specifically, are empirical and not nativistic. Children learn speech from the exemplars provided to them. No innate biases or constraints are necessary for them eventually to learn to process language as adults do.

Very specific predictions about the course of language development may be derived from the competition model. Learning occurs dependent upon the probability of form-function matches. Therefore, those forms most frequently addressed to children will be learned before rarer forms. This is known as **cue availability** and accounts for both the fact that children from English-speaking homes learn English forms and not Spanish, and less obviously, that children learn highly frequent verb forms (*is, was, were*) prior to less frequent forms. Children learning English acquire word-order forms early compared with Italian-speaking children, because word order in Italian is not a good indicator of the word's role in a sentence.

In summary, the competition model of language performance is a specific adaptation of a PDP information processing system. The language-learning mechanism within this model employs cognitive structures radically different from any previously proposed. They are not behaviorist stimulus–response associations, nor are they interrelated rule systems as suggested by linguists. Rather, they consist of multilayered networks of connections that function to interpret linguistic input and generate speech. The way PDP networks function allows predictions to be made concerning the course of language development. According to the competition model, the rate at which a particular linguistic form is mastered is determined by the nature of the form-function relations in that language system, and the way these relations are presented to children. Language learning within this system is, therefore, empirical—the only innate structure required is a powerful PDP learning mechanism.

Evaluation of the Information Processing Approach

Supporting Evidence. There is considerable evidence from research with adults that suggests the usefulness of the information processing approach in general. The application of PDP to language acquisition, namely the competition model, has some support, but it is so new that a solid body of relevant research has yet to accrue. Despite the novelty of the area, some positive findings are presented below.

PDP processes are frequently implicated in adult cognition. Semantic memory may be organized as networks of varying semantic strengths (Smith, 1978). When words are presented, they activate or prime related words. For example, after hearing the word *nurse,* people quickly recognize semantically related words, such as *woman,* and *doctor* (Meyer & Schwaneveldt, 1971), as well as phonologically related words, such as *purse* or *hearse* (Rubin, 1975). Thus, prior processing causes some spreading activation throughout the system or network of information related to the **priming** stimulus. This phenomenon can be easily demonstrated. Have a friend say the word *silk* out loud five times; then quickly answer this question: "What do cows drink?" Most people readily respond with "milk," although upon reflection they realize that cows rarely drink what they produce. The word *milk* was doubly primed, first with the similar sounds in *silk* and then with semantic association to cows. This priming subtly changes the current state of the language network, such that one particular response (*milk*) becomes more likely than any other response. Syntactic priming has been demonstrated as well (Bock, 1989). Prior exposure to passive sentences makes subsequent passive use more likely, even when topics and lexical items change.

The PDP model has been tested in a computerized simulation of the acquisition of past tense forms. Rummelhart and McClelland (1987) presented a PDP simulation with over 400 different verbs and their past tense forms. The frequency of presentation was matched to what a child might be exposed to; namely, irregular verbs like *take-took* were presented more frequently and prior to the presentation of regular verbs like *walk-walked.* Although the simulation never learned any rules per se (i.e., add *-ed* to form the past tense), the pattern of learning was remarkably similar to that found in children by Pinker (1991). The system initially used every verb correctly, then passed to an overregularization "stage," ultimately regularizing only regular verbs, and correctly producing exceptions. Any completely novel verbs were regularized. Moreover, the child's tendency to overregularize varies with verb class, making *blowed* for *blew* more common than *singed* for *sang* (Bybee & Slobin, 1982), and the

PDP simulation displayed similar patterns. Last, general PDP nets can be damaged after acquiring aspects of language, and they show performance deficits strikingly similar to those of brain-damaged human patients (Marchman, 1993; Plaut, 1995). One of the strengths of the PDP model is these very specific predictions in this domain, in contrast to the often vague predictions of linguistic theory, on the order of "overregularizations will occur and eventually disappear" (Elman, Bates, Johnson, Karmiloff-Smith, Parisi & Plunkett, 1998; Sampson, 1987, p. 878).

One of the last impediments to the PDP approach was the hierarchical organization of sentences. Connectionist networks, like children, must extract phrase structure organization (hierarchical in nature, see Chapter 5) from sentences, despite the fact that the sentences are presented one word at a time. Recently, Elman (1993) devised a network with a transitory memory structure. This network contained a separate loop of "neural nodes" that were mostly influenced by recent input and whose activity decayed rapidly in time. The system was set up to "guess" the next word in a sentential sequence. The point was to present this system with sentences like *The dog who bit the cows **was large**.* The critical bit was to show that the system could "guess" that the main verb should match the real sentence subject *dog* and not the closest sequential noun *cows*. That the network Elman (1993) devised could eventually perform this task is remarkable; however, there was more to the story. If the network was presented adultlike sentences containing the imbedded clauses it was destined to process, it did not learn the hierarchical structures required to succeed. Only if the network was presented simple, short sentences initially would it then proceed to extract appropriate clausal information from more complex sentences. As we shall see, this pattern of simple to complex language presentation mirrors exactly what children receive in real life.

The strongest data in support of the information processing approach comes from its application in the competition model. Within the competition model, the statistical properties (availability and reliability) of syntactic forms determine their rate of acquisition, so that cues that consistently signal particular meanings should be learned first. An extensive review of several candidate cues (case marking, word order, semantics) across a number of different languages (French, English, Italian, Turkish, and Hungarian) supports this prediction, virtually without exception (Bates & MacWhinney, 1989; MacWhinney, 1987). This was true even in cases where predictions were contrary to supposed "universals." For example, Pinker (1984) proposed that all children rely on word order as an initial cue to sentence meaning over other cues, such as case markings; but Turkish children, whose language has an extremely reliable case marking system, master case marking considerably sooner than word order (Slobin & Bever, 1982). Examinations of sentence processing strategies in bilinguals also provide support for the competition model (Harrington, 1987). For example, Dutch speakers acquiring English initially use valid Dutch cues to interpret English, but gradually shift to appropriate English cues with increasing exposure (MacDonald, 1987).

Contrary Evidence. Again, because the competition model is recent, not only are there few supporting data, little contrary evidence exists. However, we can identify potential problems with this approach. To the extent that this model shares assumptions with the linguistic position, it is susceptible to the same criticisms. For example, the competition model also assumes "text presentation" (no corrective feedback of language errors, Gold, 1967). Thus, the child must be endowed with extremely powerful learning mechanisms. Given the new evidence that negative evidence or corrective feedback does occur regularly (although at this point we cannot be positive that every child in every culture receives it), these learning mechanisms may be more powerful than is necessary. According to the principle of parsimony, theorists should use the simplest of the available alternative explanations, if they all describe the data equally well. Whenever information in the environment can account for children's behavior, it may be inefficient or redundant to credit them with internal processes designed to achieve identical goals. Although the competition model is based on language cues actually available to children, it is as yet woefully underspecified with respect to the conversational, social context in which those cues are embedded.

One of the factors that makes PDP networks so appealing may ultimately prove to be misleading. PDP models seductively resemble the organization of neurons in the brain. Thus, we may be tempted to adopt this model because of its superficial resemblance to the biological system, when in fact closer inspection of the operation of neurons and PDP nodes reveals vast differences (Grossberg & Stone, 1986). Sampson (1987) suggests that PDP writers "make too much" of the brain metaphor, although the strong points in favor of their theory are independent of it.

Finally, Fodor and Pylyshyn (1988) have attacked the PDP approach on theoretical grounds. They argued that PDP networks were the mere mechanism whereby linguistic rules were expressed. Although the PDP networks contain no linguistic rules, sets of universal parameters, or binding restrictions, they behave as if they did. Therefore, the PDP systems are simply uninteresting methods of linguistic expression in the same way that computer chips implement calculations of elegant mathematical equations. Further, PDP models handle well problems that can be presented all at once, such as pictures or graphics. What they handle with difficulty are problems that are presented sequentially, and natural language is just such a problem.

Social Interactionist Approach

The social interaction approach also combines many aspects of both the traditional behaviorist and linguistic positions. For example, social interactionists typically agree with linguists who stress that language has a structure and follows certain rules that make it somewhat unique from other behaviors. However, this approach shares with the behaviorists an emphasis on the role of the environment in producing such structure. Specifically, the social interactionist believes that the structure of human language may have arisen out of the social-communicative functions language plays in human relations (Bates & MacWhinney, 1982; Ninio & Snow, 1999). Conversely, a more mature linguistic structure allows more varied and sophisticated ways of socially relating to others. In Figure 7.2, the directions of possible causal relations emphasized by the behavioristic, linguistic, and social interactionist positions are outlined.

The behavioral approach views children as passive beneficiaries of the language training techniques employed by their parents. In this view, children's language development from one time to another (arrow *c* in Figure 7.2) is considered to be the exclusive result of parental action (arrow *a* in Figure 7.2). The linguistic approach sees children as active and specialized language processors, whose maturing neural systems guide development. Linguistic approaches acknowledge that although children may affect what their parents say (arrow *b* in Figure 7.2) at any one time, whatever the parents provide children in the way of language experience only triggers the maturation of children's innate tendencies. In contrast to these views, the social interactionist argues that children cue their parents (arrow *b*) into supplying the appropriate language experience (arrow *a*) that the child requires for language advancement (arrow *c*). Interactionists see children and their language environment as a dynamic system, both requiring the other for (1) efficient social communication at any point in development and (2) improving the child's linguistic skill.

Social interactionists assume that language development is equivalent to the acquisition of grammatical rules, much as linguists have suggested. They, too, search for common forms across children, cultures, and languages (Bohannon & Warren-Leubecker, 1988). On the other hand, these rules may have developed from much simpler rote associations and imitations learned within the social context (Moerk, 1991a). Therefore, although this approach tries to explain language structure, it is

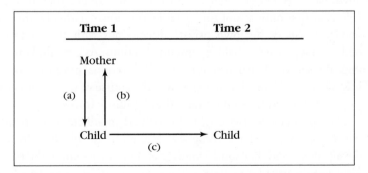

Figure 7.2

Possible directions of effects within language acquisition.

simply less committed to the form of the structure and to the time of its development than the linguistic approach.

Simultaneously, the functions of language in social communication are considered to be central throughout development. The linguistic approach attempts to abstract children's language development away from the day-to-day functions emphasized by behaviorists. Yet, the intricate grammatical structures described by linguists are useless to a child (and probably would not occur) unless they have a practical function, such as understanding and making oneself understood. Humans are such social organisms that it would be odd indeed if there were no relation between language and social skills in the acquisition of a communicative system (Bates et al., 1983). The social interactionist approach may be seen as an attempt to account for children's changing linguistic abstractions by examining how those abstractions might be derived from functioning social communication (Berko Gleason, 1977).

The competence–performance issue is considered more moderately by this approach. Since interactionists acknowledge grammatical structure, they also pursue explanations of the child's language competence. However, what children actually know about language (competence) can only be measured through what they say and understand (performance) within the context of social conversation according to social interactionists. In general, it might be said that interactionists require more performance data than do the linguists, in order to conclude that children know a particular grammatical rule. For example, interactionists realize that children's parents usually bear the burden of communication, phonetically emphasizing important content words, slowing the rate of their speech, frequently repeating themselves, and supplying critical nonverbal cues such as pointing, in order to aid communication (Berko Gleason, 1977; Ninio & Snow, 1999; Snow, 1972, 1977). Some say that parents supply a "scaffold" or supportive communicative structure (Bruner, 1978) that allows efficient communication despite the young child's primitive linguistic system. Thus, children often look much more linguistically sophisticated than they actually are (Lloyd, Baker, & Dunn, 1984). Vygotsky (1962) argued that for the young child, language is at first only a tool for social interaction. Gradually, the child begins to use language in his or her own private interactions with the environment, by talking aloud during play or verbalizing intended actions. As a result, language eventually becomes the source of structure for the child's actions, governing or directing thought. Thus, the role of language changes over the course of development from a social tool to a private tool, as the child internalizes linguistic forms.

Social interactionists might also be said to adhere to both sides of the nature–nurture controversy. They recognize that humans are physiologically specialized as language users, and that some language abilities may require the maturation of physiological systems in order to appear. Thus, interactionists agree that maturation is critical and that children cannot acquire language until a certain level of cognitive development has been attained. On the other hand, interactionists, like the behaviorists, insist that the environment, particularly the social interactive arena, is the place to look for the emergence of language (Locke, 1993). Proponents of this view insist that some specific types of experience and even training are probably necessary for children's language skills to develop. The social interactionist argues that innate linguistic mechanisms alone cannot explain the children's mastery of language and, moreover, that linguistic competence goes beyond conditioning and imitation to include nonlinguistic aspects of interaction: turn-taking, mutual gaze, joint attention, context, and cultural conventions (see Ninio & Snow, 1999). Many social interactionists point to the special nature of the speech directed to children, sometimes known as motherese, but more appropriately called *child-directed speech,* or *CDS,* as important input that may facilitate or even be required for normal language development. Thus, the innate linguistic predispositions must interact with the environment factors in order for language to develop.

Social Interactive Language Learning

As previously stated, the mother's (or other caregiver's) role in providing the child with appropriate language experience is emphasized by the interactive approach. The mother's unusual vocal behavior (CDS) is seen as important as the child's innate linguistic discriminations in explaining children's eventual ability to segment the sound stream. During the child's infancy, mothers also spend a great deal of time in face-to-face social interaction with their infants, performing the vocal behaviors described

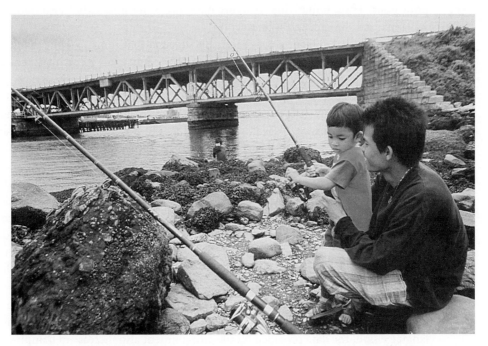

Social interactionists stress the role of parental input language in children's language development.

above. Social interactionists believe that children's maturing ability to control their vocal apparatus is assisted by watching their mothers produce the exaggerated sounds characteristic of baby talk (Field et al., 1982). Moreover, the maturing patterns of social play interaction between mothers and infants are believed to be the basis of later conversational patterns such as conversational turn-taking (Stern, Beebe, Jaffe, & Bennett, 1977).

Interactionists believe that language has an underlying structure and that children express intentions in their speech. Yet, how do children map their intentions onto the linguistic code? Many in this view suggest that children's caretakers (usually mothers) impute intentions and meaning to the child's speech regardless of what the child says. Even when a child is simply babbling, mothers will attempt to interpret the vocalizations as if they were quite meaningful. As mothers continue in their attempts to decipher these vocalizations, critical events begin to occur. These events, which Golinkoff (1983) calls *conversational bouts,* consist of meaning negotiations between the child and the mother. For example, the child might babble *glub* while hungry. The mother interprets *glub* through the present context and her knowledge of the child's past history and offers the child milk. The child continues to fuss because milk is not the object of the child's intention. The mother continues to offer different food items until the child stops fussing and concludes that the child's utterance "glub" was a request for the item that terminated the conversational bout. From there on, the mother should treat the utterance "glub" as a request for the food item that terminated the prior bout. Thus, underlying structure mapping is not innate, but negotiated or conventionalized through social interaction.

The social interaction approach also suggests that some early language may be taught by the parents and learned through rote or imitation by the children. Despite anecdotal failures to teach grammar (e.g., McNeill, 1970), parents insist on teaching children social conventions such as "bye bye" and politeness routines (Berko Gleason & Weintraub, 1976). It is not known yet whether such deliberate instruction is critical for the rest of language development, but it is believed that social use of language is assisted by such teaching. Moreover, the success of teaching social routines suggests that instruction in other forms of language might be of equal benefit.

The role of the child's language environment is stressed throughout development. It is assumed that the child's maturation and current level of grammatical skill interact with the language data provided the child to determine the further course of development (see Hirsh-Pasek & Golinkoff, 1993, 1996). Assuming that children deduce grammatical rules from the consistencies in their linguistic environment (e.g., subjects come before verbs, plurals are signaled with a terminal -s, etc.), adults make the child's task easier by pacing the complexity of the data or problem to be solved with the child's language level. That is, children who are linguistically naive will receive grammatically simple input (CDS). As the child grows older and increases in language skill, the data provided by the environment also increase in complexity. This is probably not due to any conscious effort on the part of parents to give specific language instruction, but simply an effort to facilitate communication. When the child fails to comprehend a parental utterance, the statement is usually simplified and repeated. Since the complexity of the speech addressed to the children is largely determined by cues from the children themselves (Bohannon & Marquis, 1977), one might think of language acquisition in this view as a self-paced lesson.

The parent also may have an effect upon the child independent of the interactive conversational system described above. The interactionist view of language acquisition suggests that there may be some instances when the parents provide language exemplars that are particularly salient to the child. Snow (1979, 1989) argues that the process of mapping meaning onto the language code is assisted when the code provided by the parent closely parallels the young child's attention. Not only must parents talk about things in the child's immediate environment, but they must also focus their comments upon the objects their children are attending to. It is thought that the mapping of meaning, for example, between a ball and the word *ball* is enhanced when the word is frequently used while the child is holding or playing with a ball. It is possible that the extensive occurrence of this phenomenon in infancy through early childhood is necessary for the normal development of children's vocabulary and early syntax.

In a similar fashion, children might notice the difference between their own immature sentences and more mature versions if the two closely co-occur. Nelson (1991) insists that parental recasts of their children's utterances are particularly powerful events that children use to modify their grammars into more mature versions. He argues that children's attention is focused upon the relevant aspects of the environment, and their own intentions, which together result in an utterance. For example, a child may feel thirsty, see mom open the refrigerator, want a glass of milk, and utter, "Want milk." The mother expands and recasts the child's utterance immediately in several forms, "Oh, do you want a glass of milk? Please, may I have some milk?" It is thought that the contrast between the mature and primitive forms may highlight syntactic differences for the child at a time when there is a close correspondence between the environmental context, the child's intentions, and the linguistic form that encodes those intentions and referents.

The interactive approach also recognizes the possibility that simple imitation may have important functions in language development. Although it may not be as important as the behaviorist approach insists, children may test linguistic hypotheses gained through the imitation of forms (Snow, 1978; Stine & Bohannon, 1983). Children are most likely to imitate forms that they only partially understand (Bloom, Hood, & Lightbown, 1974; Clark, 1977). This may be an interaction between the process of acquiring the form and the social-conversational role imitation plays. Stine and Bohannon (1983) argued that partially understood forms (e.g., dependent clauses) are imitated as a possible test of the grammatical rule that generates that form. At the same time, imitation is a conversational signal of partial comprehension that usually results in a recast of the full original sentence. For example, an adult tells a child, "The man who opened the door was your uncle." The child imitates, "Man who opened the door?" The parent then responds, "Yes, your uncle opened the door." It is possible that such conversational interactions, involving imitation, hypothesis testing, and recasts, combine to demonstrate new forms and their equivalent transformations.

In summary, the social interactive approach assumes that language development is the result of acquiring grammatical rules. The child is also assumed to bring a number of innate predispositions to the language-learning situation that constrain children in their search for linguistically relevant distinctions. On the other hand, the environment is believed to be almost as constrained as the children, in order to supply children with the types of language experience necessary for development. Language development is viewed as an orderly, although complex, interactive process where social interaction assists language acquisition and the acquisition of language allows more mature social interaction.

Evaluation of the Social Interactionist Perspective

Supporting Evidence.   One of the strengths of the this approach is its eclectic nature. Because the interactionist believes that language emerges from the interplay between children's linguistic and cognitive capacities and their social language environment, this position borrows from the methods and strengths of the other areas. Therefore, much of the supporting evidence for this approach has been presented previously. The point of departure of this position pivots about the role played by the language addressed to children (CDS). In contrast to other positions, the social interaction approach has sought evidence from mother–child conversations that the simplified and fine-tuned nature of CDS assists the process of acquisition.

The adult's tendency to use a special form of language apparently begins within minutes of the child's birth. Despite the infants' ability to differentially respond to speech and nonspeech stimuli (Molfese et al., 1982), child-directed speech simplifies and highlights (through differential prosodic stress) important phonological distinctions (Ferguson, 1977; Garnica, 1977). Fernald (1983) found similar cooing, repetition, and simplification in German mothers regardless of the mother's amount of experience with infants. In addition, CDS has been observed in fourteen different languages, and it is used by all adult speakers (including fathers) when addressing children (Berko Gleason & Weintraub, 1978). The role of CDS becomes even more important in light of recent research that shows that children prefer to listen to this type of speech from birth (Fernald, 1983) throughout infancy (Friedlander, 1970) and childhood (Rileigh, 1973). Moreover, DeCasper and Fifer (1980) found that infants prefer to hear their own biological mother's CDS over another mother's CDS. Clearly, infants prefer this type of speech and, if given a choice, will seek the voices of their mothers.

Several questions emerge from the data on CDS. First, what variables control the linguistic modifications observed in CDS? The answer seems to be the most obvious and intuitive—simplified and exaggerated speech is required when communicating with someone who is less linguistically sophisticated. The exact amount of simplification required for more efficient communication seems to be determined by feedback from the listener, informing the speaker of the relative success of the prior utterance. Berko Gleason (1977) argued that children rarely yield the little nods and "mm-hmms" that periodically punctuate adult conversations and mark successful communication. The lack of these listener's signals may cue a speaker to simplify.

Bohannon and his colleagues (Bohannon & Marquis, 1977; Warren-Leubecker & Bohannon, 1982, 1983) insist that listeners play a more active role in controlling the speech they hear. They have found comprehension feedback to be a powerful signal that elicits simplified speech from both adults and children as young as three years. Simply put, children are less likely to signal comprehension of longer, more complex sentences and when children signal such failures ("What?" "Huh?"), adults tend to shorten and simplify their next utterances. This pattern of conversational interaction has been observed in all but one of forty-nine adults in both English and Spanish (Bohannon, 1989). This process works equally well when the listener is a "foreigner" and understands little of the native language. The summary effect of this system seems to be a fine-tuning of the syntactic and conceptual complexity of the speech addressed to any child. Moreover, because children control the speech addressed to them, most speakers should use similar CDS, thus avoiding possible confusing variability in the linguistic environment. As children grow in their ability to comprehend more complex sentences, their success is signaled and their linguistic environment keeps pace.

An example of this process was reported by Sachs (1983), who observed her daughter, Naomi, acquiring past-tense markers. Before Naomi's spontaneous use of the past tense, Sachs found little evidence of her own use of the form when addressing her daughter. But just prior to the first appearance of -ed-marked verbs in Naomi's speech, Sachs found that her own use of that form increased markedly. Was this a random event where a mother suddenly and inexplicably chose to use the past tense when addressing her child? Obviously, it was not. The interactionist explanation suggests that Naomi's signals of noncomprehension limited the use of the form by her mother until Naomi began to struggle with a primitive concept of displacement in time (see earlier discussion of the cognitive approach). As Naomi began to signal comprehension of the few past-tense tokens used by her mother, the mother's use of the form increased. This possibly provided Naomi with the linguistic data on the past tense that were required to master the form.

Another question involves the possible benefits of CDS to the developing child. The benefits of CDS may assist with the "meaning mapping" problem addressed earlier by the linguistic approach (e.g., Gleitman & Wanner, 1982). One characteristic of CDS is that the topic of discussion is usually something concrete and the object of children's transitory attention (Cross, 1978; Tomasello & Farrar, 1986). Adults use both the direction of children's gaze and topics of the child's speech to determine conversational content. In their review of the literature, Tomasello & Farrar (1986) concluded that those mothers who spend more time talking about the object of the child's visual gaze patterns had babies who (1) used their first words earlier and (2) had larger initial vocabularies. Since the majority of semantic forms are provided when the child's attention is focused on the meaning of that form, maybe "meaning mapping" is not as mysterious as some have suggested.

A number of studies have delineated some of the features of CDS that may be important for child language acquisition (e.g., Barnes, Gutfreund, Satterly, & Wells, 1983; Cross, 1977, 1978; Newport, 1976; Newport et al., 1977). One study (Bonvillian, Raeburn, & Horan, 1979) found that young children were more successful in imitating novel sentences when the sentences were shorter in length and adults spoke them more slowly and with intonation. A second study (Furrow, Nelson, & Benedict, 1979) examined six eighteen-month-olds and their mothers over the course of nine months. They found that the mothers who used longer and more complex speech when speaking to their children had children who showed the least language gains at the end of the study. In other words, the more the mothers used CDS, the more rapidly their children acquired language. Imitation plus expansions and extensions (Barnes et al., 1983; Newport et al., 1977) are positively associated with language development, as are simple recasts (Nelson, 1991). As previously mentioned, these types of adult responses also tend to follow children's language errors (Bohannon & Stanowicz, 1988; Farrar, 1992). It is possible that adult recasts may be essential in assisting children to converge on the correct form of their native language.

Although it is unethical to deliberately delay children's language learning by experimentally manipulating the environment, there are some parents who, tragically for their children, do so of their own volition. In cases of neglect, the person who is responsible for the child generally fails to provide minimally adequate support for the child's emerging physical, emotional, and intellectual capacities. The overall rate of mother–child interaction for neglectful mothers, in comparison with control group mothers, has been shown to be much lower, with the level of maternal verbal instructional interaction particularly depressed (Bousha & Twentyman, 1984). Neglectful mothers also have been found to produce many fewer words and grammatical utterances in their speech to their young children than did a comparison group of adequately rearing mothers (Christopoulos, Bonvillian, & Crittenden, 1988).

Are there developmental consequences associated with this impoverished environment? In a study of receptive language ability (Fox, Long, & Langlois, 1988), severely **neglected children** scored much lower on measures of language comprehension than other maltreated children or control-group children. In a second study (Culp, Watkins, Lawrence, Letts, Kelly, & Rice, 1991), both the receptive and expressive language skills of neglected children were found to be quite delayed. The neglected children typically were six to nine months delayed in their development of language skills; the children identified as abused and neglected were four to eight months delayed; and the children who had been abused but not neglected were zero to two months delayed. Unlike their language skills, the levels of cognitive development of three groups of maltreated children did not differ. In light of their findings, the investigators concluded that "language development is particularly vulnerable in an environment devoid of parent–child social language exchange" (Culp et al., 1991, p. 377).

Contrary Evidence. As with the cognitive and information processing approaches, social interaction theory has outstripped data collection "to a startling degree" (Bates et al., 1983). Many of its explanations rest on untested intuitions and assumptions. Because the details of this approach have yet to be specified, true counterevidence may be difficult to find (see Valian, in press). On the other hand, some of the basic assumptions about CDS have been addressed.

Newport and colleagues (1977) questioned whether CDS was truly a simple subset of speech. They pointed out that imperatives and questions, which form a solid proportion of speech to children, are more complex than active, declarative sentences. Imperatives delete the sentence subject, and questions move parts of the verb phrase in front of the sentence subject. Although CDS is generally simpler than speech to adults, they argued, it is not a simple language. Shatz (1982) found that the form–function relations in maternal speech are not materially simplified. Hoff-Ginsberg and Shatz (1982) also argued that claims that CDS improves the child's database for language learning are theoretically inadequate because no learning mechanism is specified by this approach.

Another criticism of a strong CDS position is that not all features of CDS are found in all languages (see Bohannon & Warren-Leubecker, 1988). If CDS features are necessary for language development, shouldn't they be used with all children regardless of the native language? Further, Snow (1979) suggested that language is too important a developmental accomplishment to depend upon a single acquisition mechanism such as a precisely fine-tuned and simplified syntax. She argued that children may tolerate a fairly wide window of simplified linguistic data, some very simple sentences and some quite complex, and still acquire language normally.

Several studies (e.g., Hoff-Ginsburg, 1986) investigated the necessity of simplified speech using correlational methods. They found that the complexity of maternal speech addressed to the children was unrelated to the children's language gains. Despite the fact that these children were, on the average, older than those of Furrow and colleagues (1979), this suggests that the simplifications within CDS may not predict children's language growth in the simple, linear fashion suggested by the Furrow study (for a review, see Bohannon & Warren-Leubecker, 1988).

Although researchers have consistently documented certain features in CDS that differ from adult–adult speech patterns, the mere presence of these differences does not, in itself, suggest that CDS is necessary or even helpful to the language-learning child. Moreover, Baker and Nelson (1984) argue that it is impossible from simple correlational studies to determine "who is leading whom" in language development. For example, in much of the research on language delay in severely neglected children, it was not possible to discount the role that the children themselves played in their own neglect (Allen & Oliver, 1982). In other words, rather than the parents' neglect being the principal causal factor in their children's language delay, perhaps it was the other way around; the language impairment of children might have made them less appealing to their parents, with the consequence that their parents neglected them. Only experimental studies that manipulate the frequency of CDS features and examine the effects on child language acquisition can circumvent these problems. The experimental studies of recasts by Nelson and his colleagues represent a solution to this dilemma (see Nelson, Welsh, Camarata, & Butkovksy, 1995). These authors have shown that recasts can facilitate the acquisition of previously unused syntactic forms. Unfortunately, other features of CDS have not been experimentally examined, so conclusions regarding their effects are premature.

Another problem with CDS relates to the great variety of features that differentiate CDS from other speech registers (see Chapter 6). Even if CDS is required by the language-learning child, it is entirely possible that only a few features are really critical in this function. Most CDS studies have focused on global measures, such as mean length of utterance, or frequency of usage of particular grammatical types, and similarly general measures of child language growth. Although the sheer amount of language stimulation provided by the mother is significantly correlated with children's language growth (e.g., Bates, 1975), Bates and colleagues (1983) justifiably argued that these quantitative relationships do not prove the hypothesis that CDS teaches the child language structure. In order to test these claims, one must examine very specific types of linguistic input and relate them to specific measures of child language output. Once we have narrowed our focus in this way, we may find that some aspects of child language are quite malleable and sensitive to linguistic input, whereas others are relatively immune (e.g., Gleitman et al., 1984; Goldin-Meadow, 1982).

The correlational studies reported here are also problematic in the statistical assumption of linear relations, which has been addressed by many critics (e.g., Bates et al., 1983; Bohannon & Hirsh-Pasek, 1984). One conceptual implication of the linearity assumption is that "if some maternal input is good, then more is better" (Bates et al., 1983, p. 43). This may be true, up to a point, in that a minimal or threshold value of linguistic input is required, but additional input is irrelevant. Second, when the age range of the children studied is broad, it is inappropriate to assume that the oldest children should benefit from more CDS in the same way that the youngest children would. For example, the greatest simplification in MLU would dictate that mothers use single-word speech. Although this may be the best level of complexity to use in speech to a one-year-old (Furrow et al., 1979), it would certainly hinder further language acquisition in a four-year-old (Bohannon & Hirsh-Pasek, 1984).

In summary, despite the methodological problems involved in testing its fundamental assertions, the social interactionist approach seems to hold some promise. It employs the empirical perspective of the behaviorists by acknowledging the importance of environmental sources of language data. It also recognizes children as specialized language processors who must not only acquire the language code, but, in turn, must teach it to their children through conversation.

Summary and New Directions

Admittedly, no developmental psycholinguist seriously believes that magic is at the root of language acquisition, despite our frustrated attempts to identify the actual processes involved. Perhaps one of the reasons we have failed to discover simple and easily observable processes in language learning is that they do not exist, due to the importance of the phenomenon to the developing child. In other words, there is simply so much pressure placed on children to communicate successfully that there are probably many routes to the goal, and within each route, a great deal of variability may be tolerated (e.g., Snow, 1978, 1979).

The behaviorist approach probably has suffered most from an overreliance on simple principles to explain language development. Although reinforcement may explain food searching in rats, it has failed to explain the average human child's communicative competence. If the child's parents and peers do industriously shape verbal behavior, then we must have overlooked it somehow, or it must be much more subtle and indirect than the laborious tutelage performed in laboratory settings. On the other hand, some of the behaviorist mechanisms, such as imitation, continue to show promise as an integral part of the language-learning process (see Farrar, 1992). In fact, modern definitions of imitation postulate a process by which observers can learn new behaviors vicariously, through the mere observation of others' behavior. Even the most ardent nativist would agree that children need to be exposed to the language behavior of others in order to acquire it themselves. Thus, even linguists appear to espouse a general imitation model as a basic process responsible for language acquisition.

This unacknowledged agreement among the competing camps goes further. The more articulated model of imitation (Bandura & Walters, 1963) includes a process called *general disinhibition,* wherein the observing learner is more likely to perform a behavior in the general class of behavior as that observed in the model. This suggests that the learner had access to the behavior all along, and imitation merely disinhibited it, allowing the behavior to be performed. Viewed in this way, imitation seems to play a "releasing" function to innate language devices, which seems remarkably similar to the innatist position (Gleitman & Wanner, 1982) and to the "priming" effects used to support PDP models. Clearly, researchers from either camp would be perturbed at the liberties of comparison we have taken. Yet the point to be made here is far from frivolous. The behaviorist approach offers much to the concerned developmental psycholinguist. Just as Piaget (1926) argued that cognitive development is epigenetic (complex cognitive processes arise from simpler functions), it is probable that

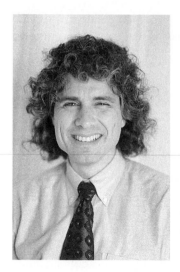
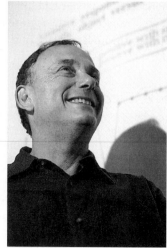
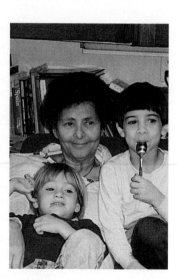

Nativists Steven Pinker (MIT), Kenneth Wexler (MIT), Lila Gleitman (UPenn).

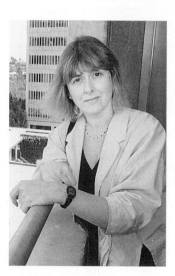
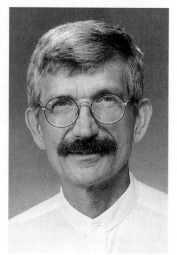

Interactionists Elizabeth Bates (UC San Diego) and Brian MacWhinney (Carnegie Mellon).

language learning at least partially depends on simpler skills such as those described by behaviorists (Moerk, 1992). Indeed, when examined closely, some of these basic principles are featured in most of the theoretical approaches. For example, Nelson's (1977) recasts could be considered a special form of imitation or modeling that comes into play as feedback to children when they make language errors (Bohannon & Stanowicz, 1988; Farrar, 1992).

The linguistic approach also suffers several maladies. The first concerns the nativism–empiricism issue and the **nominalist fallacy.** Researchers fall into this fallacy when they think that giving a phenomenon a special name sufficiently explains the phenomenon. When an observer is at a loss to explain the origin of a form in children's speech, simply labeling it as innate neither helps us determine its relation to other forms nor predict when it should appear in the developmental progression (Atkinson, 1982; Pinker, 1994). Second, the formal learnability models that have been proposed are so powerful and flexible that they can account for almost any pattern of development and hence are not falsifiable (see Morgan, 1990). But before students of developmental psycholinguistics reject the linguistic approach outright, they should reflect upon the logical nature of grammar. The internal structure of the rules used to produce and understand language will probably be discovered within the linguistic approach. As long as researchers in this approach allow children's performance data to bear upon conclusions concerning the child's language competence, then a coherent explanation that achieves Chomsky's (1965) third level of theoretical adequacy, that of psychological reality, may be achieved.

The obvious solution to the controversy between the behaviorist and linguistic approaches lies in the contribution of the various interactional approaches, each of which provides important foci for research. The cognitive approach stresses that language is only one of many complex cognitive skills that children acquire. Moreover, the structure of language and the processes involved in its learning are constrained by the nature of the child's thought at the time of acquisition. The information processing theorists emphasize cognitive processing demands of language learning. They look to the availability and reliability of linguistic cues that signal important communicative functions. It is their position that the nature of the information to be processed determines the course of development. The social interactionist approach highlights the social context in which language is learned, without which language learning seems impossible and perhaps unnecessary. This approach seeks the critical aspects of social interaction that allow normal language learning to proceed.

These varied interactional approaches seem to hold the most promise for the future, perhaps due to their eclectic natures. Recognizing the strengths of the historically earlier theoretical camps, the interactionist borrows freely from each. By avoiding a strict insistence on simple associations or strong innate mechanisms, interactionists may circumvent the more obvious pitfalls. Until language theories incorporate a general learning model that accurately specifies both the psychologically valid structure of language and the environmental variables required for children to develop language in natural settings, the language acquisition process will continue to seem mysterious and magical.

Key Words

classical conditioning	cue availability
competence	descriptive adequacy
competition model	empiricism
convergent validity	feature-blind dysphasia

functionalism
government and binding theory (gb)
grammar
imitation
language acquisition device (lad)
model adequacy
nativism
negative evidence
neglected children
nominalist fallacy
operant conditioning

parallel distributed processing (pdp)
parameter
performance
poverty of imagination
prime/priming
recast
serial processing
shaping
structuralism
text presentation
theoretical adequacy

Suggested Projects

1. Read Skinner's *Verbal Behavior.* Write a synopsis of his position on the problem of language description and acquisition. Compare Skinner's terms, such as tact, mand, and autoclitic, with traditional grammatical categories devised by linguists.

2. Select some friends to play the following games, one subject at a time. Using the figure provided (Figure 7.3), see if they can solve the puzzles you present. The figure provides a simple concept formation problem with the top set of stimuli serving as "maternal exemplars" and the bottom set of stimuli serving as opportunities for "child responses." Note that each stimulus has several features, including size (large, medium, and small), shape (circle, triangle, and square), pattern (open, vertical stripes, and horizontal stripes), and position (left, middle, and right). You begin the game by selecting one of the twelve stimulus features as "correct," without telling the "child" subject. For example, if "left" is going to be the correct "linguistic" rule, you should now point to the left-most stimulus in the top "maternal" array. The subject should then try to guess the correct form in the numbered arrays below. Various forms of language-learning assumptions can be tested:

   A. No negative evidence assumption. Regardless of what the subjects choose, act totally delighted that they chose anything at all and record their choices. Never correct the subject for a wrong stimulus choice. Offer to call Grandma to tell her the "baby" has uttered his or her first word. After several subjects, compare the resultant patterns of responses to see if they converged on the same solution (e.g., "left").

   B. Implicit negative evidence. Proceed as above; however, whenever subjects make a correct choice, point to the choice they have made and say, "That one." When the subject makes an error (e.g., any choice other than the left stimulus), point to the left stimulus and say, "That one." Never tell the subjects that they are right or wrong and act delighted that they are "speaking" (i.e., playing the game). After several subjects, compare the pattern of their

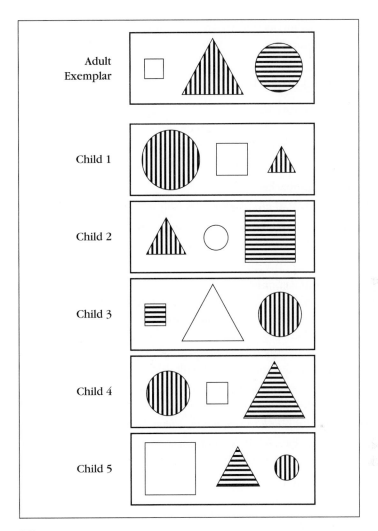

Figure 7.3

choices. Did they converge on the rule you selected? How did they do this if you never told them they were right or wrong?

Compare your data to the theoretical positions of formal language-learning theorists such as Pinker or Wexler. Read Farrar (1992) and briefly discuss the negative evidence issue in comparison to your data.

3. Record a child in normal conversation. Observe and describe as completely as possible the contextual situation in which the conversation occurred (if videotaping is possible, even better). Select at least thirty utterances by the child and analyze them according to the various theoretical perspectives: behaviorist, linguistic, cognitive,

and social interactionist. Try to account for the data that each position would consider important.

Suggested Readings

Behavioral Approaches

MacCorquodale, K. (1970). On Chomsky's review of Skinner's verbal behavior. *Journal of the Experimental Analysis of Behavior, 13,* 83–99.

Skinner, B. F. (1957). *Verbal behavior.* Englewood Cliffs, NJ: Prentice-Hall.

Linguistic Approaches

Brown, R. (1973). *A first language: The early stages.* Cambridge, MA: Harvard University Press.

Chomsky, N. (1982). *Lectures on government and binding.* New York: Foris.

Pinker, S. (1994). *The language instinct: How the mind creates language.* New York: William Morrow.

Cognitive Interactionist

Elman, J., Bates, E., Johnson, M., Karmiloff-Smith, A., Parisi, D., & Plunkett, K. (1996). *Rethinking innateness: A connectionist perspective on development.* Cambridge, MA: MIT Press/ Bradford Books.

MacWhinney, B. (1987). The competition model. In B. MacWhinney (Ed.), *Mechanisms of language acquisition* (pp. 249–308). Hillsdale, NJ: Lawrence Erlbaum.

McClelland, J., Rummelhart, D., & the PDP Research Group. (1986). *Parallel distributed processing: Explorations in the microstructure of cognition,* Vol. 2. Cambridge, MA: Bradford Books.

Piaget, J. (1926). *The language and thought of the child.* New York: Harcourt Brace Jovanovich.

Pinker, S., & Prince, A. (1988). On language and connectionism: Analysis of a parallel distributed processing model of language acquisition. *Cognition, 28,* 73–193.

Social Interactionist

Bohannon, J., & Warren-Leubecker, A. (1988). Recent developments in child-directed-speech: You've come a long way, Baby-Talk. *Language Science,* 10(1), 89–110.

Hirsh-Pasek, K., & Golinkoff, R. (1996). *The origins of grammar: Evidence from early language comprehension.* Cambridge, MA: MIT Press.

Moerk, E. L. (1983). *The mother of Eve—as a first language teacher.* Norwood, NJ: Ablex.

Moerk, E. L. (1992). *A first language taught and learned.* Baltimore: Paul H. Brookes.

References

Allen, R. E., & Oliver, J. M. (1982). The effects of child maltreatment on language development. *Child Abuse and Neglect, 6,* 299–305.

Atkinson, M. (1982). *Explanations in the study of child language development.* New York: Cambridge University Press.

Baker, N., & Nelson, K. (1984). Recasting and related conversational techniques for triggering syntactic advances by young children. *First Language, 5,* 3–22.

Bandura, A., & Harris, M. (1966). Modification of syntactic style. *Journal of Experimental Child Psychology, 66,* 341–352.

Bandura, A., & Walters, R. (1963). *Social learning and personality development.* New York: Holt, Rinehart & Winston.

Barnes, S., Gutfreund, M., Satterly, D., & Wells, G. (1983). Characteristics of adult speech which predict children's language development. *Journal of Child Language, 10,* 65–84.

Bates, E. (1975). Peer relations and the acquisition of language. In M. Lewis & L. Rosenblum (Eds.), *Friendship and peer relations.* New York: Wiley.

Bates, E. (1976). *Language and context: Studies in the acquisition of pragmatics.* New York: Academic Press.

Bates, E. (1993). Comprehension and production in early language development: Comments on Savage-Rumbaugh et al. *Monographs of the Society for Research in Child Development, Serial No. 233, 58* (3–4), 222–242.

Bates, E., Beeghly-Smith, M., Bretherton, I., & McNew, S. (1983). Social basis of language development: A reassessment. In H. Reese & L. Lipsitt (Eds.), *Advances in child development and behavior* (Vol. 16; pp. 8–75). New York: Academic Press.

Bates, E., Benigni, L., Bretherton, I., Camaioni, L., & Volterra, V. (1979). *The emergence of symbols: Cognition and communication in infancy.* New York: Academic Press.

Bates, E., Bretherton, I., & Snyder, L. (1988). *From first words to grammar: Individual differences and dissociable mechanisms.* Cambridge, UK: Cambridge University Press.

Bates, E., & MacWhinney, B. (1982). Functionalist approaches to grammar. In E. Wanner & L. Gleitman (Eds.), *Language acquisition: The state of the art* (pp. 173–218) Cambridge, UK: Cambridge University Press.

Bates, E., & MacWhinney, B. (1987). Competition, variation, and language learning. In B. MacWhinney (Ed.), *Mechanisms of language acquisition* (pp. 157–194). Hillsdale, NJ: Lawrence Erlbaum.

Bates, E., & MacWhinney, B. (1989). Functionalism and the competition model. In B. MacWhinney & E. Bates (Eds.), *The crosslinguistic study of sentence processing* (pp. 3–76). Cambridge, UK: Cambridge University Press.

Bates, E., & Snyder, L. (1985). The cognitive hypothesis in language development. In I. Uzgiris & J. McV. Hunt (Eds.), *Research with scales of psychological development in infancy.* Champaign-Urbana: University of Illinois Press.

Berko Gleason, J. (1977). Some notes on feedback. In C. E. Snow & C. A. Ferguson (Eds.), *Talking to children: Language input and acquisition.* Cambridge, UK: Cambridge University Press.

Berko Gleason, J., & Weintraub, S. (1976). The acquisition of routines in child language. *Language in Society, 5,* 129–136.

Berko Gleason, J., & Weintraub, S. (1978). Input language and the acquisition of communicative competence. In K. Nelson (Ed.), *Children's language* (Vol. 1). New York: Gardner Press.

Bever, T. G. (1970). The cognitive basis for linguistic structures. In J. Hayes (Ed.), *Cognition and the development of language.* New York: Wiley.

Bever, T. G. (1982). Some implications of the nonspecific bases of language. In E. Wanner & L. Gleitman (Eds.), *Language acquisition: The state of the art.* Cambridge, UK: Cambridge University Press.

Block, E., & Kessel, F. (1980). Determinants of the acquisition order of grammatical morphemes: A reananlysis and reinterpretation. *Journal of Child Language, 7,* 181–189.

Bloom, L. (1983). Of continuity, nature, nurture, and magic. In R. Golinkoff (Ed.), *The transition from preverbal to verbal communication.* Hillsdale, NJ: Lawrence Erlbaum.

Bloom, L., Hood, P., & Lightbown, P. (1974). Imitation in language development: If when and why? *Cognitive Psychology, 6,* 380–420.

Bloom, L., Lifter, K., & Broughton, J. (1985). The convergence of early cognition and language in the second year of life: Problems in conceptualization and measurement. In M. Barrett (Ed.), *Children's single-word speech.* Chichester, UK: Wiley.

Bloom, P. (1999). Theories of word learning: Rationalist alternatives to associationism. In W. Ritchie & T. Bhatia (Eds.), *Handbook of child language acquisition.* (pp. 249–279) New York: Academic Press.

Bock, K. (1982). Towards a cognitive psychology of syntax: Information processing contributions to sentence formulation. *Psychological Review, 89,* 1–47.

Bock, K. (1989). Syntactic persistence in language production. *Cognitive Psychology, 18,* 128–149.

Bohannon, J. N. (1982). Close encounters of the primate kind. *American Journal of Primatology, 3,* 353–358.

Bohannon, J. N. (1989). Control of adult speech in Spanish. *Acta Paedoleogica, 2(1),* 48–60.

Bohannon, J. N., & Hirsh-Pasek, K. (1984). Do children say as they're told? A new perspective on motherese. In L. Feagans, C. Garvey, & R. Golinkoff (Eds.), *The origins and growth of communication* (pp. 176–195). Norwood, NJ: Ablex.

Bohannon, J. N., MacWhinney, B., & Snow, C. E. (1990). Negative evidence revisited: Beyond learnability or who has to prove what to whom? *Developmental Psychology, 26,* 221–226.

Bohannon, J. N., & Marquis, A. (1977). Children's control of adult speech. *Child Development, 48,* 1002–1008.

Bohannon, J. N., Padgett, R., Nelson, K. E., & Mark, M. (1996). Useful evidence on negative evidence. *Developmental Psychology, 32,* 551–555.

Bohannon, J. N., & Stanowicz, L. (1988). Adult responses to children's language errors: The issue of negative evidence. *Developmental Psychology, 24,* 684–689.

Bohannon, J. N., & Stanowicz, L. (1989). Bidirectional effects of imitation: A synthesis within a cognitive model. In K. E. Nelson & G. Speidel (Eds.), *A new look at imitation in language acquisition* (pp. 122–150). Norwood, NJ: Ablex.

Bohannon, J. N., & Warren-Leubecker, A. (1988). Recent developments in child-directed-speech: You've come a long way, Baby-Talk. *Language Science, 10(1),* 89–110.

Bonvillian, J. D., Orlansky, M. D., Novack, L. L., & Folven, R. J. (1983). Early sign language and cognitive development. In D. Rogers & J. A. Sloboda (Eds.), *The acquisition of symbolic skills.* New York: Plenum Press.

Bonvillian, J. D., Raeburn, V. P., & Horan, E. A. (1979). Talking to children: The effects of rate, intonation, and length on children's sentence imitation. *Journal of Child Language, 6,* 459–467.

Bousha, D. M., & Twentyman, C. T. (1984). Mother-child interactional style in abuse, neglect, and control groups: Naturalistic observations in the home. *Journal of Abnormal Psychology, 93,* 106–114.

Bowerman, M. (1973). Structural relationships in children's utterances: Syntactic or semantic? In T. Moore (Ed.), *Cognitive development and the acquisition of language.* New York: Academic Press.

Bowerman, M. (1982). Reorganizational processes in lexical and syntactic development. In E. Wanner & L. Gleitman (Eds.), *Language acquisition: The state of the art.* Cambridge, UK: Cambridge University Press.

Branigan, G. (1979). Some reasons why some successive single word utterances are not. *Journal of Child Language, 6,* 411–421.

Brown, R. (1973). *A first language: The early stages.* Cambridge, MA: Harvard University Press.

Brown, R., & Bellugi, U. (1964). Three processes in the child's acquisition of syntax. *Harvard Education Review, 34,* 133–151.

Brown, R., & Hanlon, C. (1970). Derivational complexity and the order of acquisition in child speech. In R. Brown (Ed.), *Psycholinguistics* (pp. 155–207). New York: Free Press.

Bruner, J. (1978). The role of dialogue in language acquisition. In A. Sinclair, R. Jarvella, & W. Levelt (Eds.), *The child's conception of language.* New York: Springer-Verlag.

Butcher, C., Mylander, C., & Goldin-Meadow, S. (1991). Displaced communication in a self-styled gesture system: Pointing at the nonpresent. *Cognitive Development, 6,* 315–342.

Bybee, J., & Slobin, D. (1982). Rules and schemas in the development and use of the English past tense. *Language, 58,* 265–289.

Case, R. (1980). Intellectual development in infancy: A neo-Piagetian interpretation. Paper presented at the International Conference for Infant Studies, New Haven, CT.

Chomsky, C. (1969). *The acquisition of syntax in children from 5 to 10.* Cambridge, MA: MIT Press.

Chomsky, N. (1957). *Syntactic structures.* The Hague: Mouton.

Chomsky, N. (1965). *Aspects of a theory of syntax.* Cambridge, MA: MIT Press.

Chomsky, N. (1982). *Lectures on government and binding.* New York: Foris.

Chomsky, N. (1988). *Language and problems of knowledge.* Cambridge, MA: MIT Press.

Chomsky, N. (1999). On the nature, use and acquisition of language. In W. Ritchie & T. Bhatia (Eds.), *Handbook of child language acquisition.* New York: Academic Press.

Christopoulos, C., Bonvillian, J. D., & Crittenden, P. M. (1988). Maternal language input and child maltreatment. *Infant Mental Health Journal, 9,* 272–286.

Clark, E. (1977). Strategies and the mapping problem in first language acquisition. In J. MacNamara (Ed.), *Language learning and thought.* New York: Academic Press.

Clifton, C., & Odum, P. (1966). Similarity relations among certain English sentence constructions. *Psychological Monographs, 80,* 1–35.

Condon, W., & Sander, L. (1974). Synchrony demonstrated between movements of neonates and adult speech. *Child Development, 45,* 465–472.

Corrigan, R. (1978). Language development as related to stage six object permanence development. *Journal of Child Language, 5,* 173–190.

Cromer, J. (1987). Language growth with experience without feedback. *Journal of Psycholinguistic Research, 16,* 223–231.

Cross, T. (1977). Mothers' speech adjustments: The contribution of selected child listener variables. In C. E. Snow & C. A. Ferguson (Eds.), *Talking to children: Language input and acquisition.* Cambridge, UK: Cambridge University Press.

Cross, T. (1978). Mother's speech and its association with rate of linguistic development in young children. In N. Waterson & C. Snow (Eds.), *The development of communication.* New York: Wiley.

Culp, R. E., Watkins, R. V., Lawrence, H., Letts, D., Kelly, D. J., & Rice, M. L. (1991). Maltreated children's language and speech development: abused, neglected, and abused and neglected. *First Language, 11,* 377–389.

Curtiss, S. (1981). Dissociations between language and cognition: Cases and implications. *Journal of Autism and Developmental Disorders, 11,* 15–30.

Curtiss, S., Yamada, J., & Fromkin, V. (1979). *How independent is language?* Paper presented at the Conference on Human Development, Alexandria, VA.

DeCasper, A., & Fifer, W. (1980). Of human bonding. *Science, 208,* 1174–1176.

Derwing, B. (1973). *Transformational grammar as a theory of language acquisition.* Cambridge, UK: Cambridge University Press.

de Villiers, P., & de Villiers, J. (1972). Early judgments of semantic and syntactic acceptability by children. *Journal of Psycholinguistic Research, 1,* 299–310.

Eimas, P. D., Siqueland, E. R., Jusczyk, P., & Vigorito, J. (1971). Speech perception in infants. *Science, 171,* 303–306.

Elman, J. (1993). Learning and development in neural networks: The importance of starting small. *Cognition, 48(1),* 71–99.

Elman, J. L. (1999). The emergence of language: A conspiracy theory. In B. MacWhinney (Ed.), *The emergence of language* (pp. 1–27). Mahwah, NJ: Lawrence Erlbaum Associates.

Elman, J., Bates, E., Johnson, M., Karmiloff-Smith, A., Parisi, D., & Plunkett, K. (1996). *Rethinking innateness: A connectionist perspective on development.* Cambridge, MA: MIT Press/Bradford Books.

Ervin-Tripp, S. (1971). An overview of theories of grammatical development. In D. Slobin (Ed.), *The ontogenesis of grammar.* New York: Academic Press.

Farrar, J. (1992). Negative evidence and grammatical morpheme acquisition. *Developmental Psychology, 28,* 90–98.

Fenson, L., & Ramsey, D. (1980). Decentration and integration of the child's play in the second year. *Child Development, 51,* 171–178.

Ferguson, C. A. (1977). Baby talk as a simplified register. In C. E. Snow & C. A. Ferguson (Eds.), *Talking to children: Language input and acquisition.* Cambridge, UK: Cambridge University Press.

Fernald, A. (1983). The sound of meaning in early mother-infant interaction. In L. Feagans, K. Garvey, & R. Golinkoff (Eds.), *The origins and growth of communication.* Norwood, NJ: Ablex Publishing.

Field, T., Woodson, R., Greenberg, R., & Cohen, D. (1982). Discrimination and imitation of facial expressions by neonates. *Science, 218,* 179–181.

Fodor, J., & Pylyshyn, Z. (1988). Connectionism and cognitive architecture: A critical analysis. *Cognition, 28,* 3–71.

Fox, L., Long, S., & Langlois, A. (1988). Patterns of language comprehension deficit in abused and neglected children. *Journal of Speech and Hearing Disorders, 53,* 239–244.

Friedlander, B. (1970). Receptive language development in infancy. *Merrill-Palmer Quarterly, 16,* 7–51.

Furrow, D., Nelson, K., & Benedict, H. (1979). Mothers' speech to children and syntactic development: Some simple relationships. *Journal of Child Language, 6,* 423–442.

Garnica, O. (1977). Some prosodic and paralinguistic features of speech to young children. In C. E. Snow & C. A. Ferguson (Eds.), *Talking to children: Language input and acquisition.* Cambridge, UK: Cambridge University Press.

Garrett, M., Bever, T., & Fodor, J. (1966). The active use of grammar in speech perception. *Perception and psychophysics,* 1, 30–32.

Gleitman, L., & Gillette, J. (1999). The role of syntax in verb learning. In W. Ritchie & T. Bhatia (Eds.), *Handbook of child language acquisition* (pp. 280–297). New York: Academic Press.

Gleitman, L., Gleitman, H., & Shipley, E. (1972). The emergence of the child as grammarian. *Cognition,* 1, 137–164.

Gleitman, L., Newport, E., & Gleitman, H. (1984). The current status of the motherese hypothesis. *Journal of Child Language, 11,* 43–79.

Gleitman, L., & Wanner, E. (1982). Language acquisition: The state of the state of the art. In E. Wanner & L. Gleitman (Eds.), *Language acquisition: The state of the art.* Cambridge, UK: Cambridge University Press.

Gold, E. (1967). Language identification in the limit. *Information and Control, 10,* 447–474.

Goldin-Meadow, S. (1982). The resilience of recursion: A study of a communication system developed without a conventional language model. In E. Wanner & L. Gleitman (Eds.), *Language acquisition: The state of the art.* Cambridge, UK: Cambridge University Press.

Goldin-Meadow, S., Butcher, C., Mylander, C., & Dodge, M. (1994). Nouns and verbs in a self-styled gesture system: What's in a name? *Cognitive Psychology, 27,* 259–319.

Goldin-Meadow, S., & Feldman, H. (1977). The development of language-like communication without a language model. *Science, 197,* 401–403.

Goldin-Meadow, S., & Mylander, C. (1984). Gestural communications in deaf children: The effects and non-effects of parental input on language development. *Monographs of the Society for Research in Child Development, 49*(3–4, serial No. 207).

Goldin-Meadow, S., & Mylander, C. (1990). Beyond the input given: The child's role in the-acquisition of language. *Language, 66,* 323–355.

Golinkoff, R. (1983). The preverbal negotiation of failed messages: Insights into the transition period. In R. Golinkoff (Ed.), *The transition from preverbal to verbal communication.* Hillsdale, NJ: Lawrence Erlbaum.

Gopnik, A. (1984). The acquisition of "gone" and the development of the object concept. *Journal of Child Language, 11,* 273–292.

Gopnik, A., & Meltzoff, A. (1987). Semantic and cognitive development in 15- to 21-month-old children. *Journal of Child Language, 11,* 495–513.

Gopnik, M. (1990). Feature-blind grammar and dysphasia. *Nature, 334* (6268), 715.

Gopnik, M., & Crago, M. D. (1991). Familial aggregation of a developmental language disorder. *Cognition, 39,* 1–50.

Gough, P. (1966). The verification of sentences: The effects of delay of evidence and sentence length. *Journal of Verbal Learning and Verbal Behavior, 5,* 492–496.

Grossberg, S., & Stone, G. (1986). Neural dynamics of word recognition and recall: Attentional priming, learning, and resonance. *Psychological Review, 93,* 46–74.

Hakuta, K. (1977). Word order and particles in the acquisition of Japanese. *Papers and Reports on Child Language Development*(Stanford University), No. 13, 110–117.

Halpern, E., & Aviezer, L. (1976). *Psycholinguistic skills and sensorimotor development within Piaget's theoretical framework.* Paper presented at the 21st International Congress of Psychology, Paris.

Harrington, M. (1987). Processing transfer: Language-specific processing strategies as a source of interlanguage variation. Applied Psycholinguistics, 8, 351–378.

Hirsh-Pasek, K., & Golinkoff, R. (1993). Skeletal supports for grammatical learning: What the infant brings to the language learning task. In C. Rovee-Collier & L. Lipsitt (Eds.), *Advances in infancy research* (Vol. 8). Norwood, NJ: Ablex.

Hirsh-Pasek, K., & Golinkoff, R. (1996) *The origins of grammar.* Cambridge, MA: Cambridge University Press.

Hirsh-Pasek, K., Nelson, D., Jusczyk, P., Cassidy, K., Druss, B., & Kennedy, L. (1987). Clauses are perceptual units for young infants. *Cognition, 26,* 269–286.

Hirsh-Pasek, K., Treiman, R., & Schneiderman, M. (1984). Brown and Hanlon revisited: Mother's sensitivity to ungrammatical forms. *Journal of Child Language, 11,* 81–88.

Hoff-Ginsberg, E. (1986). Function and structure in maternal speech: Their relation to the child's development of syntax. *Developmental Psychology, 22,* 155–163.

Hoff-Ginsberg, E., & Shatz, M. (1982). Linguistic input and the child's acquisition of language. *Psychological Bulletin, 92,* 3–26.

Ingram, D. (1981). The transition from early symbols to syntax. In R. Schiefelbusch & D. D. Bricker (Eds.), *Early language: Acquisition and intervention.* Baltimore, MD: University Park Press.

Johnson, J., & Newport, E. (1989). Critical period effects in second language learning: The influence of maturational state on the acquisition of English as a second language. *Cognitive Psychology, 21,* 60–99.

Kandel, E., Schwartz, J., & Jessell, T. (Eds.). (1995). *Essentials of neural science and behavior.* Norwalk, CT: Appleton & Lange.

Katz, J. (1972). *Semantic theory.* New York: Harper & Row.

Krashen, S. (1975). The critical period for language acquisition and its possible basis. *Annals of the New York Academy of Sciences, 263,* 211–224.

Kuhl, P. K. (1993). Early linguistic experience and phonetic perception: Implications for theories of development of speech perception. *Journal of Phonetics, 21,* 125–139.

Landau, B., & Gleitman, L. (1985). *Language and experience: Evidence from the blind child.* Cambridge, MA: Harvard University Press.

Lenneberg, E. (1967). *Biological foundations of language.* New York: Wiley.

Levitt, A., & Uttman, J. (1992). From babbling towards the sound system of English and French: A longitudinal two-case study. *Journal of Child Language. 19,* 19–49.

Liebert, R., Odum, R., Hill, J., & Huff, R. (1969). The effects of age and role familiarity on the production of modeled language construction. *Developmental Psychology, 1,* 108–112.

Lloyd, P., Baker, E., & Dunn, J. (1984). Children's awareness of communication. In L. Feagans, C. Garvey, & R. Golinkoff (Eds.), *The origins and growth of communication.* Norwood, NJ: Ablex.

Locke, J. L. (1993). *The child's path to spoken language.* Cambridge, MA: Harvard University Press.

Lovaas, O. I. (1977). *The autistic child: Language development through behavior modification.* New York: Irvington Publishers.

Lovaas, O. I. (1987). Behavioral treatment and normal educational and intellectual functioning in young autistic children. *Journal of Consulting and Clinical Psychology, 55,* 3–9.

Lust, B. C. (1999). Universal grammar: The strong continuity hypothesis in first language acquisition. In W. C. Ritchie & T. K. Bhatia (Eds.), *Handbook of child language acquisition* (pp. 111–155). San Diego: Academy Press.

MacDonald, J. (1987). Sentence interpretation in bilingual speakers of English and Dutch. *Applied Psycholinguistics, 8,* 379–414.

MacWhinney, B. (Ed.). (1987). *Mechanisms of language acquisition.* Hillsdale, NJ: Lawrence Erlbaum.

MacWhinney, B. (1989). Competition and teachability. In M. Rice & R. Schiefelbusch (Eds.), *The teachability of language* (pp. 63–104). Baltimore: Paul H. Brookes.

Marchman, V. (1993). Constraints on plasticity in a connectionist model of the English past tense. *Journal of Cognitive Neuroscience. 5(2),* 215–234.

McClelland, J., & Rummelhart, D. (1981). An interactive activation model of context effects in letter perception: An account of the basic findings. *Psychological Review, 88,* 375–402.

McClelland, J., Rummelhart, D., & the PDP Research Group. (1986). *Parallel distributed processing: Explorations in the microstructure of cognition* (Vol. 2.), Cambridge, MA: Bradford.

McNeill, D. (1966). Developmental psycholinguistics. In F. Smith & G. Miller (Eds.), *The genesis of language.* Cambridge, MA: MIT Press.

McNeill, D. (1970). *The acquisition of language: The study of developmental linguistics.* New York: Harper & Row.

McShane, L. (1979). The development of naming. *Linguistics, 17,* 879–905.

Menn, L., & Obler, L. K. (Eds.). (1990). *Agrammatic aphasia: Cross-language narrative sourcebook.* Philadelphia: John Benjamins.

Menyuk, P. (1977). *Language and maturation.* Cambridge, MA: MIT Press.

Meyer, D., & Schwaneveldt, R. (1971). Facilitation in recognizing pairs of words: Evidence of a dependence between retrieval operations. *Psychological Review, 90,* 227–234.

Miller, G. (1965). Some preliminaries to psycholinguistics. *American Psychologist, 20 ,* 15–20.

Moerk, E. L. (1975). Verbal interactions between children and their mothers during the preschool years. *Developmental Psychology, 11,* 788–794.

Moerk, E. L. (1983). *The mother of Eve—as a first language teacher.* Norwood, NJ: Ablex.

Moerk, E. L. (1985). A differential interactive analysis of language teaching and learning. *Discourse Processes, 8,* 113–142.

Moerk, E. L. (1989). The LAD was a lady and the tasks were ill-defined. *Developmental Review, 9,* 21–57.

Moerk, E. L. (1991a). *Language training and learning: Processes and products.* Baltimore: Paul H. Brookes.

Moerk, E. L. (1991b). Positive evidence on negative evidence. *First Language, 11,* 219–251.

Moerk, E. L. (1992). *A first language taught and learned.* Baltimore: Paul H. Brookes.

Molfese, D. (1977). Infant cerebral asymmetry. In S. Segalowitz & F. Gruber (Eds.), *Language development and neurological theory.* New York: Academic Press.

Molfese, D., Molfese, V., & Carrell, P. (1982). Early language development. In B. Wolman (Ed.), *Handbook of developmental psychology.* Englewood Cliffs, NJ: Prentice-Hall.

Molfese, V. J. (1989). *Perinatal risk and infant development.* New York: Guilford Press.

Morgan, J. (1986). *From simple input to complex grammars.* Cambridge, MA: MIT Press.

Morgan, J. (1990). Input, innateness, and induction in language acquisition. *Developmental Psychobiology, 23,* 661–678.

Morgan, J., Bonamo, K. M., & Travis, L. L. (1995). Negative evidence on negative evidence. *Developmental Psychology, 31,* 180–197.

Mowrer, O. H. (1960). *Learning theory and the symbolic processes.* New York: Wiley.

Nelson, K. (1973). Structure and stategy in learning to talk. *Monographs of the Society for Research in Child Development, 38* (1–2, Serial No. 149).

Nelson, K. E. (1977). Facilitating children's acquisition of syntax. *Developmental Psychology, 13,* 101–107.

Nelson, K. (1981). Acquisition of words by first-language learners. In H. Winitz (Ed.), *Annals of the New York Academy of Sciences, 379,* 148–160.

Nelson, K. E. (1991). On differentiated language learning models and differentiated interventions. In N. A. Krasnegor (Ed.), *Biological and behavioral determinants of language development.* Hillsdale, NJ: Lawrence Erlbaum Associates.

Nelson, K. E., Denninger, M., Bonvillian, J., Kaplan, B., & Baker, N. (1983). Maternal input adjustments and non-adjustments as related to children's linguistic advances and language acquisition theories. In A. D. Pelligrini & T. D. Yawkey (Eds.), *The development of oral and written languages: Readings in developmental and applied linguistics.* New York: Ablex.

Nelson, K. E., Welsh, J., Camarata, S., & Butkovsky, L. (1995). Available input for language-impaired children and younger children of matched language levels. *First Language, 15,* 1–17.

Newport, E. (1976). Motherese: The speech of mothers to young children. In N. Castellan, D. Pisoni, & G. Potts (Eds.), *Cognitive theory* (Vol. 2). Hillsdale, NJ: Lawrence Erlbaum.

Newport, E. (1986, October). The effect of maturational state on the acquisition of language. Paper presented at Boston University Conference on Language Development, Boston.

Newport, E., Gleitman, L., & Gleitman, H. (1977). Mother I'd rather do it myself: Some effects and non-effects of motherese. In C. E. Snow & C. A. Ferguson (Eds.), *Talking to children: Language input and acquisition.* Cambridge, UK: Cambridge University Press.

Ninio, A., & Snow, C. (1999). The development of pragmatics: Learning to use language appropriately. In W. Ritchie & T. Bhatia (Eds.), *Handbook of child language acquisition.* (pp. 347–386). New York: Academic Press.

Osgood, C. (1953). *Method and theory in experimental psychology.* New York: Oxford University Press.

Osgood, C. (1963). On understanding and creating sentences. *American Psychologist, 18,* 735–751.

Palermo, D. (1978). *The psychology of language.* Glenview, IL: Scott, Foresman.

Palermo, D., & Eberhart, V. (1968). On the learning of morphological rules: An experimental analogy. *Journal of Verbal Learning and Verbal Behavior, 7,* 337–344.

Penner, S. (1987). Parental responses to grammatical and ungrammatical child utterances. *Child Development, 58,* 376–384.

Piaget, J. (1926). *The language and thought of the child.* New York: Harcourt Brace Jovanovich.

Piaget, J. (1954). *The origins of intelligence.* New York: Basic Books.

Piaget, J. (1962). *Play, dreams, and imitation in childhood.* New York: Norton. (Original work published 1945)

Piaget, J. (1963). *The origins of intelligence in children.* New York: Norton. (Original work published 1936)

Pinker, S. (1984). *Language learnability and language development* Cambridge, MA: Harvard University Press.

Pinker, S. (1987). The bootstrapping problem in language acquisition. In B. MacWhinney (Ed.), *Mechanisms of language acquisition.* Hillsdale, NJ: Erlbaum.

Pinker, S. (1989). *Learnability and cognition.* Cambridge, MA: MIT Press.

Pinker, S. (1991). Rules of language. *Science, 253,* 530–535.

Pinker, S. (1994). The language instinct: How the mind creates language. New York: Morrow.

Pinker, S., & Prince, A. (1988). On language and connectionism: Analysis of a parallel distributed processing model of language acquisition. *Cognition, 28,* 73–193.

Plaut, D. (1995). Double dissociation without modularity: Evidence from connectionist neuropsychology. *Journal of Clinical and Experimental Neuropsychology, 17* (2), 291–321.

Rheingold, H., & Joseph J. (1977, March). *Speech to newborns by nursery personnel.* Paper presented at the meeting of the Society for Research in Child Development, New Orleans.

Rileigh, K. (1973). Children's selective listening to stories: Familiarity effects involving vocabulary, syntax, and intonation. *Psychological Reports, 33,* 255–266.

Ritchie, W., & Bhatia, T. (1999). Child language development: Introduction, foundations, and overview. In In W. Ritchie & T. Bhatia (Eds.), *Handbook of child language acquisition.* (pp. 1–33). New York: Academic Press.

Roeper, T. (1988). Grammatical principles of first language acquisition: Theory and evidence. In F. J. Newmeyer (Ed.), *Linguistics: The Cambridge Survey: Vol. II. Linguistic theory: Extensions and implications.* Cambridge, UK: Cambridge University Press.

Rubin, D. (1975). Within word structure in the tip-of-the-tongue phenomenon. *Journal of Verbal Learning and Verbal Behavior, 13,* 392–397.

Rummelhart, D., & McClelland, J. (1987). Learning the past tense of English verbs: Implicit rules or parallel distributed processing. In B. MacWhinney (Ed.), *Mechanisms of language acquisition* (pp.195–248). Cambridge, MA: MIT Press.

Sachs, J. (1967). Recognition memory for syntactic and semantic aspects of connected discourse. *Perception and Psychophysics, 2,* 437–442.

Sachs, J. (1983). Talking about the there and then: The emergence of displaced reference in parent-child discourse. In K. Nelson (Ed.), *Children's language,* Vol. 4 (pp. 1–28). Hillsdale, NJ: Lawrence Erlbaum.

Sachs, J., Bard, B., & Johnson, M. L. (1981). Language learning with restricted input: Case studies of two hearing children of deaf parents. *Applied Psycholinguistics, 2*(I), 33–54.

Sachs, J., & Johnson, M. L. (1976). Language development in a hearing child of deaf parents. In W. von Raffler Engel & Y. Lebrun (Eds.), *Baby talk and infant speech* (pp. 240–245). Lisse, The Netherlands: Swets & Zeitlinger.

Sailor, W. (1971). Reinforcement and generalization of productive plural allomorphs in two retarded children. *Journal of Applied Behavior Analysis, 4,* 305–310.

Salzinger, K. (1959). Experimental manipulation of verbal behavior. *Journal of General Psychology, 61,* 65–94.

Sampson, G. (1987). Review of parallel distributed processing: Explorations in the microstructure of cognition, Vol. 1: Foundations, by D. Rummelhart, J. McClelland, & the PDP Research Group, *Language, 63,* 871–886.

Savin, H., & Perchonock, E. (1965). Grammatical structure and immediate recall of English sentences. *Journal of Verbal Learning and Verbal Behavior, 4,* 348–353.

Saxton, M., Gallaway, C., & Backley, P. (1999). *Negative evidence and negative feedback: Longer-term effects on the grammaticality of child speech.* Paper presented at the VIIIth International Congress for the Study of Child Language, San Sebastian, Spain.

Saxton, M., Kulcsar, B., Marshall, G., & Rupra, M. (1998). Longer-term effects of corrective input: an experimental approach. *Journal of Child Language, 25,* 701–721.

Segal, E. (1977). Toward a coherent psychology of language. In W. K. Honig & J. E. R. Staddon (Eds.), *Handbook of operant behavior.* Englewood Cliffs, NJ: Prentice-Hall.

Shatz, M. (1982). On mechanisms of language acquisition: Can features of the communicative environment account for development? In E. Wanner & L. Gleitman (Eds.), *Language acquisition: The state of the art.* Cambridge, UK: Cambridge University Press.

Singleton, J. L., Morford, J. P., & Goldin-Meadow, S. (1993). Once is not enough: Standards of well-formedness in manual communication created over three timespans. *Language, 69,* 638–715.

Sinclair-deZwart, H. (1969). Developmental psycholinguistics. In D. Elkind & J. Flavell (Eds.), *Studies in cognitive development: Essays in honor of Jean Piaget.* New York: Oxford University Press.

Sinclair-deZwart, H. (1973). Language acquisition and cognitive development. In T. Moore (Ed.), *Cognitive development and the acquisition of language.* New York: Academic Press.

Skinner, B. F. (1957). *Verbal behavior.* Englewood Cliffs, NJ: Prentice-Hall.

Slobin, D. (1966). The acquisition of Russian as a native language. In F. Smith & G. A. Miller (Eds.), *The genesis of language: A psycholinguistic approach.* Cambridge, MA: MIT Press.

Slobin, D. (1979). *Psycholinguistics* (2nd ed.). Glenview, IL: Scott, Foresman.

Slobin, D. (1982). Universal and particular in the acquisition of language. In E. Wanner & L. Gleitman (Eds.), *Language acquisition: The state of the art.* Cambridge, UK: Cambridge University Press.

Slobin, D. (1986). Crosslinguistic evidence for the language-making capacity. In D. Slobin (Ed.), *The crosslinguistic study of language acquisition* (Vol 2.). Hillsdale, NJ: Lawrence Erlbaum.

Slobin, D., & Bever, T. (1982). Children use canonical sentence schemas: A cross-linguistic study of word order and inflections. *Cognition, 12,* 229–265.

Smith, E. (1978). Theories of semantic memory. In W. K. Estes (Ed.), *Handbook of learning and cognitive processes* (Vol. 6). Hillsdale, NJ: Lawrence Erlbaum.

Snow, C. E. (1972). Mother's speech to children learning language. *Child Development, 43,* 549–565.

Snow, C. E. (1977). Mothers' speech research: From input to interaction. In C. E. Snow & C. A. Ferguson (Eds.), *Talking to children: Language input and acquisition.* Cambridge, UK: Cambridge University Press.

Snow, C. E. (1978). The conversational context of language acquisition. In R. Campbell & P. Smith (Eds.), *Recent advances in the psychology of language* (Vol. 4a). New York: Plenum Press.

Snow, C. E. (1979). The role of social interaction in language acquisition. In W. A. Collins (Ed.), *Minnesota symposia on child psychology* (Vol. 12). Hillsdale, NJ: Lawrence Erlbaum.

Snow, C. E. (1989). Understanding social interaction and language acquisition: Sentences are not enough. In M. Bornstein & J. Bruner (Eds.), *Interaction in human development* (pp. 83–104). Hillsdale, NJ: Lawrence Erlbaum.

Speidel, G. E., & Nelson, K. E. (Eds.). (1984). *The many faces of imitation in language learning.* New York: Springer-Verlag.

Staats, A. (1971). Linguistic-mentalistic theory versus an explanatory S-R learning theory of language development. In D. Slobin (Ed.), *The ontogenesis of grammar.* New York: Academic Press.

Staats, A., Staats, C., & Crawford, H. (1962). First-order conditioning of meaning and the parallel conditioning of a GSR. *Journal of General Psychology, 67,* 167–195.

Staats, C., & Staats, A. (1957). Meaning established by classical conditioning. *Journal of Experimental Psychology, 54,* 74–80.

Steckol, K., & Leonard, L. (1981). Sensorimotor development and the use of prelinguistic performatives. *Journal of Speech and Hearing Research, 24,* 262–269.

Stern, D., Beebe, B., Jaffe, J., & Bennett, S. (1977). The infant's stimulus world during social interaction: A study of caregiver behaviors with particular reference to repetition and timing. In H. Schaffer (Ed.), *Studies in mother-infant interaction.* New York: Academic Press.

Stine, E. L., & Bohannon, J. N. (1983). Imitation, interactions and acquisition. *Journal of Child Language, 10,* 589–604.

Terrace, H., & Bever, T. (1976). What may be learned from studying language in the chimpanzee? *Annals of the New York Academy of Sciences, 280,* 579–588.

Tomasello, M., & Farrar, J. (1986). Joint attention and early language. *Child Development, 57,* 1454–1463.

Umiker-Sebeok, J., & Sebeok, T. (1980). Introduction: Questioning apes. In T. Sebeok & J. Umiker-Sebeok (Eds.), *Speaking of apes: A critical anthology of two-way communication with man.* New York: Plenum Press.

Valian, V. (1999). Input and language acquisition. In W. Ritchie & T. Bhatia (Eds.), *Handbook of child language acquisition* (pp. 497–530). New York: Academic Press.

Valian, V. (in press). *Input and innateness: Controversies in language acquisition.* Cambridge, MA: MIT Press.

Vygotsky, L. S. (1962). *Thought and language.* Cambridge, MA: MIT Press.

Warren-Leubecker, A., & Bohannon, J. (1982). The effects of expectation and feedback on speech to foreigners. *Journal of Psycholinguistic Research, 11,* 207–215.

Warren-Leubecker, A., & Bohannon, J. (1983). The effects of verbal feedback and listener type on the speech of preschool children. *Journal of Experimental Child Psychology, 35,* 540–548.

Warren-Leubecker, A., & Bohannon, J. (1984). Intonation patterns in child-directed speech: Mother-father differences. *Child Development, 55,* 1541–1548.

Watson, J. (1924). *Behaviorism.* Chicago: University of Chicago Press.

Wexler, K. (1982). A principal theory for language acquisition. In E. Wanner & L. Gleitman (Eds.), *Language acquisition: The state of the art.* Cambridge, UK: Cambridge University Press.

Wexler, K. (1999). Maturation and growth of grammar. In W. Ritchie & T. Bhatia (Eds.), *Handbook of child language acquisition* (pp. 55–110). New York: Academic Press.

Wexler, K., & Culicover, P. (1980). *Formal principles of language acquisition.* Cambridge, MA: MIT Press.

Whitehurst, G. (1982). Language development. In B. Wolman (Ed.), *Handbook of developmental psychology.* Englewood Cliffs, NJ: Prentice-Hall.

Whitehurst, G., & Novak, G. (1973). Modeling, imitation training, and the acquisition of sentence phrases. *Journal of Experimental Child Psychology, 16,* 332–335.

Whitehurst, G., & Vasta, R. (1975). Is language acquired through imitation? *Journal of Psycholinguistic Research, 4,* 37–59.

Zimmerman, B., & Whitehurst, G. (1979). Structure and function: A comparison of two views of the development of language and cognition. In G. Whitehurst & B. Zimmerman (Eds.), *The functions of language and cognition.* New York: Academic Press.

Chapter 8

Individual Differences: Implications for the Study of Language Acquisition

Beverly A. Goldfield
Rhode Island College

Catherine E. Snow
Harvard Graduate School of Education

At eighteen months, Johanna has a substantial vocabulary of single words that label important objects and entities in her world. She can, for example, talk about food (*banana, apple, cheese*), clothing (*sock, shoes, hat,*) animals (*birdie, cat*), household items (*keys, light*), and toys (*dolly, ball*). Nonnominals are fewer: *hi, bye-bye, up, down, no.* Many of her words are learned and used in the course of naming games that she plays with her parents. Bath time elicits *nose, teeth, eyes, ears, face, hair, belly.* Picture books are also enjoyed as opportunities for displaying Johanna's word knowledge.

Eighteen-month-old Caitlin also has words for things to eat, wear, and play with. However, her lexicon includes many nonnominals (e.g., *there, pretty, nice, yuck, ouch, no, bye-bye, uhoh, down, up*) and quite a few phrases (e.g., *let's go, bless you, sit down, hey you guys, lemme see*), some of which may be attributed to the presence and influence of an older sibling. Caitlin produces these phrases with appropriate melodic (e.g., *where are you?*) or emphatic (*don't touch!*) intonation. Like Johanna, she enjoys picture books, but this context elicits more "conversation" than labeling. On one such occasion, Caitlin sat with Mom and a familiar book, turned to a favorite page, and delivered a prosodically varied but unintelligible twenty-seven-second discourse, embellished with the pauses, gesticulations, and gathering momentum of a narrative.

Johanna and Caitlin have each made considerable progress since first words appeared at about twelve months of age. They talk about familiar persons, entities, and events, and have some words in common. However, there are considerable individual differences in these early lexicons. In the past twenty-five years, researchers have noticed variability in other beginning language learners. These studies have grappled with the problem of how best to describe such differences. Are Johanna and Caitlin acquiring different kinds of words, using language for different purposes, or segmenting the speech they hear in different ways? Other questions concern where such differences might originate. Do children attend to different aspects of their environment, or exploit different learning or processing mechanisms? Or are these differences rooted in characteristics of the language that caregivers use?

These issues have only begun to be explored for children learning English. We will need further evidence from other languages to sort out the array of problems that varied languages present and the array of solutions that individuals bring to the task of learning to talk. These solutions, moreover, carry with them implications for a number of recent theoretical proposals, such as whether early lexical development is related to grammar and the extent to which noun-learning and learning principles that apply to object labels are the most prominent features of early lexical development.

This chapter begins by tracing the relatively brief history of individual differences research, examines variation at different levels of language learning, and considers how data on individual differences may inform the current theoretical debate.

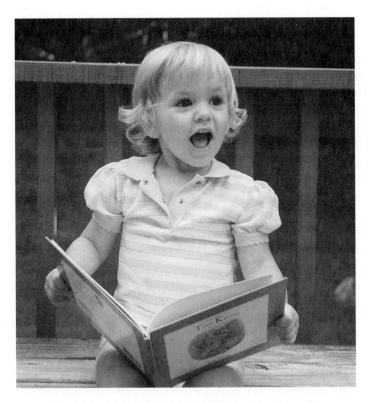

Picture books elicit labels from some children and animated conversation from others.

The History of Individual Differences in Child Language Research

Although the topic of individual differences currently generates considerable interest among child language researchers, this has not always been the case. Previous language development texts would scarcely have mentioned the topic, much less devoted an entire chapter to its discussion. This change can best be understood by considering the history of child language research.

Interest in individual differences followed almost two decades of research committed to documenting universal patterns of acquisition. Even though researchers during this period typically reported (and dismissed as unimportant) variations in the *rate* of language development, they placed greater emphasis on *similarities* among children in the sequence of development. At one level, emphasis on commonalities among language learners grew out of a practical need for basic information about the nature and sequence of development. Another contributing factor, however, was the influence of linguistic theory on child language research. In the early 1960s Chomsky's (1957) theory of **transformational syntax** offered a new and coherent way of accounting for structural principles of adult linguistic competence that cut across inter- and intralinguistic diversity. For the next ten years the kinds of questions asked and the methods used to study child language were direct outcomes of applying the new theory to problems of acquisition. Child language research focused on questions of *structure,* with the intent of documenting the *rules* governing children's early sentences; for example, *stages* were hypothesized to characterize the acquisition of *negative sentences,* of *wh-questions* (Bellugi, 1967), and of *noun* and *verb inflections* (Cazden, 1968).

The focus on linguistic universals during this period carried with it certain assumptions about the methods that could be used to investigate child language. For instance, since all normally developing children were thought to construct similar rule systems, longitudinal study of a single child or a few children was a typical research paradigm (e.g., Braine, 1963; Brown, 1973; Miller & Ervin, 1964). Many studies looked cross-linguistically for common structures and stages of acquisition (e.g., Bowerman, 1973; Slobin, 1968). While this paradigm guided much research and outlined the major dimensions of language development, it also biased us toward seeing shared patterns of development in the data. Children in some studies were selected for inclusion because of the ease with which the researcher could understand and record their speech (e.g., Brown, 1973). Children with less clear articulation or "messy," jargonlike strings in their early speech were less likely to be included (Peters, 1983). Similarly, utterances that appeared to be advanced, imitative, or nonrule-generated in an otherwise predictable corpus of child utterances were often relegated to the anomalous or miscellaneous category and were excluded from further study.

Several factors are responsible for the paradigm change represented by the current interest in variation in the pattern of language acquisition for individual children. First, linguistic theory grew more attentive to *semantic* and *pragmatic aspects* of adult language, and child language research also began to shift away from an exclusive emphasis on syntax. In the 1970s investigators became interested in the *meanings* of early words and sentences and in the ways in which language was used before the onset of word combinations. As the scope of child language research broadened, departures from a universal acquisition sequence began to be noticed and accorded some significance. Using larger samples of children to study the *meaning* and *function* as well as the *form* of early language, investigators have since observed that children vary along all three dimensions.

Another factor contributing to increased reports of variation is the attention now paid to children and child utterances previously excluded from study. Children with poor articulation and early jargonlike sentences have begun to appear in the literature (Adamson & Tomasello, 1984; Peters, 1977, 1983). Some investigators have made deliberate methodological decisions not to select children on the basis of a priori decisions about the representativeness of their language or language environment (Bloom, 1993; Lieven, 1980).

We also have the benefit of recent studies of children from *diverse language communities* (e.g., Slobin, 1985, 1992, 1997) and *varied cultural* and *socioeconomic groups* (e.g., Bloom, 1993; Heath, 1983; Lieven, Pine, & Barnes, 1992; Lifter & Bloom, 1989; Miller, 1982). The finding that some children, more than others, imitate the language they hear and that such imitation is selective (Bloom, Hood, & Lightbown, 1974; Clark, 1974, 1976; Snow, 1981, 1983, 1989) has encouraged researchers to consider how imitative utterances may help children induce the rules of language structure, in addition to serving as a means of conducting a conversation with limited linguistic resources.

Finally, reports of individual differences among children acquiring a second language (Fillmore, 1979; Hatch, 1974) have been an impetus for similar work in first language research. The variation reported among second language learners is striking and has provided investigators with clues to the kinds of strategies that younger and less advanced first language learners may likewise employ.

Serious attention to individual differences began in the 1970s, with a few studies that reported variation in children's first words (Dore, 1974; Nelson, 1973) and early sentences (Bloom, Lightbown, & Hood, 1975; Starr, 1975). Since then, research into individual differences has explored one or more of the following questions: (1) In what *ways* does language-learning vary? (2) What *factors* contribute to individual differences? and (3) What are the *implications* of individual differences for understanding the process of acquisition, for devising an adequate theory of language development, and for clarifying the complex interdependence of cognitive, social, and linguistic factors in development?

Individual Differences in Early Words

Nelson's (1973) study of early lexical development was the first to draw attention to variability among young language learners. Nelson collected diary data on the productive vocabularies of eighteen children (seven boys and eleven girls). The first fifty words of each child were assigned to form classes (nominals, action words, modifiers, personal-social items, function words) based on content or the child's first use of a word. Nelson found that all of the children acquired words for familiar people, animals, food, toys, vehicles, and household objects. The children varied, however, in the proportion of nominals in their vocabulary. Ten "**referential**" children had early lexicons that were dominated by words for *objects*. These children moved predictably from single words to a two-word stage. A sudden spurt of new words near the fifty-word level often preceded the appearance of word combinations. An early preference for object labels was positively related to talk about objects and negatively related to talk about self in a follow-up speech sample at twenty-four months of age.

Eight **expressive** children followed a different route. They had fewer object labels but more pronouns and function words than the first group. They also acquired many more personal-social expressions, which were usually longer than a single word. From early on, these children used phrases such as "go away," "stop it," "don't do it," and "I want it." Their transition into syntactic combinations was less clear and not marked by a rapid increase in new vocabulary items.

Although there was no difference in the age at which the two groups acquired fifty words, children in the referential group included both early and late talkers who tended to learn words at a faster rate than children in the expressive group, who evidenced a slower, steadier rate of acquisition.

Nelson argued that these differences reflected the children's differing hypotheses about how language is used. Children with referential language were learning to talk about and categorize the objects in their environment. Children with expressive speech were more socially oriented and were acquiring the means to talk about themselves and others.

Although Nelson introduced an important new approach to the study of language development, subsequent research has pointed out a number of problems with the original referential-expressive distinction. These include (1) the use of parental report as a source of data, (2) the composition of the early lexicon versus the frequency with which children use individual words, and (3) the categories and criteria used to define the kinds of words children acquire.

Parental reports have been a valuable source of child language data for as long as philosophers and psychologists have observed and recorded development. Parents are with their children in varied contexts in and out of the home and are typically the child's earliest and most consistent conversational partners. However, research comparing spontaneous and elicited speech with parental diary records finds that parents report more nouns and fewer verbs than children use (e.g., Bates, Bretherton, & Snyder, 1988; Benedict, 1979; Pine, 1992b; Tardif, Gelman, & Xu, 1999). This discrepancy may be due to bias on the part of English-speaking parents to notice and report words for objects. On the other hand, even young language learners may know a number of labels that they have rather limited opportunities to use. Words such as *lion, moon,* and *peas* may be evoked during book reading, bedtime, and dinner, respectively, but are less likely to occur in a recorded play session. In any case, the extent to which a child's lexicon is judged to be "referential" or "expressive" can be expected to vary with how the researcher obtains information on the child's vocabulary.

A second problematic area concerns how frequently children actually use the various words that they know. Even in cases where nouns account for about half of children's reported vocabulary, they may be used less often than other words (Pine, 1992b). Three children observed by Lieven (1980), for example, acquired more nominals than any other word class, and were thus similar to Nelson's referential speakers. However, Jane used general nominals more frequently than other types of words, whereas Kate used almost as many personal-social words as general nominals. Beth, on the other hand, used many more names for people, nonclassifiables (ambiguous words such as *there*), and action words than the other two children. Thus, frequency of usage may suggest a different pattern than does the distribution of different word types in the child's lexicon.

A third problem concerns the kinds of criteria used to classify children's words. Nelson's original classification scheme is a mixture of formal and functional characteristics. Nominals, for example, were defined as "words used to refer to the 'thing world'" that could be used to label or demand. However, it appears that some nominals could be classified otherwise, based on the child's reported use of the word. Thus, Nelson states that *door* could be classified as a nominal if the child used the word when simply touching it, or as an action word if the child appeared to want to go outside. This confounding of formal and functional criteria has led to some confusion in how to interpret the referential and expressive distinction. Do children with more referential speech more often talk about objects? Do children with more expressive speech more often use language for social purposes? Without independent observational evidence of how children are actually using their words, we cannot confirm Nelson's suggestion that the referential/expressive distinction reflects children's differing hypotheses about the functions of language.

Subsequent research has looked directly at functional differences in children's early speech. Dore (1974) examined how two children used their single-word utterances in videotaped conversations with their mothers and nursery school teachers. One child used clearly articulated single words to label, repeat, and practice, and her speech involved others 26 percent of the time. The second child produced fewer words but used prosodic features to communicate in more ways. His utterances included others 63 percent of the time. Dore suggests that the first child's language was **code-oriented,** concerned with *representing* things in the environment. The second child was **message-oriented,** more often using language to manipulate the *social* situation. Thus, Dore finds some support for Nelson's hypothesized functional differences, but it is not clear if his two subjects also differed with respect to the kinds of words (e.g., nominals versus personal-social words) they used.

Pine (1992a), on the other hand, collected diary data on the first 100 words of seven children and coded audiotaped speech samples for various functions, including attention, labeling, description, demand, and protest. Although children varied considerably in the proportion of common nouns in their lexicon (a range of 28 percent to 54 percent at 50 words, and 35 percent to 67 percent at 100 words), there was no relationship between referential vocabulary and any functional category at either vocabulary level.

Bowerman (1976) also points out that word usage may *shift* over time. She cites an example from Ferrier (1975), who reports that her daughter initially used *phew* expressively, to greet her mother in the morning. The word was originally an imitation of her mother's own routine comment on the odor she invariably encountered on these occasions. The same word was later used by her daughter referentially, as a name for diapers, clean or soiled.

Thus, although children may vary in the kinds of words they acquire, there is no consistent support for the notion that children with relatively more nouns use language in more naming and fewer social contexts. Many, if not most, early words serve a variety of functions, and the *distribution, function,* and *frequency* of word usage are related but separable aspects of early lexical development.

A number of studies have subsequently confirmed some version of the referential/expressive distinction in children's first words. Some children acquire relatively more common nouns (e.g., Bretherton, McNew, Snyder, & Bates, 1983; Lieven et al., 1992; Pine & Lieven, 1990), or words that label and describe the properties of objects (Goldfield, 1985/86, 1987), whereas other children acquire many words to describe their own actions and states and use more phrases (Goldfield, 1985/86, 1987; Lieven et al., 1992). It is important to note, however, that the referential/expressive dimension is not a dichotomy, but rather a continuum along which individual children vary. Most children appear to acquire a relative balance of referential and expressive language; only a few children acquire a distribution extreme enough to be called a distinct style or strategy. A close examination of the extremes, however, should help us to disentangle the possible mechanisms and processes that contribute to early lexical development for all children (Figure 8.1).

Segmenting the Speech Stream

The difficulties inherent in describing children's early speech in terms of formal and/or functional characteristics have led researchers to alternative ways of conceptualizing individual differences. The tendency of some children to acquire longer, phraselike utterances during the "single-word" stage suggests that children may differ with respect to the length of the linguistic units that they segment from adult speech. A sample of such phrasal speech can be found in our introductory depiction of Caitlin's early language. Note that Caitlin's phrases are two and three words in length, but the individual words do not occur alone, suggesting that the entire "package" has been learned as a whole. Moreover, she typically produces these phrases with adultlike intonation. (For a more thorough description of Caitlin's language, see Goldfield, 1985/86).

A distinction that may be related to these differing segmentation strategies occurs in children's early *phonological* systems as well. Ferguson (1979), for example, has described cautious versus risk-taking approaches. Some children's early utterances seem to be generated on the basis of an elegant and orderly set of phonological rules, such that the child-form of any adult word is highly predictable. Such children (e.g., Smith's subject Amahl, 1973) either apply their rule system consistently to imitated as well as to spontaneous forms or else resist imitating words that would constitute violations of the restrictions on their output. Other children, in contrast, operate with fairly sloppy phonological systems, showing alternation among several ways of producing most words and applying their phonological rules optionally. Typically, the children with sloppy phonological systems incorporate imitated (and thus progressive) forms into their lexicon quite easily and may be more likely to show improvement in production as a result of direct modeling (Macken, 1978).

Although segmentation may be facilitated by the shorter utterances, exaggerated intonation, pauses, repetitions, and stress patterns of child-directed talk, children must build their lexicons from the raw material of connected speech. The units that they select may thus be single words or longer phrases. A number of studies report children who orient to syllables and segments and others who attend to prosodic tunes that unify larger sequences of speech (Echols, 1993; Klein, 1978; Lieven, 1989; Peters, 1977, 1983). Seth and Daniel represent these differing strategies:

> ...formulaic children, like Seth, pay attention to "horizontal" information such as the number of syllables, stress, intonation patterns....word-oriented children, like Daniel, pay more attention to the vertical segmental information contained in single (usually

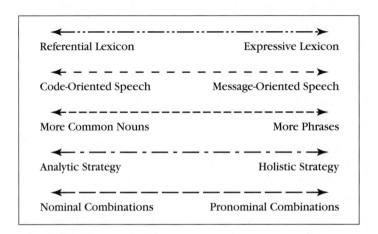

Figure 8.1

Some dimensions of individual differences in early language development.

stressed) syllables focusing on the details of consonants and vowels. (Peters & Menn, 1993, p. 745)

Plunkett (1993) suggests that articulatory fluency and articulatory precision are inversely related in early speech. Phrasal speech represents segmentation that over-shoots a target adult word. Such expressions tend to be produced fluently but with less precise articulation of the individual phonetic segments. Articulatory precision is the outcome of an alternate strategy that undershoots the adult target word by focusing on accurate production of sublexical units. Variation in perceptual acuity, in verbal memory, and/or in characteristics of the input may influence the kinds of linguistic units that are perceptually salient and likely to be used. The sounds learners attend to may be the sounds that they hear often and know they can produce, resulting in a kind of "articulatory filter" that may by unique to each child (Vihman, 1993).

Lieven and colleagues (1992) have coined the term "frozen phrases" for phrasal speech that appears before true word combinations. They defined frozen phrases as utterances containing two or more words that had not previously occurred as single units in the child's speech. They examined the number of common nouns, personal-social words, and frozen phrases in a sample of twelve children who were observed longitudinally using parent word diaries and periodic audio samples of the children's speech. They found that personal-social words declined as vocabulary increased, suggesting that such words may not be a stable defining characteristic of expressive style. On the other hand, the proportion of common nouns and frozen phrases in children's lexicons remained stable when the first fifty words were compared to the second fifty, and the two measures were negatively correlated at both vocabulary levels. This pattern of results suggests that frozen phrases and common nouns may more precisely define two approaches to early lexical development. Moreover, there was no significant correlation between either measure and age at which fifty and 100 words were acquired, suggesting that neither strategy affords an advantage at this level of development.

Peters (1977, 1983) describes how the child she observed acquired both phrasal speech marked by stress and intonation, and more clearly articulated single words. She termed these two kinds of speech *gestalt* and *analytic,* respectively. However, as Pine and Lieven (1993) point out, the segmentation of phrases from adult speech is also an analytic process. What differs is the length of the unit that children extract from the speech that they hear. The occurrence of phrasal units in children's early speech raises a number of questions about the relationship between the lexicon and syntax. We will return to this topic after first reviewing the evidence for individual differences in early syntactic development.

Individual Differences in Early Sentences

Two years after Nelson's study of variability in early words, Bloom and colleagues (1975) reported that children also differ in the early stages of multiword speech.

Bloom and her colleagues found that the sentences of the four children they observed had similar content (they talked about a common set of semantic categories such as recurrence, negation, actions, and states) that emerged in a similar order. However, the form of their early sentences differed.

All four children used a *pivot strategy* to encode negation and nonexistence (*no + X, no more + X*) and recurrence (*more + X, 'nother + X*). This strategy consisted of combining one of a small class of *function words* and any one of a larger, varying set of *content words*. Eric and Peter used this same approach to express action, location, and possession by combining all-purpose pronouns with content words. They produced utterances such as *I finish, play it, sit here,* and *my truck.* During this same period Kathryn and Gia expressed the same semantic relations by combining content words, as in *Gia push, touch milk, sweater chair,* and *Kathryn sock.*

Bloom, Lightbown, and Hood (1975) claim that the children were using two different combinatorial strategies. The pronominal approach used by the two boys allowed them to begin encoding relationships between objects and events without relying on specific lexical items. Since they used a varied lexicon in single-word utterances and in sentences with *no* and *more*, their strategy could not be attributed to simply not knowing enough labels. The two girls, on the other hand, preferred to talk about the same meanings using specific nouns. When MLU approached 2.5, the two systems began to overlap. Children using a **pronominal strategy** combined more content words, whereas the **nominal** children incorporated more pronouns into their utterances.

The child observed by Goldfield (1982) also exhibited an early pronominal style, but close examination of her multiword speech over time revealed that a few specific patterns accounted for the relative dominance of pronouns. For example, the roles of agent and possessor were initially limited to the child herself and encoded by pronouns *I* and *my,* respectively. These semantic roles later broadened to include others, and in these cases nominals were used to encode the constituent. Earliest action utterances (*I'll do it, I found it*) were initially rote phrases. Later action utterances took the form of agent + action + *it* and appeared to have evolved from the earlier pattern. Combinatorial patterns specific to individual children have also been observed in the cross-linguistic literature (Braine, 1976).

We will present more evidence for varied approaches to early syntax in the next section, which reviews those studies that have looked at the stability of individual differences in children who have been observed from early words to first sentences.

Stability of Individual Differences

The variation we have seen in strategies children use for segmenting the speech they hear, for expressing early meanings, and for introducing structure into their language may simply represent different entry points into the language system, or may be early signs of differences that persist across development. Do children with a preference for object labels tend to develop a nominal strategy for their early word combinations? Do children with relatively more expressive speech prefer a pronominal approach?

There is some evidence that children's early *lexical preferences* are reflected in the form of their first word combinations. Nelson (1975) followed the later language development of her original referential-expressive sample. Using transcripts of speech recorded when the children were twenty-four and thirty months of age, she found that referential speakers began with a high proportion of nouns in early sentences. With increasing MLU, the use of pronouns increased while nouns decreased for these children. Children from the original expressive group began with a balance of noun and pronoun use. Pronoun use changed very little for this group, but nouns increased with advanced MLU.

Functional differences that extend from single words to word combinations have also been reported. Starr (1975) observed twelve children from one to two-and-a-half years of age. She found that children who preferred to label objects in single-word speech tended to produce two-word sentences encoding object-attribute relations. A second group of children described objects less frequently but used more interjections (conventional social responses such as *hi, bye, ouch*) and made more self-references (e.g., *want ball*) in their early sentences.

Similarly, Lieven (1980) reports that early sentences of the three children she observed appeared to derive from characteristics of their single-word speech. For one child both single words and early constructions (e.g., *there, mommy, there Julian,* and *there mommy*) were used to gain adult attention rather than to convey reference. The other two children were more likely to describe attributes and actions of people and things in both their single- and multiple-word utterances.

As we saw earlier, some children, such as Caitlin, acquire a number of phrases in the early stages of learning to talk. Nelson's expressive speakers produced *go away, stop it, don't do it, I want it.* Such phrases are the result of segmenting larger units from adult speech. It is not clear, however, how these early units are related to later grammatical development. Some research suggests that early phrasal speech is unrelated to later analyzed productions. Bates and colleagues (1988) followed twenty-seven children from first words to early sentences. A number of observational and parent interview measures were used to assess language progress when children were ten, thirteen, twenty, and twenty-eight months of age. Bates and colleagues report that an "analytic" style, which included high levels of comprehension and flexible noun production at thirteen months, predicted advanced grammatical development at twenty-eight months. Variables that suggested an early "rote" or "holistic" style, on the other hand, were unrelated to later grammatical progress.

This line of research has been criticized by Pine and Lieven (1990, 1993), who argue that cross-sectional, age-related measures of individual differences confound strategy with variation due to differences in developmental level. Because the proportion of nouns increases as vocabulary totals rise, children assessed at the same age but different vocabulary levels will differ in the number of nouns in their lexicon, regardless of their particular style or strategy. Thus, assessments of individual differences should be based on comparable vocabulary totals (as was the case for Nelson's original study).

However, using controlled vocabulary levels, Bates, Marchman, Thal, Fenson, Dale, Reznick, Reilly, and Hartung (1993) continue to find evidence that early phrasal speech is unrelated to later grammatical development, whereas Pine and Lieven (1993) argue that early frozen phrases predict later productive word combinations. The apparent discrepancy, however, may be due in part to differences in age and the measures used to assess both style differences and grammatical progress. Bates and her colleagues (1993) used data from 228 children whose parents completed a checklist assessing vocabulary and grammar at twenty months, which was repeated six months later. They found no relationship between the number of closed-class words (prepositions, articles, auxiliary verbs, question words, pronouns, quantifiers, and connectives) that children used at twenty months, and the extent to which parents judged that children's sentences included words and inflections that indicate grammatical complexity (prepositions, articles, auxiliary verbs, copulas, modals, possessives, plurals, and tense markers) at twenty-six months. Thus, their analysis found no continuity between grammatical words that may appear in early phrasal speech and a related set of words and inflections that play a role in later sentence construction.

Pine and Lieven (1993), on the other hand, looked at data from seven children, who were observed using maternal report and periodic audio recordings, from eleven to twenty months of age. They found that the proportion of frozen phrases children used was positively related to the number of productive word combinations, in contrast to the proportion of common nouns, which was unrelated to sentence production. This analysis, then, finds continuity between early phrasal speech and the frequency and pattern of word combinations. Thus, the two studies are concerned with somewhat different aspects of grammar at two different periods of development.

Children's acquisition of frozen phrases has led researchers to reconsider the processes that underlie early syntactic development. Phrasal speech allows some children to derive combinatorial patterns by segmenting phrases into frames with slots that can then be filled with other lexical items (Pine & Lieven, 1993). Peters (1977, 1983) also suggests that phrasal utterances may be stored, retrieved, and used as single lexical items that are later analyzed and broken down into productive components. She suggests the term *fission* for the eventual breakdown of phrasal speech, as distinguished from the complementary process of building sentences by combining units, which she calls *fusion.* Individual children may favor one or the other approach as their entry into syntax: one that begins with single words and combines them to build phrases, or one that proceeds from whole phrases to component parts, with the parts later recombined in novel utterances. Detailed longitudinal analyses reveal that children formulate many of their early sentences by building up distributional patterns around specific lexical items (e.g., *want x, there's a x, what's x doing*) rather than by applying more general semantic (e.g., agent + action) or syntactic (e.g., verb + object) relations (Lieven, Pine, & Baldwin, 1997; Tomasello, 1992). That is, children first isolate individual segments and look for patterns in what comes before or after. Children differ, however, in the size of the items (words, formulae, or partially analyzed phrases) that they isolate and combine (Thal & Bates, 1988).

The tendency to imitate adult speech is another dimension of variation that predicts some stability across language levels. Children who have a strong tendency to imitate prosodic patterns may, as a result, acquire phrasal units as well as single words during the one-word stage, produce more high-frequency items of low semantic value (such as pronouns) during the early sentence stage, and have messier phonological systems all along. Relationships between imitativeness and the tendency to be expressive, to produce longer utterances, and to show high levels of unintelligibility have been reported (Bloom et al., 1974; Ferguson & Farwell, 1975; Nelson, 1973), but other studies have found that children with referential language imitate more and suggest that these differences lie more in what children imitate than in how much. Whereas children with expressive speech imitate large units and social expressions, children with referential language tend to imitate object labels, particularly those they do not already know (Leonard, Schwartz, Folger, Newhoff, & Wilcox, 1979; Nelson, Baker, Denninger, Bonvillian, & Kaplan, 1985).

The evidence that individual preferences in language learning are somewhat stable over the toddler period raises the possibility that more extended longitudinal studies would find even more substantial stability. For example, do children show the same preferences if faced with the task of learning a second language later in childhood, or when faced with language-related tasks such as learning to read? Bates's daughter Julia, who had been a highly referential child in learning English, was reported to adopt a much more holistic and expressive strategy in acquiring Italian, but it must be noted that she was exposed to Italian during large group interactions quite different from the primarily dyadic social circumstances in which she learned English. Bussis, Chittenden, Amarel, and Klausner (1984) found that early readers seemed to split into two groups with styles reminiscent of those described by Wolf and Gardner (1979) for language acquisition: dramatists and patterners. The **dramatists** used more meaning-driven reading strategies, often previewing texts and studying illustrations to get a sense of the content before reading, skipping easily over passages they couldn't read, and sometimes making up substitute passages for bits they could not read. The **patterners,** on the other hand, were highly faithful to the text, sounding out unknown words carefully, and building for themselves highly sequenced text representations. Long-term longitudinal studies may help us sort out some day whether, indeed, the young language learners who prefer conservative, data-gathering, analytic strategies persist in the use of these strategies for second language learning and for reading, while their more risk-taking holistic peers maintain their preferred strategies across age as well.

Sources of Variation

Given that the individual differences we have described above exist and are robust, the question that arises is what might explain them. Do they reflect child factors—for example, sociability, preceptual processing mechanisms, or cognitive style? Do they perhaps reflect differences in how caregivers interact with or talk to children? Do they represent preparation for differences that characterize the range of different languages? In other words, is the learner of English who concentrates on single words just revealing an expectation that her language will be one like Chinese, with little morphology, whereas the more holistic learner who includes syllabic slots where adults produce affixes is expecting a language more like Turkish or Polish?

Child Factors

Perhaps the most obvious difference among child language learners is in rate of learning. Some children begin talking close to their first birthday, while others wait another six months or more before words appear. Most children acquire their first words slowly and sporadically. In this early stage, words may be learned case by case, with each case an independent relationship between sound pattern and referent(s). However, as the lexicon nears fifty words, a "critical mass" is reached and children may understand that "all things can be named" (Goldfield & Reznick, 1990, 1996); that is, children may require a sufficient number of words in store to abstract the nature of words as related parts of a conventional linguistic system. With this insight, the child is motivated to deliberately and systematically acquire and use the words and, eventually, the syntactic rules of the language community. The result is a "vocabulary spurt" in which rate of word learning accelerates dramatically (Goldfield & Reznick, 1990, 1996; Reznick & Goldfield, 1992). By eighteen months, the average child has a vocabulary of about seventy-five words, although perfectly normal two-year-olds may have far fewer (Fenson, Dale, Reznick, Bates, Thal, & Pethick, 1994).

There is considerable evidence, however, that the kinds of style or strategy differences that we have described are not simply the result of observing children with differing rates of development. Children with relatively more referential or expressive speech achieve language milestones at the same age (Hampson & Nelson, 1993; Nelson, 1973; Pine & Lieven, 1990), and there appears to be no clear advantage for either style when correlated with later vocabulary or grammatical measures (Bates et al., 1993; Hampson & Nelson, 1993).

As we noted earlier, children may be differentially sensitive to the prosodic tunes that unify whole phrases or to the syllables and segments that make up single words. The source of these differences may be found in developmental asymmetries in the multiple mechanisms that support language acquisition. That is, differences in the rate at which attention, perception, and memory mature and are available to parse, store, and analyze the input stream may affect the size and form of the linguistic units children produce. Bates and colleagues (1993) and others have noted that younger learners must approach the problem of language acquisition with less memory capacity and fewer analytic skills than older learners—thus perhaps throwing themselves into production rather than comprehension and often producing forms they do not fully understand. On the other hand, there is the possibility that some children are more cautious, apprehensive about making mistakes, and disinclined to talk—in short, shy. Shy children have been shown to talk less and less complexly in a way that remains stable through kindergarten and first grade (Evans, 1993). Horgan (1981) also suggests that differences between younger and older language learners may be a function of their tendency to be cautious or to take risks. Fifteen pairs of children were matched on MLU but differed in age by at least six months. The faster (younger) learners tended to use more nouns and more complex noun phrases and to talk more about people and things. These children also tended to make more grammatical errors. The slower (older) learners used fewer and less elaborate noun phrases but more and more complex verb phrases. These same children, however, were more advanced on comprehension tasks.

Horgan suggests that the slower children were more cautious language learners, with good receptive abilities but a more guarded approach to displaying their verbal skills. They may also have attended more to the details of language structure, as evidenced by their use of more auxiliaries and more kinds of constructions. The faster children, with their more frequent errors, were "more willing to take risks" (Horgan, 1981, p. 636), especially with the finer points of grammatical structure. Their attention was focused instead on describing the objects and people in their environment. Similar differences in the tendency to take risks with new syntactic forms versus to proceed cautiously until mastery is achieved have been found for children observed by Kuczaj and Maratsos (1983) and by Ramer (1976).

We do not yet have the longitudinal data that would provide the basis for claiming that slow starters at language acquisition turn out to be the children called shy, but it is clear that such shy children are likely to be slower second-language learners (Fillmore, 1979), as well as less obviously competent communicators in their first language.

Other child factors to consider include Nelson's (1973) proposal that differences in children's prelinguistic conceptual organization contribute to their early preferences for a referential or expressive vocabulary. She hypothesized that some babies organize their world around objects, whereas others focus on people. Children's differing hypotheses about what language is for (to organize and categorize objects or to talk about self and others) derive from these differing organizations of experience. Mothers of referential children more often reported that their children favored manipulative toys, supporting the notion that preexistent cognitive differences may influence children's speech style.

Subsequent studies of children's language and play have not found consistent support for linguistic differences that map onto object and social preferences. On the one hand, there is evidence that children who acquire more referential speech are more attentive to toys (Rosenblatt, 1977) and excel at object manipulation and spatial constructions (Wolf & Gardner, 1979). Similarly, children with more noun + noun combinations have higher levels of performance on object categorization tasks (Shore, Dixon, & Bauer, 1995). Children with more expressive speech have been found to orient more toward adults (Rosenblatt, 1977) and to engage in more social-symbolic (e.g., puppets and toy telephones) play (Wolf & Gardner, 1979).

Goldfield (1985/86, 1987), however, suggests that episodes of *shared attention* to objects may contribute more to the acquisition of referential language than the sheer quantity of object or social behavior. Goldfield observed twelve children during play sessions in the home at twelve, fifteen, and eighteen months of age. Mothers kept a diary record of the children's first fifty words. Children who acquired relatively more nominals did not differ from their less referential peers on measures of time in toy play or frequency of social behaviors. Children with more nominals, however, more often initiated episodes of joint attention to objects by showing, giving, or bringing toys to their mother. Children with more expressive speech, on the other hand, were not necessarily less interested in objects nor more sociable than their peers. These children were more likely to interrupt or leave their toy play to seek social attention, rather than to share or show a toy. Differences in the use of objects to mediate social interaction may, in turn, influence the language parents address to children. Child pointing typically elicits a maternal label (Masur, 1982), and children who more frequently point to objects acquire more nouns (Goldfield, 1990).

Input Factors

Children learn to talk in the course of their interactions with any number of conversational partners, including parents, day-care providers, siblings, and peers. Each social contact provides a unique source of language variance. It is likely that Crystal learned some phrasal speech from her older brother (e.g., *lemme see, you know what*), and other researchers have noted that laterborns tend to acquire more phrasal speech (Nelson et al., 1985; Pine, 1995). Day care offers even more varied language models. Most of the available research on individual differences has focused on the speech of mothers who have been the child's primary caregiver.

Although adult speech to children shares many features, there are also clear differences in how parents talk to children and encourage their children to talk. Stable differences have been noted in maternal conversational style, including mothers' preferred use of language to direct behavior, elicit conversation, or instruct their children (Olsen-Fulero, 1982). Moreover, at least some aspects of maternal style are related to children's acquisition of referential or expressive speech.

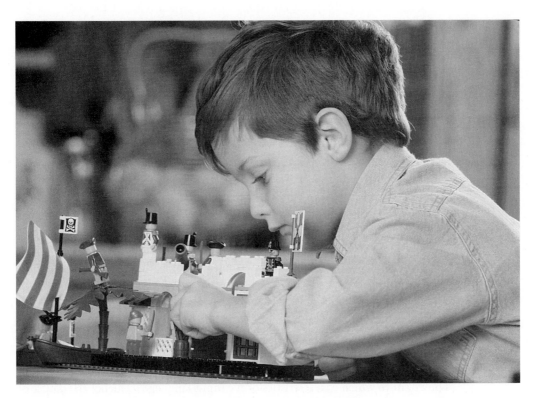

Patterners are interested in the physical properties of the world of objects.

Expressive language features, including fewer nouns, more social expressions, and more verbs are related to maternal speech that refers to persons or that directs the child's behavior in some way (Della Corte, Benedict, & Klein, 1983; Furrow & Nelson, 1984; Goldfield, 1985/86, 1987; Nelson, 1973; Pine, 1994). Referential language, on the other hand, is associated with maternal utterances that refer to and describe objects and that request and reinforce names for things (Brown, 1973; Della Corte et al., 1983; Furrow & Nelson, 1984; Goldfield, 1985/86, 1987; Hampson, 1988; Nelson & Bonvillian, 1972). Although the simple frequency of nouns in maternal talk is unrelated to children's speech style (Furrow & Nelson, 1984; Nelson, 1973), maternal descriptions that include nouns are related to the proportion of nouns in the first fifty words (Pine, 1994). It is important, then, to consider specific linguistic forms, such as nouns, in relation to the pragmatic focus (what parents talk about and for what purpose) of parental speech.

These correlations cannot tell us the extent to which parental speech affects child language, or vice versa. They do suggest, though, that mothers of children with referential or expressive speech are seeking out different opportunities for interaction and conversation. A good deal of children's referential language, for example, may originate in certain *routinized naming games.* Dore (1974) found that most of the labeling and repeating of the code-oriented baby he observed occurred in verbal routines established by the caregiver:

> M's mother set up routines in which she would pick up one item, label it, and encourage her daughter to imitate the label. There were animal-naming routines…utensil-naming and people-naming routines also occurred frequently. (p. 348)

Nelson (1973) also observed that 28 percent of the first fifty words acquired by referential children referred to body parts, almost surely learned in this kind of routine, whereas none of the expressive children had acquired labels for parts of the body. Expressive children, on the other hand, learn many conventional social expressions (e.g., *hi, bye, please, thank you, let's go,* and *oh dear*) that typically mark events such as arrivals, departures, and exchanges. Mothers of children with more expressive speech tend to use many such stereotypical utterances (Lieven, 1980; Nelson, 1973; Plunkett, 1993). Urwin (1978) observed that the parents of two visually handicapped children differed in the activities they organized and the language they used with their children. The parents of one child utilized his limited vision by encouraging attention to and labeling of objects, whereas the parents of a totally blind child more often engaged him in physical activities and social games. The latter child's early utterances were dominated by requests for and expressions of these games and routines.

The extent to which characteristics of the input language influence the course of acquisition has received mixed empirical support and continues to provoke theoretical debate. Recently, Hampson and Nelson (1993) demonstrated a relationship between maternal language at thirteen months and child grammar at twenty months when children were grouped on the basis of their language style. They found a significant, positive relationship between nouns in maternal speech and child MLU only for those children with more than 40 percent nouns in their spontaneous speech. No such relationship was found for children with more expressive speech (40 percent or fewer nouns). The two groups had similar numbers of early and late talkers at thirteen months and did not differ on MLU at twenty months. Thus, children with differing approaches to learning to talk may make differential use of selected aspects of the input. This suggests that it is crucial to consider individual differences, and the extent to which child strategy and caregiver speech style overlap, in studies that examine the efficacy of the input for acquisition.

Linguistic Factors

Children may start learning language with their own preferences and tendencies, and caregivers may emphasize certain aspects of language or provide richer input about some domains than others. In addition, though, languages differ from one another in the problems they pose to the learner. These differences may interact with learner and input factors to exaggerate individual differences.

Each language can be seen as, in effect, exploiting in its own particular way the capacities for elaboration, generalization, and rule learning that human beings possess. Both prosodic tune and segmentation into words are relatively accessible to English language learners. Slavic languages such as Polish, however, challenge speakers to learn a couple of dozen noun endings, including markings for six cases that in singular have distinct forms for masculine, feminine, and neuter (Smoczynska, 1985). This patterning is made more complex by its **synthetic** character, that is, that a particular suffix that reflects the synthesis of, for example, masculine, singular, and genitive might have no phonetic relation to the feminine singular genitive or the masculine singular dative. Since nouns in Slavic are never produced without suffixed case and gender markings, it may be almost inevitable that children choose a risk-taking strategy that leads to many errors, since they cannot learn the entire paradigm instantly. Turkish, on the other hand, also is characterized by many suffixes, but they are **agglutinated** rather than synthetic, that is, added on in a predictable sequence. Turkish learners may benefit from a tendency to use a prosodic strategy that incorporates dummy syllables for the affixes not yet learned, as that strategy creates precisely the slots into which the to-be-learned material must fit.

Unfortunately, the data on acquisition of languages other than English are relatively sparse, lacking in the large sample studies that make seeking individual differences feasible. Both word and tune babies have been observed for Danish (Plunkett, 1993), German (Stern & Stern, 1928), and Norwegian (Simonsen, 1990). Holistic, prosodic learners are also found in Hebrew (Berman, 1985), Hungarian (MacWhinney, 1985), French (E. V. Clark, 1985), Italian (Cipriani, Chilosi, Bottari, & Poli, 1990), and Portugese (Scarpa, 1990). As was the case for Peters' (1977) subject, Minh, the German tune baby observed by Elsen (1996) used some referential speech during naming routines and when looking at picture books. Many languages use intonation to signal differences in meaning (e.g., the difference between a statement and a yes-no question), suggesting that this is an individual style that is common and perhaps equally compatible with all languages. The tendency of some children learning English to seize upon whole words rather than on morphological modifications of words raises the question what such children would do if they were learning Inuktitut or Hebrew, where "words" as such can hardly be identified through the massive morphological changes that every shift in meaning imposes. Cross-linguistic analyses have also yielded more diversified patterns than those identified for English speakers. Three patterns (emphasizing nouns vs. phrases and fillers vs. verbs, adjectives, and grammatical words) have been observed for French language learners at twenty months of age (Bassano, Maillochon, & Eme, 1998).

Languages also differ in the ease with which children may extract specific parts of speech such as nouns or verbs. In English, nouns may be more salient than verbs because children hear them at the beginning and end of SVO sentences and nouns occur with fewer grammatical inflections than verbs; pragmatic factors also favor nouns over verbs in production (Goldfield, 1993, 1998). Japanese, Korean, and Mandarin Chinese, on the other hand, are languages that highlight verbs by frequently deleting nominal referents and positioning verbs at the ends of sentences (Clancy, 1985; Rispoli, 1989; Tanouye, 1979; Tardif, 1996). These interlinguistic differences appear to have consequences for language learners. As we have seen, children learning English differ in their emphasis on nouns in the first fifty words; nevertheless, noun learning is a prominent aspect of vocabulary acquisition, and the proportion of nouns typically increases between fifty and two hundred words (Bates et al., 1993). In contrast, Japanese, Korean, and Mandarin learners typically start with a higher percentage of verbs than nouns (Clancy, 1985; Gopnik & Choi, 1991, 1995)—thus, highly referential children acquiring these languages may have absolute levels of nouns much lower than relatively expressive children learning English! Italian shares some characteristics of pro-drop languages that highlight verbs, but Italian verbs are more morphologically complex and variable, and, unlike Mandarin, Italian is not a null object language. Overall, the input to Italian children is more like English than Mandarin, and, like English learners, children learning Italian produce more nouns but fewer verbs than Mandarin speakers (Tardif, Shatz, & Naigles, 1997).

Context: The Interaction of Child, Caregiver, and Language

As we have seen, both child and caregiver factors predict differences in children's approach to the problems that varied languages present to them. The challenge for research is to understand how available learning mechanisms interact with environmental supports. One approach is to consider that language is learned and used as part of a myriad of contexts that make up the daily life of children and their conversational partners. As Nelson (1981) has observed, the context in which language is used will determine the form and function of the input. Episodes of *joint object attention,* for example, are associated with more child labels and more maternal comments (Tomasello & Farrar, 1986; Tomasello & Todd, 1983). Book reading may be a particularly effective context for acquiring object labels (Ninio, 1980; Ninio & Bruner, 1978). Other situations in the child's life—eating, dressing, playing with siblings and peers, playing with toys, rough-and-tumble playing, and listening to and singing nursery rhymes and songs—provide quite different contexts for input and acquisition. Each context, then, provides a unique opportunity to learn some aspect of language: whole words or phrases, object labels or words for actions and states, labeling or demanding, prosodic or segmental accuracy. Thus, as the range of contexts varies, opportunities for language learning will differ for individual children.

The interests of both child and caregiver, moreover, will influence the kinds of contexts that make up the daily events and routines of a particular mother–child pair. Goldfield (1987) found that children's lexical differences were best predicted by a combination of child and caregiver variables. More referential language was acquired by children who more often used objects to elicit maternal attention and who had mothers who more often labeled and described toys. Johanna was the most referential child in this sample. She gave clear evidence that shared attention to objects was a familiar and enjoyable interactive context. During the play sessions, almost half (48%) of her attempts to engage her mother involved showing or giving a toy. Moreover, her mother's speech clearly and consistently supported the extraction and acquisition of single words that named objects. Talk about toys was the largest category of maternal speech (41%), and her mother highlighted names for things during all types of play, from bookreading (*egg in the hole book/look/see the tree*) to ball games (*ayy it's a ball*) and pretend play (*here's a woman—you can put the woman in the truck*). Nouns made up 76 percent or Johanna's first fifty words, and only one of these was a phrase (*get you*).

Other children may experience relatively more contexts in which the focus is on the child's behavior, performance, or nontoy play. Caitlin, a child with highly expressive speech, included a toy in only 18 percent of her social initiations. She was more likely to pause in her play to look and smile at her mother. Caitlin's mother, moreover, often engaged her baby in social play, using conversational formulae and routines more than any other mother in the sample. Almost half (48%) of her utterances were questions and directives used to prompt her daughter's performance and to engage her participation in shared play. Sixty-one percent of Caitlin's first fifty words consisted of expressive speech, and many of these, as we pointed out earlier, were phrases.

Most children, however, are likely to learn a more balanced mix of nouns, phrases, and expressive speech, acquired through participation in a range of contexts. Peters (1983) observed that Minh's use of analytic and gestalt language was often tied to specific contexts. One-word utterances were likely in situations such as naming pictures in a book, whereas gestalt language was often copied from songs and storybook rhymes.

Implications of Individual Differences for a Theory of Language Acquisition

The fact of individual differences in language acquisition has implications for theories and methods in the study of language development. Early studies in the modern era of language research assumed that universal aspects of acquisition were the proper object of study and that phenomena that varied across children were trivial. Thus, small sample studies were the norm, and no attempt was made to select children who represented the range of possible approaches to acquisition. We see now that individual differences can tell us about the processes by which children extract information from the linguistic interactions in which they participate. Assessing the extent and type of individual differences helps us construct a theory of how children learn, rather than just a description of what they know. Moreover, emphasis on the study of

English learners has limited the data we report and the theories we construct. English is a language with relatively impoverished morphology and little opportunity to exploit word order variation in simple sentences. Thus, the range of normal variation in approaches to language may be limited by the characteristics of English, and we are in danger of thinking that characteristics of English learners (e.g., a tendency to start with nouns) are in fact universal for all language learners.

Children such as Johanna, whose early language consists of clearly articulated single words that are predominantly nouns, are well represented in the bulk of language development research. Cross-linguistic studies, however, reveal that nonnominals figure more prominently in the early speech of children learning languages other than English. Italian children appear to learn fewer nouns than their English-speaking peers (Camaioni & Longobardi, 1995), and Japanese, Mandarin, and Korean speakers are precocious verb learners (Clancy, 1985; Gopnik & Choi, 1991, 1995; Tardif, 1996). Because English speakers (parents, children, and researchers) value nouns, much of our research efforts have been limited to understanding the principles that govern the acquisition of object labels (see, for example, Golinkoff, Mervis, & Hirsh-Pasek, 1994; Markman, 1989; Mervis, Golinkoff, & Bertrand, 1994). The emphasis on nouns may be misleading. For example, unlike nouns, nonostensive rather than ostensive contexts appear to be more conducive to the acquisition of verbs (Goldfield, 1998; Tomasello & Kruger, 1992). By limiting our explanations of word-learning to nouns, we may be missing many of the cognitive and linguistic resources that children bring to the task of learning to talk.

Expressive speakers such as Caitlin, who acquire numerous phrases, appear less frequently in the literature. However, the early use of phrasal utterances may be more common than has been previously acknowledged. Longer, expressive phrases occur throughout the one-word period (Branigan, 1977; Lieven et al., 1992; Stokes & Holden, 1980; Thomas, 1979). Lieven, Pine, and Barnes suggest that research would reveal more nonreferential children if samples were more often expanded to include a wider range of social backgrounds. Five out of twelve children in their sample of families from varied socioeconomic groups had twenty-five or more phrases in their first one hundred words. Attention to phrasal speech has resulted in improved methodologies and criteria for determining the length and productivity of children's linguistic units (Lieven et al., 1997; Plunkett, 1993). Connectionist models have also revealed neural networks that segment units larger than single words from connected "speech." These models demonstrate how dramatic differences in output may emerge from small differences in the learner (i.e., network) and/or in the input (Elman, 1990) and offer a potentially valuable methodological tool for exploring the kinds of interactions that are likely to underlie the variability in language form and function that we have described.

Interest in children's use of phrasal speech is especially important in view of the fact that a significant proportion of everyday adult speech may consist of phrases stored and retrieved as a whole. These formulae consists of idioms (e.g., *kick the bucket*), collocations (e.g., *sheer/pure coincidence*), adjuncts (e.g., *by and large*), sentence frames (e.g., *please pass the x*), and standard situational utterances (e.g., *can I help you?*) (Becker, 1975; Nattinger & DeCarrico, 1992; Pawley & Snyder, 1983). Wray (1998) argues that formulae perform important sociolinguistic functions that ease the burden of constructing utterances from scratch each time we have something to say, especially in the course of communicatively predictable situations. To date, syntactic theory has focused almost entirely on rule-generated constructions and has neglected to address the processes by which children acquire, store, and produce the full range of communicatively effective utterances.

Methods for collecting data on language acquisition have been developed on the assumption that all children go about it much the same way. Thus, many analyses of children's spontaneous speech are based on utterances elicited in the context of play with toys, usually a set of novel toys provided by the experimenter. Children who rely on imitation and routine contexts as sources of their utterances may be relatively disadvantaged in this novel situation and need to be observed during more familiar daily events. Similarly, phrasal speech may be more consistently elicited during interactions with an older sibling.

It is also important to note that different cultures vary in the degree to which they encourage and support various child tendencies. The highly referential child is appropriate and rewarding to a middle-class American mother who sees naming as a sensible and intelligent way to use language, but not to a Kaluli mother, who would view naming as "talking to no purpose" (Schieffelin, 1986). The skill of imitation may be relatively little valued by American mothers, but it is crucial for children whose caregivers instruct them to repeat modeled utterances as a way both to learn and to function socially, as do Kaluli (Schieffelin, 1986), Kwara'ae (Watson-Gegeo & Gegeo, 1986), and Basotho (Demuth, 1986) mothers. The existence of cultural variation in the language-learning environment has been proposed by many as an argument against a strong environmental influence on language acquisition; we see variation instead as a fact that must be understood, in the light of information from studies of individual differences, as evidence that children have many mechanisms available for the acquisition of language that are differentially exploited in different cultural and linguistic contexts.

Summary

It is important to reiterate that even though individual differences in styles or strategies for language acquisition are striking, the differences observed may reflect preferences or tendencies rather than dichotomies. Children who are classified as highly *imitative* produce many nonimitated utterances. *Pronominal* children produce some nominal word combinations. *Referential* children are not incapable of socially expressive speech. Language acquisition is a remarkably buffered process with a high rate of success; clearly, most children control many different strategies and mechanisms that contribute to language development.

We are left with the question of where the differences originate. It has been suggested that children's varying approaches to language and other cognitive problem areas reflect basic *temperamental* differences—for example, in risk-taking tendencies—or in asymmetries in how information is processed. Such hypotheses await further, more interdisciplinary investigations to test them adequately. Hardy-Brown (1983), for example, suggests that we employ research designs from the field of behavioral genetics to disentangle the effects of heredity and environment on individual differences in rate and style of acquisition. These methodologies would include adoption studies, which assess the cognitive and linguistic abilities of both birth and adoptive parents and compare these measures to the child's developing linguistic skills. Meanwhile, the fact of individual differences has implications not only for theory, but for *research* and *educational practice* as well. We can apply what we know about individual differences to amend and improve our methods of *collecting language data, intervening* with children at risk for language delay or deviance, and *teaching* reading and foreign languages.

Finally, the recognition that there are many ways to learn a language and that normally developing children may differ from one another in how they accomplish the task should help us to think more creatively about *therapy, intervention,* and *education.* A single therapeutic or educational method is unlikely to work for all children, and the failure of one method does not imply that success is impossible. The delayed or language-handicapped child, like the normally developing child, may exploit or avoid imitation, may search cautiously for rules or recklessly try out utterances, may be more easily involved in social games, or may demand a referential vocabulary. All of these preferences are compatible with successful language acquisition, and all can be utilized by therapists, teachers, and parents.

Key Words

agglutinated	patterner
analytic style	pronominal strategy
code-oriented	referential
dramatist	rote/holistic style
expressive	synthetic
message-oriented	transformational syntax
nominal strategy	

Suggested Projects

1. Analyze the speech of one child with two different adults, one familiar and one unfamiliar, in a variety of situations, to determine how much intrachild variability occurs on percentage of imitative utterances, use of pronouns, and use of object- versus social-oriented utterances.

2. Find parents of three children aged fourteen to eighteen months. Administer the MacArthur Communicative Development Inventory to the parents, and interview them about their impressions of their children's "language learning style," to determine, for example, if the children started to talk using a lot of jargon babbling or with clear words, if they were cautious comprehenders or reckless producers with lots of errors, or if they were highly or minimally imitative. Use the look-up tables in Bates and colleagues (1993) to see where the children score on referentiality. If time permits, tape and transcribe about twenty minutes of parent–child interaction (enough to get about 100 child utterances) and analyze the child talk for the dimensions of individual differences discussed in this chapter.

3. Record the interactions of three different caregiver–child pairs (children should be about the same age and/or vocabulary level). Code parental speech for its communicative intent (e.g., descriptions vs. behavioral directives as used by Pine, 1994). Do the parents differ on these dimensions?

Suggested Readings

Bates, E., Bretherton, I., & Snyder, L. (1988). *From first words to grammar: Individual differences and dissociable mechanisms.* Cambridge, UK: Cambridge University Press.

Lieven, E. V. M. (1996). Variation in a crosslinguistic context. In D. Slobin (Ed.), *The crosslinguistic study of language acquisition, Volume 5: Expanding the contexts.* Hillsdale, NJ: Lawrence Erlbaum.

Nelson, K. (1981). Individual differences in language development: Implications for development and language. *Developmental Psychology, 17,* 170–187.

Peters, A. (1983). *The units of language acquisition.* Cambridge, UK: Cambridge University Press.

Shore, C. M. (1995). *Individual differences in language development.* Thousand Oaks, CA: Sage.

References

Adamson, L. B., & Tomasello, M. (1984). An "expressive" child's language development. *Infant Behavior and Development, 7,* 4.

Bassano, D., Maillochon, I., & Eme, E. (1998). Developmental changes and variability in the early lexicon: A study of French children's naturalistic productions. *Journal of Child Language, 25,* 493–531.

Bates, E., Bretherton, I., & Snyder, L. (1988). *From first words to grammar: Individual differences and dissociable mechanisms.* Cambridge, UK: Cambridge University Press.

Bates, E., Marchman, V., Thal, D., Fenson, L., Dale, P., Reznick, J. S., Reilly, J., & Hartung, J. (1993). Developmental and stylistic variation in the composition of early vocabulary. *Journal of Child Language, 21,* 85–123.

Becker, J. (1975). *The phrasal lexicon.* BBN Report no. 3081, AI Report no. 28. Cambridge, MA: Bolt, Baranek, & Newman.

Bellugi, U. (1967). *The acquisition of negation.* Unpublished doctoral dissertation, Harvard University.

Benedict, H. (1979). Early lexical development: Comprehension and production. *Journal of Child Language, 6,* 183–200.

Berman, R. A. (1985). The acquisition of Hebrew. In D. I. Slobin (Ed.), *The crosslinguistic study of language acquisition: Vol. 1. The data.* Hillsdale, NJ: Lawrence Erlbaum.

Bloom, L. (1993). *The transition from infancy to language: Acquiring the power of expression.* Cambridge, UK: Cambridge University Press.

Bloom, L., Hood, L., & Lightbown, P. (1974). Imitation in language development: If, when and why. *Cognitive Psychology, 6,* 380–420.

Bloom, L., Lightbown, P., & Hood, L. (1975). Structure and variation in child language. *Monographs of the Society for Research in Child Development, 40.*

Bowerman, M. (1973). *Early syntactic development: A cross-linguistic study with special reference to Finnish.* London: Cambridge University Press.

Bowerman, M. (1976). Semantic factors in the acquisition of rules for word use and sentence construction. In D. Morehead & A. Morehead (Eds.), *Directions in normal and deficient child language.* Baltimore: University Park Press.

Braine, M. D. S. (1963). The ontogeny of English phrase structure: The first phase. *Language, 39,* 1–13.

Braine, M. D. S. (1976). Children's first word combinations. *Monographs of the Society for Research in Child Development, 41.*

Branigan, G. (1977, September 30). *If this kid is in the one-word period, how come he's saying whole sentences?* Paper presented at the Second Annual Boston University Conference on Language Development, Boston.

Bretherton, I., McNew, S., Snyder, L., & Bates, E. (1983). Individual differences at 20 months: Analytic and holistic strategies in language acquisition. *Journal of Child Language, 10,* 293–320.

Brown, R. (1973). *A first language.* Cambridge, MA: Harvard University Press.

Bussis, A. M., Chittenden, E. A., Amarel, M., & Klausner, E. (1984). *Inquiry into meaning: An investigation of learning to read.* Hillsdale, NJ: Lawrence Erlbaum.

Camaioni, L., & Longobardi, E. (1995). Nature and stability of individual differences in early lexical development of Italian speaking children. *First Language, 15,* 203–218.

Cazden, C. (1968). The acquisition of noun and verb inflections. *Child Development, 39,* 433–438.

Chomsky, N. (1957). *Syntactic structures.* The Hague: Mouton.

Cipriani, P., Cholosi, A. M., Bottari, P., & Poli, P. (1990, July). *Some data on transitional phenomena in the acquisition of Italian.* Paper presented at the 5th International Congress for the Study of Child Language, Budapest.

Clancy, P. M. (1985). The acquisition of Japanese. In D. I. Slobin (Ed.), *The cross-linguistic study of language acquisition, Vol. 1: The data.* Hillsdale, NJ: Lawrence Erlbaum.

Clark, E. V. (1985). The acquisition of Romance, with special reference to French. In D. J. Slobin (Ed.), *The crosslinguistic study of language acquisition: Vol. 1. The data.* Hillsdale, NJ: Lawrence Erlbaum.

Clark, R. (1974). Performing without competence. *Journal of Child Language, 1,* 1–10.

Clark, R. (1976). What's the use of imitation? *Journal of Child Language, 4,* 341–358.

Della Corte, M., Benedict, H., & Klein, D. (1983). The relationship of pragmatic dimensions of mothers' speech to the referential-expressive distinction. *Journal of Child Language, 10,* 35–44.

Demuth, K. (1986). Prompting routines in the language socialization of Basotho children. In B. Schieffelin & E. Ochs (Eds.), *Language socialization across cultures.* New York: Cambridge University Press.

Dore, J. (1974). A pragmatic description of early language development. *Journal of Psycholinguistic Research, 4,* 343–351.

Echols, C. H. (1993). A perceptually based model of children's earliest productions. *Cognition, 46,* 245–296.

Elman, J. L. (1990). Finding structure in time. *Cognitive Science, 14,* 179–211.

Elsen, H. (1996). Two routes to language: stylistic variation in one child. *First Language, 16,* 141–158.

Evans, M. A. (1993). Communicative competence as a dimension of shyness. In K. H. Rubin & J. B. Asendorpf (Eds.), *Social withdrawal, inhibition, and shyness in childhood.* Hillsdale, NJ: Lawrence Erlbaum.

Fenson, L., Dale, P., Reznick, J. S., Bates, E., Thal, D., & Pethick, S. (1994). Variability in early communicative development. *Monographs of the Society for Research in Child Development, 59.*

Ferguson, C. A. (1979). Phonology as an individual access system: Some data from language acquisition. In C. J. Fillmore, D. Kempler, & W. S.-Y. Wang (Eds.), *Individual differences in language ability and language behavior.* New York: Academic Press.

Ferguson, C. A., & Farwell, C. (1975). Words and sounds in early language acquisition. *Language, 51,* 419–439.

Ferrier, L. J. (1975, September). *Dependency and appropriateness in early language development.* Paper presented at the Third International Child Language Symposium, London.

Fillmore, L. W. (1979). Individual differences in second language acquisition. In C. J. Fillmore, D. Kempler, & W S.-Y. Wang (Eds.), *Individual differences in language ability and language behavior.* New York: Academic Press.

Furrow, D., & Nelson, K. (1984). Environmental correlates of individual differences in language acquisition. *Journal of Child Language, 11,* 523–534.

Goldfield, B. (1982, October 9). *Intra-individual variation: Patterns of nominal and pronominal combinations.* Paper presented at the Seventh Annual Boston University Conference on Language Development, Boston.

Goldfield, B. (1985/86). Referential and expressive language: A study of two mother-child dyads. *First Language, 6,* 119–131.

Goldfield, B. (1987). The contributions of child and caregiver to referential and expressive language. *Applied Psycholinguistics, 8,* 267–280.

Goldfield, B. A. (1990). Pointing, naming, and talk about objects: Referential behavior in children and mothers. *First Language, 10,* 231–242.

Goldfield, B. A. (1993). Noun bias in maternal speech to one-year-olds. *Journal of Child Language, 20,* 85–99.

Goldfield, B. A. (1998). Why nouns before verbs? The view from pragmatics. *Proceedings of the Boston University Conference on Language Development.* Somerville, MA: Cascadilla Press.

Goldfield, B. A., & Reznick, J. S. (1990). Early lexical acquisition: Rate, content, and the vocabulary spurt. *Journal of Child Language, 17,* 171–183.

Goldfield, B. A., & Reznick, J. S. (1996). Measuring the vocabulary spurt: A reply to Mervis and Bertrand. *Journal of Child Language, 23* (1), 241–246.

Golinkoff, R. M., Mervis, C. B., & Hirsh-Pasek, K. (1994). Early object labels: The case for lexical principles. *Journal of Child Language, 21,* 125–155.

Gopnik, A., & Choi, S. (1991). Do linguistic differences lead to cognitive differences? A cross-linguistic study of semantic and cognitive development. *First Language, 11,* 199–215.

Gopnik, A., & Choi, S. (1995). Names, relational words, and cognitive development in English and Korean speakers: Nouns are not always learned before verbs. In M. Tomasello & W. E. Merriman (Eds.), *Beyond names for things.* Hillsdale, NJ: Lawrence Erlbaum.

Hampson, J. (1988). Individual differences in style of language acquisition in relation to social networks. In S. Salzinger, J. Antrobus, & M. Hammer (Eds.), *Social networks of children, adolescents, and college students.* Hillsdale, NJ: Lawrence Erlbaum.

Hampson, J., & Nelson, K. (1993). The relation of maternal language to variation in rate and style of language acquisition. *Journal of Child Language, 20,* 313–342.

Hardy-Brown, K. (1983). Universals and individual differences: Disentangling two approaches to the study of language acquisition. *Developmental Psychology, 19,* 610–624.

Hatch, E. (1974). Second language learning-universals? *Working Papers on Bilingualism, 3,* 1–18.

Heath, S. B. (1983). *Ways with words: Language, life, and work in communities and classrooms.* Cambridge, UK: Cambridge University Press.

Horgan, D. (1981). Rate of language acquisition and noun emphasis. *Journal of Psycholinguistic Research, 10,* 629–640.

Klein, H. B. (1978). *The relationship between perceptual strategies and production strategies in learning the phonology of early lexical items.* Bloomington: Indiana University Linguistics Club.

Kuczaj, S. A. & Maratsos, M. P. (1983). The initial verbs of yes-no questions: A different kind of general grammatical category. *Developmental Psychology, 19,* 440–443.

Leonard, L., Schwartz, R., Folger, M., Newhoff, M., & Wilcox, M. (1979). Children's imitations of lexical items. *Child Development, 59,* 19–27.

Lieven, E. V. M. (1980). *Language development in young children.* Unpublished doctoral dissertation, Cambridge University.

Lieven, E. V. M. (1989). The linguistic implications of early and systematic variation in child language development. *Proceedings of the Berkeley Linguistic Society, 25,* 203–214.

Lieven, E. V. M., Pine, J. M., & Baldwin, G. (1997). Lexically based learning and early grammatical development. *Journal of Child Language, 24,* 187–219.

Lieven, E. V. M., Pine, J. M., & Barnes, H. D. (1992). Individual differences in early vocabulary development: Redefining the referential-expressive distinction. *Journal of Child Language, 19,* 287–310.

Lifter, K., & Bloom, L. (1989). Object knowledge and the emergence of language. *Infant Behavior and Development, 12,* 395–423.

Macken, M. (1978). Permitted complexity in phonological development: One child's acquisition of Spanish consonants. *Lingua, 44,* 219–253.

MacWhinney, B. (1985). Hungarian language acquisition as an exemplification of a general model of language development. In D. I. Slobin (Ed.), *The crosslinguistic study of language acquisition: Vol. 2. Theoretical issues.* Hillsdale, NJ: Lawrence Erlbaum.

Markman, E. M. (1989). *Categorization and naming in children: Problems of induction.* Cambridge, MA: Bradford/MIT Press.

Masur, E. F. (1982). Mothers' responses to infants' object-related gestures: Influences on lexical development. *Journal of Child Language, 9,* 23–30.

Mervis, C. B., Golinkoff, R. M., & Bertrand, J. (1994). Two-year-olds readily learn multiple labels for the same basic-level category. *Child Development, 65,* 1163–1177.

Miller, P. J. (1982). *Amy, Wendy, and Beth: Language learning in South Baltimore.* Austin: University of Texas Press.

Miller, W., & Ervin, S. (1964). The development of grammar in child language. In U. Bellugi & R. Brown (Eds.), The acquisition of language (pp. 9–34). *Monographs of the Society for Research in Child Development, 29* (Serial No. 92).

Nattinger, J. R. & DeCarrico, J. S. (1992). *Lexical phrases and language teaching.* Oxford: Oxford University Press.

Nelson, K. (1973). Structure and strategy in learning to talk. *Monographs of the Society for Research in Child Development, 38.*

Nelson, K. (1975). The nominal shift in semantic-syntactic development. *Cognitive Psychology, 7,* 461–479.

Nelson, K. (1981). Individual differences in language development: Implications for development and language. *Developmental Psychology, 17,* 170–187.

Nelson, K. E., Baker, N., Denninger, M., Bonvillian, J., & Kaplan, B. (1985). Cookie versus do-it-again: Imitative-referential and personal-social-syntactic-initiating language styles in young children. *Linguistics, 23,* 433–454.

Nelson, K. E., & Bonvillian, J. D. (1972). Concepts and words in the 18-month-old: Acquiring concept names under controlled conditions. *Cognition, 2,* 435–450.

Ninio, A. (1980). Picture book reading in mother-infant dyads belonging to two subgroups in Israel. *Child Development, 51,* 587–590.

Ninio, A., & Bruner, J. (1978). The achievement and antecedents of labeling. *Journal of Child Language, 5,* 1–15.

Olsen-Fulero, L. (1982). Style and stability in mother conversational behavior: A study of individual differences. *Journal of Child Language, 9,* 543–564.

Pawley, A. & Snyder, F. H. (1983). Two puzzles for linguistic theory: Nativelike selection and nativelike fluency. In J. C. Richards & R. W. Schmidt (Eds.), *Language and communication.* New York: Longman.

Peters, A. M. (1977). Language learning strategies: Does the whole equal the sum of the parts? *Language, 53,* 560–573.

Peters, A. M. (1983). *The units of language acquisition.* Cambridge, UK: Cambridge University Press.

Peters, A. M., & Menn, L. (1993). False starts and filler syllables: Ways to learn grammatical morphemes. *Language, 69*(4), 742–777.

Pine, J. M. (1992a). The functional basis of referentiality: Evidence from children's spontaneous speech. *First Language, 12,* 39–55.

Pine, J. M. (1992b). How referential are "referential" children? Relationships between maternal-report and observational measures of vocabulary composition and usage. *Journal of Child Language, 19,* 75–86.

Pine, J. M. (1994). Environmental correlates of variation in lexical style: Interactional style and the structure of the input. *Applied Psycholinguistics, 15,* 355–370.

Pine, J. M. (1995). Variation in vocabulary development as a function of birth order. *Child Development, 66,* 272–281.

Pine, J. M., & Lieven, E. V. M. (1990). Referential style at thirteen months: Why age-defined cross-sectional measures are inappropriate for the study of strategy differences in early language development. *Journal of Child Language, 17,* 625–631.

Pine, J. M., & Lieven, E. V. M. (1993). Reanalyzing rote-learned phrases: Individual differences in the transition to multi-word speech. *Journal of Child Language, 20,* 551–571.

Plunkett, K. (1993). Lexical segmentation and vocabulary growth in early language acquisition. *Journal of Child Language, 20,* 43–60.

Ramer, A. L. (1976). Syntactic styles in emerging language. *Journal of Child Language, 3,* 49–62.

Reznick, J. S., & Goldfield, B. A. (1992). Rapid change in lexical development in comprehension and production. *Developmental Psychology, 28,* 406–413.

Rispoli, M. (1989). Encounters with Japanese verbs: Caregiver sentences and the categorization of transitive and intransitive action verbs. *First Language, 9,* 57–80.

Rosenblatt, D. (1977). Developmental trends in infant play. In B. Tizard & D. Harvey (Eds.), *Biology of play.* London: William Heinemann Medical Books.

Scarpa, E. (1990). Prosodic strategies for the production of long utterances. Unpublished manuscript, University of Campinas, Brazil.

Schieffelin, B. (1986). *How Kaluli children learn what to say, what to do, and how to feel.* New York: Cambridge University Press.

Shore, C., Dixon, W., & Bauer, P. (1995). Measures of linguistic and non-linguistic knowledge of objects in the second year. *First Language, 15,* 189–202.

Simonsen, H. G. (1990). *Child phonology: System and variation in three Norwegian children and one Samoan child.* Doctoral dissertation: Department of Linguistics and Philosophy, University of Oslo.

Slobin, D. I. (1968). *Early grammatical development in several languages, with special attention to Soviet research* (Working Paper No. 11). Berkeley: University of California, Language-Behavior Research Laboratory.

Slobin, D. I. (1985). *The cross-linguistic study of language acquisition, Vol. 1* Hillsdale, NJ: Lawrence Erlbaum.

Slobin, D. I. (1992). *The crosslinguistic study of language acquisition, Vol. 3.* Hillsdale, NJ: Lawrence Erlbaum.

Slobin, D. I. (1997). *The crosslinguistic study of language acquisition, Vol. 5: Expanding the contexts.* Hillsdale, NJ: Lawrence Erlbaum.

Smith, N. (1973). *The acquisition of phonology: A case study.* London: Cambridge University Press.

Smoczynska, M. (1985). The acquisition of Polish. In D. I. Slobin (Ed.), *The crosslinguistic study of language acquisition, Volume 1.* Hillsdale, NJ: Lawrence Erlbaum.

Snow, C. E. (1981). The uses of imitation. *Journal of Child Language, 8,* 205–212.

Snow, C. E. (1983). Saying it again: The role of expanded and deferred imitations in language acquisition. In K. E. Nelson (Ed.), *Child language* (Vol. 4). Hillsdale, NJ: Lawrence Erlbaum.

Snow, C. E. (1989). Imitativeness: A trait or a skill? In G. Speidel & K. E. Nelson (Eds.), *The many faces of imitation in language learning.* New York: Springer-Verlag.

Starr, S. (1975). The relationship of single words to two-word sentences. *Child Development, 46,* 701–708.

Stern, C. & Stern, W. (1928). *Die kindersprache.* Leipzig, Germany.

Stokes, W. T., & Holden, S. (1980, October). Individual patterns in early language development: Is there a one-word period? Paper presented at the Fifth Annual Boston University Conference on Language Development, Boston.

Tanouye, E. K. (1979). The acquisition of verbs in Japanese children. *Papers and Reports on Child Language Development, 17* (Department of Linguistics, Stanford University), 49–56.

Tardif, T. (1996). Nouns are not always learned before verbs: Evidence from Mandarin speakers' early vocabularies. *Developmental Psychology, 32*(3), 492–504.

Tardif, T., Gelman, S. A., & Xu, F. (1999). Putting the "noun bias" in context: A comparison of English and Mandarin. *Child Development, 70*(3), 620–635.

Tardif, T., Shatz, M. & Naigles, L.(1997). Caregiver speech and children's use of nouns versus verbs: A comparison of English, Italian, and Mandarin. *Journal of Child Language, 24,* 535–565.

Thal, D., & Bates, E. (1988). *Relationships between language and cognition: Evidence from linguistically precocious children.* Paper presented to the Annual Convention of the American Speech-Language-Hearing Association, Boston.

Thomas, E. (1979). *It's all routine: A redefinition of routines as a central factor in language acquisition.* Paper presented at the Fourth Annual Boston University Conference on Language Development, Boston.

Tomasello, M. (1992). *First verbs: A case study of early grammatical development.* Cambridge, UK: Cambridge University Press.

Tomasello, M., & Farrar, M. J. (1986). Joint attention and early language. *Child Development, 57,* 1454–1463.

Tomasello, M., & Kruger, A. C. (1992). Joint attention on actions: Acquiring verbs in ostensive and nonostensive contexts. *Journal of Child Language, 19,* 311–333.

Tomasello, M., & Todd, J. (1983). Joint attention and lexical acquisition style. *First Language, 4,* 197–212.

Urwin, C. (1978). The development of communication between blind infants and their parents. In A. Lock (Ed.), *Action, gesture, and symbol.* New York: Academic Press.

Vihman, M. M. (1993). Variable paths to early word production. *Journal of Phonetics, 21,* 61–82.

Watson-Gegeo, K., & Gegeo, D. (1986). Calling-out and repeating routines in Kwara'ae children's language socialization. In B. Schieffelin & E. Ochs (Eds.), *Language socialization across cultures.* New York: Cambridge University Press.

Wolf, D., & Gardner, H. (1979). Style and sequence in symbolic play. In M. Franklin & N. Smith (Eds.), *Early symbolization.* Hillsdale, NJ: Lawrence Erlbaum.

Wray, A. (1998). Protolanguage as a holistic system for social interaction. *Language and Communication, 18,* 47–67.

Chapter 9

Atypical Language Development

Nan Bernstein Ratner
University of Maryland

Not all children acquire language easily and well. In this chapter, we examine some major causes and patterns of language delay and disorder in children. The study of childhood language disorders is important for a number of reasons. First, the case of individuals who fail to learn language normally allows us to evaluate possible prerequisites for the normal acquisition process. For instance, when a mentally retarded child does not learn to use language rapidly or appropriately, we may test hypotheses about the possible role that cognitive development plays in language development. Conversely, cases in which cognition is grossly impaired, but language appears more typical may cause us to question the relationship between cognition and language. The role of sufficient access to adult input in fostering language learning is highlighted when we examine patterns of language difficulty experienced by deaf children. Children who fail to master grammatical rules in the absence of deficits in other areas of functioning invite us to consider whether language is a discrete "module" of human ability. Thus, theories of normal language acquisition must be able to predict how the process might be disrupted to produce a variety of child language learning disorders (Leonard, 1998).

Second, the study of language disorders in children represents one attempt to apply findings about the normal language acquisition process to a practical problem: What can be done to aid children who experience difficulty in learning and using language? By examining the specific patterns of delay and disorder certain children encounter during their language development and by reviewing what we already know about the sequence and nature of normal language development, we can more effectively target our attempts to remediate their difficulties.

As we learn more about the factors that may play a role in hindering children's language development, we hope to discover that certain disorders are preventable or respond best if intervention occurs very early in the child's life (U.S. Department of Education, 1987). In other words, if we find that certain environmental or physical factors predispose children to communicative disorder, we may begin to address how we can reduce the number of children who display long-term difficulty with language skills.

Some researchers have estimated that 8 to 10 percent of school-aged children demonstrate patterns of communicative development that may be termed "delayed" or "disordered" (Silva, 1980). In this chapter, we describe some major patterns of language disturbance. In each case, we review what is known about affected children's development, how current theory attempts to explain the nature of their communicative difficulty, and what can be done to aid such children in improving their language skills. These major syndromes of language disorder involve children with *hearing impairment, mental retardation, autism,* and *specific language impairment.* While the chapter discusses them separately, it is worthwhile to appreciate that many of the behaviors of concern, and many of the approaches to treatment, cross the boundaries between these categories of disorder. Finally, we will note some conditions that lead to difficulty in producing speech, as opposed to language. Such *speech disorders* include delayed or deviant articulation and stuttering.

Communicative Development and Severe Hearing Impairment

The Effects of Sensory Deprivation

We know that it is necessary to be exposed to linguistic models in order to learn a language. We instinctively know this because we recognize that we learn only the language or languages we hear spoken around us, rather than any possible human language. At a deeper level, however, we become aware that if certain conditions limit linguistic exposure, language development may be severely hindered. Such is the case with significant **hearing impairment.** Over one million children in the United States are hearing-impaired (Tye-Murray, 1998). Children who are born with hearing impairment that limits their perception of sounds to those exceeding 60 **decibels** (dB), or about the intensity level of a baby's cry, generally will not be able to develop spontaneous oral language that approximates that of normal children. Children born with profound losses exceeding 90 dB are considered functionally deaf and will not develop speech and language skills spontaneously (without educational and therapeutic intervention; Carney & Moeller, 1998). Just as importantly, such children will eventually demonstrate language comprehension difficulties, even when the mode of language presentation (e.g., writing) bypasses their problems of auditory reception.

Hearing losses vary in severity and type. It is possible for hearing to be impaired such that only small subtleties (such as whispering) might be missed; it is also possible for hearing impairment to be severe enough to limit reception of almost all important linguistic and environmental information. Generally, the extent to which a child is handicapped by hearing loss depends upon the severity of the loss, the conditions causing the loss, the utility of hearing aids in restoring some hearing ability, and the age at which the hearing loss occurred. However, relatively large losses are not required for negative impacts on linguistic development: Even the fluctuating hearing loss of **otitis media** (middle ear infection with effusion) has been associated with lowered speech and language outcomes in children (Roberts & Wallace, 1997).

While amplification may provide the child with the ability to hear some otherwise inaudible sounds, it cannot restore normal hearing function, especially in cases of severe and profound loss. Even recent positive clinical experience with **cochlear implants,** which are capable of directly stimulating the auditory nerve to restore a sense of hearing, does not suggest that deafness can be fully overcome by assistive devices. However, evidence of the benefits and safety of cochlear implants continues to grow, especially when children with implants receive strong oral educational support (Staller, Beiter, & Brimacombe, 1994; Tait & Lutman, 1994). A later section specifically evaluates the impact of recent advances in cochlear implantation.

Losses that are **congenital** (present at birth) or that occur **prelingually** (before the child has learned language skills, the period when the majority of significant hearing losses in children occur) are much more disruptive of the language acquisition process than are losses acquired later in life (see Scheetz, 1993, for a discussion of hearing measurement and impairment). Children who have had access to the ambient language, even for a short while, demonstrate a higher level of linguistic achievement than those who have not had such exposure. Additionally, there is some suggestion that the **etiology** (cause) of the hearing loss may affect a child's linguistic progress. Hearing impairment may arise from a large number of genetic and environmental causes, and approximately 30 percent of children with significant hearing loss have other concomitant disabilities that may affect their ability to master speech and language skills (Tye-Murray, 1998).

It is important to understand how severe hearing impairment limits the child's access to linguistic input. Not all conversations occur face to face, and the deaf child misses those that take place out of his or her line of sight. We probably underestimate the degree to which we gain important linguistic insight from language interchanges that occur around us. Thus, even if the deaf child can focus on a speaker's face during conversation, **lipreading** (also called **speechreading**) does not automatically guarantee successful interpretation of the conversation. Many sounds are made in the back of the mouth and are not easily visible on the lips, such as velars and liquids.

Additionally, there are many sounds in English and in other languages that resemble one another on the lips but are acoustically distinct, such as /p/, /b/, and /m/. Since approximately 90 percent of deaf children are born to hearing parents (Tye-Murray, 1998), this means that the parents and their young child do not share a mutually intelligible communication system in the crucial early years of language development. Cases of deaf children of deaf parents who use sign language as a preferred method of communication—and thus can include the children in their language system from birth—provide an interesting comparison situation that we address later. Cases of deaf children raised in nonsigning households who develop rudimentary sign languages (Goldin-Meadow & Mylander, 1998) are rare, although of tremendous theoretical interest, and are more relevant to discussion of theories of the innate component of language acquisition (see Chapter 7) than to this section, since such children do not achieve mastery of any extant human language.

As we survey the historical impairments associated with profound hearing loss, even when children are fitted with **amplification** (hearing aids) and provided with extensive **aural rehabilitation,** we note that recent developments in cochlear implant technology (discussed below) appear to offer the potential for significantly lessening the impact of deafness. At the end of this section, we address the promise of cochlear implants—and the perhaps surprising degree of controversy that they have provoked.

Phonological Development

To an observer, the articulation of a deaf child may be the most evident manifestation of his or her disability. Many deaf children's speech is rated as quite unintelligible (Quigley & King, 1982; Tye-Murray, 1998), despite years of speech training. Certain classes of sounds (especially high-frequency sibilants and less visible phonemes) are likely to be omitted or misarticulated. Sounds at the ends of words and those embedded in consonant clusters are also likely to be missed by the hearing-impaired child. The speech of hearing-impaired children is also characterized by distinctive patterns of prosody that distinguish it from the speech of those with normal hearing; it lacks the fluid coarticulation patterns that are seen in normal conversational speech (Tye-Murray, 1998). Speech intelligibility in hearing impairment appears to be predictable on the basis of the severity and configuration of the child's hearing loss (Wolk & Schildruth, 1986). Recent research suggests that young cochlear implant users achieve greater intelligibility than children using conventional hearing aids (Tye-Murray, 1998).

Language Development

The deaf child's problems in acquiring and using the syntactic and semantic aspects of the language and in using such skills to develop proficiency in reading and writing are much more significant factors in his or her ability to succeed educationally and vocationally than is his or her typical articulation disability. Although Allen (1986) reports that deaf children's reading achievement improved somewhat in the decade between 1974 and 1983, deaf students appear to gain only two grade equivalents during their secondary school years. Furthermore, repeated surveys of the reading abilities of older deaf children and adults suggest that their reading ability may never surpass that of third-grade hearing children (Allen, 1986). LaSasso and Mobley (1997) suggest that, despite changes in educational approaches to deafness, including the development of various amplification devices and manually coded English systems, reading levels of deaf students have not changed appreciably for over eighty years. Additionally, Quigley and King (1982) suggest that refined analysis of the receptive grammatical abilities of deaf students indicates that they are less capable readers under certain circumstances than hearing children with equivalent standardized reading achievement scores. Such reading and writing inadequacies can be directly attributed to their limited exposure to the language. Chapter 10 reminds us that mastery of reading and writing is inextricably linked to knowledge of the oral language system, a system to which the deaf child has impeded access. As noted in a later section, cochlear implant technology may provide an answer to this chronic problem: Children using implants have recently been shown to demonstrate a higher level of reading achievement than children using conventional hearing aids.

Lexical Development

Some of the deaf child's problems with both oral and written language are due to depressed vocabulary skills (LaSasso & Davey, 1987; Quigley & Paul, 1984). As deVilliers (1991) observes, overt classroom instruction is simply insufficient in its ability to provide deaf students with the roughly 3,000 words per year that a hearing child acquires by merely overhearing or reading new words in context. It has been estimated that deaf adults tend to have lexical abilities more typical of a normally hearing fourth grader (Tye-Murray, 1998). Although data continue to emerge regarding the effectiveness of cochlear implants in addressing the vocabulary deficits of deaf children, in 1995, Dawson, Blamey, Dettman, Barker, and Clark reported that, "the number of children actually achieving age-appropriate language skills still form [sic] a small proportion" of cochlear implant recipients.

Grammatical Development

Delineation of the types of syntactic structures that pose particular problems for deaf students has been made possible by a series of classic studies carried out by Quigley and his coworkers (Power & Quigley, 1973; Quigley, Montanelli, & Wilbur, 1976; Quigley, Smith, & Wilbur, 1974; Quigley, Wilbur, & Montanelli, 1974, 1976; Wilbur, Montanelli, & Quigley, 1976). In general, deaf students have trouble comprehending many of the same structures that are troublesome for normally developing children: constructions that violate typical subject-verb-object (S-V-O) patterns in English, such as passives and embedded clauses. Deaf children, however, also have particular problems with modals, verb auxiliaries, infinitives, and gerunds. The deaf child's incomplete grasp of English syntax is made more apparent by errors observed in the following typical writing samples:

> We went to family camp today. She will be good family camp dog food. Boy went family fun dog friend car look. The played outuroor camp family good eat afternoon. The played eat fun camp after home. We perttey fun camp after home. The will week fun camp after car. We family will eat and aftmoon. [ten-year-old male, Performance IQ of 129, born deaf, Better Ear Average of 100 dB (ASA).]

> I really like { } college. The reason that is good for me. Also they have many students that I know. That school is good for me and keep my mind up and keep busy. they

have good education in { }. Maybe I will try for A.A. class next year. Now I am taking M.B.T. class this year. Also that M.B.T. is good for in the future. that M.B.T. is the best pay and it is hard work. There is many different jobs in the U.S.A. I am not sure what I want like plumbing, electric, or building. I hope that I an succeful in the future Also I want my family proud of me what I am doing this. (Scheetz, 1993)

Everyone is packing the food in the basket for a picnic. They are very exciting to go to the picnic for their pleasure. A girl gives a sandwich to a little dog to eat. Father carries a bat to play with his girl & boy. Then they have everythings in the car what they want.

After a while the car is leaving out but one boy saw his little dog alone. He told his father to stop to see the dog. He went out of a car. Everyone is laughing. He pats his dog and brings him in the car to go with them too. Then they arrive at a picnic. Mother cooks the food for them. A girl put any dishes on the picnic table. Father and a boy play a softball. Everyone is enjoying today for a picnic. [eighteen-year-old female, Performance IQ of 97, born deaf, Better Ear Average 100 dB (ASA).] (Quigley & King, 1982, pp. 444–445)

Table 9.1 displays some representative patterns of ungrammatical English usage found in the writings of deaf students. While some of the errors resemble those made in the speech of young, normally developing children—such as failure to invert subject and auxiliary for question formation or omission of the copula (the verb *to be*) in sentences—many are unique to hearing-impaired children.

DeVilliers (1991) observes that the repetitive style and overuse of simple sentence types that characterize the writing samples of deaf children may reflect dependence upon classroom drill for the development of syntactic proficiency. Such instruction typically focuses on the grammar of simple sentences. The emphasis upon simple sentence structures affects reading as well as writing ability. Complex sentences are much more common in textual materials than in spoken conversation, and reading proficiency rests upon ability to understand such advanced structures (Perera, 1984). Gormley and Sarachan-Deily (1987) found that deaf children often mastered spelling and punctuation conventions, while possessing poor control over syntax, especially pronominal reference. While ability to construct written narrative improves over the school years, the writing of older hearing-impaired students often lacks the more sophisticated elements found in secondary school efforts (Yoshinaga-Itano, Snyder, & Mayberry, 1996).

Educational Approaches to the Development of Language in Deaf Children

The majority of deaf children are born into hearing families, and thus are not exposed to **American Sign Language (ASL)** early in life. Historically, these children were

Table 9.1   **Examples of Distinct Syntactic Structures Generated by Deaf Children**

Structural Environment in Which Structure Occurs	Description of Structures	Example Sentences
Verb system	Verb deletion	the cat under the table.
	Be or *have* deletion	John sick. The girl a ball.
	Be–have confusion	Jim have sick.
	Incorrect pairing of auxiliary with verb markers	Tom has pushing the wagon.
	By deletion (passive voice)	The boy was pushed the girl.
Negation conjunction	Negative outside the sentence	Beth made candy no.
	Marking only first verb	Beth threw the ball and Jean catch it.
	Conjunction deletion	Joe bought ate the apple.
Complemention	Extra *for*	For to play baseball is fun.
	Extra *to* in POSS-ing complement	John goes to fishing.
	Infinitive in place of gerund	John goes to fish.
	Incorrectly inflected infinitive	Bill like to played baseball.
	Unmarked infinitive without *to*	Jim wanted go.
Relativization	NPs where *whose* is required	I helped the boy's mother was sick.
	Copying of referent	John saw the boy who the boy kicked the ball.
Question formation	Copying	Who a boy gave you a ball?
	Failure to apply subject–auxiliary inversion	Who the baby did love?
	Incorrect inversion	Who TV watched?
Question formation, negation	Overgeneralization of contraction rule	I amn't tired. Bill willn't go.
Relativization, conjunction	Object–object deletion	John chased the girl and he scared. (John chased the girl and he scared the girl.)
	Object–subject deletion	The dog chased the girl had on a red dress. (The dog chased the girl. The girl had on a red dress.)
All types of sentences	Forced subject–verb–object pattern	The boy pushed the girl. (The boy was pushed by the girl.)

Source: From "The Language Structure of Deaf Children" by S. Quigley, B. Power, and M. Steinkamp, 1977, *Volta Review 79*, p. 80. Copyright 1977 by the Alexander Graham Bell Association for the Deaf, Washington, DC. Reprinted by permission.

exposed primarily to oral language models, although this trend has changed over the past two decades (Mindel & Vernon, 1987). Proponents of an **oralist approach to deaf education** have believed that deaf children are best served by instruction in lip-reading, in maximum use of residual hearing (through amplification and auditory training), and in articulation to improve their speech.

A number of **sign systems** (Wilbur, 1987) have been developed to further the linguistic and educational development of the deaf child. These **manual approaches to deaf education** hope to improve the educational outlook of hearing-impaired children, many of whom did not appear to be able to succeed in oral programs. In general, these artificial systems attempt to convey manual representations of English sentence structure. That is, the systems translate words and grammatical morphemes used in spoken English into easily visible hand configurations and gestures. Use of **manually coded English** in combination with speech is called **total communication,** a popular educational approach (Quigley & Paul, 1987). Lou (1988) surveys the history of deaf education in the United States over the past century, and excellent overviews of the half-dozen most commonly used sign systems are provided in Bochner and Albertini (1988), Quigley and King (1982), Tye-Murray (1998) and Wilbur (1987). Most of the systems share some common features: They generally adapt some American Sign Language (**ASL** or **Ameslan**) signs for vocabulary items, invent new signs to convey grammatical concepts not expressed by discrete signs in ASL (such as articles, auxiliary verbs, and bound affixes for pluralization and tense and number agreement), and produce sentences that duplicate the syntactic structure of English. The result tends to resemble what might occur if one attempted to speak a foreign oral language, such as French, simply by placing French lexical items into an English grammatical framework (i.e., "*mon frère's voiture*" rather than "*la voiture de mon frère*" for the phrase "my brother's car"). For example, the sentence "*The* boy *is* eat*ing*" contains a number of elements not found in ASL (those in italics). While sign systems typically have invented new signs for those elements and would sign the phrase as written, the ASL version would more closely resemble "*Boy eat-eat-eat*" in English; reduplicated movement in ASL signals the progressive aspect, and the article is not necessary.

One manual system is distinct in its orientation: **Cued speech,** used by relatively few deaf children and their teachers/parents, utilizes handshapes near the mouth to disambiguate lipreading. Sign systems such as the ones mentioned above are now an integral part of the curriculum for many if not most hearing-impaired children (Quigley & Paul, 1987). Mindel and Vernon (1987) estimate that 95 percent of students with severe or profound hearing impairment utilize some form of manual communication system in their educational settings. The use of sign systems at home by parents is usually highly encouraged in the hope that they may aid deaf students to appreciate the rules that govern correct language use. However, both parents and teachers may find it difficult to communicate fluently in what is, to them, a foreign language, and there is evidence that many adults fail to include a number of the important grammatical features of English in the signed input, thus limiting the child's exposure to the language (Rudser, 1988; M. Swisher, 1985). This problem has been identified as a major need in the development of more effective early intervention initiatives (Moeller & Luettke-Stahlman, 1990).

At this point in time, neither ASL nor particular manual systems have gained recognition as the most effective vehicle for supporting acquisition of English skills in deaf children. There is some evidence to suggest that knowing ASL as a first language may aid deaf children in developing better skills with the English language, in much the same way that knowing a first language provides a basis for learning others. Moores (1987) observes that a subset of more linguistically proficient deaf students come from deaf households. Geers and Schick (1988) found that children with hearing-impaired parents who were learning manually coded English outperformed their peers with normal-hearing parents. However, orally educated children of hearing parents also often perform better educationally than the manually educated children of hearing parents, suggesting that parental proficiency with the input language is important to the child's development of linguistic skills.

As Quigley and King (1982) point out, intensive exposure both at school and at home to systems that parallel English may have the potential to be even more facilitative of linguistic progress if parents and teachers can develop good proficiency with the systems. However, any communicative system that maximizes the opportunity for fully developed language interaction between deaf children and those around them is likely to improve their progress in mastering language. Parental SES and active involvement in the child's educational programming also appear to positively affect the development of language proficiency (Moores, 1987).

Deaf and hearing-impaired students continue to experience a high degree of functional disability, regardless of educational approach (Karchmer & Allen, 1999). Some highly intensive oral programs report good English proficiency for their graduates (Geers & Moog, 1987), as do some total communication programs (Delaney, Stuckless, & Walter, 1984; Moores, 1987) and mainstreaming programs (Pflaster, 1980). After surveying their own and previous data, Musselman, Lindsay, and Wilson (1988) concluded that the nature of the hearing loss and the child's intellectual ability had a greater effect on his or her educational success than did many of the educational programming variables they examined. While there was some suggestion that children in total communication programs had both somewhat better receptive language ability and richer mother–child interaction but that orally educated children had better spoken language, the authors warn that at the present time "unequivocal statements about the value of particular approaches or the consequences of not following one approach or another are unwarranted" (p. 87). Moreover, they reported that "one clear conclusion that can be drawn is that no approach has succeeded in reversing the effects on language of severe and profound hearing impairment."

However, Strong and Prinz (1997) recently completed a study that correlated students' abilities to use ASL with literacy levels, regardless of whether ASL had been learned from deaf parents. Such data would suggest that acquisition of ASL, a natural language, supports second language skills in English more strongly than does an artificial system modeled on English. Despite such encouraging findings, Carney and Moeller (1998) note that the "paucity of studies in this area suggests that few analyses of treatment effectiveness, efficiency and effects are available regarding communication modality." Currently, researchers, teachers, and parents must grapple with matching individual students' needs and abilities to their educational programs—what works for one student may not be as effective as an alternate approach for another student. Carney and Moeller (1998) conclude that "there is no consensus of 'one treatment' that is applicable to all children with hearing loss, whether this treatment consists of the use of a sensory aid, a communication modality, or a type of academic curriculum."

Acquisition of ASL as a First Language

Many of the relatively few deaf children who are born to deaf parents grow up learning ASL as their first language. American Sign Language is a distinct language within the scope of the world's languages, with its own syntactic, semantic, and configurational rules. Klima and Bellugi (1979), Newport and Meier (1985), and Wilbur (1987) provide excellent descriptions of its grammar. ASL is not based upon English grammar and has rules for expressing S-V-O relationships, tense, pluralization, and so on that are different from the rules for these concepts in English. American Sign Language, like other sign languages of the world, is not transparently meaningful to speakers of English or other sign languages. That is, one cannot easily follow an ASL conversation without knowing the specific rules of ASL. As we discuss more fully in the next section, the language development of children learning ASL from birth closely parallels patterns observed in children acquiring oral languages (Newport & Meier, 1985).

The acquisition of ASL by such children [and by some hearing children exposed to both oral and signed language by one hearing-impaired and one normal hearing parent (Jones & Quigley, 1979; Prinz & Prinz, 1981)] essentially confirms that the language disability demonstrated by hearing-impaired children is one that stems from deficient input rather than other possible causes. That is, children learning ASL as a first language generally develop their first signed words at approximately the same age or even earlier than children who are acquiring oral language (Bonvillian, Orlansky, & Novack, 1983; McIntire, 1977; Wilbur & Jones, 1974). Such a phenomenon suggests that first-word production in speaking children may be constrained by the relatively less rapid development of oral as opposed to manual dexterity in children. However, Pettito (1991) contests the claim that sign usage emerges at an earlier age than verbal language.

There are marked similarities in the courses of ASL and oral language development. The two-word stage in early ASL usage is characterized by semantic relationships similar to those seen in early spoken language productions (Newport & Meier, 1985). Overregularizations of grammatical features and overextensions of vocabulary meaning are noted (Schlesinger & Meadow, 1972). However, accelerated use of vocabulary and combinatorial language may be observed when ASL-using infants are compared to oral language learning infants of similar ages (Bonvillian et al., 1983; McIntire, 1977).

Sign Language and the Brain

Chapter 1 surveys the neurological substrates that underlie oral language development and use. What happens when a child learns a visual, rather than an auditory language? Research suggests that, when visual input has linguistic significance, as do signs for a native deaf signer, such input is processed by areas identified for the processing of spoken languages, in the dominant (normally left) hemisphere, even though the nondominant hemisphere is normally activated during visuospatial tasks (McGuire, Robertson, Thacker, David, Kitson, Frackowiak, & Frith, 1997). However, because a language such as ASL does require some visuospatial processing not required by oral languages, deaf signers recruit both the left and right hemisphere during tasks of sentence processing (Bavelier, Corina, Jezzard, Clark, Karni, Lalwani, Rauschecker, Braun, Turner, & Neville, 1998). Brain damage also affects linguistic processing in deaf signers in ways predicted from study of hearing individuals (Hickock, Wilson, Clark, Klima, Kritchevsky, & Bellugi, 1999).

Cochlear Implants: A Controversial New Frontier in the Rehabilitation of Deaf Children

Ten years after Musselman and colleagues (1988) doubted that any therapeutic approach could effectively surmount the impact of severe hearing loss, there are suggestions that cochlear implant technology may significantly reduce the handicaps of hearing impairment in young children. Cochlear implants, first used with hearing-impaired adults over a decade ago, are implantable prostheses that stimulate the auditory nerve directly, bypassing defects in the integrity of the inner ear, the source of congenital sensorineural hearing loss. With the advent of newer devices, approval for implantation in

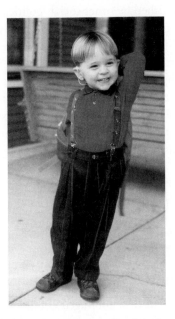

Cochlear implant technology has improved the speech and language skills of many children with severe hearing impairment.

young children, and the opportunity to observe children's progress over a relatively long time frame, the linguistic gains of the increasingly larger number of children receiving implants have become clearly evident (Miyamoto, Kirk, Svirsky & Sehgal, 1999; Robbins, Bollard, & Green, 1999; Tomblin, Spencer, Flock, Tyler, & Gantz, 1999). Observed progress greatly exceeds that seen in children wearing conventional aids and is seen as soon as two years post-implant (Tomblin et al., 1999). Francis, Koch, Wyatt, and Niparko (1999) report extremely favorable rates of mainstreaming (regular classroom inclusion) for implanted children, while Spencer and Tomblin (1999) report that many children with implants are reading at grade level, something rarely achieved by children with conventional aids. Robinson (1998) suggests that early implantation yields more favorable outcomes, perhaps because children older than age five have less plastic neurolinguistic capacity than children implanted earlier.

Cochlear implants are not without their critics. Crouch (1997) and Lane and Bahan (1998) note that, while language development is facilitated by cochlear implantation, it is not clear that implanted children successfully segue into mainstream hearing society. Further, because most deafness is not genetically transmitted, the sign languages of the world and Deaf culture are maintained rather uniquely as systems that are transferred and learned through peer-group membership, rather than passed by adults to children, as are other languages. Cochlear implantation has the potential to endanger sign languages, which are rich, full-fledged linguistic systems, and Deaf culture, in much the same way that other oral languages and cultures have been endangered and extinguished by other social, political, and economic factors.

In closing, we note that, whatever approach is used to improve the communication abilities of children with significant hearing impairment, early identification of the hearing loss is crucial (Yoshinaga-Itano, Sedey, Coulter, & Mehl, 1998). Children who are identified by six months of age, regardless of eventual therapeutic management, fare much better than do children whose hearing losses go undetected until later. Thus, the recent campaign for Universal Newborn Screening has important ramifications for improving the negative consequences usually associated with profound hearing impairment.

Mental Retardation and Communicative Development

Cognitive Disability and the Language Acquisition Process

Approximately 2 percent of school-aged children demonstrate some degree of cognitive or mental impairment (U.S. Department of Education, 1987). A good definition of normal intellectual ability is difficult to arrive at, and despite increasing dissatisfaction with the use of intelligence quotients (IQ) to measure mental development, they continue to be used to define and describe this population (Smith & Polloway, 1979). In 1992, the American Association on Mental Retardation (AAMR) redefined **mental retardation (MR)**, adding criteria that combine evidence of subaverage general intellectual functioning with depressed levels of adaptive behaviors that limit functions in areas such as "communication, self-care, home living, social skills, community use, self-direction, health and safety, functional academics, leisure and work" (AAMR, 1992). Mental retardation of a mild nature may be indicated by IQ performance falling between 53 and 70; moderate degrees of retardation by IQ scores of approximately 36 to 51; severe retardation by IQ scores between 20 and 35; and profound retardation by scores falling below IQ 20; most individuals with mental retardation are classified as mildly retarded (Owens, 1999). The majority of children with measured IQs falling below 50 will demonstrate severe language problems, and children with higher IQs may still experience language disability.

Mental retardation may result from a number of discrete etiologies; however, it is currently unclear whether most etiological subgroups of children with developmental retardation demonstrate differing patterns of linguistic impairment (Owens, 1999). The two subgroups whose distinct profiles have been analyzed most intensively have been **Down syndrome (DS)** and **Fragile X syndrome.** DS seems to be characterized by relatively weaker linguistic performance than might be expected from mental age (Fisch, Holden, Carpenter, Howard-Peebles, Maddalena, Pandya, & Nance, 1999), while Fragile X appears to result in fewer problems with language (relative to mental age), at the expense of impaired articulation and fluency (Dykens, Hodapp, & Leckman, 1994). Most major etiologies of MR appear to be characterized by abnormalities in the neuroanatomy of the hippocampus and cerebellum that affect attention, memory, and sequential information processing (Pulsifer, 1996).

The relationship between cognitive development and linguistic development in typically developing children is still a matter of intense inquiry (see Chapters 2 and 7). Miller and Chapman (1984) point out that our current understanding of cognitive prerequisites for language development does not strongly support the practice of teaching specific cognitive skills for the purpose of readying children with MR for language acquisition. Additionally, it may be that children with mental retardation demonstrate profiles of language use and ability that do not stem purely from cognitive deficits at all but rather from a cognitive orientation that results in patterns of social and motivational behaviors distinct from those of normally developing children (Kamhi & Johnston, 1982). Rosenberg (1982) suggests that the quality of passivity may best account for the slow acquisition of both cognitive and linguistic skills in most children with mental retardation.

Williams syndrome (WS) is a rare condition in which cognition is impaired but language appears intact or even precocious (Bellugi, Marks, Bihrle, & Sabo, 1988), thus weakening easy interpretation of the relationship between mental retardation and language ability. Lexical development in WS appears to be exceptionally strong. Other rare cases of supposed dissociations between cognition and language in individuals with functional MR have been reported (Smith & Tsimpli, 1995). However, Karmiloff-Smith, Grant, Berthoud, Davies, Howlin, and Udwin (1997) argue that while morpho-syntax is less impaired in WS than in other etiologies of MR, it is still quite impaired. Such an observation weakens the argument for a dissociation between cognition and language, or modularity of the language faculty (see Chapter 7), although such unusual cases of poor cognition and relatively spared language continue to spur active debate.

Owens (1997) proposes a multifaceted model of the language deficit in MR, using an information-processing schema. In this model, he notes that while children with MR appear to have adequate attentional capacity, they appear to have more trouble than typical peers in attending to the relevent stimuli in the immediate environment. Further, as input stimuli are processed, the child with MR is less able to use efficient organizational strategies to aid in storage and retrieval of linguistic information. Examples of such strategies would be to create associations to enable items to be remembered together or place concepts into categories to facilitate retrieval. Applying stored knowledge to new situations requires transfer, or generalization, an area that is particularly weak in most individuals with MR. Finally, children with MR have depressed **short-term** and **long-term memory abilities** (Owens, 1999). There seems to be evidence to suggest that auditory information is less well remembered than visual information, and that nonlinguistic input is remembered more than that containing linguistic information. Finally, auditory linguistic deficits are more evident in children with Down syndrome than in children having other forms of mental retardation (Marcell & Weeks, 1988).

Fowler (1990) suggests that the slow rate of language development in children with MR, particularly those with Down syndrome, leaves such children with minimal language skills as the sensitive period for language acquisition draws to a close and the capacity for first language learning diminishes (see Chapters 7 and 11). This may explain the finding that children with MR seem to follow a path of linguistic development that seems similar to that seen in typically developing children below a mental age of 10 years, while patterns of language ability seem to become qualitatively different from that seen in typical development after this level has been reached (Weiss, Weisz, & Bromfield, 1986). However, Chapman (1999) noted continued development of language abilities in Down syndrome adolescents, partial evidence against the critical period hypothesis.

Language Development

It is evident that children who are mentally retarded typically demonstrate depressed language ability when compared with typically developing children of the same chronological age. However, researchers are more concerned with discovering the specific patterns of language production and comprehension that characterize this population and identifying possible factors that predict mastery of certain linguistic skills. Both questions have important implications for aiding the development of more adequate linguistic ability in individuals with mental retardation.

Examination of patterns of linguistic development has yielded increasing evidence that suggests that children with diagnoses of mental retardation demonstrate language skills best described as *delayed* rather than *deviant*. That is, their patterns of language production and comprehension closely resemble those seen in younger, typically developing children. Rosenberg (1982) summarizes the general linguistic profile of the child with mental retardation:

> In comparison to nonretarded individuals in the same CA range, language development in the mentally retarded shows the following characteristics: later onset, slower progress, lower final level of achievement, retardation in all aspects of language functioning, but similar stages of acquisition. Thus it appears that the developmental lag hypothesis describes not only nonlinguistic cognitive development in the mentally retarded but linguistic cognitive development as well. (p. 339)

In general, **mental ages (MAs)** are a fairly good predictor of language abilities in children with mental retardation; however, differences may be seen between children with and without mental retardation having identical MAs and even between cognitively impaired children matched for MA in their global language profiles (Kamhi & Johnston, 1982; Lobato, Barrera, & Feldman, 1981, Miller, 1999). Additionally, there are some indications that this population experiences relatively disproportionate difficulty with morphosyntactic skills (at least in English) (Chapman, 1999; McLeavey, Toomey, & Dempsey, 1982) and less relative difficulty with pragmatic linguistic abilities (Abbeduto & Rosenberg, 1987; Bedrosian & Prutting, 1978) than would be expected from general estimates of their linguistic development. A lengthy review by Barrett and Diniz (1989) concludes that early lexical development begins at similar mental ages for children with and without mental retardation. However, children who are retarded soon begin to lag behind, showing a depressed rate of vocabulary learning. Additionally, children with Down syndrome appear to show delays in syntactic development that exceed delays in lexical acquisition (Chapman, 1995, 1999; Fowler, 1990). In general, children with Down syndrome show poorer linguistic ability overall than children having similar mental ages, but with differing etiologies of retardation (Kernan & Sabsay, 1996).

Teaching Language to Children with Mental Retardation

Owens (1999) summarizes some of the relevant considerations and approaches to language intervention with children who are mentally retarded. **Generalization** of language skills outside the clinical setting to spontaneous everyday usage may be particularly troublesome for this group of children (Guess, Keogh, & Sailor, 1978; Salzberg & Villani, 1983), whether the generalization requires either minimal or substantial differences between known instances and novel circumstances. McLean and Snyder-McLean (1978) suggest that therapy will be most effective with this group, as with other groups of language-handicapped children, if it is pragmatic in orientation, emphasizing functional communication as a primary goal. In other words, careful attention should be paid to selecting vocabulary and syntax needed to communicate in the daily environment. Chapman's (1999) Child Talk model similarly stresses instruction that contextualizes language goals through the practice of everyday routines and scripts. The predictability of such contexts for language use maximizes generalization and reduces memory demands, a weakness for this population.

In severe cases of communicative impairment, the use of **augmentative communication systems** or devices may be suggested (for reviews of considerations in such a therapeutic approach, see Glennon & DeCoste, 1997; Owens, 1997; Reichle & Karlan, 1988; Romski, Lloyd, & Sevcik, 1988). Examples of such alternatives to oral communication are the use of **communication boards,** which allow children to select symbols or pictures to communicate with others (Cohen & Shane, 1982), and the use of sign systems, discussed previously (see Wilbur, 1987, for a discussion of using sign systems with communicatively handicapped persons who are not deaf). While not symbolically or cognitively less complex than spoken language, sign systems may provide somewhat of a "teachability" advantage; that is, the child's hands may be shaped and his or her production reinforced more easily than attempts at intelligible vocalizations. Miller (1999) notes that many children supported in early intervention through nonverbal systems later progress to oral communication.

Chapman (1999) stresses that language intervention should continue for children with Down syndrome through the adolescent years, because documented progress can be made throughout this time period. At the other end of the spectrum, Miller (1999) argues that children with Down syndrome should automatically be enrolled in language intervention programs as soon as possible, without regard to standardized assessments that can only be completed at older ages, because the negative impact of DS on language development is so robustly documented.

Parent counseling may facilitate language gains, as in other disorders. For instance, Down syndrome is diagnosed early, unlike some other etiologies of MR, which permits early intervention that focuses on facilitative parent–child interactions. Research suggests that children whose mothers maintain joint attention with their toddlers and follow their children's leads in structuring language around child-selected toys show greater gains in receptive language than do Down syndrome children whose mothers do not show such patterns of interaction (Harris, Kasari, & Sigman, 1996).

Autism

General Characteristics

Kanner (1943, 1946) first described a small group of children who displayed extremely aberrant patterns of communicative interaction. Since then, an autistic syndrome has been defined and the following criteria for the diagnosis of **autism** have been established (Rutter & Schopler, 1987; Simmons & Tymchuk, 1973):

1. The child demonstrates a striking deficit in the ability to establish and maintain social relationships; he or she shows a marked lack of responsiveness to those around him or her and displays **gaze aversion** (avoidance of eye contact with others) and a lack of desire for physical contact, among other socially inappropriate behaviors.

2. The child's language is characterized by an extremely slow course of development and by **echolalia** (repetition of the speech of others); in almost half of all diagnosed cases, expressive language ability is essentially absent (*mutism*). In addition, available language is not used for social communication. Expressive speech is often characterized by *flat or inappropriate prosodic contour.* There appears to be a unique pattern of pronoun errors: The autistic child often interchanges *you* and *I.*

3. The child demonstrates an obsession with sameness in his or her environment, engages in **ritualistic behavior,** and is apparently incapable of dealing with changes in daily routine.

4. The child displays inabilities to play independently or cooperatively and may be incapable of performing self-care activities.

5. The child often evidences intellectual impairment. Freeman and Ritvo (1977) and Rutter (1979) suggest that almost three-quarters of autistic children may be classified as mentally retarded.

In the past, an additional criterion for the diagnosis of autism was onset of symptoms prior to thirty months of age. Recently, this criterion has been eliminated, as evidence of a wider age of onset has become apparent (Long, 1994; Prizant & Wetherby, 1994). However, most parents become concerned and seek professional advice for their children's behaviors before age two, usually on the basis of both language delay and abnormal interpersonal behaviors (De Giacomo & Fombonne, 1998). Some children with autism appear to develop language normally, but appear to regress in communicative ability (Lord & Paul, 1997). A differential diagnosis of autism must distinguish it from mental retardation and childhood schizophrenia, two other childhood conditions leading to similar behavior patterns in children (Long, 1994). Moreover, it has become evident that autism lies at one end of a spectrum of childhood disorders with overlapping characteristics. Because autistic behaviors appear to lie on a continuum, the *American Psychiatric Association Diagnostic and Statistical Manual on Mental Disorders* (DSM-IV, 1996) now links autism with a milder condition called **Pervasive Developmental Disorder (PDD).**

Causation

When first described years ago, autism was presumed by many to have its origins in a disturbance of the parent–child relationship; since then, there has been growing agreement that the disorder probably has an *organic* (physical) basis (Wetherby, 1984); both autism and PDD appear to be caused, in part, by genetic factors (Szatmari, Jones, Zweigenbaum, & MacLean, 1998; Trottier, Srivastava, & Walker, 1999), while a proportion of cases are linked to congenital rubella (Trottier et al., 1999). The precise nature of the underlying neuropsychological deficit is still, however, a matter of great dispute. One model suggests that many of the symptoms of autism can be explained by an underlying disturbance in sensory processing and modulation (Ornitz, 1989). Courchesne, Yeung-Courchesne, Press, Hesselink, and Jernigan (1988) discovered underdevelopment of cerebellar structures in a sample of autistic patients who underwent magnetic resonance scanning; a variety of cerebral cortical differences have also been found across studies comparing individuals with autism to nonautistic subjects (Rumsey, 1996).

Rumsey (1996) points out that while many studies found that autistic children demonstrate abnormal neurophysiological findings, there has been great inconsistency in the types of deficits noted. Deb and Thompson (1998) concur. Owens (1999) summarizes the available data to estimate that approximately 65 percent of persons with autism show some abnormality of brain patterning (see Rapin & Katzman, 1998, for additional review). While studies may detect such differences between the neurological function of autistic and nonautistic individuals, the subtle differences that have been reported do not readily predict why autistic children demonstrate the particular behaviors that they do. That is, we do not currently have adequate models of the relationships between specific aspects of neurological function and human behavior. How does one locate the neurological substrates of such a cognitive inability, and how would such an impairment produce the specific social, linguistic, and cognitive symptoms that so classically describe autism?

Theory of Mind

Tager-Flusberg (1999b) notes that many of the behaviors seen in autism can be attributed to the rather unique failure of autistic children to develop what is called a **"theory of mind"**—understanding the intentions and mental states of others in their environment. People may be seen merely as a "means for meeting a behavioral goal," a concept illustrated when an autistic child uses an adult's arm as a tool to reach things beyond his or her own grasp, rather than requesting help. Normal toddlers map the meanings of novel words in conversation partially by following the eye gaze of the speaker to determine reference. Baron-Cohen, Baldwin, and Crowson (1997) observe that children with autism follow a less productive strategy, perhaps as a reflection of limited theory of mind: They scan only their own visual field when presented with novel words to be learned.

Language

Tager-Flusberg (1999a, 1999b) and Lord and Paul (1997) present excellent surveys of the communicative deficit in autism. According to some estimates, half of the autistic population never develops expressive language at all (Bailey, Phillips, & Rutter, 1996).

Researchers have examined the language of those children who do acquire some language skills in detail in an attempt to ascertain whether their communicative difficulties stem from impairment of isolated linguistic skills or from more global patterns of either linguistic or cognitive deficiency. In this light, some have noted that children with autism may display relatively uneven language abilities. For example, Baltaxe and Simmons (1981) suggest that phonological development in autism appears to exceed accomplishments noted in other areas of language knowledge and use. Similarly, the lexicon appears relatively well-developed in autism (Tager-Flusberg, 1999b), although mental state verbs requiring the child to understand abstract mental processes may be absent. Syntactic development is delayed, but normal in patterning, showing a reliance on a relatively narrow range of grammatical constructions and lowered usage of forms that initiate social interaction, such as questions.

Most observers have viewed the language deficits in autism as lying primarily in the pragmatic or social domains (Laughton & Hasenstab, 1986; Rutter & Schopler, 1987; Tager-Flusberg, 1981). Pragmatic abnormalities in communicative development precede the appearance of oral language. Children with autism apparently do not engage in prelinguistic conversations with their caretakers (using body movement, facial expression, or babbling) as do typically developing children. However, since the disorder is usually diagnosed after the first year of life, early linguistic development of autistic children is not well understood (Lord & Paul, 1997). A failure to engage in joint attention with caretakers is characteristic and children who are more responsive to mothers' attempts to establish joint attention have a more positive prognosis for the establishment of expressive language (Sigman & Ruskin, 1999). Even the most linguistically adept individuals with autism have extreme difficulty in using language to establish or maintain joint interaction (Negri, 1992; Wetherby, 1986). Van Meter, Fein, Morris, Waterhouse, and Allen (1997) concur that the pattern of development witnessed in autism appears more deviant than delayed. Wilkinson (1998) notes that classic autistic behaviors illustrate a form-function dissociation: Language development is not spurred by the drive to socialize (Locke, 1993), and emerging forms are not used in the service of social interaction.

Perhaps surprisingly, some children with autism may demonstrate **hyperlexia** (Aram, 1997), a condition in which a child appears to have precocious reading ability. However, such ability is confined to mastery of the alphabet and excellent whole word recognition, with limited comprehension of true text.

Echolalia

The echolalic behavior of children with autism is particularly fascinating. Echolalia is the act of repeating language heard in the speech of others. It may take a number of forms. *Immediate echolalia* occurs relatively soon after the model has been presented. Many typically developing children may repeat a caretaker's utterance before responding, perhaps as a review of what they have just heard. *Delayed echolalia,* on the other hand, is the repetition of utterances or phrases hours, days, or even weeks after the model was first heard. It is particularly common in the speech of echolalic children with autism. Additionally, one can also speak of echolalia as being either exact or mitigated in nature; mitigated repetitions contain minor changes in structure from the original model. An estimated 75 percent of verbal autistic children demonstrate echolalic speech at one time or another (Ricks & Wing, 1975).

Echolalia potentially provides us with an opportunity to answer some questions about the nature of the language deficit in autism. For example, one can ask if echolalic speech, even if structurally and/or semantically inappropriate to a given situation, contains some elements of pragmatic appropriateness. We can illustrate the problem in the following way. Chris, a four-year-old boy with autism, was having great difficulty in performing a task for his teacher. Frustrated, he swept the puzzle pieces to the floor and yelled, "Chrissy, eat your oatmeal, or I'll spank you!" His mother later reported that Chris had been throwing his cereal on the floor that morning, which had prompted her to threaten him to get him to stop, using exactly those words. Was Chris's utterance totally inappropriate to the situation?

Many researchers have also noted that a great deal of autistic echolalia is somewhat mitigated. Since children's abilities to repeat adult models have often been viewed as an estimate of their own grammatical capacity (Menyuk, 1969; Slobin, 1968), it can be argued that changes that children with autism make in their echolalic renditions of utterances may provide some insight into the degree to which language input is being processed rather than simply stored for playback as unanalyzed wholes.

There is some evidence that echolalia is more likely to occur when children with autism show signs of comprehension difficulty (Paccia & Curcio, 1982) and that its frequency in an autistic child's speech is likely to diminish as he or she develops more spontaneous communicative speech (Howlin, 1982). Baltaxe and Simmons (1977) analyzed echolalic utterances in the bedtime soliloquies of a child with autism. They noted patterns of utterance breakdown, constituent replacement, and phrase recombination similar to those reported for a normal child by Weir (1962). They hypothesized that such behavior reflected knowledge of some basic linguistic rules and structures. Additionally, they suggested that although normal children appear to build up longer utterances from small linguistic units, children with autism may attempt to master language by gradually breaking down long, relatively unanalyzed strings into smaller syntactic components.

After comparing patterns of performance on imitation tasks by children who were typically developing, mentally retarded, and autistic, Tager-Flusberg and Calkins (1990) suggested that autistic children may imitate to maintain a conversational role, rather than to foster their grammatical development. They found no evidence that imitated utterances were appreciably longer or more advanced than autistic children's spontaneous speech. Tager-Flusberg and Calkins also advanced the possibility that imitation might aid lexical and phonological development.

Treatment

Prizant and Wetherby (1994) report that early intervention with children who are autistic can be very effective and that a number of children receiving intensive services early in life can achieve normal functioning by kindergarten. Rogers (1998) surveys treatment outcome studies in autism and concludes that while various approaches appear to produce positive outcomes, there is no single approach to treating autism that yet meets strict criteria for treatment efficacy. Tiegerman-Farber (1997) notes that *operant* training procedures were commonly used in the past for children with autism, perhaps as an outgrowth of the treatment of their concomitant behavioral problems (Lovaas, 1977). However, as many clinicians begin to emphasize language function over language form (pragmatic over syntactic considerations in language use), shifts have occurred to other approaches (Prizant & Wetherby, 1994). Prizant and Wetherby (1998) provide an excellent overview of the continuum of intervention approaches used in autism, from traditional behavioral treatments to approaches that focus on "milieu" teaching, in which children's communicative goals are selected, trained, and reinforced using more naturalistic settings. A typical problem in the educational management of some children with autism is instituting the notion of interpersonal interaction—the child appears to have little use for language because he or she has little use for interaction with others in general.

There is some dispute as to whether the echolalic speech of verbal autistic children should be extinguished as inappropriate or used as a springboard for more spontaneous language use. Prizant and Duchan (1981) noted that the echolalic utterances of the children they studied often appeared to serve important pragmatic functions, such as turn-taking, requesting, and self-regulation. As such, echolalia may be evidence of a desire to communicate that should be reinforced. Scherer and Olswang (1989) demonstrated the efficacy of the clinician's expansion of autistic children's spontaneous and imitative speech in teaching early semantic combinations.

Some clinicians and educators have attempted to train children with autism in the use of sign systems. Fay and Mermelstein (1982) suggest that while a number of individual cases of success have been reported, no widespread consensus about the utility of such an approach can yet be documented. Additionally, they note that it is not clear why such an approach should work when the teaching of oral language has failed. Kuder (1997), Tiegerman-Farber (1997), and Wetherby (1998) provide overviews of approaches and therapeutic considerations in teaching language to children with autism. Prizant and Wetherby (1987) indicate that when autistic children are taught how to communicate more effectively, their use of aggressive or socially inappropriate behaviors may diminish. Thus, language use is not only a symptom of the autistic syndrome, but an important tool in its management.

The long-term prognosis for children diagnosed with autism has not been promising (Ballaban-Gil, Rapin, Tuchman, & Shinnar, 1996). Only those with relatively high IQ, successful language acquisition (and a subset of relatively high functioning children diagnosed with Asperger syndrome) appear to have the likelihood of achieving functional independence later in life (Nordin & Gillberg, 1998).

Facilitated Communication

One of the most controversial recent developments in treating children with autism is the use of **facilitated communication (FC)**. Between the third (1993) and fourth (1996) edition of this text, over seventy articles on the use of facilitated communication appeared in the literature. In facilitated communication, an aide provides physical support of the forearm or hand of the person with autism in order to aid the autistic person's ability to point or type (see Crossley, 1992; Negri, 1992, for historical review). While developed to aid individuals with cerebral palsy, facilitated communication appears to enable some children with autism to spontaneously generate typed messages of great linguistic complexity, and occasionally, of great emotional content (Biklen, 1993; Biklen, Morton, Gold, Berrigan, & Swaminathan, 1992). The controversy over the utility and implications of FC revolve around a large number of issues (Duchan, 1993). A major dispute is whether messages produced under FC conditions represent the generative output of the autistic child or are influenced, albeit subconsciously, by the facilitator (aide). Fried-Oken, Paul, and Fay (1995) and Yoder (1995) note that a large number of studies have failed to support the validity of FC and suggest that in controlled studies, correct target productions cannot be obtained from the FC user if the aide does not know the question or right answer.

A second major concern over the use of FC with autistic individuals is determining how facilitated language can be explained within a model of the underlying deficit in autism. Why are such individuals able to show such literacy and interpersonal communicative intent under conditions of quite minimal physical support when language knowledge and social skills are not evident under other conditions (Duchan, 1993)?

What is the status of facilitated communication now? While a number of reports continue to emerge supporting facilitated communication (Cardinal, Hanson, & Wakeham, 1996; Sheehan & Matuozzi, 1996; Weiss, Wagner, & Bauman, 1996), the fervor surrounding this approach to encouraging language output from autistic children has subsided considerably. As a larger number of reports began to question the validity of FC study findings (Beck & Pirovano, 1996; Bomba, O'Donnell, Markowitz, & Holmes, 1996; Montee, Miltenberger, Wittrock, Watkins, Rheinberger, & Stackhaus, 1995), some professional groups and educators have publicly refused to endorse FC as an efficacious component of therapy for autistic children (American Academy of Pediatrics, 1998; American Speech-Language-Hearing Association, 1995; Huebner & Emery, 1998).

Though this section has addressed the specific problems of autistic children, many children who show emotional and behavioral disorders demonstrate concomitant speech and language problems. For more on this topic, see Prizant, Audet, Burke,

Hummel, Maher, and Theadore (1990), who surveyed the broader population of children who display both psychiatric and communicative impairments.

Specific Language Impairment

General Identity and Prevalence

The largest proportion of children who demonstrate language delay or disorder are not hearing impaired, cognitively impaired, or autistic. Moreover, they show no gross signs of brain dysfunction, although minor brain dysfunction may be suspected (Rapin, 1977) or probable (Miller, 1991). Such children demonstrate language impairment as their single obvious developmental disability. For this reason, they are often given the diagnosis of **specific language impairment (SLI).** As Leonard (1998) points out, the diagnosis of SLI is one of exclusion; that is, alternative explanations for the child's failure to learn language have been sought and not found. Estimates of the number of children who may be classified as SLI have historically varied between 1 and 3 percent of the preschool population (Leske, 1979; Stevenson & Richman, 1976). However, a more recent, large-scale study (Tomblin, 1996) found that, of over 6,000 five-year-old children, over 7 percent could be considered specifically language-impaired, based on actual linguistic and nonlinguistic test performance.

Not all studies that have examined children with SLI have used the same criteria to identify the disorder. This fact has confounded interpretation of the many studies that have examined such children's functioning (Fletcher & Ingham, 1995; McCauley & Demetras, 1990; Miller, 1991). Currently, the primary criteria for identification of SLI include the following (Leonard, 1998): language test scores falling below 1.25 standard deviations from the mean, a performance IQ of at least 85, normal hearing as assessed by screening at conventional levels, a negative recent history of otitis media (see the section on hearing impairment), no evidence of obvious neurological disfunction, intact oral-motor structure and function, and grossly normal patterns of social interaction.

Language Profiles of Children with Specific Language Impairment

In general, studies of the language abilities of SLI children seem to suggest that their linguistic development is best characterized as *delayed* in quality rather than disordered, though this characterization is still disputable (Leonard, 1989; Miller, 1991). That is, SLI children appear to use structures and strategies similar to those employed by younger, normal children in most cases. However, this term should not be taken to imply that the SLI child can be expected to "outgrow" his or her language problem, simply achieving major milestones at later ages. While a certain number of children with early diagnoses of SLI appear to resolve themselves (Bishop & Adams, 1990), a growing body of evidence suggests that a large proportion of the SLI population do not "catch up"; rather, they demonstrate continued language problems and are at risk for reading and general educational failure (Aram, Ekelman, & Nation, 1984; Beitchman, Wilson, Brownlie, Walters, & Lancee, 1996; Catts, Hu, Larrivee, & Swank, 1994; Silva, Williams, & McGee, 1987; Stevenson, 1984; Tallal, 1987). The evidence increasingly suggests that the language-delayed preschooler of today may well become the *learning-disabled* student of tomorrow. Padgett (1988) and others estimate that over half of all language-delayed preschoolers eventually show depressed reading achievement. Johnson, Beitchman, Young, Escobar, Atkinson, Wilson, Brownlie, Douglas, Taback, Lam, and Wang (1999) recently completed intensive study of a cohort of Canadian speech and language-impaired children followed for over fourteen years. Their findings suggest that while children with specific language impairment have a more favorable long-term prognosis than language-impaired children who have documented cognitive or neurological disorders, many still demonstrated deficits in linguistic and academic achievement as young adults. The authors also noted the troubling finding that children with histories of early language difficulties were less likely to receive early intervention than those with articulation disorders (see section later in this chapter), perhaps because language deficiencies are less obvious to parents, teachers, and specialists than difficulties in pronunciation.

Many investigators have noted that subsets of the SLI population may be identified on the basis of relative areas of strength and weakness. Silva and colleagues (1987) describe children who show primary deficits in language production, language comprehension, or both production and comprehension. Aram and Nation (1982) and Bates and Thal (1991) also caution that children may show uneven language proficiency.

Lexicon

It sometimes appears that SLI children perform less well at all language tasks than their normal language peers (see Figure 9.1). Some studies suggest that their language development is delayed from the outset, with emergence of a core single-word vocabulary trailing behind expectations by almost a full year (Trauner, Wulfeck, Tallal, & Hesselink, 1995). Recent work has specifically targeted a subpopulation of toddlers (about 10 to 15% of all young children) who show relatively good comprehension but poor expressive vocabulary and lack of combinatorial speech at age two (Rescorla, 1989). A fairly high proportion of such **early language delay (ELD)** or *"late-talking"* children continue to demonstrate language and articulation delays as they mature (Rescorla & Schwartz, 1990; Scarborough & Dobrich, 1990), although some "late bloomers" catch up to their peers in language performance (Paul, 1991). Leonard's

> *Mother:*   Do you know how to drive a truck?
> *Child:*   No way!
> *Mother:*   No way?
> *Child:*   Oh me get big me grow up me mailman?
> *Mother:*   When you grow up and get big, can you be a mailman?…would you bring me the mail? How many letters?
> *Child:*   Lots.
> *Child:*   Me take some my big big big bag.
> *Mother:*   You're gonna bring them in your big big big bag?
> *Child:*   Yes. Me bring my truck.… Me bring soda truck.
> *Mother:*   You'll drive in a soda truck? You know, dogs bark at mailmen. What will you do when dogs bark at you?
> *Child:*   No me come in.
> *Mother:*   You won't come in?
> *Child:*   No.
> (SLI child at age 2;11 (Gleason, 1993, p. 101).
>
> *Troy:*   This the fireperson. This the bell (indicating the fire alarm).
> *Mother:*   Does the bell ring in an emergency?
> *Troy:*   No. The bell, it has…the car come out.
> *Mother:*   The cars come out when the bell rings?
> *Troy:*   (Nods) The telephone do that, too!
> (SLI child at age 4;7 (Plante & Beeson, 1999)
>
> "So a circus was there and they had these other hands.he had these other people in it/so he first got in a train/and so he didn't get in the train cause he could fly/so he/Mr. Tyler.he was happy/he didn't care if the train was broke down/and so this little guy, Timothy, a little mouse, he gets on and they found a boat/so they sailed on the boat/and so hippopotomus/no/the elephant had to go up in a tiny bed/so the bed broke down and they try to (unintelligible) hippopotomus up there…"
> (A 9-year-old with SLI, retelling the story of *Dumbo* (Nelson, 1998))

Figure 9.1
Some examples of conversation from children with SLI.

(1998) review of the available data suggest that from one-quarter to one-half of late talkers may progress to a diagnosis of SLI by school age.

Older children with SLI continue to be slow "word mappers" (Rice, 1987), although possible reasons for this problem are not clear (Dollaghan, 1987; Leonard, 1998). Such children appear to require more presentations of novel words to learn them under experimental conditions (Rice, Oetting, Marquis, Bode, & Pae, 1994) and seem to rely on a smaller expressive lexicon and a higher proportion of *"general* all-purpose" *(GAP)* nouns and verbs, such as *thing* or *do* than their nonimpaired peers. Other researchers find children with SLI to be generally slower and less accurate when faced with naming tasks (Lahey & Edwards, 1999). A subset of children with SLI are described as **anomic;** that is, they experience marked difficulty in retrieving words for common concepts that they do seem to comprehend (German & Simon, 1991; Kail & Leonard, 1986). This **confrontation naming** or **word retrieval** problem may result in speech characterized by **circumlocutions,** or efforts to get around the blockage. A mother of one SLI child reported that her son requested "something round and English (an English muffin)" for his breakfast; another SLI child labeled pictures on an articulation test in the following manner: "on my brother's pants *(zipper)*" and "you eat breakfast with it *(spoon)*."

Morphosyntax

However, the vast majority of children with SLI are not identified on the basis of lexical performance; rather, they are identified by their failure to achieve normal syntactic production with or without accompanying deficits in comprehension (Leonard, 1998; Watkins, 1994). Their abilities to use grammatical morphemes and to utilize a wide array of simple and complex sentence structures are particularly depressed when compared to those of normal peers. In children learning English, this morphological deficit is quite striking. Specific structures that the child with SLI may have difficulty mastering include plurals, possessives, tense markers, articles, auxiliary verbs, the copula (verb *to be*), prepositions, and complementizers *(to)* in structures such as "I need *to go* now." (For an extremely thorough review, see Leonard, 1998).

Such difficulties are apparent even when children with SLI are matched to children having similar **"language age" (LA)** as measured by mean length of utterance (MLU), which is a measure of length of utterance in morphemes (see Chapter 5). Thus, even at matched utterance lengths, children with SLI include fewer grammatical inflections than their typically developing peers. Further, verb and noun morphology are much more poorly developed than one would predict given the size of the child's lexicon (Leonard, Miller, & Gerber, 1999).

Children with SLI are more likely to omit grammatical morphemes (in English), than misuse them or misplace them. Among the inflections listed above showing the most significant impairment are verb inflections, and agreement in the use of the copula and auxiliary *be,* and the auxiliary verb *do.* Confusion of case in the use of pronouns (e.g., *me* for *I*) is also common (Loeb, 1994). Figure 9.1 provides language samples from some children with SLI.

As children with SLI grow, their morphological deficits may become less obvious, while problems in the use of advanced sentence structures and narrative coherence become more apparent, as the third sample in Figure 9.1 illustrates (Bernstein & Tiegerman-Farber, 1997; Leonard, 1998; Nelson, 1998; Plante & Beeson, 1999). It is at this point that specific language impairment begins to greatly impact school achievement, as deficits in language abilities affect the child's ability to master text reading, writing assignments, and discourse.

Pragmatics

One might expect that a child who has problems with expressive language and who may also have subtle comprehension deficits will experience difficulty in many social situations. Thus, it is not surprising that many children with SLI appear to experience difficulty with a range of pragmatic functions (Craig, 1995; Donahue, 1987; Leonard, 1998), although pragmatic deficits in these children are less pervasively seen across studies than those involving morphosyntax. Children with SLI may produce less appropriate requests or respond less appropriately to the requests of others (Brinton & Fujiki, 1982; Prinz & Ferrier, 1983) or display less sensitivity to their conversational partners' needs for information or clarification (Donahue, Pearl, & Bryan, 1980; Spekman, 1981). Children with SLI are less adept at entering or guiding conversations (Bryan, Donahue, Pearl, & Sturm, 1981; Craig & Washington, 1993), display depressed narrative abilities (Roth & Spekman, 1986), and are less persuasive speakers (Donahue, 1981).

Some children with SLI additionally demonstrate a tendency to interpret language very literally, a pattern with pragmatic consequences. Wood (1982) describes the child standing in the front of the room who, when cautioned by his teacher, "John, the children can't see the board," replied, "Oh, what's the matter with their eyes?" (p. 71). One child with SLI responded to the subtle indirect request for sharing implied by "Your snack looks good" by responding, "Yes, and it tastes good, too!" Thus, a tendency toward literal interpretation will lead a child to ignore the intent behind many conversational gambits. Further, children with shallow knowledge of word meaning may alienate peers unintentionally. For example, Brinton & Fujiki (1995) report one child who used the term *liar* to refer to anyone who said something inaccurate, regardless of intent to deceive.

Because pragmatic deficits appear to be exacerbated when children are in a group setting (Leonard, 1998), it is not surprising that the classroom peers of children with SLI are less likely to pick them as preferred classmates (Gertner, Rice, & Hadley, 1994). As Donahue (1987) points out, it is unclear whether pragmatic and syntactic deficits arise separately in such children, whether their pragmatic deficits may be attributable to subtle linguistic deficiencies, or whether pragmatic deficiency actually constrains the development or display of certain syntactic skills. Evidence exists to support each position in part, and it may well be that different SLI children demonstrate different patterns of relative pragmatic-syntactic disorder. Fey (1986) and Leonard (1998) present a similar, though distinct viewpoint. These researchers argue that children may differ both in their relative degrees of structural impairment and in their social-conversational tendencies. Fey notes that some children appear to maximize limited syntactic and lexical skills in attempts to be conversationally adequate.

Other children appear to be responsive but nonassertive. And still a third subgroup of children seems to be somewhat conversationally unresponsive to those around them.

Concomitant Problems

A number of SLI children also demonstrate articulation disorders in concert with their language difficulties (Paul & Shriberg, 1982; Tallal, Ross, & Curtiss, 1989). From an opposite perspective, Shriberg, Kwiatkowski, Best, Hengst, and Terselic-Weber (1986) found that a high proportion of children referred for articulation problems demonstrated concurrent language disorder. This is not surprising, given the delayed profiles of phonological development seen in many toddlers with early language delay (Bernstein Ratner, 1994; Paul & Jennings, 1992; Rescorla & Bernstein Ratner, 1996).

As noted earlier, many children with specific language impairment continue to have difficulties with aspects of language as they mature into adolescence and adulthood (Tomblin, Freese, & Records, 1992; Weiner, 1985). At these later points in development, their problems are less obvious. Adolescents and adults with language problems may use and be able to process less sophisticated syntax, rather than making obvious grammatical errors (Loban, 1976). They may have difficulty with ambiguous words and sentences, figurative and metaphorical language, and following the essential gist of stories or lectures (Reed, 1994; Wallach & Butler, 1994).

Causative Explanations

A few researchers have proposed that SLI children merely represent the low end of the normal distribution of language talents in children (Leonard, 1991a). In this sense, they might be viewed as no more disordered than are children who lack musical or artistic prowess, if these differing abilities are considered examples of "multiple intelligences" (Gardner, 1983).

However, there is a broader consensus that SLI reflects underlying brain dysfunction at some level, even though it may not be grossly manifest (see MRI studies by Cohen, Campbell, & Yaghmai, 1989; Gauger, Lombardino, & Leonard, 1997; Plante, 1991; Stefanatos, Green, & Ratcliff, 1989; L. Swisher, 1985; Tallal, 1987). In fact, there is a body of evidence that suggests that the term SLI may in fact be a misnomer because SLI children do, upon close examination, appear more likely to have motor deficits and/or subtle cognitive deficits (King, Jones, & Lasky, 1982; Stark & Tallal, 1981). If we do assume that language impairment arises from brain dysfunction, it should not be inconceivable that such children might display varied patterns of linguistic and nonlinguistic performance, depending upon the extent and location of this hypothetical cerebral damage.

In many cases, there appears to be a familial, genetic component to SLI (Plante, Shenkman, & Clark, 1996; Rice, Haney, & Wexler, 1998; Tallal et al., 1989; Tomblin & Buckwalter, 1994). One family with an extremely high level of transmission of a particular profile of SLI has been scrutinized very intensively for clues to the genetic transmission of the disorder (see Crago & Gopnik, 1994). But this assumption does not necessarily explain how such dysfunction disrupts the normal acquisition and use of linguistic abilities, nor why many children come from families with no apparent history of SLI.

Models of SLI

Understanding what mechanism(s) underlie the behavioral profiles seen in SLI has great importance. If we can determine what causes the child to have difficulty learning language, we can develop more specific methods of early identification and effective treatment. Further, understanding why some children find language learning so difficult can inform models that attempt to explain normal language acquisition, since a model that predicts successful acquisition should also be able to predict conditions under which less than optimal development will occur (Leonard, 1998).

The list of candidate models for SLI has grown rapidly in recent years. Leonard (1998) lists at least four viable accounts of how SLI might arise. Among them are the following:

- SLI children suffer from underlying *deficits in the temporal processing of auditory signals.* Tallal and her coworkers (Tallal & Piercy, 1973, 1974, 1975; Tallal & Stark, 1981) demonstrated that SLI children have difficulty in processing rapid acoustic events. More recently, they have extended their findings to a treatment protocol that has produced impressive (and controversial) results (Mezernich, Jenkins, Johnston, Schreiner, Miller, & Tallal, 1996; Tallal, Miller, Bedi, Byma, Wang, Nagarajan, Schreiner, Jenkins, & Mezernich, 1996). Children in the treatment studies were given practice with speech stimuli that were selectively lengthened and amplified, with gradual fading to normal values. Many children participating in this intervention protocol (now available commercially) have made large gains on standardized measures of language administered pre- and post-treatment, although functional gains have not been as well documented. The major controversy regarding this account and treatment approach centers around the limits of a temporal processing deficit to explain the broad range of impairment seen in SLI (Studdert-Kennedy & Mody, 1995), and the large test gains that accompanied relatively narrow and short-term training in speech perception.

- SLI children have *difficulty processing grammatical morphology with low phonetic substance, or salience* (the *"Surface Hypothesis,"* Leonard, 1992, 1998). In comparing data from English-, Italian-, and Hebrew-speaking SLI children, Leonard observed some common patterns of language formulation that suggest that SLI children are limited in their ability to process low phonetic substance (short, unstressed) or sparsely represented (infrequent) morphemes in all three languages. Usage of such morphemes may be additionally conditioned by their perceived contributions to meaning. Leonard, McGregor, and Allen (1992) noted that children with SLI often have difficulty using morphological markers that are short and unstressed and carry little phonetic substance, whereas similarly low-substance forms that do not carry morphological information are not as troublesome. For instance, a child may use and perceive the [s] that is the last sound in *box* more effectively than the [s] that is used to mark the plural in *rocks.* Some authors also question whether SLI reflects true deficits in linguistic knowledge or is the result of competing linguistic stresses on a somewhat fragile and limited language system. Leonard and his colleagues observe that many children with SLI can spontaneously produce difficult forms in some limited contexts, but not in others. They suggest that, when overloaded, the child's system cannot fully meet all demands, and some aspects of communication are executed imperfectly. When one aspect of a linguistic task is very stressful (e.g., the required syntax is complex), other aspects of the child's production are more likely to contain errors (in phonology or fluency, for instance).

- Children with SLI have *immature/incomplete grammatical knowledge.* Views of SLI as the product of diminished or fluctuating capacity contrasts with the hypothesis that children with SLI have different underlying grammatical rule systems, in which certain features of the grammar are missing or undeveloped. Such accounts seem most appealing when a child's difficulty with apparently diverse linguistic forms can be accounted for by positing that a single concept affecting many structures is missing from the child's grammar. One specific proposal, the *"Extended Optional Infinitive"* account (Rice & Wexler, 1995), suggests that children with SLI remain "stalled" in a normal developmental phase during which children learning English appear to believe that marking of tense in main clauses is optional. Such an approach to the grammar would result in both deficient use of verb morphology and inappropriate assignment of case to pronouns, both of which are distinguishing characteristics of SLI. A second proposal from Gopnik and her colleagues, following study of their unique family containing a high saturation of individuals with SLI, is that SLI results from an inability to induce rules of the grammar without resort to overt instruction or rote memorization of grammatical forms (Crago & Gopnik, 1994). Both of these "last resort" approaches would lead individuals with SLI to incomplete knowledge and use of appropriate morphosyntax. Van der Lely, Rosen, and McClelland (1998) also present the case of a child with SLI whose difficulties with grammar cannot be attributed to weaknesses in other domains, thus suggesting a grammar-specific deficit in some children with SLI.

- Children with SLI have *generally slowed processing ability,* which leads to difficulties that include, but transcend, language. The so-called *"Generalized*

Slowing Hypothesis" (Kail, 1994) follows work that suggests that SLI children need about one-third more time to execute a range of perceptual and motor functions. Such slowing might contribute to, or interact with, other proposals that suggest that SLI is the outcome of limited processing capacity in some children. The underlying limit may be one of slowed capacity, as advanced above, or of limits on processing "space," or vulnerability to competing demands on the system. A related hypothesis is that SLI may be at least partially due to *deficits in memory,* specifically **phonological working memory** (Gathercole & Baddeley, 1993). Evidence for such a deficit comes from work by Montgomery (1995a, 1995b) and others that shows a disadvantage for children with SLI on non-word repetition tasks that vary in stimulus length, thus taxing phonological memory capacity.

How Does One Choose Among Competing Theories of SLI?

Bishop (1997) notes potential approaches for determining the most optimal account of the deficits that lead to the symptoms of SLI. Among them are:

- Experimental study of language learning and processing under conditions hypothesized to stress limited capacity in SLI.
- Longitudinal study, in which early deficit patterns are observed and then followed prospectively to determine later impacts on speech and language functioning.
- Computer modeling of impairment.
- The results of intervention studies that attempt to remediate or bypass hypothetical sources of language-learning impairment.

Is SLI Universal?

Yet another approach to evaluating theories of SLI is to examine how well they predict language impairment in differing languages. While it is obvious that children learning any language can show specific language impairment, growing interest has been expressed in comparing patterns of language disability in SLI children from different language communities (Leonard, 1992, 1998). This cross-linguistic approach to the study of specific language impairment, initiated by Leonard, Sabbadini, Volterra, and Leonard (1988) and Clahsen (1989), has the potential to greatly improve our understanding of the basic deficit in SLI. Leonard (1998) summarizes data from Italian, Spanish, German, French, Hebrew, Dutch, Swedish, Croatian, Hungarian, Japanese, Greek, and Inuktitut (an Eskimo-Aleut language). (Leonard wryly notes that children with SLI faced with the task of learning affix-rich Inuktitut may be faced with the task of mastering more morphological affixes than there are current speakers of this endangered language!) SLI in additional language communities is being described each year.

One immediate outcome of such studies is an understanding that, although SLI may manifest itself most obviously in English as a failure in the use of inflectional morphology, it looks quite different in other languages, particularly those in which inflectional endings on verbs are pervasive and do not permit the child to hypothesize that a bare verb stem is an acceptable word of the language. That is, a child learning English knows that *play* is a word, just as *plays* and *played* are words. A child learning Spanish would never presume that the root of the verb "to play" (*jugar*) could be legally used in conversation. One can say *jugo, jugas, jugamos,* and so on, but one cannot, under any circumstances, say *jug-*. Thus, the nature of the language to be learned will create different "problem spaces" for children with SLI in different language communities of the world. Leonard (1998) notes that,

> Children with SLI look first and foremost like speakers of the...language to which they are exposed.... Relative to normally developing peers, children with SLI acquiring each language will look rather weak in language ability. However, the characteristics of language that most sharply distinguish children with SLI from age or MLU controls will not be the same from one language to the next...if there is a universal feature of SLI, apart from generally slow and poor language learning, it is well hidden. (p. 117)

While the actual mechanisms responsible for deficient language development in SLI children have yet to be discovered, work has begun to identify certain factors that may place children at risk for language delay and disorder. Current research suggests that a variety of factors, some of which are amenable to preventive measures, may predispose certain children to language and learning disability. As noted earlier, there is increased understanding of genetic risk factors. Other factors have also been implicated in the etiology of SLI, such as ingestion of toxic substances by the child or mother (e.g., alcohol, drugs, or lead) (Weinberg, 1997), and bouts of otitis media (middle-ear infections) in early childhood (Friel-Patti & Finitzo, 1990).

Language Intervention with Children Who Are Specifically Language Impaired

In a retrospective analysis of reported treatment approaches to SLI, Nye, Foster, and Seaman (1987) noted that language intervention with such children definitely has the potential to improve their syntactic skills substantially, although success in remediating pragmatic deficits appears to be much more limited. In terms of specific therapeutic techniques, **modeling** was reported to be most effective and general "language stimulation" least effective (Nye et al., 1987). In a subsequent analysis, Law (1997) suggested that **imitation, recasting,** and **expansion** are effective approaches to language intervention in this population. Figure 9.2 provides some examples of these techniques used in treating grammatical impairment in SLI (as well as in the other

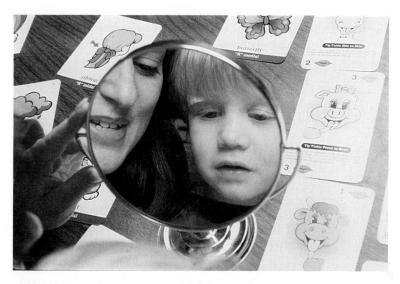

Therapy helps children with speech and hearing impairments overcome problems with phonology, grammar, and word knowledge.

disorders discussed in this chapter). Most of these are adapted in some way from patterns shown to influence language growth in typically developing children. Connell (1987) found that, while normal children learned an invented experimental morpheme most quickly through modeling procedures (see Figure 9.3 for an example of this technique), SLI children made more rapid progress when taught to imitate their clinician. He concluded that SLI children may differ from normal children not only in the amount of language knowledge they have mastered but also in the ways in which they most efficiently learn language. Nelson, Camarata, Welsh, Butkovsky, and Camarata (1996) found just the opposite: that both children with SLI and younger, language-matched peers were more likely to learn a target structure under conversational recast conditions, rather than by imitation. Most researchers agree that children with SLI need more exposure to language targets than their nonimpaired peers to learn them. In a series of studies, Rice (1991) and her colleagues found that SLI children were poor *"incidental learners."* Unlike normal children, SLI subjects learned few new words merely by hearing them embedded in a novel cartoon show.

A key problem facing SLI and other language-impaired children is that of generalization. Normal children find it very easy to create new sentences by analogy to the large variety of grammatical examples they have heard; most language-disordered children do not. This is the crux of the challenge for language teachers—to teach children to be able to create utterances they have not specifically been taught to say. Even explicit explanation of a grammatical rule does not help some children with SLI acquire and use a new language structure (see Figure 9.4). Swisher, Restrepo, Plante, and Lowell (1995) concur

In each of the following cases, we will assume that the target form to be learned by the child is either a copular or an auxiliary be *form. Setting: The child and the therapist are engaged in play with clay. (Adapted from Bernstein & Tiegerman-Farber (1997) and Leonard (1998)).*

Approach	Explanation	Example
Imitation	Child is asked to repeat model presented by therapist.	Clinician: I am rolling the clay. You are, too. Say, "I am rolling." Child: I am rolling.
	Gradually, the request for imitation may be faded to include only a question prompt.	Clinician: I am rolling the clay. I am rolling. What are you doing? Child: I am rolling.
Modeling	Adult models a target form; child takes turns creating utterances having the target form.	Clinician: I am rolling the clay. I am pounding the clay. I am stretching the clay. What are you doing? Child: I am smushing clay.
Focused stimulation	Child is exposed to a large number of exemplars of the target form or word; the child may then be asked questions requiring use of the target form or word.	Clinician: Here is green clay. Let's make vegetables. Lettuce is green. Cabbage is green. A pea is green. A green bean is green. Cucumber is green. Here, you make a tomato (hands child green clay). Child: No. Tomato is red. Clinician: That's right. Tomato is red. (hands child red clay)
Conversational recasting	The adult responds to the child's spontaneous language by rephrasing to include the target form.	Child: This green clay. Clinician: That's right. This is green clay. It is green.
Expansion	The adult responds to the child's spontaneous language by including additional information.	(Similar to recasting, but a broader set of targets are used; the child's utterances are expanded to include new elements.) Child: This clay no good. Clinician: This clay isn't any good. It is too dry.
Scaffolding	The adult provides structure for the child's attempts. Gradually, this structure is faded to allow the child to produce the target on his own.	Clinician: Look at these snakes I made. This one is very big. This one is very small. And this one is… Child: Skinny! Clinician: Right. This one is skinny. And this one… Child: is fat!

Figure 9.2

Some approaches to treatment of language impairment.

Clinician: This doll is the father. This is the mother. This is the boy, and this is the girl. They are going to get up and get ready to go to work and school. The doll, Harlan, is going to try to guess what they're doing. He's going to talk in a special way. You listen to Harlan's questions. Later, you'll get a chance to guess just like Harlan.

(The barrier is placed between the child and the materials that will be manipulated by the clinician. Harlan takes a position on the child's side.)

Clinician: Ding-a-ling-a-ling.

   Harlan: Is the alarm going off?

Clinician: Nope.

   Harlan: The boy waking up?

Clinician: Use your special talk.

   Harlan: Is the boy waking up?

Clinician: No, he isn't.

   Harlan: Is the father getting up?

Clinician: Yes, he is. (Remove barrier and shows father getting out of bed.) I wonder what he is gonna do now? (Makes a sound like flowing water.)

   Harlan: He turning on the water?

Clinician: I didn't hear your special talk.

   Harlan: Is he turning on the water?

Clinician: Yes, he is. Do you know why?

   Harlan: Is he taking a bath/taking a shower/brushing his teeth?

Clinician: Yes, he is. Mother is doing something now.

   Harlan: Is she getting up?, etc.

Next, the child gets a turn to ask questions using "special talk."

Figure 9.3

A sample training sequence to illustrate a modeling procedure. Note: This procedure exemplifies a way in which a realistic need to communicate can be created in a structured setting. The target structure is the use of auxiliary is *in questions. Materials include several dolls representing family members, toy bedroom, bathroom, and kitchen furniture, and a large doll or puppet to be used as a model.* (From *Language intervention with young children* (p. 178) by M. Fey. © 1986, Allyn and Bacon. Reprinted by permission).

with Connell (1987) that some children with SLI have "unique learning style(s)." Numerous specific procedures and discussion about approaches to language remediation with young language-disordered children may be found in Fey (1986), Leonard (1998), Nelson (1998), Owens (1999), and Paul (1995), among others. Nelson (1998) additionally discusses intervention with older children with SLI. Rice (1991) provides a classroom model for SLI remediation with preschoolers; while Merritt and Culatta (1998)

Under the *explicit-rule condition,* the "rule" governing the expression of the novel bound morpheme was stated for the child after the larger version of the figure was introduced on Day 1, before it was reintroduced on Day 2, and as part of the feedback that followed requests to name the larger figure. Examples follow with the "rule" underlined:

Day 1:

"Finally, he reached the mud house and knocked on the door, knock, knock. The door opened. It was a pimu. <u>The pimu was a big creature. When it is small you say pim, but when it's big you have to say [u], pimu.</u>"
"He is a pim. What is he (other figure)?"
(Child responds: "pimu")

Day 2:

"Remember these creatures? <u>For the small one, you say pim, but for the big one you have to say [u], pimu.</u>"
Feedback:
"This is a pim. What is this?"
(Child responds: "pimu")
"Yes, <u>for the big one, you say [u], pimu.</u>"

Under the *implicit-rule condition,* a "filler" statement that paraphrased earlier-presented information was included after the first response to the larger figure on Day 1, and before the figure was reintroduced on Day 2. Examples follow with the "filler" underlined:

Day 1:

"Finally, he reached the mud house and knocked on the door, knock, knock. The door opened. It was a pimu."
"He is a pim. What is he (other figure)?"
(Child responds: "pimu")
"<u>The pimu was sad because he lost his favorite magical object.</u>"

Day 2:

"He is a pim. What is he (other figure)?"
(Child responds: "pimu")
"<u>The pim and the pimu were very good friends.</u> He is a pim. What is he?"
Feedback:
"This is a pim. What is this?"
(Child responds: "pimu")
"Yes, it is a pimu."

Figure 9.4

Even **explicit** *instruction (first example) in a fictitious "grammatical rule" does not help some children with specific language impairment to learn effectively. In fact, some children with SLI learned less effectively than did typically developing children when the rule was explicitly stated.* (From L. Swisher, M. Restrepo, F. Plante, & S. Lowell, Effect of implicit and explicit rule presentation on bound-morpheme generalizations in specific language impairment. *Journal of Speech and Hearing Research, 38,* 1995. © American Speech-Language-Hearing Association. Reprinted by permission.)

and Wallach and Butler (1994) discuss classroom-based intervention for school-aged children and adolescents with SLI. Following principles detailed in the **learnability** literature (Pinker, 1984, 1989), theoretical issues underlying the "teachability" of language are discussed in Rice and Schiefelbusch (1989) and Rice (1991). Leonard (1998) notes that

> It is fair to conclude that we have not reached a point of knowing which approaches are the most effective for teaching particular target forms…(or) which children benefit most from particular treatment approaches…. (However,) as we have seen, most treatment approaches result in demonstrable gains. (p. 204)

Atypical Speech Development

We have described in some detail four major forms of language disorders. There are, in addition, many conditions that lead to atypical speech development. Speech disorders constitute another field of inquiry altogether, and we mention them here only briefly. As in the case of disordered language development, disordered speech development may evolve both from known organic causes and syndromes or from unknown etiology. For instance, significant hearing impairment in children typically results in poor articulation ability; motor disorders in children, such as cerebral palsy, often affect the ability to articulate normally. Children with **cerebral palsy** often demonstrate problems with respiratory support for speech and difficulty producing or controlling the rapid movements of the larynx, jaw, tongue, and lips necessary for the normal rapid rate of conversational speech (see Davis, 1997; Dabney, Lipton & Miller, 1997, and Hardy, 1983, for a general discussion). It is important to point out

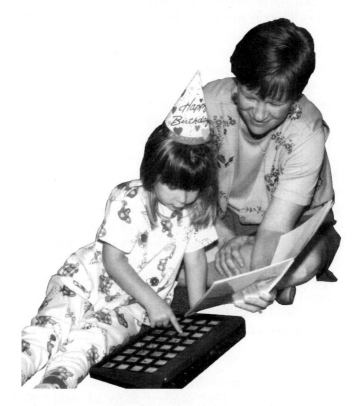

Advances in technology have allowed children with severe motor impairment to communicate effectively.

that in many cases of cerebral palsy, receptive language ability and intellectual functioning are relatively unimpaired, although recent trends in the survival rate for at-risk infants have increased both the rate of cerebral palsy and the rate of concomitant disorders (Hack & Fanaroff, 1999; Lorenz, Wooliever, Jetton, & Paneth, 1998).

Cleft palate is a condition in which various facial structures, particularly the hard and soft palates, fail to develop properly during the first trimester of gestation. A typical result is the inability to control the intra-oral air pressure necessary for normal speech development. Air leaks cut through the palatal defect and the nostrils, producing a nasal speech quality and an inability to produce certain classes of phonemes, such as sibilants and high-pressure stops and fricatives (e.g., /p/, /b/, /f/, /v/). Like the child with cerebral palsy, the child with cleft-palate speech often mistakenly elicits listener perceptions of linguistic or cognitive deficiency. The vast majority of cleft-palate children, however, possess normal linguistic and intellectual ability. Cleft-palate speech can usually be substantially improved by a combination of surgical and speech therapy intervention (Blakeley & Brockman, 1995; Moeller & Starr, 1993).

A large proportion of speech disorders in children have traditionally been termed **functional articulation disorders** (i.e., their etiology is unknown, just as in the case of SLI). There is growing evidence that **chronic otitis media** (middle ear infections) may predispose some children to delayed or disordered speech development, but this possible etiological factor has yet to be firmly established (Paden, 1994). At one point, problems with **auditory discrimination** were suspected in this population; that is, it was hypothesized that children did not articulate sounds properly because they could not discriminate the difference between their defective productions and the correct model. However, this theory has been criticized by a number of researchers (see Locke, 1980, for discussion), who find that the majority of articulation-disordered children appear to have normal perceptual abilities.

In general, children whose articulation development is perceived to be either slow or defective demonstrate phonological patterns similar to those exhibited by younger, normal children (see Chapter 3). Thus, phonemes that emerge late in normal child phonology may be missing or misarticulated in the speech of articulation-impaired children. Additionally, phonological processes common in very young children's word productions—such as consonant cluster reduction, final consonant deletion or devoicing, stopping of continuant sounds, or gliding of liquids—may persist in the speech of older, speech-disordered children (Leonard, 1995; Shriberg, 1991). A number of articulation-disordered children appear to have concurrent language problems (Shriberg et al., 1986). Additionally, syntax and phonology may interact to create varying degrees of difficulty with both articulation and grammar for individual children (Paul & Shriberg, 1982).

Articulation therapy can be effective in remediating articulation disorders of unknown etiology (Gierut, 1998; Shriberg & Kwiatkowski, 1987). Some children are aided by a "semantic" approach; for example, they would be made aware that failure to include final consonants results in inability to distinguish among words in the language (e.g., *bead, beat, beach, beak*). Other children are helped by direct instructions regarding placement of the articulators for the correct production of problematic sounds. For instance, an /s/ can be produced if the child is told to say /t/, then gradually slide the tongue back. Other approaches exist as well. Overviews of the major issues involved in assessing and remediating children's articulation disorders are provided by Bernthal and Bankson (1998), Elbert and Gierut (1986), Newman, Creaghead, and Secord (1989), and Stoel-Gammon and Dunn (1984).

Childhood Stuttering

A small percentage of children fail to develop normal fluency skills. As with language and articulation ability, fluent speech evolves over the course of child development. Thus, even normal children demonstrate a tendency to hesitate, to repeat or prolong sounds, syllables, and words, or to insert fillers such as *um* and *well* between words in utterances. This behavior is most obvious during the period of most rapid progress in language acquisition, usually between the ages of two and four years; because such disfluency is normal, it is called **developmental disfluency** and is not considered to be a problem. Starkweather (1987) provides a comprehensive overview of changes in these tendencies during childhood.

However, some children's fluency appears to differ both quantitatively and qualitatively from that seen in normal development; children may demonstrate greater degrees of disfluency, such as more than ten repeated words, syllables, or sounds per hundred words (Adams, 1984). More of their disfluencies are part-word repetitions than one would expect in normal child speech. There are likely to be more repetitions of a repeated segment than in normal speech. Most children occasionally repeat a syllable or word once, such as "but-but I don't want to," but the stuttering child may produce "b-b-b-but I don't want to." Prolonged segments are of excessive duration, and the quality of the prolongation appears tense. Finally, as the child continues to experience difficulty in producing fluent utterances, he or she may begin to demonstrate signs of self-awareness and frustration. Such symptoms of clinical stuttering most typically emerge just prior to three years of age (Yairi, Ambrose, Paden, & Throneberg, 1996).

As with many of the disorders surveyed in this chapter, the cause of **stuttering** is presently not known. Developmental stuttering is a puzzling disorder when viewed against others covered in this chapter, because stuttering emerges after the child has experienced successful speech and language development. Moreover, the extreme discomfort and struggle seen when very young stuttering children experience disfluency is incompatible with levels of self-monitoring for speech that are characteristic of children this age, and distinctly different from the relative unconcern demonstrated by other groups of children with deficient speech and language skills (Bernstein Ratner, 1997).

There is some suggestion that there may be a genetic predisposition to develop stuttering (Yairi, Ambrose, & Cox, 1999). Additionally, some research concludes that stutterers show less well-defined lateralization of brain functions (Fox, Ingham, Ingham, Hirsch, Downs, Martin, Jerabek, Grass, & Lancaster, 1996; Salmelin, Schnitzler, Schmitz, Jancke, Witte, & Freund, 1998; Watson & Freeman, 1997). Some investigators have posited that stuttering may result from problems in motor planning or coordination (Kent, 1982; Zimmerman, 1980). Because of known linguistic influences on the frequency and location of stuttering in children's speech (Bernstein Ratner, 1997), other researchers have either posited an underlying linguistic basis for stuttering (Perkins, Kent, & Curlee, 1991) or suggested that stuttering reflects an inability of the child's system to deal with simultaneous language formulation and motor speech production demands (Neilson & Neilson, 1987; Starkweather, 1987).

More than half of all children who stutter as preschoolers recover before the age of seven, many within a relatively short time after onset of symptoms (Curlee & Yairi, 1997). For those children who continue to experience difficulty in producing fluent speech, therapy can be extremely helpful in both teaching more fluent speech style and helping to avoid the development of counterproductive responses to the fear of stuttering, such as speaking fears and distracting ancillary behaviors. Guitar (1998) provides guidelines for the diagnosis and treatment of fluency disorders in children.

Evaluation of Suspected Speech and Language Disorders in Children

Parents are usually the first to suspect that a child may not be developing language skills normally. The child may not have begun to use understandable words by eighteen months of age, although other children they know began to acquire language as early as nine months or one year of age. Or the child may not appear to hear well. Or she may appear to use sentence structures that seem too immature for her age.

How does one determine whether a child's communicative development appears normal or disturbed? What is the difference between individual variation (Chapter 8) and atypical variation that places the child at a communicative disadvantage? Evaluation of the communicative competence of children with suspected language disorders is the task of **speech-language pathologists.** Before appraising the child's language skills, hearing acuity is usually evaluated by an **audiologist** to ensure that the child will be able to comply with assessment demands and to rule out hearing impairment as the possible basis for the suspected speech-language delay.

A variety of assessment devices and procedures exists to aid in the identification of children who will need therapeutic intervention to develop adequate communication skills. A number of articulation tests (e.g., the *Goldman-Fristoe Test of Articulation,* 1986, and the *Khan-Lewis Phonological Analysis,* 1987) compare both the number and pattern of a child's articulation errors against expected performance for her age. The measurement of a child's language skills may be both theoretically and practically more difficult, however (Lund & Duchan, 1993; McCauley & Swisher, 1984; Nelson, 1998). It is difficult to appraise the full range of morphological, syntactic, and pragmatic skills needed to be an effective and age-appropriate communicator in the limited time of a diagnostic session.

Because language skills encompass such a large and varied domain, tests of language ability in children are extremely numerous and diverse, and we cannot easily describe them in this chapter. Bernstein and Tiegerman-Farber (1997), Lund and Duchan (1993), and Nelson (1998) provide extensive overview descriptions of many of the commonly used tests of child language ability. We will note that many tests of language performance can be faulted for limited **content validity**—they are able to sample only a small range of possible language skills and usually do so in ways that do not duplicate real-world communicative situations. Additionally, most standardized language tests are not designed to evaluate the performance of children younger than three years. There has been increased interest in the use of parental report measures, which appear to reliably identify language-delayed and normal children as young as twenty to twenty-four months (Dale, 1991; Rescorla, 1989). Such measures utilize parental estimates of specific vocabulary, grammatical morphemes, and sentence patterns used by the child, rather than actual samples of the child's speech.

It is widely acknowledged that structured tests of language comprehension and production should be supplemented by structural and pragmatic analysis of spontaneous language samples. Miller (1981), Nelson (1993), Owens (1999), Scarborough (1990), and MacWhinney (1995) all provide guidelines for syntactic evaluation of spontaneous language; Lund and Duchan (1993) and Roth and Spekman (1984) additionally suggest procedures for assessing the degree to which children appear to be pragmatically competent. These are more time-consuming appraisal techniques, but yield a more complete and representative picture of a child's expressive grammatical ability.

Summary

While the vast majority of children appear to master language skills easily, other children may be comparatively slow language learners and, in some cases, fail to acquire normal adultlike language abilities. Four major conditions adversely affect both the speed and success of language learning. Hearing impairment limits the child's exposure to a sufficiently large and intelligible language model. Mental retardation is usually accompanied by a slower rate of language development and less proficient final language ability, although it is not clear whether cognitively impaired children's problems with language stem directly from specific cognitive skill deficiencies or from other, more global patterns of behavior.

Autistic children's language is often described as severely deviant in quality, demonstrating a lack of pragmatic appropriateness as well as structural deficiencies. The nature of the underlying deficit in autism has yet to be determined; however, analysis of the striking language patterns seen in autistic children may help to answer questions about the origins of the aberrant behaviors of this unusual syndrome.

The largest proportion of language-impaired children appear to have weak or delayed language skills when compared to their peers, but they do not suffer from obvious neurological, cognitive, or perceptual impairment. These specifically language-impaired children are thought to demonstrate poor ability to abstract and learn language rules and skills. Many children showing such a pattern of depressed language functioning during early development apparently also go on to experience difficulty with academic skills during their school years.

Language impairment—which affects the child's ability to use the lexicon, syntax, and pragmatic systems of language—needs to be differentiated from speech impairment, which affects the child's ability to articulate the phonological component of language. Some speech impairment is due to defects in oral structure (such as cleft palate); other forms may be due to problems in motor coordination of the structures necessary for speech production (such as in the case of cerebral palsy). Still other children may misarticulate because they do not hear language models correctly (in the case of hearing impairment). However, many children demonstrate delayed patterns of articulation development that are not easily explained by these considerations.

Finally, while all children are occasionally disfluent during the language-learning years, some children demonstrate patterns of sound and syllable repetition, prolongation of sounds, and tense pauses between sounds and words in utterances that lead them to be perceived as children who stutter. The cause of stuttering is, like so many of the disorders we have considered in this chapter, basically unknown, although motor planning (or timing disturbance) and linguistic encoding difficulty are two of the more commonly considered current approaches to its understanding and treatment.

Treatment of children with communicative handicaps is most effective when it considers the normal sequence of language development and attempts to integrate current beliefs about environmentally facilitating factors in normal language acquisition into the therapeutic process. Success in speech and language teaching appears to be guided in large part by knowledge of when children are ready to learn certain skills, given what they already seem to know. Additionally, the degree to which the language skills being taught can be made pragmatically relevant to everyday communicative needs is extremely important. Finally, the manner in which linguistic skills are introduced and reinforced appears extremely important, although current research does not indicate a single most effective way to teach language skills to children. When all is said and done, we are still better able to identify language disability in children than rectify it. Continued research into the bases of impairment in the differing populations of communicatively disordered children is crucial to the improvement of methods for overcoming their linguistic handicaps.

Key Words

American Sign Language (ASL, Ameslan)	auditory discrimination
amplification	augmentative communication system
anomic	aural rehabilitation
audiologist	autism

cerebral palsy
chronic otitis media
circumlocutions
cleft palate
cochlear implant
communication boards
confrontation naming
congenital
content validity
cued speech
decibel
developmental disfluency
Down syndrome (DS)
early language delay (ELD)
echolalia
etiology
expansion
Extended Optional Infinitive Account
    of SLI
facilitated communication (FC)
Fragile X syndrome
functional articulation disorders
gaze aversion
generalization
Generalized Slowing Hypothesis
hearing impairment
hyperlexia
imitation

language age (LA)
learnability
lipreading (speechreading)
long-term memory abilities
manual approach to deaf education
manually coded English
mental age (MA)
mental retardation (MR)
modeling
oralist approach to deaf education
otitis media
Pervasive Developmental Disorder
    (PDD)
phonological working memory
prelingual hearing impairment
recasting
ritualistic behavior
short-term memory abilities
sign system
specific language impairment (SLI)
speech-language pathologist
stuttering
Surface Hypothesis model of SLI
theory of mind
total communication
Williams syndrome (WS)
word retrieval

Suggested Projects

1. View the evening news or another television program with the sound off. Attempt to transcribe what the speakers are saying and to summarize the content of the news stories or program plot. How successful are you? Write a paper that discusses the degree to which a lack of auditory information makes following spoken conversation difficult.

2. View a videotape of the movie *Children of a Lesser God;* turn off the sound. How easy is it to follow the signing of the deaf actors when the oral narration is missing? Some people claim that sign languages are *transparent,* that they can be easily interpreted without knowing the specific rules for using a given sign language. Discuss your experience. Do you agree or disagree?

3. Arrange a discussion of the relative merits of cochlear implants, even if they endanger the viability of the sign languages used around the world. Should all children with profound hearing losses be outfitted with cochlear implants?

4. Try to arrange a visit to a school or class that has children who are hearing-impaired, cognitively impaired, autistic, or language-delayed. Write up and share your observations with others in your class. Be sure to address the children's patterns of communicative ability, as well as the techniques that are being used to remediate and augment their language skills.

5. If you can, arrange to observe a speech-language pathologist's therapeutic interaction with a communicatively impaired child. (Many universities operate speech-language and hearing clinics, as do many hospitals and schools. Additionally, some pathologists work in individual practice.) In a short report, summarize your impressions of the child's communicative problem. Then discuss and analyze the techniques used by the pathologist to teach a particular language skill.

6. Some authors referenced in this chapter suggest that we can gain understanding of children's communicative disorders through the use of computer models that have been designed to mimic the varying hypothetical limitations on language processing by disordered children. What limits might apply to the utility of such models in understanding children's communicative behavior?

Suggested Readings

Bernstein, D., & Tiegerman-Farber, E. (1997). *Language and communication disorders in children* (4th ed.). Boston: Allyn & Bacon.

Bernthal, J., & Bankson, N. (1998). *Articulation and phonological disorders* (3rd edition). Englewood Cliffs, NJ: Prentice-Hall.

Bishop, D. (1997). *Uncommon understanding: Development and disorders of language comprehension in children.* East Sussex: Psychology Press.

Bloodstein, O. (1995). *A handbook on stuttering.* San Diego: Singular Press.

Chapman, R. (1995). Language development in children and adolescents with Down syndrome. In P. Fletcher & B. MacWhinney (Eds.), *Handbook of child language.* Cambridge, MA: Basil Blackwell.

Donahue, M. (1987). Interactions between linguistic and pragmatic development in learning-disabled children: Three views of the state of the union. In S. Rosenberg (Ed.), *Advances in applied psycholinguistics: Vol. 1. Disorders of first-language development.* Cambridge: Cambridge University Press.

Duchan, J. (1993). Issues raised by facilitated communication for theorizing and research on autism. *Journal of Speech and Hearing Research, 36,* 1108–1119.

Fey, M. (1986). *Language intervention with young children.* San Diego: College-Hill Press.

Glennon, S., & DeCoste, D. (1997). *Handbook of augmentative and alternative communication.* San Diego: Singular Press.

Guitar, B. (1998). *Stuttering: An integrated approach to its nature and treatment.* Baltimore: Williams & Wilkins.

Klima, E., & Bellugi, U. (1979). *The signs of language.* Cambridge, MA: Harvard University Press.

Lahey, M. (1988). *Language disorders and language development.* New York: Macmillan.

Leonard, L. (1992). The use of morphology by children with specific language impairment: evidence from three languages. In R. Chapman (Ed.), *Processes in language acquisition and disorders.* St. Louis: Mosby Year Book.

Leonard, L. (1998). *Children with specific language impairment.* Cambridge, MA: MIT Press.

Lord, C., & Paul, R. (1997). Language and communication in autism. In D. J. Cohen & F. Volknar (Eds.), *Handbook of autism and PDD* (2nd ed.; pp. 195–225). New York: Wiley.

Miller, J. (1991). Research on language disorders in children: A progress report. In J. Miller (Ed.), *Research on child language disorders: A decade of progress.* Austin, TX: Pro-Ed.

Miller, J., Leddy, M., & Leavitt, L. (1999). *Improving the communication of people with Down syndrome.* Baltimore: Brookes.

Minifie, F. (Ed.) (1994). *Introduction to communication sciences and disorders.* San Diego: Singular.

Nelson, N. W. (1998). *Childhood language disorders in context: Infancy through adolescence* (second edition). New York: Macmillan.

Owens, R. (1999). *Language disorders: A functional approach to assessment and intervention.* Boston: Allyn & Bacon.

Paul, R. (1995). *Language disorders in children.* New York: Mosby.

Quigley, S., & Paul, P. (1987). Deafness and language development. In S. Rosenberg (Ed.), *Advances in applied psycholinguistics: Vol. 1. Disorders of first language development.* Cambridge: Cambridge University Press.

Reed, V. (1994). *An introduction to children with language disorders* (2nd ed.). New York: Merrill.

Tager-Flusberg, H. (1999). Understanding the language and communicative impairments in autism. In L. Glidden (Ed.), *International review of research on mental retardation.* New York: Academic Press.

Wallach, G., & Butler, K. (1994). *Language learning disabilities in school-age children and adolescents.* New York: Merrill.

Watkins, R., & M. Rice (Eds.) (1994). *Specific language impairments in children.* Baltimore: Brookes.

Wilbur, R. B. (1987). *American Sign Language: Linguistic and applied dimensions.* San Diego: College-Hill Press.

References

Abbeduto, L., & Rosenberg, S. (1987). Linguistic communication and mental retardation. In S. Rosenberg (Ed.), *Advances in applied psycholinguistics: Vol. 1. Disorders of first-language development.* Cambridge, UK: Cambridge University Press.

Adams, M. (1984). The young stutterer: Diagnosis, treatment and assessment of progress. In W. Perkins (Ed.), *Stuttering disorders.* New York: Thieme-Stratton.

Allen, T. (1986). Patterns of academic achievement among hearing-impaired students. In A. Schildroth & M. Karchmer (Eds.), *Deaf children in America*. Austin, TX: Pro-Ed.

American Academy of Pediatrics, Committee on Children with Disabilities. (1998). Auditory integration training and facilitated communication for autism. *Pediatrics, 102* (2 pt. 1), 341–433.

American Association on Mental Retardation (1992). *Mental retardation: Definition, classification and systems of support*. (9th ed.). Washington, DC: Author.

American Psychiatric Association (1996). *Diagnostic and statistical manual of mental disorders* (4th ed.). Washington, DC: Author.

American Speech-Language-Hearing Association (1995). Facilitated communication. *Asha, 37* (Suppl.), 14, 22.

Aram, D. (1997). Hyperlexia: Reading without meaning in young children. *Topics in Language Disorders, 17,* 1–13.

Aram, D., Ekelman, B., & Nation, J. (1984). Preschoolers with language disorders: 10 years later. *Journal of Speech and Hearing Research, 27,* 232–244.

Aram, D., & Nation, J. (1982). *Child language disorders*. St. Louis, MO: C. V. Mosby.

Bailey, A., Phillips, W. & Rutter, M. (1996). Autism: Toward an integration of clinical, genetic, neuropsychological and neurobiological perspectives. *Journal of Child Psychology and Psychiatry, 37,* 89–126.

Ballaban-Gil, K., Rapin, I., Tuchman, R. & Shinnar, S. (1996). Longitudinal examination of the behavioral, language, and social changes in a population of adolescents and young adults with autistic disorder. *Pediatric Neurology, 15,* 217–23.

Baltaxe, C., & Simmons, J. (1977). Bedtime soliloquies and linguistic competence in autism. *Journal of Speech and Hearing Disorders, 42,* 376–393.

Baltaxe, C., & Simmons, J. (1981). Disorders of language in childhood psychosis: Current concepts and approaches. In J. Darby (Ed.), *Speech evaluation in psychiatry*. New York: Grune & Stratton.

Baron-Cohen, S., Baldwin, D., & Crowson, M. (1997). Do children with autism use the speaker's direction of gaze strategy to crack the code of language? *Child Development, 68,* 48–57.

Barrett, M., & Diniz, F. (1989). Lexical development in mentally handicapped children. In M. Beveridge, G. Conti-Ramsden, & I. Leudar (Eds.), *Language and communication in mentally handicapped people*. London: Chapman and Hall.

Bates, E., & Thal, D. (1991). Associations and dissociations in language development. In J. Miller (Ed.), *Research on child language disorders: A decade of progress*. Austin, TX: Pro-Ed.

Bavalier, D., Corina, D., Jezzard, P., Clark, V., Karni, A., Lalwani, A., Rauschecker, J., Braun, A., Turner, R. & Neville, H. (1998). Hemispheric specialization for English and ASL: Left invariance—right variability. *Neuroreport, 11,* 1537–42.

Beck, A., & Pirovano, C. (1996). Facilitated communicators' performance on a task of receptive language. *Journal of Autism and Developmental Disorders, 26,* 497–512.

Bedrosian, J., & Prutting, C. (1978). Communicative performance of mentally retarded adults in four conversational settings. *Journal of Speech and Hearing Research, 21,* 79–95.

Beitchman, J., Wilson, B., Brownlie, E., Walters, H., & Lancee, W. (1996). Long-term consistency in speech/language profiles: I. Developmental and academic outcomes. *Journal of the American Academy of Child and Adolescent Psychiatry, 35,* 804–814.

Bellugi, U., Marks, S., Bihrle, A., & Sabo, H. (1988). Dissociation between language and cognitive functions in Williams syndrome. In D. Bishop & K. Mogford (Eds.), *Language development in exceptional circumstances* (pp. 177–189). London: Churchill Livingstone.

Bernstein, D., & Tiegerman-Farber, E. (1997). *Language and communication disorders in children* (4th ed.). Boston: Allyn & Bacon.

Bernstein Ratner, N. (1994). Phonological analysis of child speech. In J. Sokolov & C. Snow (Eds.), *Handbook of research in language development using CHILDES* (pp. 324–372). Hillsdale, NJ: Erlbaum.

Bernstein Ratner, N. (1997). Stuttering: a psycholinguistic perspective. In R. Curlee & G. Siegel (Eds.), *Nature and treatment of stuttering: New directions* (2nd ed.) (pp. 99–127). Boston: Allyn & Bacon.

Bernthal, J., & Bankson, N. (1998). *Articulation and phonological disorders* (4th ed.) Boston: Allyn & Bacon.

Bicklen, D. (1993). *Communication unbound.* New York: Columbia University Press.

Biklen, D., Morton, M., Gold, D., Berrigan, C., & Swaminathan, S. (1992). Facilitated communication: Implications for individuals with autism. *Topics in Language Disorders, 12* (4), 1–28.

Bishop, D. (1997). *Uncommon understanding: Development and disorders of language comprehension in children.* East Sussex: Psychology Press.

Bishop, D., & Adams, C. (1990). A prospective study of the relationship between specific language impairment, phonological disorders and reading retardation. *Journal of Child Psychology and Psychiatry, 31,* 1027–1050.

Blakely, R., & Brockman, J. (1995). Normal speech and hearing by age 5 as a goal for children with cleft palate: A demonstration project. *American Journal of Speech-Language Pathology, 4,* 25–32.

Bochner, J., & Albertini, J. (1988). Language varieties in the deaf population and their acquisition by children and adults. In M. Strong (Ed.), *Language learning and deafness.* Cambridge: Cambridge University Press.

Bomba, C., O'Donnell, L., Markowitz, C., & Holmes, D. (1996). Evaluating the impact of facilitated communication on the communicative competence of fourteen students with autism. *Journal of Autism and Developmental Disorders, 26,* 43–58.

Bonvillian, J., Orlansky, M., & Novack, L. (1983). Developmental milestones: Sign language acquisition and motor development. *Child Development, 54,* 1435–1445.

Brinton, B., & Fujiki, M. (1982). A comparison of request-request sequences in the discourse of normal and language disordered children. *Journal of Speech and Hearing Disorders, 47,* 57–62.

Brinton, B., & Fujiki, M. (1995). Conversational interaction with children with language impairment. In M. Fey, J. Windsor, & S. Warren (Eds.), *Language intervention: Preschool through the primary school years* (pp. 183–212). Baltimore: Brookes.

Bryan, T., Donahue, M., Pearl, R., & Sturm, C. (1981). Learning disabled children's conversational skills. *Learning Disability Quarterly, 4,* 250–259.

Cardinal, D., Hanson, D., & Wakeham, J. (1996). Investigation of authorship in facilitated communication. *Mental Retardation, 34,* 231–42.

Carney, A., & Moeller, M. P. (1998). Treatment efficacy: hearing loss in children. *Journal of Speech, Language and Hearing Research, 41,* S61–85.

Catts, H., Hu, C-F., Larrivee, L., & Swank, L. (1994). Early identification of reading disabilities in children with speech-language impairments. In R. Watkins & M. Rice (Eds.), *Specific language impairments in children*. Baltimore: Brookes.

Chapman, R. (1995). Language development in children and adolescents with Down syndrome. In P. Fletcher & B. MacWhinney (Eds.), *Handbook of child language*. Cambridge, MA: Basil Blackwell.

Chapman, R. (1999). Language development in children and adolescents with Down syndrome. In J. Miller, M. Leddy & L. Leavitt (Eds.), *Improving the communication of people with Down syndrome*. (pp. 41–60). Baltimore: Brookes.

Clahsen, H. (1989). The grammatical characterization of developmental dysphasia. *Linguistics, 27,* 897–904.

Cohen, C., & Shane, H. (1982). An overview of augmentative communication. In N. Lass, L. McReynolds, J. Northern, & D. Yoder (Eds.), *Speech, language and hearing*. Philadelphia: Saunders.

Cohen, M., Campbell, R., & Yaghmai, F. (1989). Neuropathological abnormalities in developmental dysphasia. *Annals of Neurology, 25,* 567–570.

Connell, P. (1987). An effect of modeling and imitation teaching procedures on children with and without specific language impairment. *Journal of Speech and Hearing Research, 30,* 105–113.

Courchesne, E., Yeung-Courchesne, B., Press, G., Hesselink, J., & Jernigan, T. (1988). Hypoplasia of cerebellar vermal lobules VI and VII in autism. *New England Journal of Medicine, 318,* 1349–1354.

Crago, M., & Gopnik, M. (1994). From families to phenotypes: Theoretical and clinical implications of research into the genetic basis of specific language impairment. In R. Watkins & M. Rice (Eds.), *Specific language impairments in children* (pp. 35–51). Baltimore: Brookes.

Craig, H. (1995). Pragmatic impairments. In P. Fletcher & B. MacWhinney (Eds.), *The handbook of child language*. Cambridge, MA: Basil Blackwell.

Craig, H., & Washington, J. (1993). The access behaviors of children with specific language impairment. *Journal of Speech and Hearing Research, 36,* 322–337.

Crossley, R. (1992). Lending a hand: A personal account of the development of facilitated communication training. *American Journal of Speech-Language Pathology, 1*(3), 15–18.

Crouch, R. (1997). Letting the deaf be deaf: Reconsidering the use of cochlear implants in prelingually deaf children. *Hastings Center Reports, 27,* 14–21.

Curlee, R., & Yairi, E. (1997). Early intervention with early childhood stuttering: A critical examination of the data. *American Journal of Speech-Language Pathology, 6,* 8–18.

Dabney, K., Lipton, G., & Miller, F. (1997). Cerebral palsy. *Current Opinion in Pediatrics, 9,* 81–88.

Dale, P. (1991). The validity of a parent report measure of vocabulary and syntax at 24 months. *Journal of Speech and Hearing Research, 34,* 565–571.

Davis, D. (1997). Review of cerebral palsy, Part I: Description, incidence and etiology. *Neonatal Network, 16,* 7–12.

Dawson, P., Blamey, P., Dettman, S., Barker, E., & Clark, G. (1995). A clinical report on receptive vocabulary skills in cochlear implant users. *Ear and Hearing, 16,* 287–294.

Deb, S., & Thompson, B. (1998). Neuroimaging in autism. *British Journal of Psychiatry, 173,* 299–302.

De Giacomo, A., & Fombonne, E. (1998). Parental recognition of developmental abnormalities in autism. *European Child and Adolescent Psychiatry, 7,* 131–136.

Delaney, M., Stuckless, E., & Walter, G. (1984). Total communication effects: A longitudinal study of a school for the deaf in transition. *American Annals of the Deaf, 129,* 481–486.

deVilliers, P. (1991). English literacy development in deaf children. In J. Miller (Ed.), *Research on child language disorders: A decade of progress.* Austin, TX: Pro-Ed.

Dollaghan, C. (1987). Fast mapping in normal and language-impaired children. *Journal of Speech and Hearing Disorders, 52,* 218–222.

Donahue, M. (1981). Requesting strategies of learning disabled children. *Applied Psycholinguistics, 2,* 213–234.

Donahue, M. (1987). Interactions between linguistic and pragmatic development in learning-disabled children: Three views of the state of the union. In S. Rosenberg (Ed.), *Advances in applied psycholinguistics: Vol. 1. Disorders of the first-language development.* Cambridge, UK: Cambridge University Press.

Donahue, M., Pearl, R., & Bryan, T. (1980). Conversational competence in learning-disabled children: Responses to inadequate messages. *Applied Psycholinguistics, 1,* 387–403.

Duchan, J. (1993). Issues raised by facilitated communication for theorizing and research on autism. *Journal of Speech and Hearing Research, 36,* 1108–1119.

Dykens, E., Hodapp, R., & Leckman, J. (1994). *Behavior and development in Fragile X syndrome.* Thousand Oaks, CA: Sage.

Elbert, M., & Gierut, J. (1986). *Handbook of clinical phonology: Approaches to assessment and treatment.* San Diego: College-Hill Press.

Fay, D., & Mermelstein, R. (1982). Language in infantile autism. In S. Rosenberg (Ed.), *Handbook of applied psycholinguistics: Major thrusts of research and theory.* Hillsdale, NJ: Lawrence Erlbaum.

Fay, W., & Schuler, A. (1980). *Emerging language in autistic children.* Baltimore: University Park Press.

Fey, M. (1986). *Language intervention with young children.* San Diego: College-Hill Press.

Fisch, G., Holden, J., Howard-Peebles, P., Maddalena, A., Pandya, A., & Nance, W. (1999). Age-related language characteristics of children and adolescents with fragile X syndrome. *American Journal of Medical Genetics, 83,* 253–256.

Fletcher, P., & Ingham, R. (1995). Grammatical impairment. In P. Fletcher & B. MacWhinney (Eds.), *The handbook of child language.* Cambridge, MA: Basil Blackwell.

Fowler, A. (1990). Language abilities in children with Down syndrome: Evidence for a specific syntactic delay. In D. Cichetti & M. Beeghly (Eds.), *Children with Down syndrome: A developmental perspective* (pp. 302–328). New York: Cambridge University Press.

Fox, P., Ingham, R., Ingham, J., Hirsch, T., Downs, J., Martin, C., Jerabek, P., Glass, T., & Lancaster, J. (1996). A PET study of the neural systems of stuttering. *Nature, 382,* 158–161.

Francis, H., Koch, M., Wyatt, J., & Niparko, J. (1999). Trends in educational placement and cost-benefit considerations in children with cochlear implants. *Archives of Otolaryngology and Head and Neck Surgery, 125,* 499–505.

Freeman, B., & Ritvo, E. (1977). Diagnostic and evaluation systems: Helping the advocate cope with the "state of the art." In J. Budde (Ed.), *Advocacy and autism.* Lawrence: University of Kansas Press.

Fried-Oken, M., Paul, R., & Fay, W. (1995). Questions concerning facilitated communication: Response to Duchan. *Journal of Speech and Hearing Research, 38,* 200–202.

Friel-Patti, S., & Finitzo, T. (1990). Language learning in a prospective study of otitis media with effusion in the first two years of life. *Journal of Speech and Hearing Research, 33,* 188–194.

Gardner, H. (1983). *Frames of mind: The theory of multiple intelligences.* New York: Basic Books.

Gathercole, V., & Baddeley, A. (1993). *Working memory and language.* Hillsdale, NJ: Erlbaum.

Gauger, L., Lombardino, L., & Leonard, C. (1997). Brain morphology in children with specific language impairment. *Journal of Speech, Language and Hearing Research, 40,* 1272–1285.

Geers, A., & Moog, J. (1987). Predicting spoken language acquisition of profoundly hearing-impaired children. *Journal of Speech and Hearing Disorders, 52,* 84–94.

Geers, A., & Moog, J. (1994). Spoken language results: vocabulary, syntax and communication. *Volta Review, 96*(5), 131–150.

Geers, A., & Schick, B. (1988). Acquisition of spoken and signed English by hearing-impaired children of hearing-impaired or hearing parents. *Journal of Speech and Hearing Disorders, 53,* 136–143.

German, D., & Simon, E. (1991). Analysis of children's word finding skills in discourse. *Journal of Speech and Hearing Research, 34,* 309–316.

Gertner, B., Rice, M., & Hadley, P. (1994). The influence of communicative competence on peer preferences in a preschool classroom. *Journal of Speech and Hearing Research, 37,* 913–923.

Gierut, J. (1998). Treatment efficacy: Functional phonological disorders in children. *Journal of Speech, Language, and Hearing Research, 41,* 585–600.

Gleason, P. (1993) *Psycholinguistics: Instructor's manual.* Fort Worth: Harcourt Brace Jovanovich.

Glennon, S., & DeCoste, D. (1997) *Handbook of augmentative and alternative communication.* San Diego: Singular.

Goldin-Meadow, S., & Mylander, C. (1998). Spontaneous sign systems created by deaf children in two cultures. *Nature, 391,* 279–81.

Goldman, R., & Fristoe, M. (1986). *The Goldman-Fristoe Test of Articulation.* Circle Pines, MN: American Guidance Service.

Gormley, K., & Sarachan-Deily, A. (1987). Evaluating hearing-impaired students' writing: A practical approach. *Volta Review, 89,* 157–170.

Guess, E., Keogh, W., & Sailor, W. (1978). Generalization of speech and language behavior: Measurement and training tactics. In R. Schiefelbusch (Ed.), *Bases of language intervention.* Baltimore: University Park Press.

Guitar, B. (1998). *Stuttering: An integrated approach to its nature and treatment.* Baltimore: Williams and Wilkins.

Hack, M., & Faranoff, A. (1999). Outcomes of children of extremely low birthweight and gestational age in the 1990s. *Early Human Development, 53,* 193–218.

Hardy, J. (1983). *Cerebral palsy.* Englewood Cliffs, NJ: Prentice-Hall.

Harris, S., Kasari, C., & Sigman, M. (1996). Joint attention and language gains in children with Down syndrome. *American Journal of Mental Retardation, 100,* 608–619.

Hickock, G., Wilson, M., Clark, K., Klima, E., Kritchevsky, M., & Bellugi, U. (1999). Discourse deficits following right hemisphere damage in deaf signers. *Brain and Language, 66,* 233–248.

Howlin, P. (1982). Echolalic and spontaneous phrase speech in autistic children. *Journal of Child Psychology and Psychiatry, 23,* 281–293.

Huebner, R., & Emery, L. (1998). Social psychological analysis of facilitated communication: implications for education. *Mental Retardation, 36,* 259–68.

Johnson, C., Beitchman, J., Young, A., Escobar, M., Atkinson, L., Wilson, B., Brownlie, E., Douglas, L., Taback, N, Lam, I., & Wang, M. (1999). Fourteen-year follow-up of children with and without speech/language impairments: Speech/language stability and outcomes. *Journal of Speech, Language and Hearing Research, 42,*(3), 744–760.

Jones, M., & Quigley, S. (1979). The acquisition of question formation in English and American Sign Language by two hearing children of deaf parents. *Journal of Speech and Hearing Disorders, 44,* 196–208.

Kail, R. (1994). A method of studying the generalized slowing hypothesis in children with specific language impairment. *Journal of Speech and Hearing Research, 37,* 418–421.

Kail, R., & Leonard, L. (1986). Word-finding abilities in language-impaired children. *ASHA Monographs, 25.* Rockville, MD: American Speech, Language and Hearing Association.

Kamhi, A., & Johnston, J. (1982). Towards an understanding of retarded children's linguistic deficiencies. *Journal of Speech and Hearing Research, 25,* 435–445.

Kanner, L. (1943). Autistic disturbances of affective contact. *The Nervous Child, 2,* 217–250.

Kanner, L. (1946). Irrelevant and metaphorical language in early infantile autism. *American Journal of Psychiatry, 103,* 242–246.

Karchmer, M. & Allen, T. (1999). The functional assessment of deaf and hard of hearing students. *American Annals of the Deaf, 144,* 68–77.

Karmiloff-Smith, A., Grant, J., Berthoud, I., Davies, M., Howlin, P., & Udwin, O. (1997). Language and Williams syndrome: how intact is "intact"? *Child Development, 68,* 246–62.

Kent, R. (1982). Stuttering as a temporal programming disorder. In R. Curlee & W. Perkins (Eds.), *Nature and treatment of stuttering: New directions.* San Diego: College-Hill Press.

Kernan, K., & Sabsay, S. (1996). Linguistic and cognitive ability of adults with Down syndrome and mental retardation of unknown etiology. *Journal of Communication Disorders, 29,* 401–422.

Khan, L., & Lewis, N. (1987). *Khan-Lewis Phonological Analysis.* Circle Pines, MN: American Guidance Service.

King, R., Jones, C., & Lasky, E. (1982). In retrospect: A fifteen year follow-up report of speech-language disordered children. *Language, Speech and Hearing Services in the Schools, 13,* 24–32.

Klima, E., & Bellugi, U. (1979). *The signs of language.* Cambridge, MA: Harvard University Press.

Kuder, S. (1997). *Teaching students with language and communication disabilities.* Boston: Allyn & Bacon.

Lahey, M., & Edwards, J. (1999). Naming errors of children with specific language impairment. *Journal of Speech, Language and Hearing Research, 42,* 195–205.

Lane, H., & Bahan, B. (1998). Ethics of cochlear implantation in young children: A review and reply from a Deaf-World perspective. *Otolaryngology and Head and Neck Surgery, 119,* 297–313.

LaSasso, C., & Davey, B. (1987). The relationship between lexical knowledge and reading comprehension for prelingually, profoundly hearing-impaired students. *Volta Review, 89,* 211–220.

LaSasso, C., & Mobley, S. (1997). National survey of reading instruction for deaf or hard-of-hearing students in the U.S. *Volta Review, 99,* 31–59.

Laughton, J., & Hasenstab, M. (1986). *The language learning process: Implications for management of disorders.* Rockville, MD: Aspen.

Law, J. (1997). Evaluating intervention for language impaired children: A review of the literature. *European Journal of Disorders of Communication, 32,* 1–14.

Leonard, L. (1975). Facilitating linguistic skills in children with specific language impairment. *Applied Psycholinguistics, 2,* 89–118.

Leonard, L. (1989). Language learnability and specific language impairment in children. *Applied Psycholinguistics, 10,* 179–202.

Leonard, L. (1991a). Specific language impairment as a clinical category. *Language, Speech and Hearing Services in Schools, 22,* 66–68.

Leonard, L. (1991b). The cross-linguistic study of language-impaired children. In J. Miller (Ed.), *Research on child language disorders: A decade of progress.* Austin, TX: Pro-Ed.

Leonard, L. (1992). The use of morphology by children with specific language impairment: Evidence from three languages. In R. Chapman (Ed.), *Processes in language acquisition and disorders.* St. Louis: Mosby Year Book.

Leonard, L. (1995). Phonological impairment. In P. Fletcher & B. MacWhinney (Eds.), *The handbook of child language.* Cambridge, MA: Basil Blackwell.

Leonard, L. (1998). *Children with specific language impairment.* Cambridge, MA: MIT Press.

Leonard, L., McGregor, K., & Allen, G. (1992). Grammatical morphology and speech perception in children with specific language impairment. *Journal of Speech and Hearing Research, 35,* 1076–1085.

Leonard, L., Miller, C., & Gerber, E. (1999). Grammatical morphology and the lexicon in children with specific language impairment. *Journal of Speech, Language and Hearing Research, 42,* 678–689.

Leonard, L., Sabbadini, L., Volterra, V., & Leonard, J. (1988). Some influences on the grammar of English- and Italian-speaking children with specific language impairment. *Applied Psycholinguistics, 9,* 39–57.

Leske, C. (1979). *Incidence and prevalence in communication disorders.* Report to the National Advisory Neurological and Communicative Disorders and Stroke Council (Report No. 79–1914). Washington, DC: National Institutes of Health.

Loban, W. (1976). *Language development: Kindergarten through grade 12.* Urbana, IL: National Council of Teachers of English.

Lobato, D., Barrera, R., & Feldman, R. (1981). Sensorimotor functioning and prelinguistic communication of severely and profoundly retarded individuals. *American Journal of Mental Deficiency, 85,* 489–496.

Locke, J. (1980). The inference of speech perception in the phonologically disordered child: Part I. A rationale, some criteria, the conventional tests. Part II. Some clinically novel procedures, their use, some findings. *Journal of Speech and Hearing Disorders, 45,* 431–468.

Locke, J. (1993). *The child's path to spoken language.* Cambridge, MA: Harvard University Press.

Loeb, D. (1994). Pronoun case errors of children with and without specific language impairment: Evidence from a longitudinal elicited imitation task. Paper at Stanford Child Language Research Forum.

Long, S. (1994). Language and children with autism. In V. Reed (Ed.), *An introduction to children with language disorders* (2nd ed.). New York: Merrill.

Lord, C., & Paul, R. (1997). Language and communication in autism. In D. Cohen & F. Volknas (Eds.), *Handbook of autism and pervasive developmental disorder* (2nd ed.; pp. 195–225). New York: Wiley.

Lorenz, J., Wooliever, D., Jetton, J., & Paneth, N. (1998). A quantitative review of mortality and developmental disability in extremely premature newborns. *Archives of Pediatric and Adolescent Medicine, 152,* 425–435.

Lou, M. (1988). The history of language use in the education of the deaf in the United States. In M. Strong (Ed.), *Language learning and deafness.* Cambridge, UK: Cambridge University Press.

Lovaas, O. (1977). *The autistic child: Language development through behavior modification.* New York: Irvington.

Lund, N., & Duchan, J. (1993). *Assessing children's language in naturalistic contexts* (2nd ed.). Englewood Cliffs, NJ: Prentice-Hall.

MacWhinney, B. (1995). *The CHILDES Project: Computational tools for analyzing talk* (2nd ed.). Hillsdale, NJ: Erlbaum.

Marcell, M., & Weeks, S. (1988). Short-term memory difficulties and Down's syndrome. *Journal of Mental Deficiency Research, 32,* 153–162.

McCauley, R., & Demetras, M. (1990). The identification of language impairment in the selection of specifically language-impaired subjects. *Journal of Speech and Hearing Disorders, 55,* 468–475.

McCauley, R., & Swisher, L. (1984). Use and misuse of norm-referenced tests in clinical assessment: A hypothetical case. *Journal of Speech and Hearing Disorders, 49,* 338–348.

McGuire, P., Robertson, D., Thacker, A., David, A., Kitson, N., Frackowiak, R. & Frith, C. (1997). Neural correlates of thinking in sign language. *Neuroreport, 8,* 695–698.

McIntire, M. (1977). The acquisition of American Sign Language hand configurations. *Sign Language Studies, 16,* 247–266.

McLean, J., & Snyder-McLean, L. (1978). *A transactional approach to early language training.* Columbus, OH: Merrill/Macmillan.

McLeavey, B., Toomey, J., & Dempsey, P. (1982). Nonretarded and mentally retarded children's control over syntactic structures. *American Journal of Mental Deficiency, 86,* 485–494.

Menyuk, P. (1969). *Sentences children use.* Cambridge, MA: MIT Press.

Merritt, D., & Culatta, B. (1998). *Language intervention in the classroom.* San Diego: Singular Press.

Mezernich, M., Jenkins, W., Johnston, P., Schreiner, C., Miller, S., & Tallal, P. (1996). Temporal processing deficits of language-learning impaired children ameliorated by training. *Science, 271,* 77–81.

Miller, J. (1981). *Assessing language production in children: Experimental procedures.* Baltimore: University Park Press.

Miller, J. (1991). Research on language disorders in children: A progress report. In J. Miner (Ed.), *Research on child language disorders: A decade of progress.* Austin, TX: Pro-Ed.

Miller, J. (1999). Profiles of language development in children with Down syndrome. In J. Miller, M. Leddy, & L. Leavitt (Eds.), *Improving the communication of people with Down syndrome* (pp. 11–40). Baltimore: Brookes.

Miller, J., & Chapman, R. (1984). Disorders of communication: Investigating the development of language of mentally retarded children. *American Journal of Mental Deficiency, 88,* 536–545.

Mindel, E., & Vernon, M. (1987). *They grow in silence.* Boston: College-Hill Press.

Miyamoto, R., Kirk, K., Svirsky, M., & Sehgal, S. (1999). Communication skills in pediatric cochlear implant recipients. *Acta Otolaryngologica, 119,* 219–224.

Moeller, K. & Starr, C. (1993). *Cleft palate: Interdisciplinary issues and treatment.* Austin: Pro-Ed.

Moeller, M., & Luettke-Stahlman, B. (1990). Parents' use of Signing Exact English: A descriptive analysis. *Journal of Speech and Hearing Disorders, 55,* 327–338.

Montee, B., Miltenberger, R., Wittrock, D., Watkins, N., Rheinberger, A., & Stackhaus, J. (1995). An experimental analysis of facilitated communication. *Journal of Applied Behavior Analysis, 28,* 189–200.

Montgomery, J. (1995a). Examination of phonological working memory in specifically language-impaired children. *Applied Psycholinguistics, 16,* 355–378.

Montgomery, J. (1995b). Sentence comprehension in children with specific language impairment: The role of phonological working memory. *Journal of Speech and Hearing Research, 38,* 187–199.

Moores, D. (1987). *Factors predictive of literacy in deaf adolescents.* NIH–NINCDS–83–19. NIH Report.

Musselman, C., Lindsay, P., & Wilson, A. (1988). An evaluation of trends in preschool programming for hearing-impaired children. *Journal of Speech and Hearing Disorders, 53,* 71–88.

Negri, N. (1992). Individuals with autism: Language acquisition with restricted social and emotional knowledge. In R. Chapman (Ed.), *Processes in language acquisition and disorders.* St. Louis: Mosby.

Neilson, M., & Neilson, P. (1987). Speech motor control and stuttering: a computation model of adaptive sensory-motor processing. *Speech Communication, 6,* 325–333.

Nelson, K., Camarata, S., Welsh, J., Butkovsky, L., & Camarata, M. (1996). Effects of initiative and conversational recasting treatment on the acquisition of grammar in children with specific language impairment and younger language-normal children. *Journal of Speech and Hearing Research, 39,* 850–859.

Nelson, L., Kamhi, A., & Appel, K. (1987). Cognitive strengths and weaknesses in language-impaired children: One more look. *Journal of Speech and Hearing Disorders, 52,* 36–43.

Nelson, N. W. (1993). *Childhood language disorders in context: Infancy through adolescence.* New York: Macmillan.

Nelson, N. W. (1998). *Childhood language disorders in context: Infancy through adolescence* (2nd ed.). Boston: Allyn & Bacon.

Newman, P., Creaghead, N., & Secord, W. (1989). *Assessment and remediation of articulatory and phonological disorders* (2nd ed.). Columbus, OH: Merrill/Macmillan.

Newport, E., & Meier, R. (1985). The acquisition of American Sign Language. In D. Slobin (Ed.). *The cross-linguistic study of language acquisition. Volume 1* (pp. 881–938). Hillsdale, NJ: Lawrence Erlbaum.

Nordin, V., & Gillberg, C. (1998). The long-term course of autistic disorders: Update on follow-up studies. *Acta Psychiatrica Scandinavia, 2,* 99–108.

Nye, C., Foster, S., & Seaman, D. (1987). Effectiveness of language intervention with the language-learning disabled. *Journal of Speech and Hearing Disorders, 53,* 348–357.

Ornitz, E. (1989). Autism at the interface between sensory and information processing. In G. Dawson (Ed.), *Autism: Nature, diagnosis and treatment* (pp. 174–207). New York: Guilford Press.

Owens, R. (1997). Mental retardation: Difference or delay? In D. Bernstein & E. Tiegerman-Farber (Eds.), *Language and communication disorder in children* (4th ed.). Columbus, OH: Merrill/Macmillan.

Owens, R. (1999). *Language disorders: A functional approach to assessment and intervention* (3rd ed.). Boston: Allyn & Bacon.

Paccia, J., & Curcio, F. (1982). Language processing and forms of immediate echolalia in autistic children. *Journal of Speech and Hearing Research, 25,* 42–47.

Paden, E. (1994). Otitis media and disordered phonologies: Some concerns and cautions. *Topics in Language Disorders, 14,* 72–83.

Padgett, S. (1988). Speech- and language-impaired three and four year olds: A five-year follow-up study. In R. Masland & M. Masland (Eds.), *Preschool prevention of reading failure.* Parkton, MD: York Press.

Palinscar, A., Brown, A., & Campione, J. (1994). Models and practices of dynamic assessment. In G. Wallach & K. Butler (Eds.), *Language learning disabilities in school-age children and adolescents.* New York: Merrill.

Paul, R. (1991). Profiles of toddlers with slow expressive language development. *Topics in Language Disorders, 11,* 1–13.

Paul, R. (1995). *Language disorders from infancy through adolescence.* New York: Mosby.

Paul, R., & Jennings, P. (1992). Phonological behaviors in toddlers with slow expressive language development. *Journal of Speech and Hearing Research, 35,* 99–107.

Paul, R., & Shriberg, L. (1982). Associations between phonology and syntax in speech-delayed children. *Journal of Speech and Hearing Research, 25,* 536–547.

Perera, K. (1984). *Children's writing and reading.* Oxford: Blackwell.

Perkins, W., Kent, R., & Curlee, R. (1991). A theory of neuropsycholinguistic function in stuttering. *Journal of Speech and Hearing Research, 34,* 734–752.

Pettito, L. (1991). Babbling in the manual mode: Evidence for the ontogeny of language. *Science, 251,* 1493–1496.

Pflaster, G. (1980). A factor analysis of variables related to academic performance of hearing-impaired children in regular classes. *Volta Review, 82,* 71–84.

Pinker, S. (1984). *Language learnability and language development.* Cambridge, MA: Harvard University Press.

Pinker, S. (1989). Learnability paradox in verb lexicon acquisition. In M. Rice & R. Schiefelbush (Eds.), *The teachability of language.* Baltimore: Brookes.

Plante, E. (1991). MRI findings in the parents and siblings of specifically language-impaired boys. *Brain and Language, 41,* 67–80.

Plante, E., & Beeson, P. (1999). *Communication and communication disorders: A clinical introduction.* Boston: Allyn & Bacon.

Plante, E., Shenkman, K., & Clark, M. (1996). Classification of adults for family studies of developmental language disorders. *Journal of Speech and Hearing Research, 39,* 661–667.

Power, D., & Quigley, S. (1973). Deaf children's acquisition of the passive voice. *Journal of Speech and Hearing Research, 16,* 5–11.

Prinz, P., & Ferrier, L. (1983). "Can you give me that one?": The comprehension, production and judgment of directives by language-impaired children. *Journal of Speech and Hearing Disorders, 48,* 44–54.

Prinz, R., & Prinz, E. (1981). Acquisition of ASL and spoken English by a hearing child of a deaf mother and a hearing father: Phase II. Early combinatorial patterns. *Sign Language Studies, 30,* 78–88.

Prizant, B., Audet, L., Burke, G., Hummel, L., Maher, S., & Theadore, G. (1990). Communication disorders and emotional/behavioral disorders in children and adolescents. *Journal of Speech and Hearing Disorders, 55,* 179–192.

Prizant, B., & Duchan, J. (1981). The functions of echolalia in autistic children. *Journal of Speech and Hearing Disorders, 46,* 241–249.

Prizant, B., & Wetherby, A. (1987). Communicative intent: A framework for understanding social-communicative behavior in autism. *Journal of the American Academy of Child and Adolescent Psychiatry, 26,* 472–479.

Prizant, B., & Wetherby, A. (1994). Providing services to children with autism (ages 0 to 2 years) and their families. In K. Butler (Ed.), *Early intervention: Working with infants and toddlers.* Gaithersburg, MD: Aspen Publishers.

Prizant, B., & Wetherby, A. (1998). Understanding the continuum of discrete-trial traditional behavioral to social-pragmatic developmental approaches in communication enhancement for young children with autism/PDD. *Seminars in Speech and Language, 19,* 329–352.

Pulsifer, M. (1996). The neuropsychology of mental retardation. *Journal of the International Neuropsychological Society, 2,* 159–176.

Quigley, S., & King, C. (1982) The language development of deaf children and youth. In S. Rosenberg (Ed.), *Handbook of applied psycholinguistics: Major thrusts of research and theory* (pp. 429–476). Hillsdale, NJ: Lawrence Erlbaum.

Quigley, S., Montanelli, D., & Wilbur, R. B. (1976). Some aspects of the verb system in the language of deaf students. *Journal of Speech and Hearing Research, 19,* 536–550.

Quigley, S., & Paul, P. (1984). *Language and deafness.* Austin, TX: Pro-Ed.

Quigley, S., & Paul, P. (1987). Deafness and language development. In S. Rosenberg (Ed.), *Advances in applied psycholinguistics: Vol. 1. Disorders of first language development.* Cambridge, UK: Cambridge University Press.

Quigley, S., Smith, N., & Wilbur, R. B. (1974). Comprehension of relativized sentences by deaf students. *Journal of Speech and Hearing Research, 17,* 325–341.

Quigley, S., Wilbur, R. B., & Montanelli, D. (1974). Question formation in the language of deaf students. *Journal of Speech and Hearing Research, 17,* 699–713.

Quigley, S., Wilbur, R. B., & Montanelli, D. (1976). Complement structures in the language of deaf students. *Journal of Speech and Hearing Research, 19,* 448–457.

Rapin, I. (1977). Language disability in children. In M. Blaw, I. Rapin, & M. Kinsbourne (Eds.), *Topics in child neurology.* Toronto: Spectrum.

Rapin, I., & Katzman, R. (1998). Neurobiology of autism. *Annals of Neurology, 43,* 7–14.

Rawlings, B., & Jensema, C. (1977). *Two studies of the families of hearing impaired children.* Washington, DC: Office of Demographic Studies.

Reed, V. (1994). *An introduction to children with language disorders* (2nd ed.). New York: Merrill.

Reichle, J., & Karlan, G. (1988). Selecting augmentative communication interventions: A critique of candidacy criteria and a proposed alternative. In R. Schiefelbusch & L. Lloyd (Eds.), *Language perspectives: Acquisition, retardation and intervention* (2nd ed.). Austin, TX: Pro-Ed.

Rescorla, L. (1989). The language development survey: A screening tool for delayed language in toddlers. *Journal of Speech and Hearing Disorders, 54,* 587–599.

Rescorla, L., & Bernstein Ratner, N. (1996). Phonetic profiles of toddlers with Specific Expressive Language Impairment (SLI-E). *Journal of Speech and Hearing Research, 39*(1), 153–165.

Rescorla, L., & Schwartz, E. (1990). Outcome of toddlers with specific expressive language delay. *Applied Psycholinguistics, 11,* 393–407.

Rice, M. (1987). Preschool children's fast mapping of words: Robust for most, fragile for some. Paper presented at the Fourth Congress of the International Association for the Study of Child Language, Lund, Sweden.

Rice, M. (1991). Children with specific language impairment: Toward a model of teachability. In N. A. Krasnegor, D. M. Rumbaugh, R. L. Schiefelbusch, & M. Studdert-Kennedy (Eds.), *Biobehavorial foundations of language development* (pp. 447–480). Hillsdale, NJ: Erlbaum.

Rice, M., Haney, K., & Wexler, K. (1998). Family histories of children with SLI who show extended optional infinitives. *Journal of Speech, Language, Hearing Research, 41,* 419–433.

Rice, M., Oetting, J., Marquis, J., Bode, J., & Pae, S. (1994). Frequency of input effects on word comprehension of children with specific language impairment. *Journal of Speech and Hearing Research, 37,* 106–122.

Rice, M., & Schiefelbusch, R. (Eds.). (1989). *The teachability of language.* Baltimore: Brookes.

Rice, M., & Wexler, K. (1995). Extended optional infinitive (EOI) account of specific language impairment. In D. MacLaughlin & S. McEwen (Eds.), *Proceedings of the 19th Annual Boston University Conference on Language Development, 2,* 451–462. Somerville, MA: Cascadilla Press.

Ricks, D., & Wing, L. (1975). Language, communication and the use of symbols in normal and autistic children. *Journal of Autism and Childhood Schizophrenia, 5,* 191–221.

Robbins, A., Bollard, P., & Green, J. (1999). Language development in children implanted with the CLARION cochlear implant. *Annals of Otology, Rhinology and Laryngology, Supplement, 177,* 113–118.

Roberts, J., & Wallace, I. (1997). Language and otitis media. In J. Roberts, I. Wallace & F. Henderson (Eds.), *Otitis media in young children: Medical, developmental and educational considerations* (pp. 133–162). Baltimore: Brookes.

Robinson, K. (1998). Implications of developmental plasticity for the language acquisition of deaf children with cochlear implants. *International Journal of Pediatric Otorhinolaryngology, 46,* 71–80.

Rogers, S. (1998). Empirically supported comprehensive treatments for young children with autism. *Journal of Clinical Child Psychology, 27,* 168–179.

Romski, M., Lloyd, L., & Sevcik, R. (1988). Augmentative and alternative communication issues. In R. Schiefelbusch & L. Lloyd (Eds.), *Language perspectives: Acquisition, retardation and intervention* (2nd ed.). Austin, TX: Pro-Ed.

Rosenberg, S. (1982). The language of the mentally retarded. In S. Rosenberg (Ed.), *Handbook of applied psycholinguistics: Major thrusts of research and theory.* Hillsdale, NJ: Lawrence Erlbaum.

Roth, F., & Spekman, N. (1984). Assessing the pragmatic abilities of children: Part 1. An organizational framework and assessment parameters. Part II. Guidelines, considerations and specific evaluation procedures. *Journal of Speech and Hearing Disorders, 49,* 2–17.

Roth, F., & Spekman, N. (1986). Narrative discourse: Spontaneously generated stories of learning-disabled and normally achieving students. *Journal of Speech and Hearing Disorders, 51,* 8–23.

Rudser, S. (1988). Sign language instruction and its implications for the deaf. In M. Strong (Ed.), *Language learning and deafness.* Cambridge, UK: Cambridge University Press.

Rumsey, J. (1996). Neuroimaging studies of autism. In G. Lyon & J. Rumsey (Eds.), *Neuroimaging: A window into the neurological foundations of learning and behavior in children.* Baltimore: Brookes.

Rutter, M. (1979). Language, cognition and autism. In R. Katzman (Ed.), *Congenital and acquired cognitive disorders.* New York: Raven Press.

Rutter, M., & Schopler, E. (1987). Autism and pervasive developmental disorders: Concepts and diagnostic issues. *Journal of Autism and Developmental Disorders, 17,* 159–186.

Salmelin, R., Schnitzler, A., Schmitz, F., Jancke, L., Witte, O., & Freund, H. (1998). Functional organization of the auditory cortex is different in stutterers and fluent speakers. *Neuroreport, 9,* 2225–2229.

Salzberg, C., & Villani, T. (1983). Speech training by parents of Down syndrome toddlers: Generalization across settings and instructional contexts. *American Journal of Mental Deficiency, 87,* 403–413.

Scarborough, H. (1990). Index of productive syntax. *Applied Psycholinguistics, 11,* 1–22.

Scarborough, H., & Dobrich, W. (1990). Development of children with early language delay. *Journal of Speech and Hearing Research, 33,* 70–83.

Scheetz, N. (1993). *Orientation to deafness.* Boston: Allyn & Bacon.

Scherer, N., & Olswang, L. (1989). Using structured discourse as a language intervention technique with autistic children. *Journal of Speech and Hearing Disorders, 54,* 383–394.

Schlesinger, H., & Meadow, K. (1972). *Sound and sign: Childhood deafness and mental health.* Berkeley: University of California Press.

Sheehan, C., & Matuozzi, R. (1996). Investigation of the validity of facilitated communication through the disclosure of unknown information. *Mental Retardation, 34,* 94–107.

Shriberg, L. (1991). Directions for research in developmental phonological disorders. In J. Miller (Ed.), *Research on child language disorders: A decade of progress.* Austin, TX: Pro-Ed.

Shriberg, L., & Kwiatkowski, J. (1987). A retrospective study of spontaneous generalization in speech delayed children. *Language, Speech and Hearing Services in the Schools, 18,* 144–157.

Shriberg, L., Kwiatkowski, J., Best, S., Hengst, J., & Terselic-Weber, B. (1986). Characteristics of children with phonologic disorders of unknown origin. *Journal of Speech and Hearing Disorders, 51,* 140–160.

Sigman, M., & Ruskin, E. (1999). Continuity and change in the social competence of children with autism, Down syndrome and developmental delays. *Monographs of the Society for Research in Child Development, 64,* (256).

Silva, P. (1980). The prevalence, stability and significance of developmental language delay in preschool children. *Developmental Medicine and Child Neurology, 22,* 768–777.

Silva, P., Williams, S., & McGee, R. (1987). A longitudinal study of children with developmental language delay at age three: Later intelligence, reading and behavior problems. *Developmental Medicine and Child Neurology, 29,* 630–640.

Simmons, J., & Tymchuk, A. (1973). Learning deficits in childhood psychosis. *Pediatric Clinics of North America, 20,* 665–679.

Slobin, D. (1968). Imitation and grammatical development in children. In N. Endler, L. Boulter, & H. Osser (Eds.), *Contemporary issues in developmental psychology.* New York: Holt, Rinehart & Winston.

Smith, J., & Polloway, E. (1979). The dimension of adaptive behavior in mental retardation research: An analysis of recent practices. *American Journal of Mental Deficiency, 84,* 203–206.

Smith, N., & Tsimpli, I.-M. (1995). *The mind of a savant: Language learning and modularity.* Oxford: Blackwell.

Spekman, N. (1981). A study of the dyadic verbal communication abilities of learning disabled and normally achieving fourth and fifth grade boys. *Learning Disability Quarterly, 4,* 139–151.

Spencer, L., & Tomblin, J. B. (1999). Reading skills in children with multichannel cochlear implant experience. *Volta Review,* 99, 193–202.

Staller, S., Beiter, A., & Brimacombe, J. (1994). Use of the Nucleus 22 Channel cochlear implant system with children. *Volta Review, 96*(5), 15–40.

Stark, R., & Tallal, P. (1981). Selection of children with specific language deficits. *Journal of Speech and Hearing Disorders, 46,* 114–122.

Starkweather, C. W. (1987). *Fluency and stuttering.* Englewood Cliffs, NJ: Prentice-Hall.

Stefanatos, G., Green, G., & Ratcliff, G. (1989). Neurophysiological evidence of auditory channel anomalies in developmental dysphasia. *Archives of Neurology, 46,* 871–875.

Stevenson, J. (1984). Predictive value of speech and languagescreening. *Developmental Medicine and Child Neurology, 26,* 528–538.

Stevenson, J., & Richman, M. (1976). The prevalence of language delay in a population of three-year-old children and its association with general retardation. *Developmental Medicine and Child Neurology, 18,* 431–441.

Stoel-Gammon, C., & Dunn, C. (1984). *Normal and disordered phonology in children.* Baltimore: University Park Press.

Strong, M., & Prinz, P. (1997). A study of the relationship between American Sign Language and English literacy. *Journal of Deaf Studies and Deaf Education, 2,* 37–46.

Studdert-Kennedy, M., & Mody, M. (1995). Auditory temporal perception deficits in the reading-impaired: a critical review. *Psychonomic Bulletin and Review, 2,* 508–514.

Swisher, L. (1985). Language disorders in children. In J. Darby (Ed.), *Speech and language evaluation in neurology: Childhood disorders* (pp. 33–97). New York: Grune and Stratton.

Swisher, L., Restrepo, M., Plante, E., & Lowell, S. (1995). Effect of implicit and explicit "rule" presentation on bound-morpheme generalization in specific language impairment. *Journal of Speech and Hearing Research, 38,* 168–173.

Swisher, M. (1985). Characteristics of hearing mothers' manually coded English. In W. Stokoe & V. Volterra (Eds.), SLR '83: *Sign language research.* Silver Spring, MD: Linstok Press.

Szatmari, P., Jones, M., Zweigenbaum, L. & MacLean, J. (1998). Genetics of autism: Overview and new directions. *Journal of Autism and Developmental Disorders, 28,* 351–368.

Tager-Flusberg, H. (1981). On the nature of linguistic functioning in early infantile autism. *Journal of Autism and Developmental Disorders, 11,* 45–56.

Tager-Flusberg, H. (1999a). Language development in atypical children. In M. Barrett (Ed.), *The development of language* (pp. 311–348). East Sussex: Psychology Press.

Tager-Flusberg, H. (1999b). Understanding the language and communicative impairments in autism. In L. Glidden (Ed.). *International Review of Research on Mental Retardation.* New York: Academic Press.

Tager-Flusberg, H., & Calkins, S. (1990). Does imitation facilitate the acquisition of grammar? Evidence from a study of autistic, Down's syndrome and normal children. *Journal of Child Language, 17,* 591–606.

Tait, M., & Luttman, M. (1994). Comparison of early communicative behavior in young children with cochlear implants and with hearing aids. *Ear and Hearing, 15*(5), 352–361.

Tallal, P., (1987). Developmental language disorders. In *Learning disabilities: A report to the U.S. Congress.* Washington, DC: Interagency Committee on Learning Disabilities.

Tallal, P., Miller, S., Bedi, G., Byma, G., Wang, X., Nagarajan, S., Schreiner, C., Jenkins, W., & Mezernich, M. (1996). Language comprehension in language-learning impaired children improved with acoustically modified speech. *Science, 271,* 81–84.

Tallal, P., & Piercy, M. (1973). Defects of non-verbal auditory perception in children with developmental aphasia. *Nature, 241,* 468–469.

Tallal, P., & Piercy, M. (1974). Developmental aphasia: Rate of auditory processing and selective impairment of consonant perception. *Neuropsychologia, 12,* 83–93.

Tallal, P., & Piercy, M. (1975). Developmental aphasia: The perception of brief vowels and extended stop consonants. *Neuropsychologia, 13,* 69–74.

Tallal, P., Ross, R., & Curtiss, S. (1989). Familial aggregation in specific language impairment. *Journal of Speech and Hearing Disorders, 54,* 167–173.

Tallal, P., & Stark, R. (1981). Speech acoustic-cue discrimination abilities of normally developing and language-impaired children. *Journal of the Acoustical Society of America, 69,* 568–574.

Tiegerman-Farber, E. (1997). Autism: Learning to communicate. In D. Bernstein & E. Tiegerman-Farber (Eds.), *Language and communication disorders in children* (4th ed.). Boston: Allyn & Bacon.

Tomblin, B. (1996). The big picture of SLI: Results of an epidemiological study of SLI among kindergarten children. Paper presented at the Symposium on Research in Child Language Disorders, University of Wisconsin, Madison.

Tomblin, B., & Buckwalter, P. (1994). Studies of genetics of specific language impairment. In R. Watkins & M. Rice (Eds.), *Specific language impairments in children* (pp. 17–34). Baltimore, MD: Paul Brookes.

Tomblin, B., Freese, P., & Records, N. (1992). Diagnosing specific language impairment in adults for the purpose of pedigree analysis. *Journal of Speech and Hearing Research, 35,* 832–843.

Tomblin, B., Spencer, L., Flock, S., Tyler, R., & Gantz, B. (1999). A comparison of language achievement in children with cochlear implants and children using hearing aids. *Journal of Speech, Language and Hearing Research, 42,* 497–511.

Trauner, D., Wulfeck, B., Tallal, P., & Hesselink, J. (1995). Neurologic and MRI profiles of language impaired children. Technical report CND-9513, Center for Research in Language, University of California at San Diego.

Trottier, G., Srivastava, L., & Walker, C. (1999). Etiology of infantile autism: A review of recent advances in genetic and neurobiological research. *Journal of Psychiatry and Neuroscience, 24,* 103–115.

Tye-Murray, N. (1998). *Foundations of aural rehabilitation.* San Diego: Singular.

U.S. Department of Education. (1987). *Learning disabilities: A report to the U.S. Congress.* Washington, DC: Interagency Committee on Learning Disabilities.

van der Lely, H., Rosen, S., & McClelland, A. (1998). Evidence for a grammar-specific deficit in children. *Current Biology, 8,* 1253–1258.

Van Meter, L., Fein, D., Morris, R., Waterhouse, L., & Allen, D. (1997). Delay versus deviance in autistic social behavior. *Journal of Autism and Developmental Disorders, 27,* 557–69.

Wallach, G., & Butler, K. (1994). *Language learning disabilities in school-age children and adolescents.* New York: Merrill.

Watkins, R. (1994). Grammatical challenges for children with specific language impairments, In R. Watkins & M. Rice (Eds.), *Specific language impairments in children.* Baltimore: Brookes.

Watson, B., & Freeman, F. (1997). Brain imaging contributions. In R. Curlee & G. Siegel (Eds.), *Nature and treatment of stuttering: New directions* (2nd ed.). Boston: Allyn & Bacon.

Weinberg, N. (1997). Cognitive and behavioral deficits associated with parental alcohol use. *Journal of the American Academy of Child and Adolescent Psychiatry, 36,* 1177–86.

Weiner, P. (1985). The value of follow-up studies. *Topics in Language Disorders, 5,* 78–92.

Weir, R. (1962). *Language in the crib.* The Hague: Mouton.

Weiss, B., Weisz, J., & Bromfield, R. (1986). Performance of retarded and nonretarded persons on information processing tasks: Further tests of the similar structure hypothesis. *Psychological Bulletin, 100,* 157–175.

Weiss, M., Wagner, S., & Bauman, M. (1996). A validated case study of facilitated communication. *Mental Retardation, 34,* 220–30.

Wetherby, A. (1984). Possible neurolinguistic breakdown in autistic children. *Topics in Language Disorders, 4,* 19–33.

Wetherby, A. (1986). Ontogeny of communication functions in autism. *Journal of Autism and Developmental Disorders, 16,* 295–316.

Wetherby, A. (1998). (Ed.) Preschoolers with autism: Communication and language interventions. *Seminars in Speech and Language, 19.*

Wilbur, R. B. (1987). *American Sign Language: Linguistic and applied dimensions.* San Diego: College-Hill Press.

Wilbur, R. B., & Jones, M. (1974). Some aspects of the bilingual/bimodal acquisition of sign language and English by three hearing children of deaf parents. In M. LaGaly, R. Fox, & A. Bruck (Eds.), *Papers from the Tenth Regional Meeting of the Chicago Linguistic Society.* Chicago: Chicago Linguistic Society.

Wilbur, R. B., Montanelli, D., & Quigley, S. (1976). Pronominalization in the language of deaf students. *Journal of Speech and Hearing Research, 19,* 120–140.

Wilkinson, K. (1998). Profiles of language and communication skills in autism. *Mental retardation and developmental disabilities research reviews, 4,* 73–79.

Wolk, S., & Schildroth, A. (1986). Deaf children and speech intelligibility: A national study, In A. Schildroth & M. Karchmer (Eds.), *Deaf children in America.* San Diego: College-Hill Press.

Wood, M. L. (1982). *Language disorders in school-age children.* Englewood Cliffs, NJ: Prentice-Hall.

Yairi, E., Ambrose, N., & Cox, N. (1996). Genetics of stuttering: a critical review. *Journal of Speech and Hearing Research, 39,* 771–784.

Yairi, E., Ambrose, N., Paden, E., & Throneburg, R. (1996). Predictive factors of persistence and recovery: pathways of childhood stuttering. *Journal of Communication Disorders, 29,* 51–77.

Yoder, P. (1995). Validity of facilitated communication intervention: Response to Duchan. *Journal of Speech and Hearing Research, 38,* 202–204.

Yoshinaga-Itano, C., Sedey, A., Coulter, D., & Mehl, A. (1998). Language of early- and later-identified children with hearing loss. *Pediatrics, 102,* 1161–1171.

Yoshinaga-Itano, C., Snyder, L., & Mayberry, R. (1996). How deaf and normally hearing students convey meaning within and between written sentences. *Volta Review, 98,* 9–38.

Yuwiler, A., Geller, E., & Ritvo, E. (1976). Neurobiochemical research. In E. Ritvo (Ed.), *Autism: Diagnosis, current research and management.* New York: Spectrum.

Zimmerman, G. (1980). Stuttering: A disorder of movement. *Journal of Speech and Hearing Research, 23,* 122–136.

Chapter 10

Language and Literacy in the School Years

Richard Ely
Boston University

In the first few years of life, most children master the rudiments of their native language. This remarkable achievement appears to require little conscious effort, and it occurs in a wide variety of contexts (Gallaway & Richards, 1994). By their third birthday, children have acquired a large and varied lexicon. They string together multiword utterances, participate appropriately in conversations, and make simple jokes (Horgan, 1981). They even begin to talk about objects and events that are not present in their immediate context (Snow, 1991).

By the time children enter kindergarten, usually around age five, they have acquired a relatively sophisticated command of language, an accomplishment that has sometimes led researchers to believe that language development was essentially complete. However, major tasks still await the child, and developments that are as dramatic as those of the early years are yet to come (Nippold, 1998). This chapter will describe changes that occur during the school years. We will pay particular attention to two trends that are qualitatively different from earlier developments: The first is children's growing ability to produce connected multi-utterance language as seen, for example, in their personal narratives (Karmiloff-Smith, 1986; Peterson & McCabe, 1983). The second is children's evolving knowledge of the language system itself, reflected in their expanding metalinguistic awareness and in their acquisition of literacy (Hulme & Joshi, 1998).

Our focus on extended discourse and metalinguistic awareness is not meant to imply that development in other domains has abated. Quite the contrary, children continue to acquire greater expertise in the phonological (Vihman, 1996), semantic, syntactic (Kemper, Rice, & Chen, 1995; Leadholm & Miller, 1992), and pragmatic (Ninio & Snow, 1996) aspects of language, as has been described in earlier chapters. Taking semantic development as an example, children's vocabulary continues to grow at a rapid rate during the school years (Anglin, 1993), with approximately 3,000 new words added to their lexicon each year (Just & Carpenter, 1987; Nagy & Herman, 1987). A significant portion of these new words come from reading (Carnine, Kameenui, & Coyle, 1984; Nagy, Herman, & Anderson, 1985; Perera, 1986), a finding that illustrates the importance of literacy, as well as the manner in which literacy interacts with ongoing language development.

Lexical development is also related to world knowledge (Crais, 1990), knowledge that in most children also develops rapidly throughout the school years. Children who know more about a wide range of topics acquire new words more easily than children whose knowledge of the world is more limited. With the acquisition of new words, the breadth and depth of semantic knowledge also increases (Landauer & Dumais, 1997). And bringing the process full circle, the addition of new words to the child's lexicon is facilitated by the presence of an already rich lexicon (Robbins & Ehri, 1994). The robust growth of the lexicon throughout the school years should make it clear that the progress that was made in the early years continues. This progress serves as an important foundation for further growth and, in most instances, allows the child to acquire qualitatively new skills like reading and writing.

The chapter is organized topically. We look first at how children's interactions with peers and the media influence their language development. We then turn to a discussion of children's use of a form of multi-utterance language termed **decontextualized language**. Decontextualized language is language that refers to phenomena that are not immediately present. Examples of decontextualized language include personal narratives and explanations. Next, we consider metalinguistics, knowledge of the language system itself. Children's awareness of the rule-governed nature of the language system evolves rapidly during the school years, and we will describe some of the developments of this period.

Metalinguistic awareness is an important component of literacy, our next topic. Literacy implies fluent mastery of reading and writing. We will describe how children acquire these important skills and what happens when they find reading difficult. Both metalinguistic awareness and literacy affect, and are affected by, children's ongoing cognitive development. Finally, we will examine children's experience with bilingualism during the school years.

The notion that language development is a life-span process is a guiding principle of this book. This chapter will bring us up to the threshold of adulthood, connecting the early years of language development described in the preceding chapters to the changes that occur during adulthood that are described in Chapter 11.

Interactions with Peers and the Media

On Their Own

For most children, early experiences with language occur with an adult, usually their mother or other primary caregiver. In the first years of life, the child has the advantage

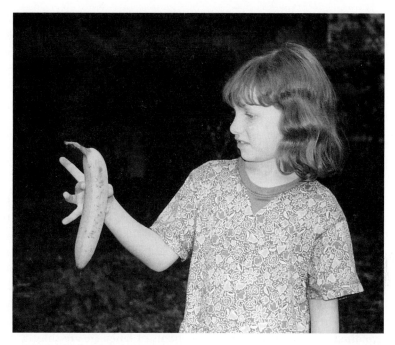

"...They're icky. They're slimy. They're gooey." Children may employ poetic devices to express their feelings of disgust.

of interacting with a helpful and knowledgeable speaker. Where the child's linguistic skill is weak or incomplete, the parent can fill in, or scaffold (Bruner, 1983). However, as children mature, they are more likely to find themselves in the company of other children, where they must fend for themselves. Peer interactions represent true testing grounds for the young child's evolving communicative competence (Preece, 1992; Rice, 1992). In time, peer interactions can become more important than parent–child interactions (Harris, 1998; Richards & Light, 1986; Whiting & Edwards, 1988). As children begin to enter the larger world, their language skills play a very important role in their social and cognitive development (Parker & Gottman, 1989; Teasley, 1995).

How well do children do on their own? What do they talk about, and how are conversations between peers different from conversations between children and adults? Although we have extensive data on early parent–child interaction, we know less about child-to-child interaction in the school years (Goodwin, 1990). In part, this lack of knowledge results from the difficulty of obtaining data from school-aged children, who have become self-conscious and susceptible to the **observer effect,** to altering their behavior because they know they are being observed (Labov, 1972).

In addition, as children enter adolescence, they use language to ally themselves with their peers or in-group, and to exclude outsiders, including curious researchers. Teenagers mark their group membership through the use of the **adolescent register.**

Adolescent registers encompass a variety of linguistic features, including distinct phonological and syntactic patterns (Beaumont, 1995; Nippold, 1993; Romaine, 1984). One striking component of the adolescent register is its lexicon, which includes slang terms (e.g., *lallies, nish, dibble, vada*) whose use is restricted to adolescents themselves. These terms are initially specific to particular eras, geographic regions, and social and cultural classes. They change rapidly, and either fall out of fashion or become absorbed into the general lexicon (Romaine, 1984).

Language Play, Verbal Humor, and Irony

Despite the difficulties associated with collecting language samples from school-aged children, researchers have documented many developments during this period. One aspect of language use that is uniquely childlike is the propensity to play with language (Dunn, 1988; Martlew, Connolly, & McCleod, 1978). In the early school years, play with language represents a sizable portion of children's language. In one study, approximately one-quarter of all utterances produced by kindergarten children contained some form of language play (Ely & McCabe, 1994). Children treat language as they would any other object, as a rich source of material that can be playfully exploited (Garvey, 1977). All components of language are subject to manipulations, and spontaneous word play and rhyming sometimes lead to the invention of new words, often nonsense words. In the following example, a child who clearly did not like bananas used repetition and partial rhyming to amplify her feelings of disgust:

> Yuck I hate bananas.
> They're icky.
> They're slimy.
> They're gooey. (Ely & McCabe, 1994, p. 26)

The almost poetic quality of this spontaneous utterance is echoed in children's more explicit attempts at creating poetry. Ann Dowker (1989; Dowker & Pinto, 1993) asked young children to generate poems in response to pictures. One boy, aged five-and-a-half, produced the following lines in response to a picture of a snowy day:

> It's a latta with a peed,
> A plappa plotty pleed.
> And there's a wop,
> A weep,
> A stop.
> And yes. No.
> Sledge.
> Fledge. (Dowker, 1989, p. 192)

These excerpts show that children have a propensity to play with the phonological features of language. Recent work suggests that this phonological play may sharpen children's linguistic skills. For example, children's early exposure to certain playful forms of language like nursery rhymes correlates positively with their later development of literacy (Bryant, Bradley, Maclean, & Crossland, 1989).

School-aged children also display a great interest in riddles and other interactive language play. **Riddles** are word games, usually structured as questions, that are dependent on phonological, morphological, lexical, or syntactic ambiguity (Pepicello & Weisberg, 1983). To solve a riddle correctly children must have some insight into the ways that words can be ambiguous. In the following examples of riddles, the first plays primarily on morphological ambiguity, the second on syntactic ambiguity (phrase structure):

> *Question:* Where did the King hide his armies?
> *Answer:* In his sleevies.
> *Question:* How is a duck like an icicle?
> *Answer:* They both grow down.

Between the ages of six and eight, children display a heightened interest in riddles (McDowell, 1979). Spontaneous riddle sessions can involve many children, each shouting out riddles as challenges, and answering riddles in turn. Table 10.1 gives examples of how children responded to a riddle. Children's ability to solve riddles varies with their knowledge of the genre itself and also with their metalinguistic development. Skill in solving riddles is also positively correlated with children's reading ability

Table 10.1   **Stages in Solving Riddles**

Target riddle: What dog keeps the best time?   Answer: A watch dog.

Level 0
Absent or minimal response: "I don't know."

Level 1
Illogical or negative attempt at explication: "Because dogs don't really have watches."

Level 2
Explanation focuses on the situation to which the language referred, not the language itself: "Because a watch dog is a kind of dog and also it keeps time."

Level 3
Incongruity is clearly attributed to the language itself: "Because, well, watch dogs are really dogs to watch and see if anybody comes in but watch dogs…It's a joke 'cause it's also another *word* for telling time."

Most six-year-olds are at level 1; most eight- and nine-year-olds perform at level 3.
(from Ely & McCabe, 1994)

(Ely & McCabe, 1994; Fowles & Glanz, 1977; Hirsh-Pasek, Gleitman, & Gleitman, 1978). Thus, language play is a marker of children's developing mastery of the language system, and also a means of acquiring linguistic knowledge.

Verbal humor represents another form of language play. Humor is a universal feature of language and culture (Apte, 1985; Kirshenblatt-Gimblett & Sherzer, 1976). To become full participants in the discourse of their community, children must become familiar with its basic forms of humor. Children's ability to both produce and appreciate verbal humor develops over time and is closely associated with their growing mastery of all aspects of language. Younger children, who have a limited appreciation of the social and situational aspects of language, are more likely than older children to find simple scatological utterances like "poo-poo head" humorous. Older children are less amused by such simple pragmatic violations and are more likely to focus on the semantic and syntactic manipulations found in conventional jokes and puns. At a later stage, adolescents are similar to adults in their comprehension and production of verbal humor.

Older children and adolescents are also known for their use of **sarcasm.** Sarcasm usually involves the use of **irony.** In using irony, a speaker intends to convey a meaning that goes beyond the literal meaning, often a meaning that is in direct opposition to the literal meaning. When the thrust of the utterance is mean or pointed, the speaker is said to be using sarcasm. For example, the comment "Nice move" said to someone who had just tripped represents a criticism, not a compliment. Although irony and sarcasm are common in everyday discourse, very young children fail to understand their true intent (Winner, 1988). The ability to understand and express irony increases with age and is initially particularly dependent on intonational cues (e.g., a sarcastic tone) (Dews et al., 1996). Only later are children able to use context to understand sarcasm (Capelli, Nakagawa, & Madden, 1990).

Verbal Aggression

There is much overlap between verbal humor and **verbal aggression.** Just as children can be playful, they can be cruel (Sluckin, 1981). Children intermingle verbal humor and verbal aggression to establish, maintain, and reorder social hierarchies (Goodwin, 1990; Labov, 1972). In a study of classroom discourse, more than 27 percent of children's utterances contained some form of verbal aggression. Verbal aggression included reprimands, harsh commands and insults ("Hold this, you jerk"), tattling ("Aaron said 'shut up' again"), rejections ("You're not my buddy, Ethan"), and criticisms (McCabe & Lipscomb, 1988). Boys were proportionally more verbally aggressive than girls, with fifth-grade boys being the most verbally aggressive; fully 40 percent of their utterances included verbal aggression.

Some forms of verbal aggression are highly structured and ritualistic. *Sounding, playing the dozens,* or *dissing* is an activity that is found predominantly among adolescent African American males (Labov, 1972), although similar behavior has been documented in female and mixed-sex groupings (Goodwin, 1990). Many of the insults are explicitly sexual; however some employ nonsexual imagery (Labov, 1972, pp. 312, 319), as in the following examples:

> Your mother so skinny, she do the hula hoop in a Applejack.
> Your mother play dice with the midnight mice.

Ritual insults build upon preceding utterances, with the goal being to outwit one's opponent by generating an insult that cannot be topped. One study of elementary school children found that frequent engagement in sounding was associated with better comprehension of figurative language (e.g., metaphors) (Ortony, Turner, & Larson-Shapiro, 1985). Unlike the verbal aggression found frequently in the speech of school-aged children, most adults go out of their way to mark their speech as nonaggressive (Deese, 1984). Thus, frequent use of verbal aggression may be a developmental stage through which many children pass on their way to becoming more circumspect adults.

Influence of the Media

School-aged children spend an extraordinary amount of their out-of-school time watching television (Anderson, Wilson, & Fielding, 1988; Williams, Haertel, Haertel, & Walberg, 1982). However, the effects of television on language development are not well known. There is some evidence that children can and do learn some language, especially vocabulary, from viewing (Rice & Woodsmall, 1988), and exposure to educational shows like *Sesame Street* can affect children's literacy development positively (Chall, 1967/1983).

Some critics of children's television believe that high levels of viewing displace more intellectually demanding activities like reading (Singer & Singer, 1990). Although data that support such a position exist, there is also some evidence that argues against such a simple formulation. For example, Csikszentmihalyi, Rathunde, and Whalen (1993) found that talented teenagers actually spent nearly twice as much time watching television as their nontalented counterparts, yet there was no significant difference in the percent of time each group of teenagers spent on reading. There was also no relation between the amount of time spent watching television and the amount of time spent studying. A more recent study of younger children found that the relationship between TV viewing and educational activities was complex (Huston, Wright, Marquis, & Green, 1999). For example, children's watching of informational and educational programming was unrelated to time spent reading. In contrast, children who watched cartoons and general audience programs were less likely to read and less likely to engage in other educational activities (e.g., art, music, puzzles).

Television both influences and is influenced by its younger audience. Television and other popular media provide models of language that many children will rarely experience personally. The models, may, of course be stereotypic rather than accurate, but they are available for imitation. For instance, young viewers who have never been to New York City have learned how young singles supposedly converse in New York City by watching the popular show *Friends.* Many white middle-class suburban youth who have had little contact with urban African Americans learn the registers of rappers through viewing music videos and listening to the lyrics of rap music. Television is an integral part of most children's development. Given that many children spend more time watching television than speaking directly with their parents or other adults, it is important that we learn more about how television interacts with language and literacy development (Rice, 1983).

Gender Differences

In Chapter 6 we saw that children as young as two or three begin to develop *genderlects* or special ways of talking associated with their gender. During the school years, gender differences in many domains become pronounced. The self-segregation by gender that begins in the preschool years often continues through adolescence, and researchers have noted differences between girls' social groups and boys' social groups (Maccoby, 1998). There are also some differences in the language of boys and girls, although researchers are not in agreement about the possible origins of gender differences. With several notable exceptions, there is little evidence that there are major biological differences underlying boys' and girls' typical language differences. Since differences between boys and girls in basic verbal abilities are small (Hyde & Linn, 1988), differential *ability* is unlikely to be responsible for the kinds of gender differences in language use that have been observed. Most of the gender differences that do exist in boys' and girls' language are more likely to be the product of socialization and context than the result of innate biological differences.

Adults have a strong influence on children's development of genderlects. Parents, especially fathers, may play an important role in the early years (Perlmann & Berko Gleason, 1994). However, during the school years, other adults, including teachers, begin to affect children's acquisition of genderlects. A dramatic demonstration of gender socialization is displayed in the following exchange drawn from an observation of a fifth-grade classroom (Sadker & Sadker, 1994, p. 43, emphasis added):

> *Stephen: (calling out):*   I think Lincoln was the best president. He held the country together during the war.
> *Teacher:*   A lot of historians would agree with you.
> *Mike:*   (seeing that nothing happened to Stephen, *calls out*): I don't. Lincoln was okay, but my Dad liked Reagan. He always said Reagan was a great president.
> *David:*   (*calling out*): Reagan? Are you kidding?
> *Teacher:*   Who do you think our best president was, Dave?
> *David:*   FDR. He saved us from the depression.
> *Max:*   (*calling out*): I don't think it's right to pick one best president. There were a lot of good ones.

Teacher: That's interesting.

Kimberly: (*calling out*): I don't think the presidents today are as good as the ones we used to have.

Teacher: Okay, Kimberly. But you forgot the rule. You're supposed to raise your hand.

In this example, when the boys interrupted, they were encouraged by the teacher; but when a girl (Kimberly) called out, the teacher chided her for not having raised her hand and waited to be called upon before speaking. The cumulative effects of years of interactions like this are likely to be profound, with boys and girls developing distinctly different notions of how to use language.

Beyond the pervasive influence of linguistic socialization by adults, children influence one another, and this peer socialization becomes more important during the school years. Furthermore, because of self-segregation by gender, peer socialization is likely to occur within same-sex groups, where, according to some theorists, boys and girls have different interactional goals: Girls seek affiliation and boys pursue power and autonomy (Gilligan, 1982; Maltz & Borker, 1982). There is evidence that in same-sex friendships, middle-class adolescent girls do show a strong preference for sharing conversation (Aukett, Ritchie, & Mill, 1988), and in these conversations adolescent girls are more likely than boys to talk about emotions and feelings (Barth & Kinder, 1988; Martin, 1997). However, in analyses of conversations between teenagers, Goodwin (1990) found that urban African American teenage girls were as likely to compete as they were to cooperate and were as interested in justice and rights (supposedly male concerns) as they were in care and responsibility.

Gender differences have been found in several other domains of language during the school years. For example, boys swear more than girls (Jay, 1992; Martin, 1997). Although it had been long been believed that boys used more slang than girls, recent evidence reveals that girls are as proficient in their use of taboo or pejorative language as are boys (de Klerk, 1992). In their personal narratives, girls are more likely than boys to quote the speech of others (Ely & McCabe, 1993; Ely, Gleason, & McCabe, 1996). This attention to language itself appears to carry over to achievements in literacy. Girls on average score higher than boys in measures of reading, writing, and spelling, and these differences persist through high school (Allred, 1990; Hedges & Nowell, 1995; Hogrebe, Nest, & Newman, 1985; Swann, 1992). It is important to recognize that these gender differences in performance may be due in part to gender differences in attitudes toward literacy. For example, some boys view reading and writing as quiet, passive activities with little intrinsic appeal, and some consider the content and subject matter of many reading and writing tasks in school to be more suitable for girls than for boys (Swann, 1992).

There are two gender differences that do have strong biological ties. First, with puberty, the size of boys' vocal tracts undergoes rapid change, leading to characteristic *voice cracking*. Postpubescent males have longer vocal cords than postpubescent females, giving adolescent and adult males the ability to speak at lower fundamental frequencies (Tanner, 1989). However, biology appears to play a lesser role in sex differences in voice pitch than would be predicted by the anatomical differences alone. Mattingly (1966) found that differences in pitch were as much stylistic, reflecting linguistic convention, as they were based on differences in vocal-tract size. As anyone who has ever taken voice lessons knows, individuals have some control over where they "place" their voice. In our gender dimorphic society, males place their voices low and females place their voices high, thus exaggerating biologically determined differences.

The second area in which a gender difference appears to have a strong biological basis is in the incidence of language disorders, particularly developmental dyslexia (impairment in learning to read; see "When Learning to Read Is Difficult," p. 434). The reported incidence of dyslexia is much greater in boys than in girls, with ratios varying between 2:1 and 5:1, although some of this difference may be due to referral bias (Shaywitz, Shaywitz, Fletcher, & Escobar, 1990). Possible biological reasons for sex differences in the incidence of reading disabilities include differences in brain lateralization and organization (see Chapters 1 and 11).

Decontextualized Language

Much of children's earliest speech is embedded in the immediate conversational context; it revolves around the child's needs and wants (Ely et al., 1992). Conversation for the sake of conversation is uncommon, as is talk about people, objects, and events that are not part of the current context. However, as children get older, they increasingly find themselves in situations in which they are speaking to conversational partners (e.g., peers, teachers) who may lack shared knowledge. In these settings, children need to learn to talk about themselves and their pasts in ways that are comprehensible and meaningful. In school settings, children are asked to describe phenomena that are not immediately present—like what they did while on vacation, or why birds migrate. In telling personal narratives about the past and in providing explanations children are using *decontextualized language*. This is language that refers to people, events, and experiences that are not part of the immediate context (Snow, 1991; Snow & Dickinson, 1991).

Decontextualized language can express two quite distinct modes of thought, the **paradigmatic mode** and the **narrative mode** (Bruner, 1986). The paradigmatic mode is scientific and logical, and the language of paradigmatic thought is consistent and noncontradictory. Many upper-grade classroom assignments, such as presentations in sciences courses, require children to think paradigmatically.

The narrative mode of thought focuses on human intentions. The language of narrative thought can be more varied, reflecting both the content of the story and also the style of the storyteller. In general, children develop some level of mastery of both modes of thought, although the respective balance will vary according to the child's culture, exposure to school, and individual circumstances.

Narratives

Narratives are stories, usually about the past. Some researchers define narratives (or a minimum narrative) as containing at least two sequential independent clauses about a single past event (Labov, 1972). Personal narratives are stories about personal experiences, often describing firsthand experiences of the storyteller. Through the telling and sharing of narratives, narrators (children and adults alike) make sense of their experiences.

The following example is part of a longer narrative told by a boy, almost four years old. He had been prompted by his mother to describe a recent visit to a fire station. Although the initial focus of the narrative was on what he saw (fire tools, a steering wheel), the key point of the narrative describes what the storyteller described as a "mistake."

> "But you know what I didn't…that was not, that I, that I think was a mistake for him to do.
> He let me wear the big heavy fire hat.
> But that was a mistake. Because when we got home I was, I was crying.
> And my eyes were starting to hurt.
> And actually my head hurt.
> And my, actually my hand and arm and elbow hurt.
> I was so sick when I got home."

In this narrative, the child has given linguistic expression to past events. He cites the wearing of a heavy fire hat as the cause of his illness and does so as part of a story. Following his narrative, his mother provided a paradigmatic explanation for what "really" happened. In her explanation, she used the word *associated* in its logical and scientific sense, to make clear that one event (wearing the fire hat) was temporally but not causally connected to another (the child's illness).

Interest in the development of children's narratives has grown in recent years (Bamberg, 1997; Berman & Slobin, 1994; Engel, 1995; Fivush & Hudson, 1990; McCabe & Peterson, 1991). During the school years most children master the ability to tell coherent narratives. Development proceeds from single-utterance narratives produced by children as young as twenty-four months to novella-length personal stories shared between adolescents.

A number of aspects of narratives show developmental change. For example, the structure of narratives has been analyzed from a variety of perspectives, including story grammar (which focuses on the structural elements and problem-solving aspects of stories; Mandler & Johnson, 1977; Stein, 1988; Stein & Albro, 1997), stanza analysis (which uses the notion of lines and groups of lines, or stanzas; Gee, 1986; Hymes, 1981), and high-point analysis (Labov, 1972; Peterson & McCabe, 1983). In high-point analysis, the story is structured around a *high point* in which the narrator emphasizes *reference,* what happened, and *evaluation,* the narrator's attitude about what happened.

In their study of a large corpus of personal narratives from children between the ages of four and nine, Peterson and McCabe (1983) found a number of age-related changes. Using high-point analysis, they found that the structure used most frequently by the youngest children (the four-year-olds) was the *leap-frog narrative,* in which the child unsystematically jumps from one event to another, often leaving out important points in the process. The following is an example of a leap-frog narrative from a four-year-old girl (Peterson & McCabe, 1983, p. 72):

Experimenter: Have you ever been to Oberlin or Cleveland, any place like that?
Child: I been, been to, to Christ Jovah's right there.
Experimenter: You've been where?
Child: Christ Jovah's house. Sometimes.
Experimenter: And?
Child: I just said, I, I said, Hi, hello, and how are you? And then, and then, they go to someplace else, and then, and then I had a party, with, with, with, with candy and…hmm…my, and my, um, I don't know.
Experimenter: And you what?
Child: I don't know what I did. I *sure* had a party.

Another common structure that was used by children between the ages of four and eight was the *chronological narrative* that takes the form of recounting a sequence of events ("and then…and then"). The most mature form of narrative, according to high-point analysis, is the *classic narrative* in which events build to a high point, are briefly suspended and evaluated, and then resolved. Classic narratives were relatively uncommon in four-year-olds, but made up about 60 percent of the narratives of eight- and nine-year-olds. The following is a classic narrative from an eight-year-old boy (the high point is in bold type):

You know Danny Smith? He's in third grade, you know, and when he was doing jumping jacks in gym, you know, his pants split and in class you know his teacher said, "Danny Smith, what are you doing?" He said, "I'm trying to split my pants the rest of the way." It was only this much, and he had it this much in class. **On the bus he was going like this, you know, splitting it more, and he was showing everybody.** We told Danny he was stupid, and he said, "No, I'm not. You guys are the stupids." (Peterson & McCabe, 1983, p. 236)

Evaluation is another important feature of high-point analysis. Evaluation describes how the narrator feels about the events being depicted and can be expressed in a number of ways, including compulsion words (*have to, must*), affect terms (*scared, funny*), and negatives (events that did not happen: *He didn't hit me*) (Peterson &

McCabe, 1983, p. 223). Children use a greater variety of evaluations with age (Peterson & McCabe, 1983). A continued emphasis on evaluation also marks the development of narratives through adolescence. In comparing narratives from preadolescent, adolescent, and adult African Americans, Labov (1972) found that evaluations increased threefold from preadolescents to adults. Interestingly, a control group of white adolescents produced narratives with rates of evaluations similar to those of the younger African American preadolescents, highlighting how narrative forms vary across cultures, a topic to which we now turn.

Narratives Across Cultures

Structural analyses that employ high-point or story-grammar perspectives may implicitly suggest that there is a universal standard for narrative form. However, examination of the personal narratives of children and adults from diverse cultures suggests that each culture has its preferred ways of telling stories (McCabe, 1996; Smoczyńska, 1992) and that the preferred way of telling stories varies from culture to culture. For example, Hispanic children's narratives focus on personal and family relationships rather than on what happened (Rodino, Gimbert, Pérez, & McCabe, 1991). Japanese children connect temporally distinct events thematically, often using a structure that reflects haiku, a culturally valued literary form (Minami & McCabe, 1990).

There is currently much theoretical and empirical support for viewing narratives as important social, cognitive, and linguistic tools for understanding and defining one's culture and one's world (Bruner, 1986; Gee, 1992). Children typically adopt the narrative style of their own community. Thus, middle- and working-class white children in North America generally tell **topic-focused narratives,** stories about a single person or event that have clear beginnings, middles, and ends. These stories often conform to the structure of classic high-point narratives.

In contrast, children from other cultures, working-class African American girls, for example, often tell what are termed **topic-associating narratives** (Michaels, 1981, 1991). Topic-associating narratives link several episodes thematically, and the episodes may involve several principal characters and shifts in time and setting. These narratives are usually longer than topic-focused narratives. Sara Michaels (1981, 1991) has documented what can happen in school when children tell stories that do not follow the conventional topic-focused formula. A topic-associating first-grade African American girl was told by her teacher that she should talk "about things that are really really very important" and "to stick with one thing" (Michaels, 1991, pp. 316, 320). The way this girl usually made sense of her world through her personal narratives was explicitly discouraged, and she was urged to adopt a narrative style that conformed to the dominant (topic-focused) genre of the classroom.

Although there is nothing intrinsically wrong with teaching students to use different speaking genres, a teacher's implicit devaluation of the narrative style of a child's indigenous culture may have negative consequences (McCabe, 1996). In a follow-up interview one year later, the African American child angrily portrayed her first-grade teacher as uninterested in what she had to say. Because this experience occurred early in her educational experience, its influence on her attitude toward teachers, school, and literacy was potentially profound (Ogbu, 1990). Many researchers now see a need for educators to recognize these potential conflicts and to provide educational environments that can nurture cultural and linguistic diversity as well as academic achievement (Gee, 1992; Gutierrez, 1995; Michaels, 1991). The need to recognize the cultural diversity of narratives extends to counseling clinicians, who, regardless of their own ethnicity, are more likely to perceive signs of psychopathology in the personal narratives of healthy African American and Latino American children than in the personal narratives of healthy European American children (Pérez & Tager-Flusberg, 1998).

Other Forms of Decontextualized Language

The ability to narrate well and to use other forms of decontextualized language is also an important precursor to literacy (Snow, 1991). Written language is itself decontextualized, often making reference to phenomena that are not part of the immediate context. Thus, the development of decontextualized language skills has important educational implications.

In addition to narratives, other forms of decontextualized language include explanations and descriptions. Explanatory talk is an important part of classroom discourse and college lectures (Beals, 1993; Lehrer, 1994). Children's initial experiences with explanatory talk are likely to occur in the home, where parents may use explanations as a way of conveying knowledge about how the world works. In the following example, a father moves beyond the immediate context (the family dinner) to impart knowledge about the world, about how water flows in rivers and lakes (Perlmann, 1984).

> *Child:*   Who's that spoon?
> *Father:*   That is the gravy spoon. All the juice from the meat runs into that little hole, you spoon it out.
> *Child:*   Isn't that running in?
> *Father:*   Well, it was running in. See all these little holes in the tracks down here.
> *Child:*   Yes.
> *Father:*   When you cut the meat, the juice runs out of the meat into that little track there. Runs down till it gets to that hole. Blu-up! Fills it right up. [Pause]. That's the way rivers and lakes work.

Evidence that decontextualized talk like this supports literacy comes from a study that found that the *length* of family mealtimes positively predicted children's literacy scores. This association, in turn, was felt to reflect children's exposure to decontextualized language (Anderson et al., 1988).

Teachers are often very explicit in their encouragement of decontextualized language. In first-grade classrooms, teachers have been noted to elicit explanations about objects (e.g., candles, board games) children had brought to sharing time by saying, "Pretend we don't know a thing about candles," or, "TELL us how to play. Pretend we're all blind and can't see the game" (Michaels, 1981, 1991). These remarks make sharing time more like the *referential communication paradigm,* in which a speaker is asked to communicate about an object that is not in view of the listener (Ricard, 1993). In this situation, effective communication requires the speaker to be clear and unambiguous about anaphoric reference (e.g., terms like *she, they*) and to avoid using inappropriate deictic terms (e.g., *this, that*). It also requires that listeners share responsibility for understanding by asking for clarification when reference is ambiguous. Children's performance in referential communication tasks develops incrementally over the school years (Lloyd, Mann, & Peers, 1998; Ricard, 1993).

Metalinguistic Development in the School Years

Throughout the school years children continue to acquire new words at a rapid rate (Anglin, 1993), as noted earlier. They learn to master ever more complex syntactic structures (Chomsky, 1969; Karmiloff-Smith, 1986), and, as we have just seen, they learn to use a variety of genres of decontextualized language. However, rapid unfolding of **metalinguistic awareness** is an especially notable characteristic of language development during the school years. As we saw in Chapter 4, metalinguistic awareness is knowledge about language itself.

For the young child, language is a transparent medium. In using language, children need have no conscious awareness of its complex rule-governed nature. In time, however, some aspects of the system become opaque (Cazden, 1976), perhaps as a result of the child's active exploration of the system through language play (Kuczaj, 1982). In addition, ongoing cognitive development influences children's understanding of the linguistic system (Karmiloff-Smith, 1987), as does exposure to literacy (Donaldson, 1978; Gibb & Randall, 1988).

At the most basic level, a precursor of metalinguistic awareness is seen in children's corrections of their own speech (Clark, 1978). However, the awareness that underlies self-correction does not necessarily include a conscious understanding of the language system itself; self-correction shows only that the child recognizes ideal models or rules and notes implicitly a discrepancy between her linguistic behavior and the model or rule. True metalinguistic awareness requires that knowledge of the language system be explicit. For example, Bialystok (1991) has shown that a sample of non-reading preschool children who knew the letters of the alphabet and who knew the sounds associated with them had no explicit knowledge that the letters *represented* the sounds, and thus did not have true metalinguistic awareness.

Metasemantic and Metasyntactic Awareness

What is a word? One aspect of metasemantic awareness that has been studied is children's development of word awareness. Bowey and Tunmer (1984) identify three components to word awareness:

1. Comprehension of the term *word*
2. An appreciation that words are units of the language system
3. Understanding that the relationships between the phonological constituents of words and their referents are arbitrary

Awareness of each of these components unfolds over the school years at varying rates. Thus, children between the ages of five and seven readily recognize content words such as *dog* or *breakfast* as words, but fail to include function words like *the* and *was* in their conception of words (Papandropoulou & Sinclair, 1974). By age ten, children have acquired a clear understanding of the use of the term *word:* "A word is something that means something, it's written with letters" (Papandropoulou & Sinclair, 1974, p. 247).

The understanding that words are units of the language system evolves over time (Bowey & Tunmer, 1984). By age seven, most children can segment words correctly, suggesting that they are able to distinguish words from smaller units (e.g., phonemes) as well as from larger units (e.g., noun phrases). Finally, children's understanding of the arbitrary nature of the relationship between the phonological form of words and their referents develops incrementally. Young children asked to produce a long word might say *train,* because trains are long objects; the distinction between word and referent is blurred. By contrast, older children clearly understand the difference between form and referent.

Another important metasemantic skill is the ability to define words. Defining words is a regular part of classroom discourse, with teachers frequently asking children what a word or term means. In addition, teachers often press children to produce formal definitions, which requires the use of the copula and a superordinate relative clause (e.g., "a bird is a kind of animal that likes to fly") (Dickinson & Snow, 1987; Snow, Cancini, Gonzales, & Shriberg, 1989). Younger children often give associative (e.g., "a clock tick tock tick tock) or functional definitions (e.g., "a knife is for cutting things"). Older children are more proficient at generating formal definitions, a proficiency that increases throughout middle childhood (Dickinson & Snow, 1987; Johnson & Anglin, 1995; Snow, 1990) and reaches near adult levels in some populations by the fourth grade (Kurland & Snow, 1997). Skill in producing formal definitions is also positively correlated with overall language ability and with reading (Snow et al., 1989).

Metasyntactic awareness is sometimes assumed to underlie children's ability to correct syntactic errors. Five-year-old children can correct ungrammatical sentences, but often their corrections reflect their propensity to correct the deviant *semantic meaning* created by the syntactic errors. When young children are asked to correct the syntax, but not the semantic meaning, of sentences that are both syntactically *and* semantically deviant (e.g., *The baby eated the typewriter*), their rates of failure are relatively high (Bialystok, 1986).

Metasyntactic awareness also includes an understanding of syntactic structure. Ferreira and Morrison (1994) studied children's developing knowledge of sentence structure. They found that even before formal schooling, five-year-olds can identify the subject of a sentence like *The mailman delivered a shiny package* about 80 percent of the time. In general, schooling may be the single most important source of explicit knowledge about syntax, since talk about terms like *subject* and *verb* is extremely rare outside of educational settings. In reviewing the evidence on metasyntactic development, including a classic cross-cultural study by Scribner and Cole (1981), Gombert (1992) argues that explicit syntactic awareness comes only through formal education in literacy skills.

Metapragmatic Awareness

Metapragmatic awareness includes an awareness of the relationship between language and the social context in which it is being used (Hickmann, 1985; Pratt & Nesdale, 1984). Common examples of metapragmatic awareness include the ability to judge referential adequacy, the ability to determine comprehensibility, and the ability to describe *explicitly* the social rules (e.g., politeness rules) governing language use.

In judging referentially inadequate messages, children five and under often blame the listener *who should have listened better,* not the speaker, for communicative failure. After age eight, children are able to identify the speaker as the source of the problem (Robinson, 1981). Similar age trends were found in a study by Hughes and Grieve (1980) in which children were asked bizarre questions like "Is red heavier than yellow?" or "Is milk bigger than water?" Beyond metaphorical interpretations, these questions require clarification of the speaker's intended meaning. Yet very few five-year-old children asked for clarification. Instead, they attempted to answer the question in a straightforward manner. By contrast, most seven-year-olds gave responses that reflected their uncertainty about the speaker's intended meaning (e.g., "Milk is heavier, isn't it?").

Metapragmatic awareness requires more than knowing how to use language in culturally appropriate ways. Children must be able to articulate the rules explicitly. In spite of the observation that younger children frequently fail to follow the social norms of language use by, for example, being verbally polite (Bates, 1976; Berko Gleason, 1973), there are some anecdotal accounts of young children's awareness of these same rules. In one such example, a kindergarten girl chastises her classmate for nagging (Ely & Berko Gleason, 1995, p. 267):

Mark: Can I pick up the turtle, John?
Teacher: Not right now.
Mark: Please, John.

Allison: No nagging. When, when he [Mark] keep telling him [the teacher] and telling him, that's nagging.

By late childhood and early adolescence, most children have a fairly solid understanding of the rules governing language use in everyday social contexts (Berko Gleason, Hay, & Cain, 1988). In fact, one feature of the adolescent register is the occasional conscious and explicit violation of pragmatic rules. Thus, the failure to exchange conventional greetings or to offer verbal thanks, particularly in settings with parents, may be more a way that adolescents linguistically mark their autonomy and independence than a sign of developmental delay.

Thus far we have described how children's interactions with their peers and the media influence language development. We have described several forms of decontextualized language and have seen how children acquire some knowledge of the language system itself. Many of these developments are relatively independent of school attendance. At this point, however, we narrow our focus in order to describe what happens to many children living in literate societies, particularly English-speaking children in North America, as they learn to read and write.

Literacy Experiences at Home

Children growing up in literate societies are exposed in varying degrees to literacy in their homes and in their communities, and this exposure can be an important introduction to formal literacy instruction. Children's earliest awareness of the function and form of literacy has been termed **emergent literacy** (Teale & Sulzby, 1986). Young children are able to recognize **environmental print** on road signs (e.g., STOP) and in familiar commercial logos (e.g., Coca-Cola and McDonald's). They also acquire some of the conventions of print, including, for example, that in written English reading proceeds from left to right, and from top to bottom, and that printed words are separated from one another by spaces.

While children are learning about the forms of literacy, they are also being exposed to some of the functions literacy serves. Although form is relatively standard across communities of English speakers (reading always proceeds from left to right), there is much greater variation in the functions of literacy. Thus, in some homes literacy may be valued and emphasized. Children growing up in homes like these may frequently encounter their parents and older siblings engaged in reading and writing for recreation or for work and may themselves be read to extensively. Children growing up in homes where literacy serves exclusively instrumental functions (e.g., reading bills and school notices; writing checks and grocery lists) may develop very different notions about its worth (Gee, 1992; Heath, 1983; Snow, Barnes, Chandler, Goodman, & Hemphill, 1991).

In addition, parents vary in the degree to which they actively encourage the development of emergent literacy. Jim Gee (1992) describes how many middle-class parents are the "*best* teachers of school based literacy" (emphasis in original) without the benefit of any formal training in educational practices.

> They [parents] engage their children in conversations and keep them on a single topic even when the children can hardly talk at all. They play alphabet games, recite nursery rhymes, read books aloud with great affect. They ask their children "What's that?" and "What's that say?" of pictures in a book they've seen a hundred times. They encourage children to pretend they can read when they can't; they let them manipulate magnetic letters on a refrigerator; and they get them to watch "Sesame Street" for hours on end. They send them to preschool and constantly relate what the children have seen or heard in books to the children's daily experience of the world. (Gee, 1992, p. 123; reference citations in original deleted)

This kind of focus on literacy communicates explicitly that competence in reading, writing, and decontextualized talk are socially and culturally valued activities. Children from these households are at a distinct advantage upon entering school, where there is much continuity between the focus on decontextualized talk at home and the dominant and valued decontextualized discourse of the classroom (Gee, 1992). Children who are not exposed to these types of preliteracy experiences are often at a severe disadvantage when they enter school (Baker, Serpell, & Sonnenschein, 1995; Heath, 1983; Michaels, 1991; Snow, Burns, & Griffin, 1998).

The degree to which home environments support literacy is of great interest, both from a theoretical and a practical perspective (Whitehurst, Arnold, Epstein, & Angell, 1994). For example, shared book reading between parents and children has long been held to be a very important introductory step to literacy (Adams, 1990; Goldfield & Snow, 1984). Shared book reading is not only an opportunity to gain knowledge about the conventions of print, it is also an opportunity for extended talk, often decontextualized talk, that is stimulated by the material being read. Different styles of interaction are associated with different longer term effects, with the best outcomes across a variety of measures being associated with an interactive, dyadic, or collaborative approach in which the child's verbal participation is encouraged (Haden, Reese, & Fivush, 1996; Sénéchal, 1997; Whitehurst et al., 1994). In addition, children's exposure to shared bookreading can be an important influence in the development of positive attitudes towards literacy (Baker, Scher, & Mackler, 1997).

Dramatic social class differences in exposure to shared book reading have been documented; working-class children typically experience only a fraction of the number of hours of shared book reading that middle-class children experience (Payne, Whitehurst, & Angell, 1994). Although the difference in the frequency of exposure to book reading may explain a portion of the observed social class differences in the acquisition of literacy skills (Wells, 1985), other factors, including socioeconomic factors, and the attitude and skills of preschoolers themselves, may also be important (Scarborough & Dobrich, 1994).

Children from economically disadvantaged homes are at greater risk for failing to acquire basic literacy skills (Chall, Jacobs, & Baldwin, 1990; Snow et al., 1998). Of course, many children from economically disadvantaged homes do learn to read and write well. Snow and her colleagues (1991) examined the relationship between the home environment and children's acquisition of literacy skills in a longitudinal study of ethnically diverse working-class families. They found that the quality of the parent–child relationship was predictive of the child's writing ability, with good relationships being positively associated with children's ability to write well. One of the most important findings was that reading comprehension appeared relatively unrelated to any of the home measures. Reading was more strongly associated with school factors such as practice with structured materials like workbooks. They note that literacy practices such as reading at home should be encouraged, and that for children, time with adults, as opposed to time with siblings and peers, is important.

Reading

Components of Reading

Reading is a complex process. It involves a number of components that in the skilled reader work together in a seamless fashion, so much so that written text appears to convey meaning almost automatically. Table 10.2 lists some of the major components that underlie skilled reading.

Letter Recognition

The first component involves detection of the features of the letters of the alphabet, leading to **letter recognition.** Texts come in a variety of different forms, from highly regular and readable print to highly variable and barely legible handwritten script. Even standard print takes a variety of forms, so that dramatically different typefaces or

---

Table 10.2   Components of Skilled Reading

- Detection of visual features of letters leading to letter recognition
- Knowledge of the grapheme-phoneme correspondence rules
- Word recognition
- Semantic knowledge
- Comprehension, interpretation

fonts produce different graphic patterns. In order to identify a letter correctly, the reader must be able to extract its defining features. For example, the letter *A* can appear in many forms (see Figure 10.1).

Grapheme–Phoneme Correspondence Rules

An understanding of the **alphabetic principle** and knowledge of **grapheme–phoneme correspondence rules** are critical components in reading a language like English. According to the alphabetic principle, letters of the alphabet represent the sounds of oral language. **Graphemes** are the actual graphic forms or elements of the writing system, the letters of the alphabet, for example. As noted in Chapter 3, phonemes are the basic sounds of a language. Thus grapheme–phoneme correspondence rules define the relationship between a letter, or combination of letters, and the sound they represent.

In a perfect alphabetic system, grapheme–phoneme correspondence rules would have three characteristics:

1. They would be simple; there would be a one-to-one correspondence between each symbol and each sound.

2. They would be transparent; the name of a grapheme and the sound it represents would be identical.

3. They would be completely regular; there would be no exceptions to the two features listed above.

Orthographic systems with nearly perfect one-to-one grapheme–phoneme relationships are termed **shallow orthographies.** Italian represents an example of a shallow orthography, and readers of Italian can use spelling as a reliable guide to pronunciation and pronunciation as a reliable guide to spelling (Perfetti, 1997). In contrast, English is considered a **deep orthography** in that the relationships between graphemes and phonemes are more variable. For example, the letter *i* sometime sounds like itself, as in the pronoun *I.* However, it can also represent many other sounds, including the /I/ of *bit,* the /iy/ of *radio,* and so on. Furthermore, graphemes

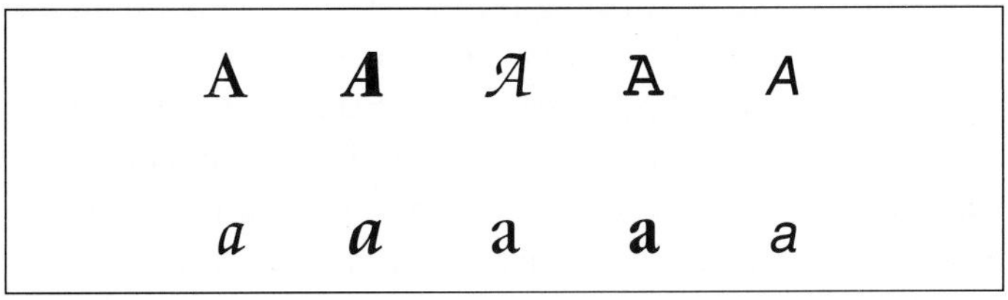

Figure 10.1

Letter detection requires recognizing many different graphic forms: Some forms of the letter **A.**

represent abstract forms, phonemes, whose actual phonetic form varies according to the other speech sounds (phonemes) with which it is combined.

To achieve fluency in reading English, the child must master these and other irregularities of the grapheme–phoneme correspondence rules (Bryne & Fielding-Barnsley, 1998). This task is particularly difficult because **segmentation** or breaking words into their constituent phonemes is not a straightforward or intrinsically intuitive skill. For example, a simple three-letter, one-syllable word like *cat* is composed of three distinct phonemes /k/, /æ/, and /t/. Although some children gain awareness of segmenting through informal instruction and exposure to texts like nursery rhymes (that often highlight segmenting through rhymes; Bryant, MacLean, & Bradley, 1990), many children require formal instruction before acquiring explicit knowledge of phonemic segmentation (Bryne & Fielding-Barnsley, 1995).

Word Recognition

The recognition of letter strings as representing conventional words in the orthography of the language defines the next component of reading, **word recognition.** Many laboratory studies of word recognition compare subjects' response time in recognizing different classes of words or letter combinations. True words (e.g., *king*) are words that follow the orthographic conventions of the language and are part of the language. Nonsense words are words that do not exist in the language (e.g., *gink*), although they are possible words because they follow conventional orthographic rules. False words are words that violate the orthographic rules (e.g., *nkgi*) and would be unlikely to be found in the language. In these *lexical decision tasks* true words are recognized more rapidly than nonsense words or false words.

Semantic Knowledge

Most of the time the word that is read is a word that is known to the reader. Its recognition stimulates a number of possible meanings based on the reader's **semantic knowledge.** Semantic knowledge refers to all the information about a word, its possible meanings, and its relations to other words and to real-world referents. (See the discussion of semantic networks in Chapter 4.) Incomplete semantic knowledge impedes comprehension of written text. As a young reader I encountered a story about a boy who lived in Washington and whose father worked in the *Cabinet.* My semantic knowledge of the word *cabinet* was limited to its meaning *cupboard.* How could a grown man fit in a cabinet, I wondered? What kind of work would he do inside a cabinet? I had a great deal of difficulty understanding an important aspect of the story, so much so that nearly forty years later I still remember how puzzled I was!

Comprehension and Interpretation

The final component of the reading process encompasses the ability to comprehend and interpret texts. Successful comprehension and interpretation depend on a number of developing skills and knowledge, including the automaticity of word recognition, vocabulary size, the capacity of working memory, and world knowledge. In order to accommodate children's developing abilities, books for young readers are age-graded, that is, designed specifically for children's evolving skill levels and knowledge bases (Baker & Freebody, 1989).

Reading Development in Children

Because reading is a complex skill, expertise in reading evolves slowly. In addition, purposes for reading change with age. Although there are a number of different models of reading development (Frith, 1985; Marsh & Desberg, 1983), we will focus on the model Jean Chall (1983, 1996) has formulated, a model that describes the stages through which children pass (see Table 10.3).

Chall's model begins with prereaders, young children in the preschool years (Stage 0) and ends with college-aged readers (Stage 5). As Table 10.3 shows, the prereader pretends to read, although she may have acquired some important concepts about the conventions of printed texts and may possess some elementary reading skills

Table 10.3 Some Features of Chall's (1983, 1996) Model of Reading Development

Stage	Age and Grade	Major Features	Method of Acquisition
0	6 months to 6 years Preschool, Kindergarten	"pretend" reading, names letters of alphabet, prints own name, recognizes some signs (e.g., Stop, Coca-cola)	exposure
1	6 to 7 years Grade 1, beginning Grade 2	learns grapheme–phoneme rules; sounds out one-syllable words; reads simple texts; reads about 600 words	direct instruction
2	7 to 8 years Grades 2 and 3	reads simple stories more fluently; consolidation of basic decoding skills, sight vocabulary and meaning; reads about 3,000 words	direct instruction
3	9 to 14 years Grades 4 to 9	reads to learn new knowledge, generally from a single perspective	reading and studying; classroom discussion; systematic study of words
4	15 to 17 years Grades 10 to 12	reads from a wide range of materials with a variety of viewpoints	reading and studying more broadly
5	18 and older	reads with self-defined purpose; reads to integrate self knowledge with knowledge of others; reading is rapid and efficient	reading even more widely; writing papers.

(Adapted from Chall, 1983, Table 5-1, pp. 85–87)

(e.g., recognizing her own name). In this stage, the child is primarily using top-down processes in making hypotheses about what reading is all about (Chall, 1983, 1996). According to **top-down models** of reading, reading is a psycholinguistic guessing game that consists of generating and testing hypotheses (Goodman, 1986; Goodman & Goodman, 1990; Smith, 1971). With the onset of formal instruction (Stage 1), bottom-up processes become important. **Bottom-up models** of reading hold that reading is largely dependent upon accurate perception of the letter strings that make up words (Gough, 1972). Stages 1 and 2 have been characterized as "learning to read." The emphasis is on mastering decoding skills, on recognizing and sounding out words. In order to facilitate this decoding process, many of the texts children read during these stages are relatively simple and contain little knowledge that is truly new.

In Chall's model, a major shift occurs between Stages 2 and 3, which normally occurs after the third grade. Where Stages 1 and 2 were characterized as "learning to read," Stages 3 through 5 have been characterized as "reading to learn." Here the focus is on extracting meaning from texts, and many of the materials children read contain new knowledge, including new words or phrases for a variety of never-before-encountered concepts. During Stages 3 through 5, reading is best characterized as interactive, with the child drawing on both bottom-up and top-down processes. At the highest level (Stage 5) the mechanics of decoding are highly **automatized** so that reading is rapid and efficient. More importantly, the goals of reading are more intellectually sophisticated than at previous stages. Now reading is a process through which readers seek to broaden their knowledge. Snow (1993a) has defined sophisticated college-level literacy as involving "the ability to read in ways adjusted to one's purpose (to enjoy light fiction, to memorize factual material, to analyze literature, to learn facts and discover ideas in texts, to judge the writer's point of view, and to incorporate information and perspectives from texts into one's own thinking but also to question and disagree with information and opinions expressed (p. 12))." Clearly, such high-level reading involves both the ability to accurately comprehend the literal meaning of text as well as the ability to reflect on the broader meaning of the text itself (Snow et al., 1998).

Approaches to Reading Instruction

Models of the stages through which skilled reading is attained have implications for reading instruction. How best to teach young children to read (and write) has been a source of controversy (Adams, 1990; Adams, Treiman, & Pressley, 1998; Chall, 1967/1983). The controversy reflects differences in theories of child development and learning, as well as the concern that some teaching methods may be associated with higher frequencies of reading failure (Flesch, 1985). Nevertheless, proponents of varying viewpoints share the same goal: They all want children to acquire a solid mastery of the basic skills of reading and writing.

There have been a number of approaches to the teaching of reading. The belief that reading is primarily a perceptual process involving vision has been largely discredited, although it was a dominant force in instruction for the early part of the century.

More recent approaches treat reading as a language-based activity (Wolf & Vellutino, 1993). Within this conceptualization, two different aspects of reading are stressed: reading for meaning and reading as decoding. According to proponents of **reading for meaning,** children should be encouraged to treat texts as sources of meaning. The function, rather than the form, of written language is stressed. Reading familiar texts (e.g., basal readers) and fostering the development of a large sight vocabulary are common features of the reading for meaning approach. Formal instruction often involves a look–say approach, in which whole words and sentences are presented to children, who are encouraged to say them aloud. Within the reading for meaning or whole word approach, when children encounter unfamiliar words, they are encouraged to use their knowledge of context (including pictures that accompany the text) to make a best guess. Thus, this approach presumes that children will use top-down processes extensively.

A currently popular variant of the reading for meaning approach is termed the **whole language** or **language experience** approach (K. S. Goodman, 1993; Y. Goodman, 1986). Presented more as a philosophy of learning than a specific instructional method, whole language models are based on a conceptualization of the child as an active learner who seeks to construct meaning from interactions with texts. According to this view, the texts that children encounter must contain complete ("whole") meaningful language. Attention to the mechanics of decoding is usually secondary to the goal of obtaining meaning from any given text.

In contrast to whole word and whole language approaches to reading instruction, **reading as decoding,** or phonics methods, emphasize bottom-up skills. These methods explicitly teach decoding, particularly grapheme–phoneme correspondence rules. Instruction focuses on acquiring fluency in naming the letters of the alphabet, segmenting and blending phonemes, and learning the grapheme–phoneme rules. Reading for comprehension and meaning are felt to be dependent on successful, rapid, and automatic decoding. Within a decoding approach, when children encounter unfamiliar words, they are encouraged to sound them out, letter by letter.

Which approach is best? This is, of course, the controversial question. Several influential analyses of the vast literature on the effects of different reading programs point to the importance of presenting most children with some formal instruction in phonics (Adams, 1990; Chall, 1983, 1996; Stahl & Miller, 1989; Snow et al., 1998). However, reading for meaning is also important. Stahl and Miller (1989) compared whole language approaches with decoding approaches. Their findings suggest that at different stages, different approaches may be beneficial. For example, reading for meaning or whole language approaches were more effective in kindergarten, where whole language classrooms appeared to replicate many of the emergent literacy practices found in middle-class homes. However, in the first grade, students in programs that emphasized decoding attained higher scores in a number of standard reading measures than students in whole language classrooms. Of particular interest was the finding that children who had had less prior literacy experience at home benefitted particularly from formal instruction in decoding skills. This finding has recently been replicated in a study of at-risk children in which explicit decoding instruction was compared to less explicit code instruction

(Foorman, Francis, Fletcher, Schat-Schneider, & Mehta, 1998). Children who had received direct code instruction were later able to read more quickly and to recognize more words than children who had experienced less explicit code instruction.

Thus, for certain children, relying on context may be problematic. This includes children who have difficulty learning to read and is illustrated by a clinical example described by Liberman and Liberman (1992). A third-grade boy who had not yet mastered the grapheme–phoneme correspondence rules, and thus could not decode unfamiliar words, encountered the following sentence: "A boy said, 'Run little girl.'" Table 10.4 lists the steps the boy employed to arrive at the incorrect reading: "A baby is running little go." In this case, the boy's lack of decoding skills impaired his ability to gain meaning from the text, and the hypotheses he generated led him astray.

When Learning to Read Is Difficult

Not all children learn to read easily. Causes of reading failure that are beyond the individual child include attending inadequate schools and living in poor neighborhoods (Snow et al., 1998). These factors reflect exposure to environments in which resources and expectations regarding literacy may be less than optimal. Other group risk factors include having limited competence in spoken English and speaking a dialect different from that used in school. These attributes place the child at risk because they often reflect a history of limited experience with the phonology of standard written English. Risk factors specific to individual children include cognitive deficits, language-specific problems, reduced preliteracy experiences, and a family history of reading problems (Snow et al., 1998). (See Chapter 9 for a discussion of atypical language development.)

One group of children who experience much difficulty in learning to read (and write) is of particular concern to educators, researchers, and parents. These children

Table 10.4 **When the Psycholinguistic Guessing Game Goes Astray: One Boy's Misreading of the Sentence: "A Boy Said: 'Run Little Girl.'"**

Words in Target Sentence	Strategies Employed by the Reader	Words "Read"
A	sight word known to reader	A
boy	unknown, uses beginning letter *b* to guess *baby*	baby
said, "Run	*said* unknown; reader jumps ahead to the next word (*run*), which he recognizes; uses the *s* in *said* and knowledge of syntax to generate *is running*	is running
little	sight word known to reader	little
girl."	unknown, uses beginning letter *g* to guess *go*	go

(From I. Y. Liberman, & A. M. Liberman. Whole language versus code emphasis: Underlying assumptions and their implications for reading. In P. Gough, L. Ehri, & R. Treiman (Eds.), *Reading Acquisition* (pp. 343–366). © 1992 Lawrence Erlbaum Associates. Reprinted with permission.)

are of average or above-average intelligence; they have no significant social-emotional or cognitive deficits; and they have received adequate instructional support. Despite these resources, they fail to achieve age-appropriate mastery of the fundamental aspects of written language and are often diagnosed as dyslexic (Shaywitz, 1996). **Dyslexia** and **developmental dyslexia** are terms used to describe reading failure in children (and adults) who are otherwise unimpaired.

Historically, dyslexia was thought to be caused by deficits in visual-perceptual processing, with spontaneous letter reversals being a classic example (e.g., treating a *b* as a *d* and a *w* as an *m*). Currently, however, visual-perceptual deficits are felt to play only a very minor role in dyslexia; the dominant view is that dyslexia is a language-specific disorder, characterized by marked deficits in linguistic processing (Morrison, 1993; Shankweiler, Crain, Katz, Fowler, et al., 1995; Stanovich, 1993; Vellutino, 1979). Although there is no consensus as to whether dyslexia is a single disorder, or a cluster of related disorders (dyslexias), it is clear that dyslexic children have significantly more problems in phonological processing than children of average reading abilities. For example, children with dyslexia perform poorly in segmenting words, in naming, and in phonological short-term memory tasks (Stanovich, 1993). The incidence of dyslexia is reported to be between 3 and 10 percent of the population, although rates vary according to the age of the population studied and the diagnostic criteria employed (Catts, 1996; Shaywitz, Escobar, Shaywitz, Fletcher, & Makuch, 1992; Shaywitz et al., 1990). Histories of reading difficulties are significantly higher than average in parents of dyslexic children (Scarborough, 1998), and there are data that suggest that dyslexia may be in part a genetic disorder (DeFries & Alarcon, 1996; Grigorenko, Wood, Meyer, Hart, Speed, Shuster, & Pauls, 1997).

Writing

In this chapter we have presented reading before writing, as is conventional. However, writing and reading are inextricably linked, and both influence and are influenced by the child's ongoing language development and metalinguistic knowledge (Adams et al., 1998; Perera, 1986). The traditional approach held that children could only learn writing through formal instruction. Writing should follow the elementary mastery of reading, because through reading children would acquire the grapheme–phoneme correspondence rules and would learn the conventions of print. Within this traditional approach, early instruction in writing often involved having children practice forming the letters of the alphabet and copying texts.

Garton and Pratt (1989) have questioned the logic of this approach. They believe that children, as active learners, acquire much information about writing even before they receive formal instruction in reading. They cite four benefits to encouraging prereading children to experiment with writing. First, children who spontaneously make writing marks on a page are actively involved in the writing process (versus passively copying letters and texts). Second, in making efforts to write what they themselves say, children begin to become aware of the relationship between written and spoken language. Third, children who, on their own, write single letters and letter strings to represent words are beginning to discover the alphabetic principle. Fourth, and finally, as children read back what they have written, however inaccurately, they are being exposed to the close relationship between writing and reading.

Development of Spelling

DOT MAK NOYS
Don't make noise.
B CYIYIT
Be quiet (Read, 1980)

In many instances, children write in order to communicate (Bissex, 1980). They want to say something *in writing* to themselves or to others. In children's earliest writing, there may be little relationship between the letter strings they write and what they intend "to say" (Bialystok, 1995). Eventually, they will be confronted with the task of mastering the conventions of standard spelling. The grapheme–phoneme correspondence rules that must be learned in order to read are the same rules that must be learned in order to spell conventionally. Children must come to recognize that the vowel sound /uw/ can take many different orthographic forms, as in the words *do, food, group, blue, knew, super,* and *fruit* (Treiman, 1993). In addition, *the letter names themselves* can be a source of confusion to beginning spellers (Treiman, Weatherston, & Berch, 1994) and children need to be able to distinguish letter names from letter sounds (McBride-Chang, 1999; Treiman, Tincoff, Rodriquez, Mouzaki, & Francis, 1998). The confusion between letter names and letter sounds explains why kindergarten children are more likely to spell the phoneme /w/ with a *y* because the name of y /wai/ begins with /w/.

Children often rely on creative or invented spelling (Read, 1986; Treiman, 1993) in their early writing. **Invented spelling** is systematic rule-governed spelling that is created (invented) by developing writers. In its early stages it is in large part phonetic, as the invented spellings children use are generally not modeled by adults or found in printed texts (Read, 1986). Children's early attempts at encoding language orthographically reveal that they are active learners who seek rational solutions to mapping the sounds of their oral language (Adams et al., 1998). For example, Read found that many young children deleted the nasals /m/, /n/, and /nj/, particularly when the nasal precedes a true consonant. As in the example above, *don't* is spelled DOT. Other examples of this strategy include spelling *monster* as MOSTR, and *New England* as NOOIGLID (Read, 1986). It appears as if children are analyzing the speech stream in a way that is qualitatively different from that of adults, often treating nasals as part of the preceding vowel instead of perceiving nasals as distinct phonemes (Treiman, Zukowski, & Richmond-Welty, 1995).

Table 10.5	Examples of One Child's Spelling Development According to Gentry and Gillet's (1993) Stage Theory of Spelling		
Stage	**Spelling**	**Translation**	**Age**
Precommunicative	EOIIVELIOE NEMLIEDN MDRMNE	(Story describing a picture of a flock of butterflies)	3 years, 3 months
Semiphonetic	HMT DPD	Humpty Dumpty	5 years, 11 months
Phonetic	I HEP UOU LEK TAS PACHERR EV DNL DEK AND DASY DEC.	I hope you like this picture of Donald Duck and Daisy Duck.	6 years, 3 months
Transitional	WONES A PON a time we BOTE a LITTEL kitten.	Once upon a time we bought a little kitten.	7 years
Conventional	When I went to the zoo, I saw lions.		7 years, 9 months

(Adapted from Gentry & Gillet, 1993, Table 3-1, p. 25. Reprinted with permission of J. Richard Gentry and Jean Wallace Gillet: *Teaching Kids to Spell* (Heinemann, A division of Reed Elsevier Inc., Portsmouth, NH, 1993))

Table 10.5 presents examples of Gentry and Gillet's (1993) stage theory of spelling. They see children as starting at a precommunicative level, moving through several phonetic stages, and finally arriving at a conventional stage. Underlying the pattern of development is a progression of strategies that children employ. They begin by using phonetics, then they look to regularities in orthographic patterns, and finally they utilize their knowledge of the origins of word roots.

Development of Writing and Genres of Writing

One form of writing that is common in the early school years is **expressive writing** (Britton, Burgess, Martin, McLeod, & Rosen, 1975). Expressive writing is informal personal writing, sometimes characterized as thinking out loud, and includes diary entries and letters to friends. Above all, expressive writing is characterized by the writer's close awareness of self and close relationship with the reader. Because it often fulfills a personal need, children need little prompting to engage in expressive writing.

A third-grader's final science project (see below) contains elements of expressive writing, seen particularly in his adoption of a first-person voice, although, as we will see, the general form of the essay is more expository than expressive:

Hi I Perry, the pituitary gland. I control other endocrine glands, growth, mother's milk production and I also control the amount of water the kidneys remove from the blood. I also tell other endocrine glands to produce their own hormones. You can come visit me at the base of the brain. Sometimes when I really get mad I give very little growth hormones. But doctors always give injections of growth hormones. I produce the hormone which controls growth. I tell the ovaries to produce a hormone called progesterone. I've heard a pituitary made a person over nine feet. Some pepole call me master gland. I'm reddish-gray. There's this relly cool feedback mechanism of mine. This makes sure that enough of each hormone circulates in the body. I also have three lobes. I forgot to tell you but I connect to the hypothalamus by a stalk. Oh and I'm the size of a pea. Bye.

Overall, the writing is generally coherent. The style is marked by a mixture of formal and informal prose, reflecting the influence of ongoing exposure to written genres of language, including science texts, as well as the child's longstanding experience with oral language. His essay also includes some fairly sophisticated technical terms (*feedback mechanism*) and rare vocabulary words (e.g., *injection* versus *shot*) that were copied down in the course of doing his research. Although *progesterone* is spelled correctly, there are several inventive spelling errors of relatively common words (e.g., *pepole, relly*). In addition, there are a number of errors of syntax, primarily omissions of function words. Nevertheless, the essay achieves what the author intended; it successfully conveys information about the pituitary gland to the reader, and does so in an engaging and, at times, humorous manner.

Despite the informal tone of the text, its overall form can be characterized as expository. **Expository writing** is organized hierarchically and is closely associated with Bruner's paradigmatic mode of thought, discussed earlier. Good expository writing requires organization, with key points and arguments presented clearly, concisely, and logically. Young children find expository writing especially difficult. Early attempts at expository often represent *knowledge telling,* in which children list ideas as they come to mind, with no clearly marked beginnings or endings, and little overall organization (Bereiter & Scardamalia, 1987). Over time, and with instruction, children may learn to revise their written work (Beal, 1990). The best writers plan what they are going to write while keeping the potential reader in mind. They are also able to put their plan into action and are able to successfully revise what they have written (Flowers & Hayes, 1980). Nevertheless, skill in expository writing develops slowly in most children and adolescents and reaches maturity only in adulthood, and then only in some writers (Applebee, Langer, Mullis, & Jenkins, 1990).

In contrast to the logical and hierarchical basis of expository writing, **narrative writing** is organized chronologically and uses a time line as its organizational basis. Written personal and fantasy narratives follow a chronological order. The developmental course of narrative writing is varied, in part because it is generally neglected in high school and in college, where most writing assignments require an expository style. Outside of creative writing courses, few older students have extensive experience in narrative writing.

Although much of children's writing takes place in school settings under the direction of teachers, writing is a social process. Writing is often shared with peers, and writing projects are sometimes set up to be collaborative (Daiute & Griffin, 1993). The social aspects of writing are not just restricted to school. As was noted in our discussion of the home-school study by Snow and her colleagues (1991), writing was associated with positive parent-child interactions. Children who have generally positive relationships with their parents may develop confidence that they have something to say in their writing. Thus, the origins of good writing may begin very early in a child's life.

Bilingualism

When my wife returned to the United States at age five, she spoke four languages. She had lived in Indonesia with her family and members of her extended household and spoke English, two dialects of Chinese, and Malay. She had even begun to master written Chinese, having attended kindergarten in a Chinese school. Her workbooks, now very faded, indicate that she showed great talent in her brush work. Today, she

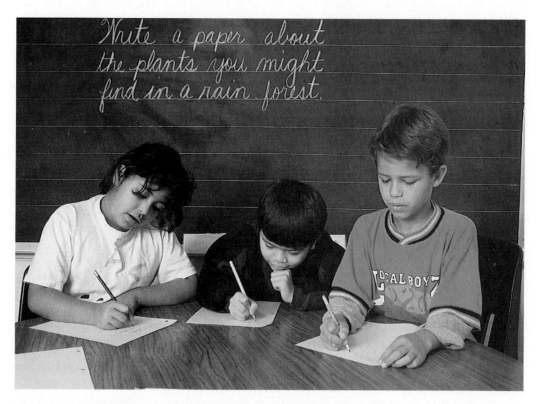

Expository writing is organized logically and hierarchically. Narrative writing follows a chronological time line.

has little knowledge of three of the four languages she spoke fluently when she was a child, and she has only a minimal command of French, a language she studied in high school and college thirty years ago. The changes she experienced in her ability to speak second languages are experienced by many multilingual children, and these changes are often accelerated by children's entry into school.

When a speaker gains a second language while retaining a first language, the process is called **additive bilingualism** (Bialystok & Hakuta, 1994). Often, the acquisition of the second language is seen as an asset, as enhancing the prestige and social and economic prowess of the speaker. Thus, a Cambodian teenager whose parents immigrated to the United States might rapidly acquire English in order to complete high school and attend college, while still remaining fluent in her native language. Her acquisition of English could occur in **submersion** settings in which she alone was surrounded by English speakers, or in **immersion** settings, in which she and other non-English speaking students received instruction in English only.

In contrast to additive bilingualism, **subtractive bilingualism** refers to the loss of fluency in one's native language that occurs when acquiring a second language. Subtractive bilingualism is also seen in children of immigrants. The language of their parents, the language of the old country, is gradually replaced by the dominant language of the new country, as the children interact and speak more and more with peers and other adults who are not speakers of their native language. In some settings, the language of the old country is even stigmatized; thus, a nine-year-old Russian immigrant might shy away from speaking Russian at home, preferring instead the language of his new schoolmates. Families who are concerned with their children's potential loss of fluency often send their children to special schools where they receive instruction in the language and culture of their parents.

Children who acquire a second language before puberty are likely to speak it with a native accent (Krashen, Long, & Scarcella, 1982). However, being younger is not necessarily an advantage in terms of the *rate* of acquisition, as older learners acquire a second language more rapidly than younger learners in untutored settings (Snow, 1983, 1987). Children growing up learning two or more languages simultaneously can do so without difficulty. Although they may show slight delays in vocabulary growth in each language because they are learning two or more lexicons, they often have more advanced metalinguistic knowledge than monolingual children. They learn at an early age about the arbitrary relation between words and their referents (Reynolds, 1990). For example, a bilingual Creole- and English-speaking Haitian child learns that the same food on her plate can be called *duri,* or it can be called *rice.*

Children who are acquiring English as a second language in a community where English is the dominant language often face the challenge of acquiring literacy in a language with which they are not fully proficient (August & Hakuta, 1997; Snow et al., 1998). As noted earlier, these children may be at risk for reading difficulties. Educators face the challenge of determining whether it is better to begin literacy instruction in the child's native language or to move directly toward promoting literacy in

English. There are some data (reviewed in Snow et al., 1998) that suggest that if children begin to master literacy in their native language, they are able to transfer literacy skills to English. This approach may be especially important for children whose proficiency in English is relatively limited.

For many monolingual English-speaking children in the United States, encounters with a second language occur exclusively in school settings. Although there is controversy as to when it is best to begin formal instruction, many high school and college students are required to complete several years of a "foreign language." Unfortunately, this is often viewed as drudgery, and many adolescents have little opportunity to use the languages they are studying outside the classroom (Snow, 1993b). Thus, most native English-speaking adolescents enter adulthood as functionally monolingual, whereas adults in the rest of the world are often bilingual or multilingual, at least to some extent.

Summary

During the school years, children's language development becomes increasingly individual. It is easier to describe the language of the typical two-year-old than it is to describe the language of the typical twelve-year-old. In this chapter, we have seen how language undergoes change and growth during the school years. For many children, these developments are positive. Ideally, they are built on extensive early experiences with oral language, including many conversations with parents and other adults, especially conversations in which decontextualized language was encouraged and supported.

Children following a positive trajectory learn to joke and tease comfortably with other children. When confronted with formal instruction in reading and writing, they may already have a basic grasp of many of the important concepts. They might already read, having inferred the alphabetic principle and the basic grapheme–phoneme correspondence rules from their many encounters with books read to them by parents. Throughout the middle school years, their ability to read and write improves rapidly. They read to learn, and through school assignments and extracurricular activities, they acquire strong foundations in the literate knowledge base of their culture. In high school, they have continued exposure to the media in order to be certain that their command of their peer group register (adolescent register) is current. They acquire a sense of gender stereotypes in language use, although they may choose not to abide by them. In addition, they are often exposed to formal foreign language instruction.

Not all children follow this pattern. Many do not have extensive emergent literacy experiences at home. Many are in poor schools where reading and writing instruction is inadequate, where literate materials like books are scarce, and where rates of reading failure are high. Even children who do learn to read and write well may have few opportunities to use their literacy skills in meaningful and satisfying ways. Many bilingual children feel pressured to suppress their native language in favor of the dominant language, and many monolingual children have trouble learning a second language.

Thus, in its extreme forms, language development in the school years can follow two opposite courses. One course represents arrested development and lost opportunities, with the progress of the early years overshadowed by stagnation, particularly in the failure to acquire a solid grasp of literate language. This developmental trajectory makes the transition to adulthood problematic. The other course represents a continuation of the dramatic developments the child experienced in the first five to six years of life. Building on these strong foundations, children following this route achieve even greater mastery of oral language and develop a strong command of written language as well. These developments in turn enhance the transition into adulthood.

Key Words

additive bilingualism
adolescent register
alphabetic principle
automaticity (automatized)
bottom-up model
decontextualized language
deep orthography
dyslexia (developmental dyslexia)
emergent literacy
environmental print
expository writing
expressive writing
grapheme
grapheme–phoneme correspondence
  rules
immersion
invented spelling
irony
letter recognition
metalinguistic awareness
narrative mode

narratives
narrative writing
observer effect
paradigmatic mode
reading as decoding
reading for meaning
riddles
sarcasm
segmentation
semantic knowledge
shallow orthography
submersion
subtractive bilingualism
top-down model
topic-associating narrative
topic-focused narrative
verbal aggression
verbal humor
whole language (language experience)
word recognition

Suggested Projects

1. Present children between the ages of five and nine with a sample of riddles. Ely and McCabe (1994), Fowles and Glanz (1977), and Pepicello and Weisberg (1983) are good sources. Use the coding scheme presented in Table 10.1 to assess

their metalinguistic development. Pay particular attention to the metalinguistic terms they use (e.g., *word, means, sounds like*).

2. Ask a group of adolescents to generate a list of slang words or expressions that are used by their age group. Then ask a thirty-year-old, a fifty-year-old, and a seventy-year-old (who ideally have had little recent contact with adolescents) if they know what the words or expressions mean. Ask your older informants to list words that were particular to their adolescence. What similarities and differences do you find?

3. Ask boys and girls of different ages how they might ask another unfamiliar child or an adult for directions—for instance, how to find a familiar landmark. See to what degree children use politeness markers (*excuse me, pardon me, thank you*) in their requests, and ask them why they did or did not include them. Ask them how they would judge the adequacy of the directions. See if you find any gender differences.

4. Peterson and McCabe (1983) developed a technique for eliciting narratives from children. When talking to their subjects, they included prompts about specific events. Example: "The other day I had to go to the doctor and get a shot. Has anything like that ever happened to you?" Using this approach, gather a small sample of narratives from children of different ages. Examine the narratives for developmental differences.

5. Find three young children between the ages of five and seven: one who does not read, one who is just learning to read, and one who reads relatively well. Using an interesting children's book, ask each child about the conventions of print (Where do you begin reading? What are the spaces between the words for? What are punctuation marks for?). Ask each child what it means to read and how you learn to read. How do the children's notions about reading compare with what we know about reading?

6. Find an interesting object (an egg beater, an animal skull) and ask children of different ages to "write anything you want" about the object for five minutes. Compare the children's performances, paying attention to their writing form. Look also for invented spelling in younger children's writing. What developmental trends do you notice?

Suggested Readings

Adams, M. J. (1990). *Beginning to read: Thinking and learning about print.* Cambridge, MA: MIT Press.

Adams, M. J., Treiman, R., & Pressley, M. (1998). Reading, writing, and literacy. In I. E. Sigel & K. A. Renninger (Eds.), *Handbook of child psychology, Vol. 4* (5th ed.; pp. 275–355). New York: Wiley.

Bamberg, M. (Ed.). (1997). *Narrative development: Six approaches.* Mahwah, NJ: Erlbaum.

Berman, R. A., & Slobin, D. I. (1994). *Relating events in narrative: A crosslinguistic developmental study.* Hillsdale, NJ: Lawrence Erlbaum.

Chall, J. S. (1996). *Stages of reading development* (2nd ed.). New York: McGraw-Hill.

Chall, J. S., Jacobs, V. A., & Baldwin, L. E. (1990). *The reading crisis: Why poor children fall behind.* Cambridge, MA: Harvard University Press.

Goodwin, M. H. (1990). *He-said-she-said: Talk as a social organization among Black children.* Bloomington, IN: Indiana University Press.

Hulme, C., & Joshi, R. M. (Eds). (1998). *Reading and spelling: Development and disorders.* Mahwah, NJ: Erlbaum.

McCabe, A. (1996). *Chameleon readers: Teaching children to appreciate all kinds of good stories.* New York: McGraw Hill.

Ninio, A., & Snow, C. E. (1996). *Pragmatic development.* Boulder, CO: Westview Press.

Perfetti, C. A., Rieben, L., & Fayol, M. (Eds). (1997). *Learning to spell: Research, theory, and practice across language.* Mahwah, NJ: Erlbaum.

Snow, C. E., Burns, M. S., & Griffin, P. (Eds.). (1998). *Preventing reading difficulties in young children.* Washington: National Academy Press.

Teale, W. H., & Sulzby, E. (Eds.). (1986). *Emergent literacy: Writing and reading.* Norwood, NJ: Ablex.

Wolf, M., & Vellutino, F. (1993). A psycholinguistic account of reading. In J. B. Gleason & N. B. Ratner (Eds.), *Psycholinguistics* (pp. 351–390). Fort Worth: Harcourt Brace Jovanovich.

References

Adams, M. J. (1990). *Beginning to read: Thinking and learning about print.* Cambridge, MA: MIT Press.

Adams, M. J., Treiman, R., & Pressley, M. (1998). Reading, writing, and literacy. In I. E. Sigel & K. A. Renninger (Eds.), *Handbook of child psychology, Vol. 4* (5th ed.; pp. 275–355). New York: Wiley.

Allred, R. A. (1990). Gender differences in spelling achievements in grades 1 through 6. *Journal of Educational Research, 83,* 187–193.

Anderson, R., Wilson, P., & Fielding, L. (1988). Growth in reading and how children spend their time outside of school. *Reading Research Quarterly, 23,* 285–303.

Anglin, J. M. (1993). Vocabulary development: A morphological analysis. *Monographs of the Society for Research in Child Development, 58* (10, Serial No. 238).

Applebee, A., Langer, J., Mullis, I., & Jenkins, L. (1990). *The writing report card, 1984–88. Findings from the nation's report card.* The National Assessment of Education Progress. Princeton, NJ: Educational Testing Service.

Apte, M. L. (1985). *Humor and laughter: An anthropological approach.* Ithaca, NY: Cornell University Press.

August, D., Hakuta, K. (Eds.). (1997). *Improving schooling for language-minority children: A research agenda. National Research Council and Institute of Medicine.* Washington, DC: National Academy Press.

Aukett, R., Ritchie, J., & Mill, K. (1988). Gender differences in friendship patterns. *Sex Roles, 19,* 57–66.

Baker, C. D., & Freebody, P. (1989). *Children's first school books: Introduction to the culture of literacy.* Cambridge, MA: Blackwell.

Baker, L., Scher, D., & Mackler, K. (1997). Home and family influences on motivations for reading. *Educational Psychologist, 32,* 69–82.

Baker, L., Serpell, R., & Sonnenschein, S. (1995). Opportunities for literacy learning in the homes of urban preschoolers. In L. M. Morrow (Ed.), *Family literacy: Connections in schools and communities* (pp. 236–252). Newark, DE: International Reading Association.

Bamberg, M. (Ed.). (1997). *Narrative development: Six approaches.* Mahwah, NJ: Erlbaum.

Barth, R. J., & Kinder, B. N. (1988). A theoretical analysis of sex differences in same-sex friendship. *Sex Roles, 19,* 349–363.

Bates, E. (1976). *Language and context: The acquisition of pragmatics.* New York: Academic Press.

Beal, C. R. (1990). The development of text evaluation and revision skills. *Child Development, 61,* 247–258.

Beals, D. E. (1993). Explanatory talk in low-income families' mealtime conversations. *Applied Psycholinguistics, 14,* 489–513.

Beaumont, S. L. (1995). Adolescent girls' conversations with mothers and friends: A matter of style. *Discourse Processes, 20,* 109–132.

Bereiter, C., & Scardamalia, M. (1987). *The psychology of written communication.* Hillsdale, NJ: Erlbaum.

Berko Gleason, J. (1973). Code switching in children's language. In T. E. Moore (Ed.), *Cognitive development and the acquisition of language* (pp. 159–167). New York: Academic Press.

Berko Gleason, J., Hay, D., & Cain, L. (1988). Social and affective determinants of language acquisition (pp. 171–186). In M. L. Rice & R. L. Schiefelbusch (Eds.), *The teachability of language.* Baltimore: Brookes.

Berman, R. A., & Slobin, D. I. (1994). *Relating events in narrative: A crosslinguistic developmental study.* Hillsdale, NJ: Erlbaum.

Bialystok, E. (1986). Factors in the growth of linguistic awareness. *Child Development, 57,* 498–510.

Bialystok, E. (1991). Letters, sounds, and symbols: Changes in children's understanding of written language. *Applied Psycholinguistics, 12,* 75–89.

Bialystok, E. (1995). Making concepts of print symbolic: Understanding how writing represents language. *First Language, 15,* 317–338.

Bialystok, E., & Hakuta, K. (1994). *In other words: The science and psychology of second-language acquisition.* New York: Basic Books.

Bissex, G. (1980). *GNYS AT WORK: A child learns to read and write.* Cambridge, MA: Harvard University Press.

Bowey, J. A., & Tunmer, W. E. (1984). Word awareness in children. In W. E. Tunmer, C. Pratt, & M. L. Herriman (Eds.), *Metalinguistic awareness in children: Theory, research, and implications* (pp. 73–91). New York: Springer-Verlag.

Britton, J., Burgess, T., Martin, N., McLeod, A, & Rosen, H. (1975). *The development of writing abilities* (pp. 11–18). London: Macmillan Education.

Bruner, J. S. (1983). *Child's talk: Learning to use language.* New York: W. W. Norton.

Bruner, J. (1986). *Actual minds, possible worlds.* Cambridge, MA: Harvard University Press.

Bryant, P. E., Bradley, L., Maclean, M. & Crossland, J. (1989). Nursery rhymes, phonological skills and reading. *Journal of Child Language, 16,* 407–428.

Bryant, P., Maclean, M., & Bradley, L. (1990). Rhyme, language, and children's reading. *Applied Psycholinguistics, 11,* 237–252.

Bryne, B., & Fielding-Barnsley, R. (1995). Evaluation of a program to teach phonemic awareness to young children. A 2- and 3-year follow up and a new preschool trial. *Journal of Educational Psychology, 87,* 488–503.

Bryne, B., & Fielding-Barnsley, R. (1998). Phonemic awareness and letter knowledge in the child's acquisitions of the alphabetic principle. *Journal of Educational Psychology, 81,* 313–321.

Capelli, C. A., Nakagawa, N., & Madden, C. M. (1990). How children understand sarcasm: The role of context and intonation. *Child Development, 61,* 1824–1841.

Carnine, D., Kameenui, E. J., & Coyle, G. (1984). Utilization of contextual information in determining the meaning of unfamiliar words. *Reading Research Quarterly, 19,* 188–204.

Catts, H. W. (1996). Defining dyslexia as a developmental language disorder: An expanded view. *Topics in Language Disorders, 16,* 14–29.

Cazden, C. B. (1976). Play with language and metalinguistic awareness: One dimension of language experience. In J. Bruner, J. Jolly & K. Sylva (Eds.), *Play: Its role in development and evolution* (pp. 603–608). New York: Basic Books.

Chall, J. S. (1967/1983). *Learning to read: The great debate.* New York: McGraw-Hill.

Chall, J. S. (1983). *Stages of reading development.* New York: McGraw-Hill.

Chall, J. S. (1996). *Stages of reading development* (2nd ed.). New York: McGraw-Hill.

Chall, J. S., Jacobs, V. A., & Baldwin, L. E. (1990). *The reading crisis: Why poor children fall behind.* Cambridge, MA: Harvard University Press.

Chomsky, C. (1969). *The acquisition of syntax in children from 5 to 10.* Cambridge, MA: MIT Press.

Clark, E. V. (1978). Awareness of language: Some evidence from what children say and do. In A. Sinclair, R. J. Jarvella, & W. J. Levelt (Eds), *The child's conception of language* (pp. 17–43). New York: Springer-Verlag.

Crais, E. R. (1990). World knowledge to word knowledge. *Topics in Language Disorders, 10* (3), 13–28.

Csikszentmihalyi, M., Rathunde, K., & Whalen, S. (1993). *Talented teenagers: The roots of success and failure.* New York: Cambridge University Press.

Daiute, C., & Griffin, T. M. (1993). The social construction of written narratives. In C. Daiute (Ed.), *The development of literacy through social interaction* (pp. 97–120). New Directions for Child Development, No. 61. San Francisco: Jossey-Bass.

Deese, J. (1984). *Thought into speech: The psychology of a language.* Englewood Cliffs, NJ: Prentice-Hall.

DeFries, J. C., & Alarcon, M. (1996). Genetics of specific reading disability. *Mental Retardation and Developmental Disabilities Research Reviews, 2,* 39–47.

de Klerk, V. (1992). How taboo are taboo words for girls? *Language in Society, 21,* 277–289.

Dews, S., Winner, E., Kaplan, J., Rosenblatt, E., Hunt, M., Lim, K., McGovern, A., Qualter, A., & Smarsh, B. (1996). Children's understanding of the meaning and functions of verbal irony. *Child Development, 67,* 3071–3085.

Dickinson, D. K., & Snow, C. E. (1987). Interrelationships among prereading and oral language skills in kindergarteners from two social classes. *Early Childhood Research Quarterly, 2,* 1–25.

Donaldson, M. (1978). *Children's minds.* New York: W. W. Norton.

Dowker, A. (1989). Rhyme and alliteration in poems elicited from young children. *Journal of Child Language, 16,* 181–202.

Dowker, A., & Pinto, G. (1993). Phonological devices in poems by English and Italian children. *Journal of Child Language, 20,* 697–706.

Dunn, J. (1988). *The beginnings of social understanding.* Cambridge, MA: Harvard University Press.

Ely, R., & Berko Gleason, J. (1995). Socialization across contexts. In P. Fletcher & B. MacWhinney (Eds.), *Handbook of child language* (pp. 251–270). Oxford: Blackwell.

Ely, R., Berko Gleason, J., & McCabe, A. (1996). "Why didn't you talk to your Mommy, Honey?"— Gender differences in talk about past talk. *Research on Language and Social Interaction, 29,* 7–25.

Ely, R., Berko Gleason, J., & Perlmann, R. Y. (1992). *Ma, I need a Mommy: First person reference in young children's discourse.* Paper presented at the Seventeenth Annual Boston University Conference on Language Development, Boston University, Boston, MA.

Ely, R., & McCabe, A. (1993). Remembered voices. *Journal of Child Language, 20,* 671–696.

Ely, R., & McCabe, A. (1994). The language play of kindergarten children. *First Language, 14,* 19–35.

Engel, S. (1995). *The stories children tell: Making sense of the narratives of children.* New York: W. H. Freeman.

Ferreira, F., & Morrison, F. J. (1994). Children's metalinguistic knowledge of syntactic constituents: Effects of age and schooling. *Developmental Psychology, 30,* 663–678.

Fivush, R., & Hudson, J. (1990). *Knowing and remembering in young children.* New York: Cambridge University Press.

Flesch, R. (1985). *Why Johnny can't read* (2nd ed.). New York: Harper and Row.

Flowers, L. S., & Hayes, J. R. (1980). The dynamics of composing: Making plans and juggling constraints. In L. Gregg & E. Steinberg (Eds.), *Cognitive processes in writing* (pp. 31–50). Hillsdale, NJ: Erlbaum.

Foorman, B. R., Francis, D. J., Fletcher, J. M., Schatschneider, C. & Mehta, P. (1998). The role of instruction in learning to read: Preventing reading failure in at-risk children. *Journal of Educational Psychology, 90,* 37–55.

Fowles, B., & Glanz, M. E. (1977). Competence and talent in verbal riddle comprehension. *Journal of Child Language, 4,* 433–452.

Frith, U. (1985). Beneath the surface of dyslexia. In K. Patterson, J. Marshall, & M. Coltheart (Eds.), *Surface dyslexia* (pp. 301–330). London: Erlbaum.

Gallaway, C., & Richards, B. J. (Eds.). (1994). *Input and interaction in language acquisition.* New York: Cambridge University Press.

Garton, A., & Pratt, C. (1989). *Learning to be literate: The development of spoken and written language.* New York: Basil Blackwell.

Garvey, C. (1977). Play with language and speech. In S. Ervin C. & Mitchell-Kernan & (Eds.), *Child discourse* (pp. 27–47). New York: Academic Press.

Gee, J. P. (1986). Units in the production of narrative discourse. *Discourse Processes, 9,* 391–422.

Gee, J. P. (1992). *The social mind: Language, ideology and social practice.* New York: Bergin & Garvey.

Gentry, J. R., & Gillet, J. W. (1993). *Teaching kids to spell.* Portsmouth, NH: Heinemann.

Gibb, C., & Randall, P. F. (1988). Metalinguistic abilities and learning to read. *Educational Research, 30,* 135–141.

Gilligan, C. (1982). *In a different voice: Psychological theory and women's development.* Cambridge, MA: Harvard University Press.

Goldfield, B. A., & Snow, C. E. (1984). Reading books with children: The mechanics of parental influences on children's reading achievement. In J. Flood (Ed.), *Understanding reading comprehension* (pp. 204–215). Newark, DE: International Reading Association.

Gombert, J. E. (1992). *Metalinguistic development.* Chicago: University of Chicago Press.

Goodman, K. S. (1986). *What's whole in whole language?* Portsmouth, NH: Heinemann.

Goodman, K. S. (1993). *Phonic phacts.* Portsmouth, NH: Heinemann.

Goodman, Y. (1986). Children coming to know literacy. In W. H. Teale & E. Sulzby (Eds.), *Emergent literacy: Writing and reading* (pp 1–14). Norwood, NJ: Ablex.

Goodman, Y. E., & Goodman, K. S. (1990). Vygotsky and the whole-language perspective. In L. C. Moll (Ed.), *Vygotsky and education: Instructional implications and applications of sociohistorical psychology.* New York: Cambridge University Press.

Goodwin, M. H. (1990). *He-said-she-said: Talk as a social organization among Black children.* Bloomington, IN: Indiana University Press.

Gough, P. B. (1972). One second of reading. In J. F. Kavanagh & I. G. Mattingly (Eds.), *Language by eye and ear* (pp. 331–358). Cambridge, MA: MIT Press.

Grigorenko, E. L., Wood, F. B., Meyer, M. S. Hart, L. A. Speed, W. C. Shuster, B. S., & Pauls, D. L. (1997). Susceptibility loci for distinct components of developmental dyslexia on chromosomes 6 and 16. *American Journal of Human Genetics, 60,* 27–39.

Gutierrez, K. D. (1995). Unpackaging academic discourse. *Discourse Processes, 19,* 21–37.

Haden, C. A., Reese, E., & Fivush, R. (1996). Mothers' extratextual comments during storybook reading: Stylistic differences over time and across texts. *Discourse Processes, 21,* 135–169.

Harris, J. R. (1998). *The nurture assumption: Why children turn out the way they do.* New York: Free Press.

Heath, S. B. (1983). *Ways with words.* New York: Cambridge University Press.

Hedges, L. V., & Nowell, A. (1995). Sex differences in mental test scores, variability, and numbers of high-scoring individuals. *Science, 269,* 41–45

Hickmann, M. (1985). Metapragmatics in child language. In E. Mertz & R. J. Parmentier (Eds.), *Semiotic mediation: Sociocultural and psychological perspectives* (pp. 177–201). New York: Academic Press.

Hirsh-Pasek, K., Gleitman, L. R., & Gleitman, H. (1978). What did the brain say to the mind? A study of the detection and report of ambiguity by young children. In R. J. Jarvella & W. J. M. Levelt (Eds.), *The child's concept of language* (pp. 97–132). New York: Springer-Verlag.

Hogrebe, M. C., Nest, S. L., & Newman, I. (1985). Are there gender differences in reading achievement? An investigation using the high school and beyond data. *Journal of Educational Psychology, 77,* 716–724.

Horgan, D. (1981). Learning to tell jokes. *Journal of Child Language, 8,* 217–224.

Hughes, M., & Grieve, R. (1980). On asking children bizarre questions. *First Language, 1,* 149–160.

Hulme, C., & Joshi, R. M. (Eds). (1998). *Reading and spelling: Development and disorders.* Mahwah, NJ: Erlbaum.

Huston, A. C., Wright, J. C., Marquis, J., & Green, S. B. (1999). How young children spend their time: Television and other activities. *Developmental Psychology, 35,* 919–925.

Hyde, J. S., & Linn, M. C. (1988). Gender differences in verbal ability: A meta-analysis. *Psychological Bulletin, 104,* 53–69.

Hymes, D. (1981). *"In vain I tried to tell you.": Essays in Native American ethnopoetics.* Philadelphia: University of Pennsylvania Press.

Jay, T. (1992). *Cursing in America.* Philadelphia: J. Benjamins.

Johnson, C. J., & Anglin, J. M. (1995). Qualitative developments in the content and form of children's definitions. *Journal of Speech and Hearing Research, 38,* 612–629.

Just, M. A., & Carpenter, P. A. (1987). *The psychology of reading and language comprehension.* Boston: Allyn & Bacon.

Karmiloff-Smith, A. (1986). Some fundamental aspects of language development after age 5. In P. Fletcher & M. Garman (Eds.), *Language acquisition: Studies in first language development* (pp. 455–474). Cambridge: Cambridge University Press.

Karmiloff-Smith, A. (1987). Function and process in comparing language and cognition. In M. Hickmann (Ed.), *Social and functional approaches to language and thought* (pp. 185–202). New York: Academic Press.

Kemper, S., Rice, K., & Chen, Y-J. (1995). Complexity metrics and growth curves for measuring grammatical development from five to ten. *First Language, 15,* 151–166.

Kirshenblatt-Gimblett, B., & Sherzer, J. (1976). Introduction. In B. Kirshenblatt-Gimblett (Ed.), *Speech play: research and resources for the study of linguistic creativity* (pp. 1–16). Philadelphia: University of Pennsylvania Press.

Krashen, S., Long, M., & Scarcella, R. (1982). Age, rate, and eventual attainment in second language acquisition. In S. Krashen, R. Scarcella, & M. Long (Eds.), *Child-adult differences in second language acquisition.* Rowley, MA: Newbury House.

Kuczaj, S. A. (1982). Language play and language acquisition. In H. Reese (Ed.), *Advances in child development and behavior* (pp. 197–232). New York: Academic Press.

Kurland, B. F., & Snow, C. E. (1997). Longitudinal measurement of growth in definitional skill. *Journal of Child Language, 24,* 603–625.

Labov, W. (1972). *Language in the inner city: Studies in the black English vernacular.* Philadelphia: University of Pennsylvania Press.

Landauer, T. K., & Dumais, S. T. (1997). A solution to Plato's problem: The latent semantic analysis theory of acquisition, induction, and representation of knowledge. *Psychological Review, 104,* 211–240.

Leadholm, B. J., & Miller, J. F. (1992). *Language sample analysis: The Wisconsin guide.* Madison, WI: Wisconsin Department of Public Instruction.

Lehrer, A. (1994). Understanding classroom lectures. *Discourse Processes, 17,* 259–281.

Liberman, I. Y., & Liberman, A. M. (1992). Whole language versus code emphasis: Underlying assumptions and their implications for reading. In P. Gough, L. Ehri, & R. Treiman (Eds.), *Reading acquisition* (pp. 343–366). Hillsdale, NJ: Erlbaum.

Lloyd, P., Mann, S., & Peers, I. (1998). The growth of speaker and listener skills from five to eleven years. *First Language, 18,* 81–103.

Maccoby, E. E. (1998). *The two sexes: Growing up apart, coming together.* Cambridge, MA: Harvard University Press.

Maltz, D. N., & Borker, R. A. (1982). A cultural approach to male-female miscommunications. In J. A. Gumperz (Ed.), *Language, interaction, and social identity* (pp. 196–216). New York: Cambridge University Press.

Mandler, J., & Johnson, N. (1977). Remembrance of things parsed: Story structure and recall. *Cognitive Psychology, 9,* 111–151.

Marsh, G., & Desberg, P. (1983). The development of strategies in the acquisition of symbolic skills. In D. A. Rogers & J. A. Sloboda (Eds.), *The acquisition of symbolic skills.* New York: Plenum.

Martin, R. (1997). "Girls don't talk about garages!": Perceptions of conversation in same- and cross-sex friendships. *Personal Relationships, 4,* 115–130.

Martlew, M., Connolly, K. J., & McCleod, C. (1978). Language use, role and context in a five-year-old. *Journal of Child Language, 5,* 81–99.

Mattingly, I. C. (1966). Speaker variation and vocal-tract size. *Journal of the Acoustical Society of America, 39,* 1219.

McBride-Chang, C. (1999). The ABCs of the ABCs: The development of letter-name and letter-sound knowledge. *Merrill-Palmer Quarterly, 45,* 285–308.

McCabe, A. (1996). *Chameleon readers: Teaching children to appreciate all kinds of good stories.* New York: McGraw Hill.

McCabe, A., & Lipscomb, T. J. (1988). Sex differences in children's verbal aggression. *Merrill-Palmer Quarterly, 34,* 389–401.

McCabe, A., & Peterson, C. (Eds.). (1991). *Developing narrative structure.* Hillsdale, NJ: Erlbaum.

McDowell, J. H. (1979). *Children's riddling.* Bloomington, Indiana: Indiana University Press.

Michaels, S. (1981). "Sharing time": Children's narrative styles and differential access to literacy. *Language in Society, 10,* 423–442.

Michaels, S. (1991). The dismantling of narrative. In A. McCabe & C. Peterson (Eds.), *Developing narrative structure* (pp. 303–351). Hillsdale, NJ: Lawrence Erlbaum.

Minami, M., & McCabe, A. (1990). Haiku as a discourse regulation device: A stanza analysis of Japanese children's personal narratives. *Language in Society, 20,* 577–599.

Morrison, F. J. (1993). Phonological processes in reading acquisition: Toward a unified conceptualization. *Developmental Review, 13,* 279–285.

Nagy, W. E., & Herman, P. A. (1987). Breadth and depth of vocabulary knowledge: Implications for acquisition and instruction. In M. McKeown & M. Curtis (Eds.), *The nature of vocabulary acquisition* (pp. 19–35). Hillsdale, NJ: Erlbaum.

Nagy, W. E., Herman, P. A., & Anderson, R. C. (1985). Learning words from context. *Reading Research Quarterly, 22,* 233–253.

Ninio, A., & Snow, C. E. (1996). *Pragmatic development.* Boulder, CO: Westview Press.

Nippold, M. A. (1993). Developmental markers in adolescent language: Syntax, semantics, and pragmatics. *Language, Speech, and Hearing Services in Schools, 24* (1), 21–28.

Nippold, M. A. (1998). *Later language development: The school-age and adolescent years.* Austin, TX: Pro-Ed.

Ogbu, J. V. (1990). Cultural model, identity, and literacy. In J. W. Stigler, R. A. Shweder, & G. Herdt (Eds.), *Cultural psychology: Essays on comparative human development* (pp. 520–541). New York: Cambridge University Press.

Ortony, A., Turner, T. J., & Larson-Shapiro, N. (1985). Cultural and instructional influences on figurative language comprehension by inner city children. *Research in the Teaching of English, 19,* 25–36.

Papandropoulou, I. & Sinclair, H. (1974). "What is a word?" Experimental study of children's ideas on grammar. *Human Development, 17,* 241–258.

Parker, J. G., & Gottman, J. M. (1989). Social and emotional development in a relational context: Friendship interaction from early childhood to adolescence. In T. J. Berndt & G. W. Ladd (Eds.), *Peer relationships in child development.* New York: Wiley.

Payne, A. C., Whitehurst, G. J., & Angell, A. L. (1994). The role of home literacy environment in the development of language ability in preschool children from low-income families. *Early Childhood Research Quarterly, 9,* 427–440.

Pepicello, W. J., & Weisberg, R. W. (1983). Linguistics and humor. In P. E. McGhee & J. H. Goldstein (Eds)., *Handbook of humor research.* New York: Springer-Verlag.

Perera, K. (1986). Language acquisition and writing. In P. Fletcher & M. Garman (Eds.), *Language acquisition: Studies in first language acquisition* (2nd ed.; pp. 494–519). Cambridge: Cambridge University Press.

Pérez, C., & Tager-Flusberg, H. (1998). Clinicians' perceptions of children's oral personal narratives. *Narrative Inquiry, 8,* 181–201.

Perfetti, C. A. (1997). The psycholinguistics of spelling and reading. In C. A. Perfetti, L. Rieben, & M. Fayol, *Learning to spell: Research, theory, and practice across languages* (pp. 21–38). Mahwah, NJ: Erlbaum.

Perlmann, R. Y. (1984). *Variations in socialization styles: Family talk at the dinner table.* Unpublished doctoral dissertation, Boston University.

Perlmann, R. Y., & Berko Gleason, J. (1994). The neglected role of fathers in children's communicative development. *Seminars in Speech and Language, 14,* 314–324.

Peterson, C., & McCabe, A. (1983). *Developmental psycholinguistics: Three ways of looking at a child's narrative.* New York: Plenum.

Pratt, C., & Nesdale, A. R. (1984). Pragmatic awareness in children. In W. E. Tunmer, C. Pratt, & M. L. Herriman (Eds.), *Metalinguistic awareness in children: Theory, research, and implications* (pp. 105–125). New York: Springer-Verlag.

Preece, A. (1992). Collaborators and critics: The nature and effects of peer interaction on children's conversational narratives. *Journal of Narrative and Life History, 2,* 277–292.

Read, C. (1980). Creative spelling by young children. In T. Shopen & J. M. Williams (Eds.), *Standards and dialects in English.* Cambridge, MA: Winthrop Publishers.

Read, C. (1986). *Children's creative spelling.* London: Routledge & Kegan Paul.

Reynolds, A. (1990). The cognitive consequences of bilingualism. In A. G. Reynolds (Ed.), *Bilingualism, multiculturalism, and second language learning: The McGill conference in honor of Wallace E. Lambert.* Hillsdale, NJ: Erlbaum.

Ricard, R. J. (1993). Conversational coordination: Collaboration for effective communication. *Applied Psycholinguistics, 14,* 387–412.

Rice, M. L. (1983). The role of television in language acquisition. *Developmental Review, 3,* 211–224.

Rice, M. L. (1992). "Don't talk to him; he's weird": The role of language in early social inter-actions. In A. Kaiser & D. Gray (Eds.), *Enhancing children's communication: The social use of language.* Baltimore: Brookes.

Rice, M. L., & Woodsmall, L. (1988). Lessons from television. Children's word learning when viewing. *Child Development, 59,* 420–429.

Richards, M., & Light, P. (Eds.). (1986). *Children of social worlds.* Cambridge: Harvard University Press.

Robbins, C., & Ehri, L. C. (1994). Reading storybooks to kindergartners helps them learn new vocabulary words. *Journal of Educational Psychology, 86,* 54–64.

Robinson, E. J. (1981). The child's understanding of inadequate messages and communication failures: A problem of ignorance or egocentrism? In W. P. Dickson (Ed.), *Children's oral communication skills.* New York: Academic Press.

Rodino, A. M., Gimbert, C., Pérez, C., & McCabe, A. (1991). *Getting your point across: Contrastive sequencing in low-income African-American and Latino children's personal narratives.* Paper presented at the Sixteenth Annual Boston University Conference on Language Development, Boston.

Romaine, S. (1984). *The language of children and adolescents—the acquisition of communicative competence.* New York: Blackwell.

Sadker, M., & Sadker, D. (1994). *Failing at fairness: How America's schools cheat girls.* New York. Charles Scribner's Sons.

Scarborough, H. S. (1998). Early identification of children at risk for reading disabilities: Phonological awareness and some other promising predictors. In B. K. Shapiro, P. J. Accardo, & A. J. Capute (Eds.), *Specific reading disability: a view of the spectrum* (pp. 77–121). Timonium, MD: York Press.

Scarborough, H. S., & Dobrich, W. (1994). On the efficacy of reading to preschoolers. *Developmental Review, 14,* 245–302.

Scribner, S., & Cole, M. (1981). *The psychology of literacy.* Cambridge, MA: Harvard University Press.

Sénéchal, M. (1997). The differential effect of storybook reading on preschoolers' acquisition of expressive and receptive vocabulary. *Journal of Child Language, 24,* 123–138.

Shankweiler, D., Crain, S., Katz, L. Fowler, A. E., et al. (1995). Cognitive profiles of reading-disabled children: Comparison of language skills in phonology, morphology, and syntax. *Psychological Science, 6,* 149–156.

Shaywitz, S. E. (1996). Dyslexia. *Scientific American, 275* (5), 98–104.

Shaywitz, S. E., Escobar, M. D., Shaywitz, B. A., Fletcher, J. M., & Makuch, R. (1992). Evidence that dyslexia may represent the lower tail of a normal distribution of reading ability. *New England Journal of Medicine, 326,* 145–150.

Shaywitz, S. E., Shaywitz, B. A., Fletcher, J. M., & Escobar, M. D. (1990). Prevalence of reading disability in boys and girls. *Journal of the American Medical Association, 264,* 998–1002.

Singer, D. G., & Singer, J. L. (1990). *The house of make-believe: Play and the developing imagination.* Cambridge, MA: Harvard University Press.

Sluckin, A. (1981). *Growing up in the playground: The social development of children.* London: Routledge & Kegan Paul.

Smith, F. (1971). *Understanding reading: A psycholinguistic analysis of reading and learning to read.* New York: Holt, Rinehart and Winston.

Smoczyńska, M. (1992). Developing narrative skills: Learning to introduce referents in Polish. *Polish Psychological Bulletin, 23,* 103–120.

Snow, C. E. (1983). Age differences in second language acquisition; Research findings and folk psychology. In K. Bailey, M. Long, & S. Peck (Eds.), *Second language acquisition studies.* Rowley, MA: Newbury House.

Snow, C. E. (1987). Relevance of the notion of a critical period to language acquisition. In M. Bornstein (Ed.), *Sensitive periods in development: An interdisciplinary perspective.* Hillsdale, NJ: Erlbaum.

Snow, C. E. (1990). The development of definitional skill. *Journal of Child Language, 17,* 697–710.

Snow, C. E. (1991). The theoretical basis for relationships between language and literacy development. *Journal of Research in Childhood Education, 6,* 5–10.

Snow, C. E. (1993a). Families as social contexts for literacy development. In C. Daiute (Ed.), *The development of literacy through social interaction* (pp. 11–24). New Directions for Child Development, No. 61. San Francisco: Jossey-Bass.

Snow, C. E. (1993b). Bilingualism and second language acquisition. In J. Berko Gleason & N. B. Ratner (Eds.), *Psycholinguistics* (pp. 391–416). Fort Worth, TX: Harcourt Brace Jovanovich.

Snow, C. E., Barnes, W. S., Chandler, J., Goodman, I. F., & Hemphill, L. (1991). *Unfulfilled expectations: Home and school influences on literacy.* Cambridge, MA: Harvard University Press.

Snow, C. E., Burns, M. S., & Griffin, P. (Eds.). (1998). *Preventing reading difficulties in young children.* Washington: National Academy Press.

Snow, C. E., Cancini, H., Gonzalez, P., & Shriberg, E. (1989). Giving formal definitions: An oral language correlate of school literacy. In D. Bloome (Ed.), *Classrooms and literacy* (pp. 233–249). Norwood, NJ: Ablex.

Snow, C. E., & Dickinson, D. K. (1991). Skills that aren't basic in a new conception of literacy. In A. Purves & E. Jennings (Eds.), *Literate systems and individual lives. Perspectives on literacy and schooling.* Albany, NY: SUNY Press.

Stahl, S. A., & Miller, P. A. (1989). Whole language and language experience approaches for beginning readers: A quantitative synthesis. *Review of Educational Research, 59,* 87–116.

Stanovich, K. E. (1993). A model for studies of reading disability. *Developmental Review, 13,* 225–245.

Stein, N. L. (1988). The development of children's storytelling skill. In M. B. Franklin & S. Barten (Eds.), *Child language: A book of readings* (pp. 282–297). New York: Oxford University Press.

Stein, N. L., & Albro, E. R. (1997). Building complexity and coherence: Children's use of goal-structured knowledge in telling stories. In M. Bamberg (Ed.), *Narrative development: Six approaches* (pp. 5–44). Mahwah, NJ: Erlbaum.

Swann, J. (1992). *Girls, boys, and language.* Cambridge, MA: Blackwell.

Tanner, J. M. (1989). *Fetus into man: Physical growth from conception to maturity* . Cambridge, MA: Harvard University Press.

Teale, W. H., & Sulzby, E. (Eds.). (1986). *Emergent literacy: Writing and reading.* Norwood, NJ: Ablex.

Teasley, S. D. (1995). The role of talk in children's peer collaborations. *Developmental Psychology, 31,* 207–220.

Treiman, R. (1993). *Beginning to spell: A study of first grade children.* New York: Oxford University Press.

Treiman, R., Tincoff, R., Rodriguez, K., Mouzaki, A., & Francis, D. J. (1998). The foundations of literacy: Learning the sounds of letters. *Child Development, 69,* 1524–1540.

Treiman, R., Weatherston, S., & Berch, D. (1994). The role of letter names in children's learning of phoneme–grapheme relations. *Applied Psycholinguistics, 15,* 97–122.

Treiman, R., Zukowski, A., & Richmond-Welty, E. D. (1995). What happened to the "n" of sink? Children's spelling of final consonant clusters. *Cognition, 55,* 1–38.

Vellutino, F. R. (1979). *Dyslexia: Theory and research.* Cambridge, MA: MIT Press.

Vihman, M. M. (1996). *Phonological development: The origins of language in the child.* Oxford: Basil Blackwell.

Vygotsky, L. S. (1978). *Mind in society: The development of higher psychological processes.* Cambridge, MA: Harvard University Press.

Vygotsky, L. S. (1986). *Thought and language.* Cambridge, MA: Harvard University Press.

Wells, G. (1985). Preschool literacy-related activities and success in school. In D. R. Olson, N. Torrance, & A. Hilyard (Eds.), *Literacy, language, and learning* (pp. 229–255). New York: Cambridge University Press.

White, H. (1980). The value of narrativity in the representation of reality. In W. J. T. Mitchell (Ed.), *On narrative* (pp. 1–49). Chicago: University of Chicago Press.

Whitehurst, G. (1997, April). Continuities and discontinuities in the move from emergent literacy to reading. In *Developmental Psychologists Contribute to Early Childhood Education.* Symposium conducted at the Society for Research in Child Development, Washington, DC.

Whitehurst, G. J., Arnold, D. S., Epstein, J. N., & Angell, A. L. (1994). A picture book reading intervention in day care and home for children from low-income families. *Developmental Psychology, 30,* 679–689.

Whiting, B. B., & Edwards, C. P. (1988). *Children of different worlds: The formation of social behavior.* Cambridge, MA: Harvard University Press.

Williams, P. A., Haertel, E. H., Haertel, G. D., & Walberg, H. J. (1982). The impact of leisure-time television on school learning: A research synthesis. *American Educational Research Journal, 19,* 19–50.

Winner, E. (1988). *The point of words: Children's understanding of metaphor and irony.* Cambridge, MA: Harvard University Press.

Wolf, M., & Vellutino, F. (1993). A psycholinguistic account of reading. In J. Berko Gleason & N. B. Ratner (Eds.), *Psycholinguistics* (pp. 351–390). Fort Worth: Harcourt Brace Jovanovich.

Chapter 11

Developments in the Adult Years

Loraine K. Obler
City University of New York

Language in Adulthood

Many of us continue to learn languages and language-related skills in adulthood. There are many business concerns that teach language skills: foreign languages, typing and word processing, coherent writing, effective speaking, and most recently, effective listening. For *bilinguals* and *polyglots,* there are programs to teach simultaneous translation. And etiquette books teach "correct" forms to use in formal social situations. However, we do not usually treat all these postchildhood language skills under the rubric of language acquisition. In this chapter we challenge that view, appreciating that the language changes of adulthood are a part of the developmental continuum.

In some sense, the language development of early childhood and even late childhood must be different from that of adulthood, however, since there is probably a *core language* all children learn, whereas the special language registers and skills of adolescence and adulthood are relatively optional—only people who need them and find themselves exposed to them have a chance to acquire them. As Grimshaw and Holden (1976, p. 41) put it, "the bulk of postchildhood learning…appears to be in the enrichment of repertoires and the acquisition of appropriateness systems."

Although little is known about language development in middle age, somewhat more work has been done over the last several decades on the language of advanced age. This research has been almost entirely on the language deficits that develop with aging. It is possible, for example, to demonstrate that elderly people as a group have more trouble on *naming tasks* after age seventy (Goodglass, 1980), perform worse on vocabulary definition subtests of the Wechsler Adult Intelligence Scale (Wechsler, 1955), and do less well on comprehension tasks in general (Bergman, 1980; Corso, 1977). These findings fit in too nicely with Western society's belief that old age is a time of decline; the research focus is unbalanced. Research must also look for changes in *linguistic strategy* and try to dissociate from one another the various levels of cognitive deficit that may underlie apparent changes in language use. For example, one would obviously want to distinguish between the poor comprehension that results from impaired hearing and the poor comprehension that results from changes in the language parts of the brain. The first is a relatively peripheral problem that can be partially remedied, whereas the second involves an essential brain-based language skill, namely the ability to understand language.

In this chapter we first consider abilities and styles acquired in adulthood that may be termed *registers*. The various forms of language we acquire to employ in social groups and at work are compared with the more explicit learning of "second" or "foreign" languages. When we turn to the language developments of advanced age, it is useful to see the way separate language subsystems change differently. At that point we also discuss what is known about changes in brain dominance for language across the lifespan. Finally, we focus on language patterns that result from brain damage in order to distinguish those changes resulting from disease from the changes linked to healthy aging.

The Language of Peer and Social Groups

Special registers are mastered starting in childhood, exploited in adolescence, and refined in adulthood for social activities and for many aspects of interpersonal relationships. One of the primary divisions in our society, of course, is that between females and males. Thus, as one grows to adulthood, one acquires gender-appropriate speech styles. Tannen (1990) has documented how women and men differ in their styles of language use. Women use language more for rapport, while men use it more for competition. Such language mechanisms as interruption and holding the floor have been studied to see how they indicate subtle differences in power (Edelsky, 1981). As a rule, for instance, males interrupt females much more than females interrupt males.

Of course, one may choose deliberately to take on speech characteristics of the other gender, and in certain situations one is expected to. For example, as women became news "anchors" on television, a certain subtype of women's language evolved, a style deemed more "listenable" than the style often associated with nonprofessional women in our society. Professional women, in general, learn to lower their *fundamental frequency* somewhat and also to lessen the range of pitch variation in their speech (Kramer, 1975). Likewise, men who participate in child rearing learn the sociolinguistic ways of talking with children and talking about children with other parents.

Bonding language serves not only to identify members within a group but also to distinguish members from outsiders. One of the experimental paradigms that demonstrates this is the **matched guise model** of Lambert (1972). Lambert used it first with respect to French-English bilinguals, but it has been used in all sorts of other situations since. In this paradigm the same speaker is recorded in two separate segments, speaking in two separate languages. Listeners are not told that they are hearing the same speaker more than once; they are simply asked to listen to each passage and to comment on various characteristics of the speaker. Thus, their responses betray the stereotypes they have about the subgroups with which the speakers can be identified. For example, in the 1972 study, French-English Canadian bilinguals judge a male to be taller, more intelligent, and more handsome when he is speaking English than when he is speaking French. And a lecturer with an upper-class pronunciation is deemed more intelligent than the same lecturer with a lower-class accent. Indeed, Romaine (1984) has demonstrated that even school-aged children are aware of social class differences in language use, and in adolescence they become more sophisticated in identifying their features and sometimes in switching between different dialects for different purposes.

Special registers are also used to create bonds among members of larger subgroups of society. In many subcultures, such as, historically, the gay community, virtual put-downs may be a part of humorous conversation (e.g., "nice car, but where do you put it when they lock the park?") (Murray, 1979, p. 215). Of course, not all members of a given community participate in ritual insults; indeed, not all members participate in the larger community's use of subdialects or registers.

Chaika (1980) has detailed the special vocabulary of bowlers, noting that in order to be considered an expert bowler, one must be able not only to bowl well but also to use special terminology and idioms. In the same article Chaika details elements of the special register used to communicate by citizen band radio. Not only do CB-radio users have a special vocabulary, they also have a phonology that is apparently free of regional dialects, and they use syntactic structures that are markedly different from standard English (e.g., "I be pushin' an 18-wheeler"). In addition, there are certain subtopics that are heavily used in the CB register: not only the obvious discussion of traffic and police patrol, but also explicit sexual topics encouraged by the anonymity of CB communication and perhaps by boredom.

Language in intimate relationships takes on quite different registers, also. Couples often develop special terminology to refer to private jokes and intimate functions, and they learn to employ language in stimulating ways at intimate times. They may also develop pet names for one another, and it is of interest to note how these evolve over time. Intimate conversations are structured differently from conversations with acquaintances or strangers, Hornstein (1983) has observed. Hornstein recorded sixty telephone conversations, one-third between close friends, one-third between strangers, and one-third between acquaintances. Even in telephone conversations the procedures used for opening a conversation and for negotiating its conclusion are distinctly different for close friends. In particular, with close friends some people feel no need to identify themselves when they call. And conversations between friends can be less goal-oriented or structured; sometimes they are simply for keeping in touch. Between strangers or even acquaintances a phone conversation needs to have a more practical purpose.

Formal social relations are maintained by a highly refined set of skills called *manners*. Through experience we learn what to say in specific adult situations and what not to say. One learns the appropriate way to congratulate someone or to express condolence. In her "Miss Manners" book and syndicated columns, Judith Martin (1983) has enjoined readers to employ conventional expressions, rather than being spontaneous. Spontaneity leads to remarks such as "I'm surprised you're able to keep yourself going like this"; she recommends "I'm terribly sorry. You have my deepest sympathy." In response to an announced pregnancy she requires "Oh, how wonderful! When is it to be?" and not "Was this planned?" or "Aren't you concerned about population growth?"

Language at Work

In Chapter 10 we discussed some of the language developments of adolescence. Entering the work force in young adulthood requires a whole new set of language skills. Consider the catalog of special language skills that much adult work requires. For many people, work involves the ability to talk on the telephone, which requires an estimation of another person's behavior even though one cannot see nonverbal responses. Other jobs require the ability to produce certain forms of scientific writing, communicative but nonemotional. The conventions of e-mailing must be differently used for business as compared to personal communications—for example, one may permit oneself to send unedited messages to friends but not to colleagues. Indeed, the ability to type has long been a requirement for many positions, and now all workers must have typing skills and advanced word-processing skills. Some jobs require knowledge of specific computer "languages."

In addition, there are special jobs that involve skills in more than one natural language. For example, there are those who prepare translations for a living. Some translate scientific texts and need a particular set of skills; others translate literary texts and need another, overlapping set of skills. Then there are the *simultaneous translators*—people who accompany monolingual officials to foreign countries and provide immediate translations of their interactions. People who work at the United Nations are responsible for translating as the delegates speak. In order to perform this work, one must have mastered at least two languages and must have the ability to listen and speak at practically the same time.

In theater performance, special language skills are required of the actors—in particular, the ability to speak memorized lines as if they were spontaneous and to use a louder than usual voice as if it were natural. Many members of the clergy employ a special meter and voice modulations in delivering their sermons (Rosenberg, 1970). Another occupation that requires extensive specialized language abilities is that of psychotherapist. Therapists and counselors must hear what their clients and patients are really saying. Sometimes they must decode a message that says one thing on the surface but means another. And therapists must learn to respond in ways that will help effect change in the client (Haley, 1963; Rosen, 1982).

Then there are professional editors, who do not necessarily create written language themselves but who take the efforts of others and mold them into effective written pieces. Good editing requires more than knowing where to use *that* and where to use *which;* it requires an ability to impose logical and artistic structure on someone else's thoughts. And there are the creative writers in our society, from the journalists to the novelists and poets. Even though certain people may have special language skills at an early age, writers develop their talents through hard work. Creative writers often attend workshops and seminars to discuss their work and improve their skills; their style may evolve over many years. Edel (1953–69) gives a picture of the novelist Henry James's development of a more elaborate or convoluted writing style during his adult years. James was undoubtedly influenced by many things, including the typewriter, which was invented during the course of his life, and his shift to dictation that accompanied it. As Gardner has pointed out (1982), dictation requires certain additional skills, such as the ability to concentrate on what one is saying.

Even in work realms that do not focus on language, there is a certain amount of *jargon* to be acquired. Best studied are the special jargons of health care, the legal field, and the political arena with its bureaucratic and administrative language. Medical jargon is used to enable health care workers to communicate effectively with one another; it may also be used to ensure their sense of expertise and power in relation to the clients who come to them without knowledge of this jargon (Elgin, 1983; Shuy, 1979). For example, what the lay person calls senility, the health care worker may call SDAT (senile dementia of the Alzheimer's type) or OBS (organic brain syndrome). Ideally, the health care worker should be able to use the appropriate jargon with colleagues but converse in lay terms with clients.

Medical jargon, it should be noted, is not mere mastery of Latin and Greek vocabulary. As Elgin points out (1983), learning to communicate as a physician includes mastering large structures of discourse and many elements of nonverbal conversations. Paget (personal communication), for example, studied the way physicians use silence in conversations with patients in order to maintain professional status. The use of professional jargon in the medical setting also lends a certain amount of dignity to procedures that are embarrassing.

Similar phenomena exist in the legal community, with initiates becoming quite fluent in the lexicon, syntax, and idioms of legal language, while lay people flounder unless translations are made. Studies of the difficulties that jurors have in understanding their instructions (Charrow, 1982) have resulted in greater awareness within the legal community of a responsibility to avoid legal jargon in dealing with the noninitiate. Similar studies of bureaucratic and administrative language (Charrow, 1982) have demonstrated that jargon can be useful for communication within a community and for preserving a sense of identity within that community, but it can be ineffective when it is not translated for people who have not had an opportunity to master it.

In addition to these particular professions, most other work situations have their own special linguistic requirements. These may be a few specialized lexical items that refer to elements of the job, or ways of creating terms—abbreviation use can become a special skill. Special items of syntax must be mastered in most jargons. And many professions require the ability to lecture, a style of discourse that demands sensitivity to the audience and redundancy that would be inappropriate if the same material were written. For certain professions in which practitioners assume that a distance must be maintained from the listener, special language skills are required to maintain a careful balance between appearing to say something but not committing oneself to it entirely.

Second Language Acquisition in Adulthood

Lenneberg (1967) argued that after puberty acquiring a new language is quite difficult. Indeed, Scovel (1969) has estimated that only 5 percent of speakers can acquire full mastery of a second language after puberty. Some researchers attribute this inability to an ego link with accent; Guiora, Brammer, and Dull (1972) maintain that individuals who have a hard time learning a second language without accent have a strong ego identification in the phonological system of their first language. Others maintain that motivation to learn a second language becomes more crucial with age; the child is motivated to learn in order to communicate, but for the adult it is more complex. Clearly, there are motivational features involved; in some cultures—such as that of French Canada, where there is great incentive to speak French like a native speaker—a substantially greater percentage of *anglophones* can sound like native speakers of French despite postpubertal acquisition. Other researchers such as Snow (1987) argue that the child has more time to devote to acquiring a language, whereas the adult is never able to focus energy solely on acquisition. Snow found the speed of language acquisition in younger children to be slower actually than that in older children and adults when syntactic abilities were compared.

Indication that brain organization for language may also influence the ability to acquire a second language comes not only from lateralization studies, but also from research on sex differences: Girls are substantially better second language learners than are boys (in U.S. studies at least). One could postulate that the greater *bilateral* organization of a first language in girls renders them better able to acquire a second language. This corresponds with work by Albert and Obler (1978) suggesting that right hemisphere abilities are involved in the early stages of second language acquisition. Also of interest are studies of exceptional second language learners. The first case identified by Novoa, Fein, and Obler (1988) happens to be a left-hander, who may have the unusual organization that suggests.

Thus, there may be a critical stage for certain aspects of language acquisition. In order to learn a first language like a native speaker, it is crucial that acquisition start before lateralization is fixed. Puberty is too late. However, in order to acquire a second language like a native speaker, there appears to be somewhat more leeway, although the majority of individuals will do substantially better before puberty. Certain individuals—perhaps those with greater bilateral organization for language—may acquire a second language with a native accent well into adulthood.

Acquisition of Adult Registers

There are some studies on the acquisition of different registers and even dialects in late childhood and adolescence but virtually none on the acquisition of register by adults. We may assume that, as with the language skills of childhood, exposure to the language in question is crucial. Probably it is best to hear the register spoken; reading it or reading about it is a poor substitute. In many ways this parallels the recommended modes for learning a second language. Hearing a social register in context should enable the listener to pick up certain meanings; the adult's ability to explicitly question other meanings is also of use. Again this is analogous to learning a second language, which, Snow (1987) points out, adults can do as well as children if they have the time to focus on it. Nevertheless, adolescents and adults have different styles from those of children because they have different cognitive structures that permit them to think about learning and to question in ways that young children cannot.

Exposure to the language is perhaps sufficient for passive use, that is, for comprehension. More exposure brings about better abilities. Sankoff (1970) demonstrated that in Papua, New Guinea, the ability to understand language spoken in a related dialect increased from adolescence through young adulthood and grew further in the thirty- to forty-year-olds (cited in Grimshaw & Holden, 1976).

In order to produce the language, some practice is necessary. No doubt there is much rehearsal of language among adolescents as well as adults, practicing what one would say in an expected situation or reviewing what one *did* say and could have said differently (Grimshaw & Holden, 1976). Additionally, adolescents' and adults' ability to criticize themselves, to observe variation in others' usage, and to select among possible styles contributes to speaking adult registers with confidence. Until recently the ability to leave a complete, concise voice-mail message was a skill honed in adulthood through practice (now children learn it, too).

Why some individuals choose (deliberately or unconsciously) to master the registers and others do not is less clear. It may be that people choose more or less to identify with the subgroups in question. And it is possible that certain people have a particular verbal talent and can acquire styles and change among them at will. Role conflict can also be involved in register choice; for example, a woman who sees herself as very feminine may not acquire the register associated with a male occupation even if she chooses to go into that occupation.

Language Developments with Advanced Age

Although it is assumed that phonology does not change with advanced age, most people believe that lexical abilities diminish (in particular, people have trouble remembering the names of things and of other people), that comprehension is impaired with age, and that discourse in the elderly tends to run on. In fact, these stereotypes are too simplistic to explain the diversity of language behaviors associated with advanced age. From recent research we learn that there are language changes that result both from direct changes in language areas of the brain and from strategies to compensate for memory or attentional deficits associated with aging. These changes may be seen across many languages (Juncos-Rabadan & Iglesias, 1994).

Phonology

Phonology does not change substantially with increasing age. Nevertheless, one way in which languages themselves change is through phonological change over time. This may occur between or within generations, so the extent to which speakers vary their phonology as they age is worth studying longitudinally. Bilingualism may also play a role. Clyne (1977) has described a woman who reverted to a heavy German accent (German was her first language) in her second language, English, with advanced age. It is unclear whether the patient was demented; if so, her language development was not indicative of healthy aging. Indeed, de Bot and Clyne (1989) have demonstrated that such behavior is not the rule for immigrants with a similar history.

Lexicon

Psychologists and psycholinguists have studied lexical items because they are quite discrete and easy to specify, unlike syntax, semantics, discourse, and pragmatics. Early studies of word associations (Riegel, 1968) suggested that older subjects had a more varied range of associations than did younger subjects. Riegel pointed out the interesting fact that in his study younger adults were more likely to choose words that fit into the same word class as the stimulus item (*table* and *chair,* for example), whereas older adults were more likely to choose words that co-occur syntactically (*sit* and *chair*). Critics of his interpretation have reminded us that the younger adults in his study had undergone more education, with its standardizing effects. Indeed, in a somewhat more recent study to verify this finding, Lovelace and Cooley (1982) did not find that older and younger adults perform differently on this free association task. They concluded that semantic networks are not likely to operate differently because of age differences *per se,* but because of differences in education level. It is worth recalling that there is development in childhood from **syntagmatic** responses in younger children to more **paradigmatic** responses in older children in similar word association studies.

When given certain sorts of lexical tasks, in particular *confrontation-naming* tasks, there is no question that some seventy-year-olds perform substantially worse than younger adults. In a confrontation-naming task subjects are shown a picture (or an object) and are asked to tell its name. In a series of studies from our laboratory (e.g., Nicholas, Obler, Albert, & Goodglass, 1985), thirty-year-olds performed somewhat worse than fifty-year-olds on confrontation-naming of both common nouns and verbs. There was a slight decline for sixty-year-olds on the average and a substantial decline among seventy-year-olds. Longitudinal study of the same subjects (Au, Joung, Nicholas, Obler, Kass, & Albert, 1995; Barth Ramsey, Nicholas, Au, Obler, & Albert, 1999) indicates scores decline several points for subject groups age fifty and older over the course of seven years. Proper nouns—the names of people—and particularly, well-known names, are particularly hard to retrieve with advancing age (Barresi, 1996; Cohen & Burke, 1993). Studies of passive access to lexicon, however, seem to show no decrement with aging. That is, if older adult subjects are not asked to produce the label for a concept but rather to recognize that label or name, they perform just as well or better than younger adult subjects. And when they are asked to define words, as on the vocabulary subtest of the Wechsler Adult Intelligence Scale, there are differential results depending on the scoring method. As Botwinick, West, and Storandt (1975) have reported, if one uses a modification of the standard scoring system and requires a single word synonym as a good definition, there are decrements with age starting at age forty. However, by the standard scoring, whereby definitions consisting of more than one word are as good as single-word synonyms, older adults perform as well as younger adults. Thus, it is clear that lexical items are not actually lost in older adults; rather, the ability to access them in order to produce them spontaneously is impaired.

With regard to this question of active and passive access to the lexicon, consider Moscovitch's study with Landowski (personal communication). They found that even though older subjects were more likely to use old-fashioned terminology, they recognized current terminology as well or as quickly as younger subjects. The methodology of that study is worth noting: They compared two word-frequency lists, the Thorndike and Lorge (1944) list created in the 1940s and the Kucera and Francis (1967) list used in the 1970s, and they looked specifically for lexical items that had changed frequency between the two lists. They found that the older adult subjects were more familiar with the 1940s words and were more likely to use them than were the younger adults. Note that Wingfield, Goodglass, Berko Gleason, Bowles, and Hyde (1988) have seen in their studies with the Boston Naming Test that older subjects may "fail" to name a picture because they use a word that is no longer common. For instance, they may call a bicycle a *wheel,* a usage that was once quite popular. However, the older adults recognized the test items as well as the younger subjects.

Older adults do not have different strategies on these tasks from those of young adults. Nicholas and her colleagues (1985) looked at whether older adults made different sorts of errors. Although the older adults did use relatively more circumlocutions of the correct items ("moving on his hands and knees, crawling" for "crawling")

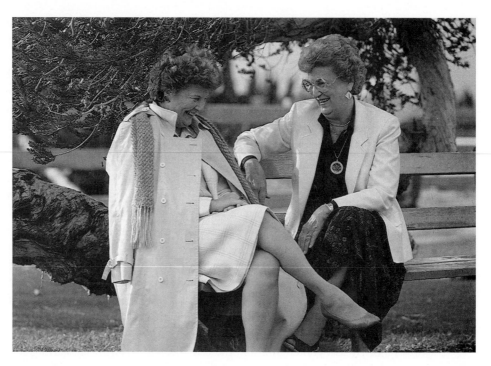

Older adults who engage in frequent conversations have better naming abilities than those who spend their time watching television.

and did tend to comment on the task more (as a way of avoiding response or buying time), it was clear that for all subjects the most common errors were semantically related items (e.g., *elevator* for *escalator*). Thus, the authors concluded that the different styles were related not to different strategies in response but to the greater difficulty of the task. It is also interesting to note that there appeared to be no distinction among different word classes; essentially the same patterns of lexical access were found for verbs, common nouns, and proper nouns.

However, individual differences on naming tasks may be explained by one's experiences in using language. Barresi, Obler, Au, and Albert (1999) have demonstrated that older adults who engage in conversation more perform somewhat better on a naming test, while those who watch television more perform significantly worse.

Some authors have argued (e.g., Goulet, Ska, & Kahn, 1994) that we do not know for sure that naming ability declines with age because no studies have considered all the necessary factors that may interact with naming abilities, such as the medications that subjects are taking or their general health status. Indeed, it would appear that the inner lexicon itself does not change structure with advanced age, except that more items can be acquired over the lifespan. Access for production may become more difficult, however, and there may be a bit of semantic degradation (Barresi, Nicholas, Connor, Obler, & Albert, submitted). The ability to access the lexicon for comprehension, too, probably does not change, although it may be stressed under speeded conditions. It is possible, however, that the ability to learn new words decreases in advanced age.

Comprehension

In Western society, virtually all people are exposed to enough noise over their lifetime that their hearing deteriorates with age. Relatively good hearing is required for comprehension of spoken language. Thus, on any comprehension test, whether testing on a low level the ability to repeat individual words or on a high level the ability to understand sentences and paragraphs, healthy older subjects will perform worse than healthy younger subjects. The questions of interest to the linguist, however, focus primarily on any change in the brain *substrate* for comprehension with advanced age and secondarily on different comprehension strategies used to deal with hearing loss.

Let us consider the question of special comprehension strategies first. It has been assumed that healthy elderly people who comprehend fairly well despite impaired hearing must have developed special strategies.

There are not likely to be general memory strategies. Although older adults benefit more from categorized materials on memory tasks than younger adults, no differences are seen across studies in their use of association strategies or imagery (Verhaeghen, Marcoen, & Goossens, 1993).

In a study conducted in Boston (Obler, Nicholas, Albert, & Woodward, 1985), it was hypothesized that older adults rely more heavily on lip reading and face reading than younger people and also that they rely more on semantics, that is, guessing what someone is saying. Neither of these hypotheses proved to be true. Face reading was tested by giving 120 healthy adults aged thirty to seventy-nine a battery of comprehension tests under two conditions. In one they saw a speaker on a TV screen at the same time they heard comprehension questions like "The lion was killed by the tiger; who died?" In the second they heard the same sorts of questions over the same earphones, but did not see the speaker's face. The same difference between the two conditions was found for all four age groups tested, suggesting that all subjects relied equally heavily on face reading, regardless of their age.

In similar fashion subjects' reliance on semantic context was tested. Subjects heard the sentences from the *Speech Perception in Noise Test* (Kalikow, Stevens, & Elliot, 1977). In half of the sentences the last word is highly predictable from the context of the earlier part of the sentence (e.g., The rose bush had prickly *thorns*); in the other half of the sentences the final word is not easily predictable from the earlier words (e.g., The boy liked to talk about *thorns*). Subjects are asked to write down the final word of each sentence, but the sentences are made harder to hear by having a babbling noise imposed over them. Naturally, scores were higher for everybody in the predictable condition than in the nonpredictable condition. But again there was no greater differential between the two conditions for the sixty- and seventy-year-old subjects than for the thirty- and fifty-year-old subjects. Older and younger adults seem to rely equally on guessing the meaning of a word from its semantic context.

In a later study, however, Obler, Fein, Nicholas, and Albert (1991) demonstrated that older adults do rely more heavily than younger adults on plausibility. That is, responding to "The doctor who helped the patient who was sick was healthy; was the doctor healthy?" was easier than "The guide who drove the tourist who was bored was excited; was the guide bored?"

Similarly, when Kahn and Till (1991) presented stories to younger and older adults, materials that conformed to expectations permitted older adults, as compared to younger adults, to interpret pronouns markedly better than materials with pronoun use that did not conform to expectations.

We cannot conclude on the basis of these studies what differences there are in comprehension strategy for younger and older adults. There may be other differences that we have not yet thought of. In fact, Bergman (1980) reviewed the literature on comprehension of synthetically distorted speech and found that older adults do worse than younger adults on both slowed-down and speeded-up speech. But it is unclear whether this is due to overall hearing impairment or whether it reflects changes in the cognitive processes of comprehension.

Actually, it is important to note that the task Bergman used was a task requiring repetition of the sentence. Thus it could be memory factors rather than strictly linguistic comprehension that cause subjects' problems in his study. Qualls, for example, has demonstrated that working memory limitations associated with advanced age are associated with poorer understanding of idioms and metaphors (Qualls, 1998, and in preparation). Moreover tasks asking for paragraph processing or recall consistently show that older adults perform worse than younger subjects in numbers of items, concepts, or themes retrieved (Cohen, 1979). In a study where older and younger adults were given texts to read for comprehension, though education helped both younger and older adults determine if the materials were internally consistent, older adults as a rule were less able than younger adults to determine that texts were internally inconsistent, particularly when the crucial inconsistent sentences were separated by at least one other sentence (Zabrucky, Moore, & Schultz, 1993). However, Kemper (1987) was able to demonstrate that certain syntactic structures posed particular difficulties for older subjects. Left-branching structures, where modifiers pile up before the structures they modify (e.g., the *tall, skinny, greedy* aristocrat) caused the greatest difficulty, as compared to right-branching structures (e.g., the aristocrat *who was tall, skinny, and greedy*). Such a finding suggests that syntactic structure at least interacts with memory load in rendering comprehension progressively difficult with increasing age.

The most provocative suggestion of different approaches to comprehension derives from a set of studies done by Warren and Warren (1966). They developed a methodology to elicit what is called the **verbal transformation effect,** in which subjects listen to a single word presented over and over on a tape loop. The phenomenon that occurs for all subjects at some time is that they think they are hearing a different word. Subjects are instructed to raise their hand whenever they think they hear something new on the tape. Of interest for our discussion is the fact that older people hear new items less frequently than younger people. Moreover, there are qualitative differences in the types of responses people of different ages are prone to make. In particular, older adults hear only real words (e.g., *stress, tress, rest*), whereas younger adults may hear words that are not English but could be in terms of phonology and morphology (e.g., *res, trest*). Young children, it should be noted, identify words that are not even possible in English (e.g., *rster*). Thus, we are led to believe that older adults may be doing the most efficient processing in terms of what is possible in a given language, without permitting themselves to be distracted by impossible sequences. This may reflect a certain **automaticity** of language processing that develops across the lifespan.

Discourse

There are a variety of popular beliefs in Western culture about discourse in the elderly: Older people tend to run on or to go off on tangents; older people tend to tell stories over and over again without realizing it; bilingual elders can no longer limit themselves to the language appropriate to the listener. According to research these beliefs hold true only for patients with brain damage or *dementia,* a disease-induced loss of intellectual function. In healthy adults language may even become more elaborate with age. Hints of this have occurred in studies referred to earlier; for example, older people are more likely than thirty-year-olds to give definitions consisting of more than one word, and older people are more likely to give comments and circumlocutions on naming tasks.

The verbosity that has been associated with normal aging, Arbuckle and Gold (1993) have demonstrated, is linked to diminished ability—evidence on neuropsychological tests—to ignore irrelevant information in working memory.

In research on written discourse in aging, Obler (1980) collected written paragraphs from healthy subjects aged thirty through seventy-nine. Subjects were all shown the same picture, the cookie theft picture from the *Boston Diagnostic Aphasia Exam* (Goodglass & Kaplan, 1972), and were asked to describe it. The fifty-year-olds were more likely to use an abbreviated style (e.g., "Boy standing on stool. Mother washing dishes"), whereas the older adults were more likely to use an elaborate style with articles and *deictics* as well as various modifying words and phrases. Moreover, they were likely to link their sentences (e.g., "The boy is standing on the stool while the mother is carefully drying dishes, unaware that the water is running over"). Thus, by word count within several categories and within each theme, one could see a development between the fifties and the seventies toward more elaborate speech. It is worth noting, however, that the thirty-year-olds resembled the seventy-year-olds in this use of elaborate speech. Thus, it may be that younger adults use an elaborate style naturally, which becomes more abbreviated in the fifties and then elaborates again near the older end of the lifespan.

Bromley (1991), however, analyzed descriptions that a sizable number (240) of adults ranging in age from twenty to eighty-six had written of themselves. When such variables as education as socioeconomic status were controlled for, age-related effects were seen for sentence complexity and length. In this study, where subjects had as long as they wanted to write their description, sentence complexity correlated with sentence length; both decreased with age.

In cultures that value tale-telling, it is the older storytellers who are considered the most skilled performers. In Obler's (1980) research in Beit Safafa, a Palestinian village outside Jerusalem, the best tale-tellers were all in their sixties and older. It is precisely the ability to use elaborate speech that makes a tale effective entertainment. This elaboration includes not only details and connections between sentences and larger units, but also personalization and an ability to create rhythm.

Some research on oral discourse shows deficits with increasing age. Kynette and Kemper (1986) found less varied syntactic use in the older subjects (aged 70 and 80) when they analyzed their spontaneous speech in a twenty-minute interview. Also, these older subjects made more actual errors than did the fifty- and sixty-year-olds in the use of morphological markers such as past tense and subject-verb agreement. Ulatowska, Cannito, Hayashi, and Fleming (1985) found intradiscourse referencing via pronouns to be less unambiguously communicative in the group aged over seventy-six as compared to middle-aged and "young-old" groups (i.e., subjects between the ages of 60 and 75). Similarly, when Kemper, Rash, Kynette, and Norman (1990) collected story-narratives from adults aged sixty to ninety, they showed that with increasing age, the stories evidenced less syntactic complexity within sentences and fewer cohesive links (like use of pronouns and conjunctions) signalling connections among sentences.

Bates, Marchman, Harris, Wulfeck, and Kritchevsky (1995) showed subjects from different age groups animated film scenarios of both simple and complex activities and found that older adults (aged 67 to 100) used the same range of syntactic structure as young-old adults (aged 50 to 66), who in turn tended to use more complex structures than college students. Thus some subtle markers of discourse may be seen to decline with age, even while overall more elaborate structures may be used in certain tasks.

Speech

Older adults' speech is slower than that of younger adults, by 20 to 25 percent (Smith, Wasowicz, & Preston 1987). They have also been reported to produce more **disfluencies,** such as stuttering, word repetition, and sentence fragments (Ehrlich, 1990) in speech, but they are able to repair speech errors as well as younger adults (McNamara, Obler, Au, & Albert, 1992).

Nonlanguage Cognitive Factors Influencing Performance

Three nonlanguage cognitive abilities have been reported to have substantial influence on language. One is **speed of processing,** the second is **inhibition,** and the third is **working memory.** Speed of processing we have referred to above: Speech elements from segments to sentences are produced at slower rates (Smith et al., 1987) and the ability to take in and repeat speeded speech is diminished (Bergman, 1980, Wingfield, Prentice,

Koh, & Little, in press). Even the ability to generate lists of words based on their starting with a certain letter, or *not* including a certain letter, is linked to basic measures of speed of processing (Bryan, Luszcz, & Crawford, 1997). Speed of reading for comprehension clearly declines with age, as well (Harris, Rogers, & Qualls, 1998).

Inhibition, in the cognitive psychology sense, means the ability to ignore irrelevant stimuli. It seems to become more difficult with advancing age (Burke, 1997). When written discourse is prepared with extraneous words written in italics, for example, and, subjects are instructed to ignore the words in italics, it is harder for older adults than younger ones to skip over the italicized words when reading aloud (Dywan & Murphy, 1996).

Working memory—the ability to keep information in mind while processing— declines with age, and this decline has been linked to comprehension problems as we mentioned above, even in studies such as that of Qualls (1998 and in preparation) on idiom comprehension.

Laterality

Lateralization for a cognitive task means that one or the other of the two halves of the brain is primarily responsible for that task. It has been known for almost a century that language is lateralized in the left hemisphere for most people. More recently, it has become clear that some visual-spatial abilities are lateralized in the right hemisphere. Brown and Jaffe (1975) have hypothesized that laterality intensifies over the lifespan. The studies of brain damage and changes in aphasia across the lifespan speak to this hypothesis. In particular, Brown and Jaffe maintain that lateralization for language in the left hemisphere develops not only during the first five years of life, but in fact during the entire lifespan. They base this claim on the different types of aphasia resulting from the same lesion to a child and to an older adult. Thus, one would expect that in advanced age left hemisphere dominance for language would be even more marked than it is in the thirties.

Several studies of lateralization have now been undertaken (Borod & Goodglass, 1980; Clark & Knowles, 1973; Johnson, Cole, Bowers, Foiles, Nakaido, Patrick, & Woliver, 1979; Obler, Woodward, & Albert, 1984) that look at language both in the visual modes and in the auditory modes. These studies suggest that there are not changes in gross lateralization. That is, the left hemisphere would appear to be dominant for language from an early age, and it becomes no more dominant in later ages.

However, there is a second element of the Brown and Jaffe hypothesis, suggesting that there might be changes *within* the left hemisphere language area for organization of language across the lifespan. This suggestion is more plausible, given our current understanding, and may shed light on increased automaticity of language use with age, as evidenced in the studies of the Warrens and their colleagues (1966).

Wingfield and colleagues (in press) remind us that the ability to process language with advancing age is remarkably spared in light of the marked declines in the underlying processes that support it, such as speed of processing, working memory, and actual cellular interconnections. We must assume, then, that older adults use conscious and unconscious strategies to compensate for the diminished underlying abilities.

Language Strategies with Aging

On naming tasks we have noted that older adults may use more words in the course of getting to a correct answer. On vocabulary tasks, where they are asked to define words, older adults also use more words (Botwinick et al., 1975). On comprehension tasks, by contrast, the two strategies tested so far have proven not to change with aging. The behavioral psychologist B. F. Skinner wrote on the ways he used language for "intellectual self-management" (Skinner, 1983). For example, when he needed to remember the name of someone, he found it helpful to recall the original use of the name and then go through the alphabet, trying each letter as the initial letter of the name. He and his wife had also developed some pragmatic routines that made it possible for him to avoid remembering names socially. For example, when he had to introduce his wife to someone whose name he had forgotten and there was a chance that the two had met previously, Skinner said to his wife, "Of course you remember...?" and she quickly interrupted, "Yes, of course. How are you?" The Skinners assumed that acquaintances may or may not have remembered meeting Mrs. Skinner but probably did not trust their own memories, either.

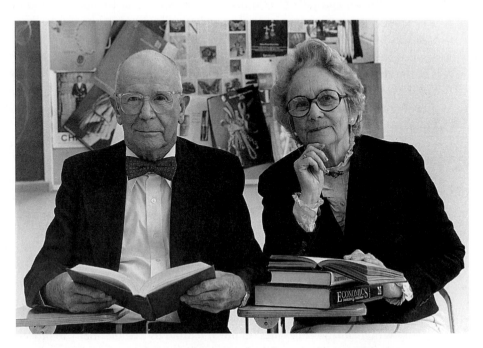

Intellectual curiosity and an openness to new ideas characterize successful aging.

Skinner also developed numerous uses of written language to facilitate diminished memory and attention: "In place of memories, memoranda" was his motto. Thus, he would carry around a notepad so that he would jot down thoughts as they occurred to him and assure that they would not be lost. He also used detailed outlines to plan papers in advance and kept a written index of what he had said so that he would not repeat himself or go off on a tangent. His general strategy was that one can do nothing about the actual accessibility of language, but one can enhance the conditions under which verbal behavior must occur. For example, he suggested a deliberate adoption of new intellectual styles and new ways of thinking to prevent being bogged down in older ones that will no longer be used as well.

Auditory verbal abilities can also be deliberately maintained. One way of keeping records of what one has said or thought is to carry around a tape recorder. Skinner also recommended setting up conversations with colleagues, since the ability to talk to a thoughtful, responsive audience helps stimulate one's own thinking. Of course, Skinner pointed out, any of these strategies would be helpful at any age, but he found them particularly useful in his old age to compensate for difficulties he would otherwise have. Skinner could write and speak articulately about these strategies, but it may be that many older people develop such strategies unconsciously—thus explaining the fact that language abilities in daily life do not appear to change substantially with age.

Adult Language and Brain Damage

Damage to the adult's brain brings about several different sorts of language and communication disturbance. In particular, we consider **aphasia** (essentially, language disturbance from left-hemisphere damage), language disturbance from right-hemisphere damage, and the language disturbance of the **dementias.**

Aphasia

Traditionally, aphasia has been divided into several major types, which have to do not with age but with the type of language disturbance a patient shows. Thus (see Table 11.1), in **Broca's aphasia** the patient produces speech with effort and *telegrammatically*, but her comprehension is relatively good. One patient with agrammatic Broca's aphasia, when asked what had happened to cause it replied, in full, "Stroke. Two years ago and et months, eight months." A second, who had been a mechanical engineer, replied, in full, "Five months ago, I, I, here and here and here (pointing to his leg, his arm and his mouth). Seven o'clock; it's, gone."

In **Wernicke's aphasia,** by contrast, production of speech is quite fluent, but comprehension is very poor. The classic Wernicke's aphasic will make paragrammatic errors, as in this example from a seventy-year-old patient, studied by Elmera Goldberg:

"I have liked to watch the doctor works on the robot." In writing, as in speech, word substitutions contribute to, but do not fully account for, the emptiness. Consider the following segments of a three-paragraph essay written for Dr. Joyce West by a fifty-six-year-old plumber who had completed eight years of education. He wrote this nearly two and a half years after his stroke:

> As I was sleeping I sort of felt a spain at my harm and my leg. They sort of stayed at the same fixed way. I did not go to do anything about it…. First I couldnt even talk to my wife. The next thing I knew I was or right. Then I went to bed all right because that what he wanted.
>
> It was not too long before that call came over me. I had to go the hospital. I was not too long to wait for my cause. They discoursed my cause for being there. They finally discovered that I had a strock…. But they discouted the streant of the strock. Well they finally got that selthed.

In **global aphasia** both comprehension and production are impaired; in **conduction aphasia** spontaneous production is all right and comprehension is relatively good, too, but the ability to repeat is impaired. In **anomic aphasia** only the ability to name items is lost. Aphasia may occur suddenly in childhood as a result of either stroke or accident (**childhood aphasia**) or children with **developmental dysphasia** may have difficulties over the course of learning language, with no sudden change in their brains. Aphasia can be seen in young adults who have suffered traumatic injuries from vehicle accidents or war wounds. However, the primary population of aphasic individuals in the Western world today is found among older adults who have suffered strokes.

There are several points to be made about how the language disturbances of aphasia relate to age. First, the ability to recover from aphasia differs substantially across the lifespan. In young children, perhaps up until the age of puberty, the recovery from even severe aphasia is likely to be nearly complete. Only with the most sophisticated testing can these subjects be seen to have language deficits (Dennis & Whitaker, 1976; Guttman, 1942). After brain damage in young adulthood, as well, there is often substantial recovery. Although there are also older adults who recover from aphasia, recovery is much less frequent in this population, and it is hard to predict which aphasic patients will recover. Patients with certain types of aphasia in the

Table 11.1   Adult Aphasia Types and Symptoms

	Comprehension	Speech
Broca's aphasia	good	effortful, nonfluent, telegrammatic
Wernicke's aphasia	poor	fluent, empty
Global aphasia	poor	virtually none
Conduction aphasia	good	only poor for repetition
Anomic aphasia	good	many circumlocutions

early stages are much more likely than other aphasics to recover, but beyond that individual differences are hard to predict.

One question to ask is whether older or younger adults recover better, either spontaneously or in response to speech therapy. There is some debate as to whether older and younger people recover differently when given speech therapy. Bartlett, Rubens, Holland, Barresi, and Satake (in preparation) report functional communication recovers variably but with no regard for age in adult aphasics over the first year post-onset. Sarno (1980) argues that if one omits all patients who are thought to have dementing diseases from a population of aphasics, recovery is not significantly related to age. However, the tendencies in all her measures are for older subjects to recover less completely than younger adults. We must not assume on the basis of these findings that there are changes in brain substrate for language with advanced age; even if older adults tend to have more limited recoveries in response to therapy, this tendency may be due to age-related changes in nonlanguage areas subserving the language areas, such as memory or learning ability.

Let us define aphasia as the explicit language disturbance resulting from localized or delimited impairment of the language areas of the brain (see Figure 1.1). For most individuals these areas are primarily in the cortex, the exterior part of the brain, and in the central area of the left hemisphere. The type of aphasia resulting from a given lesion changes markedly across the lifespan. In particular, as Brown and Jaffe (1975) and others have observed, in the young child a lesion to the posterior sections of the language area never results in a *fluent aphasia,* whereas the same lesion in an older adult almost invariably results in a fluent aphasia. (For our purposes the fluent aphasia is similar to Wernicke's, and a *nonfluent aphasia* is similar to Broca's.) In an epidemiological study of the relation between aphasia type and age, aphasic patients' charts for the past decade at the Boston Veterans Administration Medical Center were checked. Certain classic forms of aphasia clustered around different ages in advanced adulthood. In particular, the nonfluent abbreviated-language style aphasia with good comprehension evidenced a mean age of fifty-two and occurred in thirty-year-olds through sixty-year-olds, whereas the fluent aphasia with poor comprehension occurred with a mean age of sixty-three in forty-year-olds through eighty-year-olds. This finding, that Broca's aphasics are on the average a decade or more younger than Wernicke's aphasics, has been verified at numerous centers throughout the world. This effect does not seem to relate to a predilection to get strokes in different parts of the brain at different ages, since Miceli, Caltagirone, Gianotti, Masulo, Silveri, and Villa (1981) found the same pattern in aphasics whose language disorder resulted from tumors. We may tentatively speculate that there are actual changes in brain substrate organization for language throughout older adulthood as throughout the lifespan.

Right-Hemisphere Damage and Language

Until recently it was assumed that the left hemisphere was dominant for language and the right hemisphere had little if anything to do with language. Only recently has the study of various language and communication functions considered right-hemisphere damage. Although basic language skills like phonology and lexicon and syntax are not impaired when patients suffer right-hemisphere damage, the abilities to use language appropriately in broader, pragmatic senses are affected. For example, Brownell, Michel, Powelston, and Gardner (1983) studied the ability to appreciate humor and discovered that it is impaired in right-hemisphere subjects. Bloom, Borod, Obler, and Gerstman (1992) demonstrated that discourse involving emotional content was particularly impaired in patients with right-hemisphere damage.

Pragmatic aspects of discourse production are particularly impaired, such as its coherence (Bloom, Borod, Obler, & Gerstman, 1994). Foldi (1983) studied the ability to appreciate indirect discourse in brain-damaged adults. When we see a picture of a man and a boy standing by a dirty car and the man says to the boy, "That car certainly does look dirty," we understand that the man is not only commenting on the way the car looks, but he may be requesting the boy to clean it. Although the left-hemisphere-damaged subjects appropriately selected the underlying meaning, the right-hemisphere-damaged subjects were unable to appreciate such underlying pragmatic meanings.

Prosodic aspects of speech production are also impaired in right-brain-damaged patients. Intonation, for example, may be flat, conveying little emotion. The ability to appreciate prosody is also impaired (Brownell, Gardner, Prather, & Martino, 1995). (See Table 11.2 for a comparison of the language and communication problems associated with left- and right-hemisphere damage.)

Language in the Dementias

The onset of aphasia is usually sudden, particularly in the case of aphasia resulting from stroke or accident. In the case of a tumor there is a progressive onset of aphasia,

Table 11.2	**Language and Communication Problems Associated with Left- and Right-Hemisphere Damage**
Left-Hemisphere Damage	*Right-Hemisphere Damage*
• Naming problems	• Tangential speech
• Effortful speech	• Inference problems
• Phonemic and phonetic distortions	• Humor impaired
• Speech devoid of meaning	• Appreciation and production of emotion impaired
• Speech with few functors	• Prosody impaired
• Word substitutions	
• Little speech initiated	
• Comprehension problems for words and/or sentences	

but the lesion, or area of damage, is still relatively delimited. In the **dementing diseases** like Alzheimer's, by contrast, there is more widespread damage to the brain. This damage may be subtle enough in any individual location that is not revealed by our current methods of x-raying the brain. Nevertheless, after a person with one of these diseases had died, postmortem study of the brain shows changes at the cellular level that have been reflected in the progressive deterioration of cognitive abilities. These abilities include memory, problem-solving ability, and learning ability, as well as the language abilities on which we are focusing.

There are a number of diseases that include dementia. Many of them are only now beginning to be well studied from a medical viewpoint, and the neurobehavioral and neurolinguistic studies have started only in recent decades. Compared to the studies of aphasia, which have been going on for the last century, studies of dementia are in a relatively early phase. Yet, as Westerners live longer, the incidence of dementing diseases—particularly **Alzheimer's disease**—increases, since it is relatively rare before age seventy (0.6 percent), but markedly more common in individuals over age eighty-four (8.4 percent) (Hubert, Scherr, Beckett, Albert, Pilgrim, Chown, Funkenstein, & Evans, 1995). We must first distinguish among the various sorts of dementia, and then we can describe the language behaviors associated with them.

One basic distinction to be made is whether the brain structures involved in the dementia are primarily *cortical* (on the surface of the brain) or *subcortical* (beneath the surface of the brain). In diseases such as **Parkinson's disease** and *progressive supranuclear palsy*, it is predominantly subcortical structures that are impaired, whereas in diseases such as Alzheimer's disease, it is predominantly cortical structures that are impaired. Thus, it is in Alzheimer's disease in particular that we see language disturbance that mimics that of the aphasias (see Table 11.3). Specifically, the language disturbance of early Alzheimer's disease looks like anomic aphasia, where the primary deficit is in the ability to name things. By the mid to late stage, the language disturbance looks like Wernicke's aphasia: Patients produce fluent, poorly monitored speech with syntactically correct usage of some words and occasional *jargon* items (which in this terminology means nonsense words). Patients with Alzheimer's disease also have difficulty in comprehension of language and in repeating sentences that are quite long or quite improbable.

By the late stages of the disease, most patients produce little language and are sometimes taken to be mute. Other patients may produce language inappropriately—talking when no one is around and/or not talking when people are present. The language produced at this stage is almost entirely stereotypic, with nothing that is propositional. Thus, late Alzheimer's patients may look like global aphasic patients, who produce and comprehend very little language. Even in the late stages, however, some pragmatic competence remains. Patients may still maintain eye contact appropriately or respond to formulaic questions like "How are you today?" (Causino, Obler, Knoefel, & Albert, 1994).

In the early stages of the disease the ability to read may actually be better for Alzheimer's patients than the ability to understand spoken language, because spoken language requires more consistent attention. In the mid-stages, word substitutions are included (Henderson, Buckwalter, Sobel, Freed, & Diz, 1992). However, the ability to write deteriorates fairly rapidly. In the early stages, problems in writing are simply misspellings and an occasional omission or inappropriate addition of an inflectional suffix. By early-mid stages, however, the ability to read aloud is markedly better spared than the ability to read for comprehension. Until recently it has been thought that reading aloud was spared until quite late, although Patterson, Graham, and Hodges (1994) have demonstrated that even the ability to read aloud is progressively impaired starting with minimal dementia for irregularly spelled words such as *placebo*. By the later stages, however, patients produce nonsense words and incomplete sentences and eventually refuse to write altogether.

In those dementias that co-occur with subcortical disease, in particular Parkinson's disease, it is the speech faculties that are most impaired rather than underlying language abilities. Patients tend to speak very softly, and their speech is inarticulate,

Table 11.3	The Stages of Language Decline in Alzheimer's Disease

Early to Mid-Stage

Primarily naming problems

Some discourse problems

Mild comprehension problems for complex materials

Problems with repetition of long complex sentences only

Reading aloud spared; some problems with writing

Mid to Late Stage

Fluent, empty discourse

Word substitutions

Occasional jargon nonwords

Poor repetition of sentences

Impaired comprehension

Reading aloud relatively spared

Writing impaired in parallel to oral production

Bilingual subjects impaired in language choice

Late Stage

Little language produced

No comprehension testable

No repetition

One or two low-level pragmatic abilities spared

speeding up to a mumble after the first several words. When one asks these patients to write, however, or listens carefully to their oral language production, one can note certain mild errors of syntax, particularly the deletion of morphemes or the inappropriate addition of morphemes. For example, the patient may write, "The grandchildren comes around." In subcortical as in cortical impairment, the incorrect use of grammatical forms may also occur. For example, in telling us the story of Little Red Riding Hood, one patient said, "The wolf took a liking *toward* the basket," instead of "The wolf took a liking *to* the basket." Such examples suggest a certain lack of monitoring on the part of the patients and are of interest to the theoretician because they suggest that idioms are not necessarily represented in unitary fashion in the brain, but may be broken up. Further evidence of this is seen in the work of Kempler and Van Lancker (1988), who showed that for patients with Alzheimer's disease, comprehension is impaired for high-frequency idioms whose meaning is not transparent (e.g., a *blue mood*).

In addition to the broader, descriptive studies, specific studies of naming, sentence comprehension, and discourse abilities in Alzheimer's disease have been undertaken. Rochford (1971) maintained that affected subjects show primarily visual misperception errors on a naming task. Thus, they label a picture of flippers as the visually similar aprons more frequently than healthy elderly individuals do. However, Bayles and Tomoeda (1983) have shown results analogous to those found by Nicholas and colleagues (1985) for healthy subjects of all ages; as with healthy individuals, semantic substitutions are the most frequent error that demented patients make on a naming task. Thus, these results contradict earlier findings, which may have represented a particular subpopulation of Alzheimer's patients with predominantly visual-spatial difficulties rather than language difficulties.

If naming is impaired, researchers have asked, is it because the lexicon itself is losing its internal structure, or is it rather than access into the lexicon is impaired? Schwartz, Marin, and Saffran (1979, 1980) found that the demented subject they studied extensively (WLP) was able to read words aloud and demonstrate their meaning via gesture when she heard them. Nevertheless, she had trouble distinguishing pictures of dogs from those of cats in a sorting task; distinguishing pictures of birds, however, was not difficult. Thus they conclude that aspects of the linguistic lexicon and its connection to meaning are spared, but some strictly semantic categories are starting to break down. Nebes, Martin, and Horn (1984), in apparent contradiction, present evidence that certain aspects of semantic structure are still effective in mild to moderately demented patients. Verbal priming via a semantically related word (e.g., *nurse* for *doctor*) facilitates the patients' ability to read a word aloud relatively faster than an equivalent unprimed word, as it does for normals, even though overall it takes the demented patients longer in both conditions. Also, when we measured the semantic distance between the errors and their targets on a naming task, we saw that the distance was no greater for patients with Alzheimer's disease than it was for normal age-matched individuals (Nicholas, Obler, Au, & Albert, 1996). The apparent contradiction can perhaps be resolved if we consider that it is possible for some aspects of the semantic system to disintegrate while others do not, a point made quite effectively by Bayles and Kaszniak (1987).

As to comprehension, Rochon, Waters, and Caplan (1994) demonstrated that, even in the early stages of dementia of the Alzheimer's type, certain syntactic structures—primarily those with more prepositions, rather than those that are syntactically more complex—posed particular problems. Emery (1985) had earlier demonstrated problems with comprehension tasks employing syntactically complex materials. Rochon and colleagues point out that Emery's battery of tasks required the subjects to manipulate objects (for example, to show one toy hitting another), whereas Rochon and her colleagues used the presumably simpler response of having subjects choose which of two pictures appropriately represented a given sentence. Thus, they argue, their subjects showed problems with "post-interpretative processing"; they were able to process the lexical items and even the syntax, but materials with two clauses required substantially more resources for the actual matching task, thus resulting in their findings.

Aspects of pragmatic abilities break down over the course of Alzheimer's dementia. Tomoeda and Bayles (1993) studied the development of discourse over five years in three patients who entered the study in early-mid to mid-late stages of the disease. In the testing sessions, the patients actually produced more words than normals, but the total words on their picture description task declined with the progression of the disease to the late stages. Not surprisingly, the amount of information conveyed decreased across the five years of testing. In the early stages studied, conciseness was impaired, but by the later stages it became a meaningless measure.

Written discourse breaks down relatively early; oral discourse breaks down more subtly and over a longer course in Alzheimer's disease. Ehrlich, Obler, Clark, and Gerstman (1995) studied the characteristics of picture description narrative in patients with probable Alzheimer's disease and demonstrated that the amount of information to be included interacted with the complexity of the information to be produced in rendering the discourse of the patients with Alzheimer's disease both emptier and briefer. Bates and her colleagues (1995) demonstrated that patients with Alzheimer's dementia use less-complex syntax—fewer passives overall, for example, and relatively more passives that employ the word *get* (e.g., "The vase got broken)—than did age-matched controls. However, such avoidance of complex syntactic forms does not fully account for the generalized diminishment of discourse content. Presumably, working memory (and long-term memory when required) as well as diminished self-monitoring functions contribute to the impairments in discourse.

Another aspect of pragmatics that has been studied in patients with Alzheimer's disease can occur in bilingual patients who lose the ability to choose the right language to address their listener. They may also mistakenly code-switch between their two or more languages when their listener only speaks one (De Santi, Obler, Sabo-Abramson, & Goldberger, 1989; Hyltenstam & Stroud, 1989).

Since aphasia is the most studied of the language and communication disturbances resulting from brain damage, it is understandable that therapies have been developed only for aphasia. Because the incidence of dementia is increasing in Western populations as people live longer, researchers and clinicians are currently at work developing therapies to improve or at least forestall the deficits in patients who have both language disturbances and learning difficulties. This work is on the cutting edge of current research.

Of the numerous ways to study both the language changes that take place over the healthy lifespan and adult language impaired by brain damage, there is one that we have not yet touched on that provides a good conclusion: the **regression hypothesis.**

Roman Jakobson suggested in 1941 that the language deficits of aphasia occur in the reverse order of the process of development of language in childhood. In doing this, he was extending the theory of Ribot (1882), which proposed that, across a broad range of psychological skills, the first learned elements were the last to be lost, whether from brain damage or advanced age. Jakobson's hypothesis, which he presented brilliantly with regard to the phonological systems, although appealing in its symmetry, has not held up to close scrutiny (see Berko Gleason in Caramazza & Zurif, 1978, and Menn & Obler, 1990). Patients who lose the ability to produce plurals and past tenses do not have the same morphological systems as children just acquiring those inflections. For instance, a Broca's aphasic may be able to make an /-əz/ plural like *nurses* but unable to make a possessive of the same word. This is a pattern not seen in children. So acquisition of language, when studied in detail, is not the reverse of aphasia. In part, this is evident from the fact that there are different sorts of aphasia but essentially only one hierarchy for childhood acquisition of language.

Obler (1981) has suggested that dementia be considered a more appropriate field for looking at the regression hypothesis, since in dementia one sees a progressive deterioration that is more strictly a reversal of language and cognitive development than the sudden impairment of aphasia. Moreover, as with the child, in whom language development is closely linked to other cognitive development, in the patient suffering from dementia the progress of language deficits is closely linked to the progression of nonlanguage cognitive deficits. However, even with the demented patients there are more differences to be seen than similarities. In particular, these revolve around automatic abilities, which are not yet developed in the child but which may remain until a very late stage in the demented patient. Very demented patients may retain only swear words or politeness routines acquired in later childhood. Children at the one- or two-word stage are quite different from older people at these stages.

Summary

Language development after childhood can be relatively subtle. Older children continue to acquire expertise in pragmatic linguistic behaviors, such as those pertaining to power differences (e.g., gender and social class differences). Also, as adolescents and adults join different subcultures, they may acquire language registers appropriate to those subcultures. Many work situations require distinctive language use as well.

Learning a second language may occur at any age. It appears, however, that there is a sensitive period around puberty after which it is much more difficult for most people to acquire phonological proficiency in a new language.

In late adulthood, certain language changes are obvious, while other areas of language remain unchanged for the most part. Access to the lexicon becomes problematic for many elderly subjects who must search for a specific word or idiom. We can deduce, however, that the lexicon itself remains unchanged for the most part, since when they are given a word to define, the elderly can do this with the proficiency of any young adult. Learning new words continues throughout the lifespan, but it is possible that it becomes somewhat more difficult with older adulthood.

Studies of comprehension in the elderly suggest that in addition to the obvious difficulties brought on in Western society by peripheral hearing loss, there are changes in the ability to process complex materials for comprehension. Whether these are strictly linguistic changes based in the brain or whether they are secondary to memory and attentional changes remains unclear. Moreover, many elderly adults develop successful strategies to get around these problems.

The data on possible changes of discourse with aging are controversial. Some have reported increased elaborateness, while others have reported less varied and less complex syntax. In any event, discourse does not appear to suffer the same degree of decline that lexical access and comprehension manifest. Nor are changes seen for lateral brain organization for language.

Two forms of brain damage are likely to affect the elderly population in Western cultures; these result in aphasia and dementia. Of all the aphasia types, fluent aphasias (such as Wernicke's aphasia) are most likely to occur in older subjects. There is debate as to whether recovery from aphasia becomes more difficult with increasing age.

Specific language disorders associated with dementing diseases such as Alzheimer's disease have recently been described. Overall, the language and communication behavior looks similar to what is seen in the fluent aphasias; anomia in the early stages and Wernicke's aphasia in mid- to late stages. With subcortical dementias, by contrast, primarily speech and not language problems are seen. Even in the cortical dementias, where general cognitive loss accompanies the language and communication deficits, Jakobson's regression hypothesis does not hold; the quality of language changes in Alzheimer's disease is markedly different at every stage of the progressive decline from that of language in early childhood.

Key Words

Alzheimer's disease	Broca's aphasia
anomic aphasia	childhood aphasia
aphasia	conduction aphasia
automaticity	dementia

dementing disease

developmental dysphasia

disfluencies

global aphasia

inhibition

lateralization

matched guise model

paradigmatic

Parkinson's disease

regression hypothesis

speed of processing

syntagmatic

verbal transformation effect

Wernicke's aphasia

working memory

Suggested Projects

The ideal projects to be suggested from a study of lifespan development of language are longitudinal studies. In a semester or even a year it is simply not possible to see natural language change in adults, except in language learners and in a limited number of demented or aphasic patients. The following projects can give some sense of language change with time by using a cross-sectional approach or a post-hoc longitudinal approach.

1. Find an older friend who agrees that he forgets the names of things more than previously. Go through some of his photograph books and see what sort of strategies he uses when he cannot remember specific names. You could also discuss the things he has noticed that are called something different today from what they were called when he learned the names. See whether you can find which idioms have changed.

2. The next time you are the client of a professional (a physician or a lawyer or a plumber), note the words and idioms that are used that you do not understand or understand but would not use. Question the professional about these words; consider the extent to which she is able to translate and the extent to which these words are an unexplainable part of her jargon. Also observe how she feels about your questioning her use of jargon. You could also bring together a friend who is in the first year of professional school and a friend who is completing professional school or practicing in the field. Note how the two of them converse on common topics and see what differences there are in their abilities to use their professional jargon and to translate it for you as a noninitiate.

3. Find someone who wrote journals at the age of twenty and continued writing them through the age of sixth or seventy, and who is prepared to share the journals with you. Note how the language changes over the years, not only in terms of content, but also in the vocabulary and idioms used and in the form of sentences and paragraphs. A similar project would be to compare the writing styles of a poet or novelist who has produced very different works in early and late career (e.g., W. B. Yeats, W. H. Auden, Colette, Shakespeare, Racine, Plato, Drabble).

4. Spend a day with someone who has several children of different ages. Observe how the adult has developed different language registers appropriate to the age of each child. Detail what the differences are.

5. List the special language skills you have learned in college or graduate school. Consider what you have been taught and also what you have learned about constructing a composition, using speech appropriately in different classes, and acquiring the jargon of your major field.

6. If you are a member of an intimate relationship that employs creative pet names, write these down and study their development over a course of a semester.

Suggested Readings

Kemper, S. (1992). Language and aging. In F. Craik & T. Salthouse (Eds.), *The handbook of aging and cognition* (pp. 213–270). Hillsdale, NJ: Lawrence Erlbaum Associates.

Kemper, S., Rash, S., Kynette, D., & Norman, S. (1990). Telling stories: The structure of adults' narratives. *European Journal of Cognitive Psychology, 2,* 205–228.

Nicholas, M., Barth, C., Obler, L. K., Au, R., & Albert, M. L. (1997). Naming in normal aging and dementia of the Alzheimer's type. In H. Goodglass & A. Wingfield (Eds.), *Anomia: Neuroanatomical and cognitive correlates* (pp. 166–188). San Diego: Academic Press.

Nicholas, M., Connor, L., Obler, L., & Albert, M. (1998). Aging, language, and language disorders. In M. Sarno (Ed.), *Acquired aphasia* (3rd ed.; pp. 413–450). San Diego: Academic Press.

Obler, L. K., & Gjerlow, K. (1999). *Language and the brain.* Cambridge, England: Cambridge University Press.

Skinner, B. F. (1983). Intellectual self-management in old age. *American Psychologist, 38,* 239–244.

References

Albert, M. L., & Obler, L. K. (1978). *The bilingual brain: Neuropsychological and neurolinguistic aspects of bilingualism.* New York: Academic Press.

Arbuckle, T., & Gold, D. P. (1993). Aging, inhibition, and verbosity. *Journal of Gerontology: Psychological Sciences, 48,* 225–232.

Au, R., Joung, P., Nicholas, M., Obler, L., Kass, R., & Albert, M. (1995). Naming ability across the adult lifespan. *Aging and Cognition, 2,* 300–311.

Barresi, B. (1996). Proper noun and common noun learning and recall. Unpublished Ph.D. dissertation at Emerson College.

Barresi, B., Nicholas, M., Connor, L., Obler, L. K., & Albert, M. L. (Submitted). Semantic degradation and lexical access in age-related naming failures.

Barresi, B., Obler, L. K., Au, R., & Albert, M. L. (1999). Language related factors influencing naming in adulthood. In H. Hamilton (Ed.), *Old age and language: Multidisciplinary perspectives.* New York: Garland Publishing Company.

Barth Ramsey, C., Nicholas, M., Au, R., Obler, L. K., & Albert, M. L. (1999). Verb naming in normal aging. *Applied Neuropsychology, 6*(2), 57–67.

Bartlett, C., Rubens, A., Holland, A., Barresi, B., & Satake, E. (in preparation). *Recovery of functional communication in aphasia: Effects of age and severity.* Manuscript in preparation.

Bates, E., Marchman, V., Harris, C., Wulfeck, B., & Kritchevsky, M. (1995). Production of complex syntax in normal aging and Alzheimer's disease. *Language and Cognitive Processes, 10,* 487–539.

Bayles, K., & Kaszniak, A. (1987). *Communication and cognition in normal aging and dementia.* Boston: Little Brown.

Bayles, K., & Tomoeda, L. (1983). Confrontation naming impairment in dementia. *Brain and Language, 19,* 98–114.

Bergman, M. (1980). *Aging and the perception of speech.* Baltimore: University Park Press.

Berko Gleason, J. (1978). The acquisition and dissolution of the English inflectional system. In A. Caramazza & E. Zurif (Eds.), *Language acquisition and language breakdown.* Baltimore: Johns Hopkins University Press.

Bloom, R., Borod, J., Obler, L. K., & Gerstman, L. (1992). Impact of emotional content on discourse production in patients with unilateral brain damage. *Brain and Language, 42,* 153–164.

Bloom, R., Borod, J., Obler, L. K., & Gerstman, L. (1994). Suppression and facilitation of pragmatic performance. *Journal of Speech and Hearing Research.*

Borod, J., & Goodglass, H. (1980). Hemispheric specialization and development. In L. Obler & M. Albert (Eds.), *Language and communication in the elderly: Clinical, therapeutic, and experimental issues.* Lexington, MA: D.C. Heath.

Botwinick, J., West, R., & Storandt, M. (1975). Qualitative vocabulary responses and age. *Journal of Gerontology, 30,* 574–577.

Bromley, D. B. (1991). Aspects of written language production over adult life. *Psychology and Aging, 6,* 296–308.

Brown, J., & Jaffe, J. (1975). Hypothesis on cerebral dominance. *Neuropsychologia, 13,* 107–110.

Brownell, H., Gardner, H. J., Prather, P., and Martino, G. (1995). Language, communication, and the right hemisphere. In H. S. Kirshner (Ed.), *Handbook of neurological speech and language disorders* (pp. 325–349). New York: Marcel Dekker.

Brownell, H., Michel, D., Powelston, J., & Gardner, H. (1983). Surprise but not coherence: Sensitivity to verbal humor in right hemisphere patients. *Brain and Language, 18,* 20–27.

Bryan, J., Luszcz, M., & Crawford, J. (1997). Verbal knowledge and speed of information processing as mediators of age differences in verbal fluency performance among older adults. *Psychology and Aging, 12,* 473–478.

Burke, D. (1997). Language, aging, and inhibitory deficits: Evaluation of a theory. *Journal of Gerontology: Psychological Sciences, 52B,* 254–264.

Caramazza, A., & Zurif, E. (1978). *Language acquisition and language breakdown: Parallels and divergencies.* Baltimore: Johns Hopkins University Press.

Causino, M., Obler, L., Knoefel, J., & Albert, M. (1994). Spared pragmatic abilities in late-stage Alzheimer's disease. In L. K. Obler, R. Bloom, S. De Santi, & J. Ehrlich (Eds.), *Discourse in clinical populations.* Hillsdale, NJ: Lawrence Erlbaum.

Chaika, E. (1980). Jargons and language change. *Anthropological Linguistics, 22,* 77–96.

Charrow, V. (1982). Linguistic theory and the study of legal and bureaucratic language. In L. Obler & L. Menn (Eds.), *Exceptional language and linguistics.* New York: Academic Press.

Clark, L., & Knowles, J. (1973). Age differences in dichotic listening performance. *Journal of Gerontology, 28* , 173–178.

Clyne, M. (1977). Bilingualism of the elderly. *Talanya, 4,* 45–56.

Cohen, G. (1979). Language comprehension in old age. *Cognitive Psychology, 11,* 412–429.

Cohen, G., & Burke, D. (1993). Memory for proper names: A review. *Memory, 1,* 249–263.

Corso, J. (1977). Auditory perception and communication. In J. Birren & K. W. Schaie (Eds.), *The psychology of aging.* New York: Van Nostrand Reinhold.

de Bot, K., & Clyne, M. (1989). Language reversion revisited. *Studies in Second Language Acquisition, 11,* 167–177.

Dennis, M., & Whitaker, H. (1976). Language acquisition following hemi-decortication: Linguistic superiority of the left over the right hemisphere. *Brain and Language, 3,* 404–433.

De Santi, S., Obler, L., Sabo-Abramson, H., & Goldberger, J. (1989). Discourse abilities and deficits in multilingual dementia. In Y. Joanette & H. Brownell (Eds.), *Discourse abilities in brain damage: Theoretical and empirical perspectives.* New York: Springer.

Dywan, J., & Murphy, W. (1996). Aging and inhibitory control in text comprehension. *Psychology and Aging, 11,* 199–206.

Edel, L. (1953–69). *Henry James* (4 vols.). London: Hart-Davis.

Edelsky, C. (1981). Who's got the floor. *Language in Society, 10,* 383–421.

Ehrlich, J. (1990). *Influence of structure on the content of oral narrative in adults with dementia of the Alzheimer's type.* Unpublished doctoral dissertation, CUNY Graduate School.

Ehrlich, J., Obler, L., Clark, L., & Gerstman, L., (1995). Influence of structure on narrative production in adults with dementia of the Alzheimer's type. *Journal of Communication Disorders.*

Elgin, S. (1983). *The gentle art of verbal self-defense.* Englewood Cliffs, NJ: Prentice-Hall.

Emery, O. (1985). Language in aging. *Experimental Aging Research, 11,* 3–59.

Foldi, N. (1983). Sensitivity to indirect commands by right- and left-hemisphere brain-damaged adults. (Doctoral dissertation, Clark University, 1983). *Dissertation Abstracts International, 44,* 1958B.

Gardner, H. (1982). Dictated by necessity, or every man his own Boswell. In *Art, mind, and brain* (pp. 257–261). New York: Basic Books.

Goodglass, H. (1980). Naming disorders in aphasia and aging. In L. K. Obler & M. L. Albert (Eds.), *Language and communication in the elderly: Clinical, therapeutic, and experimental issues.* Lexington, MA: D.C. Heath.

Goodglass, H., & Kaplan, E. (1972). *Assessment of aphasia and related disorders.* Philadelphia: Lea and Febiger.

Goulet, P., Ska, B., & Kahn, H. (1994). Is there a decline in picture naming with advancing age? *Journal of Speech and Hearing Research, 37,* 629–644.

Grimshaw, A., & Holden, L. (1976). Postchildhood modifications of linguistic and social competence. *Social Science Research Council Items, 30,* 33–42.

Guiora, A., Brammer, R., & Dull, C. (1972). Empathy and second language learning. *Language Learning, 22,* 111–130.

Guttman, E. (1942). Aphasia in children. *Brain, 65* , 205–219.

Haley, J. (1963). *Strategies of psychotherapy.* New York: Grune & Stratton.

Harris, J., Rogers, W., & Qualls, C. (1998). Written language comprehension in younger and older adults. *Journal of Speech, Language and Hearing Research, 41,* 603–617.

Henderson, V., Buckwalter, J., Sobel, E., Freed, D., & Diz, M. (1992). The agraphia of Alzheimer's disease. *Neurology, 42,* 776–784.

Hornstein, G. (1983). Intimate conversations among women. Paper presented at the Association for Women in Psychology Conference, Seattle.

Hubert, L., Scherr, P., Beckett, L., Albert, M. S., Pilgrim, D., Chown, M., Funkenstein, H., & Evans, D. (1995). Age-specific incidence of Alzheimer's disease in a community population. *Journal of the American Medical Association, 273,* 1354–1359.

Hyltenstam, K., & Stroud, C. (1989). Bilingualism in Alzheimer's dementia: Two case studies. In K. Hyltenstam & L. K. Obler (Eds.), *Bilingualism across the lifespan: Aspects of acquisition, maturity, and loss.* Cambridge, UK: Cambridge University Press.

Jakobson, R. (1941/1968). *Child language, aphasia, and phonological universals.* The Hague: Mouton.

Johnson, R., Cole, R., Bowers, J., Foiles, S., Nakaido, A., Patrick, J., & Woliver, R. (1979). Hemispheric efficiency in middle and later adulthood. *Cortex, 15,* 109–119.

Juncos-Rabadan, O., & Iglesias, F. (1994). Decline in the elderly's language: Evidence from cross-linguistic data. *Journal of Neurolinguistics, 8,* 183–190.

Kahn, H., & Till, R. (1991). Pronoun reference and aging. *Developmental Neuropsychology, 7,* 459–475.

Kalikow, D., Stevens, K., & Elliot, L. (1977). Development of a test of speech intelligibility in noise using sentence materials with controlled word predictability. *Journal of the Acoustic Society of America, 61,* 1337–1351.

Kemper, S. (1987). Syntactic complexity and the recall of prose by middle-aged and elderly adults. *Experimental Aging Research, 13,* 47–52.

Kemper, S., Rash, S., Kynette, D., & Norman, S. (1990). Telling stories: The structure of adults' narratives. *European Journal of Cognitive Psychology, 2,* 205–228.

Kempler, D., & Van Lancker, D. (1988). Proverb and idiom comprehension in Alzheimer's disease. *Alzheimer's Disease and Associated Disorders, 2,* 38–49.

Kramer, C. (1975). Women's speech: Separate but unequal? In C. Thorne & N. Henley (Eds.), *Language and sex: Difference and dominance.* Rowley, MA: Newbury House.

Kucera, H., & Francis, W. N. (1967). *Computational analysis of present-day American English.* Providence, RI: Brown University Press.

Kynette, D., & Kemper, S. (1986). Aging and the loss of grammatical forms. *Language and Communication, 6,* 65–72.

Labov, W., & Fanshel, D. (1977). *Therapeutic discourse: Psychotherapy as conversation.* New York: Academic Press.

Lambert, W. (1972). *Language, psychology, and culture.* Palo Alto, CA: Stanford University Press.

Lenneberg, E. (1967). *Biological foundations of language.* New York: Wiley.

Lovelace, E. A., & Cooley, S. (1982). Free association of older adults to single words and conceptually related words and triads. *Journal of Gerontology, 37,* 432–437.

Martin, J. (1983, March 28). Miss Manners. *Boston Globe.*

McNamara, P., Obler, L., Au, R., & Albert, M. (1992). Speech repair processes in Alzheimer's disease, Parkinson disease and normal aging. *Brain and Language, 42,* 35–51.

Menn, L., & Obler, L. K. (Eds.). (1990). Summary chapter. *Agrammatic aphasia: A cross-language narrative sourcebook.* Amsterdam: Benjamins.

Miceli, G., Caltagirone, C., Gianotti, G., Masullo, C., Silveri, M., & Villa, G. (1981). Influence of age, sex, literacy and pathologic lesion on incidence, severity and type of aphasia. *Acta Neurologica Scandinavica, 64,* 370–382.

Murray, S. (1979). The art of gay insulting. *Anthropological Linguistics, 21,* 211–223.

Nebes, R. D., Martin, D.C., & Horn, L. C. (1984). Sparing of semantic memory in Alzheimer's disease. *Journal of Abnormal Psychology, 93,* 331–330.

Nicholas, M., Obler, L., Albert, M., & Goodglass, H. (1985). Lexical retrieval in healthy aging and in Alzheimer's dementia. *Cortex, 21,* 595–606.

Nicholas, M., Obler, L. K., Au, R., & Albert, M. L. (1996). On the nature of naming errors in aging and dementia: A study of semantic relatedness, *Brain and Language, 54,* 184–195.

Novoa, L., Fein, D., & Obler, L. (1988). A neuropsychological study of an exceptional second language learner. In L. Obler & D. Fein (Eds.), *The exceptional brain: The neuropsychology of talent and special abilities.* New York: Guilford Press.

Obler, L. (1980). Narrative discourse style in the elderly. In L. Obler & M. Albert (Eds.), *Language and communication in the elderly.* Lexington, MA: D.C. Heath.

Obler, L. (1981). Review of *Le langage des déments* by Luce Irigaray. *Brain and Language, 12,* 375–386.

Obler, L., Fein, D., Nicholas, M., & Albert, M. L. (1991). Auditory comprehension and aging: Decline in syntactic processing. *Journal of Applied Psycholinguistics, 12,* 433–452.

Obler, L., Nicholas, M., Albert, M. L., & Woodward, S. (1985). On comprehension across the adult lifespan. *Cortex, 21,* 273–280.

Obler, L., Woodward, S., & Albert, M. (1984). Lateralization in aging? *Neuropsychologia, 22,* 235–240.

Patterson, K., Graham, N., & Hodges, J. R. (1994). Reading in dementia of the Alzheimer type: A preserved ability? *Neuropsychology, 8,* 395–407.

Qualls, C. (1998). *Figurative language comprehension in younger and older African Americans.* Dissertation submitted.

Ribot, T. (1882). *Diseases of memory: An essay in the positive psychology.* London: Paul.

Riegel, K. (1968). Changes in psycholinguistic performance with age. In G. Talland (Ed.), *Human aging and behavior.* New York: Academic Press.

Rochford, G. (1971). A study of naming errors in dysphasic and in demented patients. *Neuropsychologia, 9,* 437–443.

Rochon, E., Waters, G., & Caplan, D. (1994). Sentence comprehension in patients with Alzheimer's disease. *Brain and Language, 46,* 329–349.

Romaine, S. (1984). *The language of children and adolescents: The acquisition of communicative competence.* Oxford: Blackwell.

Rosen, S. (Ed.). (1982). *My voice will go with you: The teaching tales of Milton H. Erickson.* New York: Norton.

Rosenberg, B. A. (1970). *The art of the American folk preacher.* New York: Oxford University Press.

Sankoff, G. (1970). Mutual intelligibility, bilingualism and linguistic boundaries. In *International days of sociolinguistics* (pp. 839–848). Rome: Institut Luigi Sturzo.

Sarno, M. T. (1980). Language rehabilitation outcome in the elderly aphasic patient. In L. K. Obler & M. L. Albert (Eds.), *Language and communication in the elderly: Clinical, therapeutic, and experimental issues.* Lexington, MA: D.C. Heath.

Schwartz, M., Marin, O., & Saffran, E. (1979). Dissociations of language function in dementia: A case study. *Brain and Language, 7,* 277–306.

Schwartz, M., Saffran, E., & Marin, O. (1980). Fractionating the reading process in dementia: Evidence for word specific print-to-sound associations. In M. Coltheart, K. Patterson, & J. Marshall (Eds.), *Deep dyslexia* (pp. 259–269). London: Routledge & Kegan Paul.

Scovel, T. (1969). Foreign accents, language acquisition, and cerebral dominance. *Language Learning, 19,* 245–254.

Shuy, R. (1979). Language policy in medicine: Some emerging issues. In J. Alatis & G. R. Tucker (Eds.), *Language in public life* (pp. 126–136). Washington, DC: Georgetown University Press.

Skinner, B. F. (1983). Intellectual self-management in old age. *American Psychologist, 38,* 239–244.

Smith, B., Wasowicz, J., & Preston, J. (1987). Temporal characteristics of the speech of normal elderly adults. *Journal of Speech and Hearing Research, 30,* 522–529.

Snow, C. (1987). Relevance of the notion of a critical period to language acquisition. In M. Bornstein (Ed.), *Sensitive periods in development* (pp. 183–209). Hillsdale, NJ: Lawrence Erlbaum.

Tannen, D. (1990). *You just don't understand: Women and men in conversation.* New York: William Morrow.

Thorndike, E., & Lorge, I. (1944). *The teacher's word book of 30,000 words.* New York: Teacher's College Press.

Tomoeda, C., & Bayles, K. (1993). Longitudinal effects of Alzheimer's disease on discourse production. *Alzheimer Disease and Dissociated Disorders, 7,* 223–236.

Ulatowska, H., Cannito, M., Hayashi, M., & Fleming, S. (1985). Language abilities in the elderly. In H. Ulatowska (Ed.), *The aging brain: Communication in the elderly.* San Diego: College-Hill Press.

Verhaegen, P., Marcoen, A., & Goossens, L. (1993). Facts and fiction about memory aging: A quantitative integration of research findings. *Journal of Gerontology: Psychological Sciences, 48,* 157–171.

Warren, R. M., & Warren, R. P. (1966). A comparison of speech perception in childhood, maturity, and old age by means of the verbal transformation effect. *Journal of Verbal Learning and Verbal Behavior, 5,* 142–146.

Wechsler, D. (1955). *Manual for the Wechsler Adult Intelligence Scale.* New York: Psychological Corporation.

Wingfield, A., Prentice, K., Koh, C., & Little, D. (in press). Neural change, cognitive reserve and behavioral compensation in rapid encoding and memory for spoken language in adult aging. In L. Connor & L. K. Obler, Eds. *Neurobehavior of language and cognition: Studies of normal aging and brain damage.* Boston: Kluwer Academic Publishers.

Wingfield, A., Goodglass, H., Berko Gleason, J., Bowles, N., & Hyde, M. R. (1988). *A process model for naming and its aberrations.* Unpublished manuscript.

Zabrucky, K., Moore, D., & Schultz, N. (1993). Young and old adults' ability to use different standards to evaluate understanding. *Journal of Gerontology: Psychological Sciences, 38,* 238–244.

Glossary

This glossary defines words as they are used in this book. Many of the words (i.e., *competence*, *assimilation*) are technical terms here that have very different meanings in other contexts.

additive bilingualism   Learning a second language while retaining one's original language.

adolescent register   Special forms of speech used by adolescents to mark themselves as adolescents.

affricatives/affricates   Sounds are a combination of a stop and fricative, such as the voiced sound at the beginning of *judge* or the unvoiced sound at the beginning of *church.*

African American Vernacular English (AAVE) A variety of English spoken by many African Americans that is characterized in by its phonological, syntactic, and pragmatic features.

agglutinated   Characterizes languages like Turkish, which add separate inflectional suffixes for masculine, plural, etc. in a predictable order. Contrasts with *synthetic.*

allomorph   Any one of the possible phonetic forms of a morpheme; for example, the English possessive ending, spelled *s,* has three allomorphs: /s/, /z/, and /əz/. Which allomorph is used depends on the final sound of the word.

alphabetic principle   The basic principle that underlies our orthographic system: Letters of the alphabet represent the sounds of our spoken language

alveolar   Refers to any consonant made with the tongue near or touching the alveolar ridge, behind the upper front teeth. English alveolar consonants include /t/, /d/, /n/, /s/, and /z/.

Alzheimer's disease   A progressive dementia characterized by the presence of neuronal plaques and tangles in the cerebral cortex.

American Sign Language   See *ASL*

Ameslan   See *ASL*

amplification   The use of hearing aids to improve impaired hearing ability.

analytic style   An early language acquisition strategy displayed by infants who have good comprehension and pay particular attention to individual words, rather than to phrases. Contrasts with *rote/holistic style.*

anaphora   Referring back to previous discourse through the use of pronouns, definite articles, and other linguistic devices. For example, "I saw a rainbow. *It* was beautiful."

anomia   Aphasic difficulty in producing nouns.

anomic   Without nouns. See *anomic aphasia.*

anomic aphasia   See *anomia.*

aphasia   Loss or impairment of language ability because of brain damage. Aphasic syndromes vary, depending on the site of the damage.

arcuate fasciculus   A band of subcortical fibers connecting Broca's area and Wernicke's area in the left hemisphere of the human brain. See *conduction aphasia.*

articulatory phonetics   The study of the types of sound waves produced by different shapes of the vocal tract when making speech sounds. This knowledge allows scientists to synthesize speech by reproducing the acoustic patterns.

ASL   American Sign Language. A complete language, related historically to French, this is the manual language used by the deaf community in the United States.

assimilation   Changing a sound in a word to make it more similar to an adjacent or nearby sound in that word or a neighboring word, e.g., *Assimilation* leads us to pronounce "greenbeans" as "greembeans."

audiologist   A professional who has the training and equipment to test the auditory acuity of a subject. If a child does not appear to be acquiring language in typical fashion, one of the first steps is to have her hearing tested by an *audiologist.*

auditory discrimination   The process of hearing accurately the individual sounds of language—for instance, the ability to hear the difference between *sat* and *fat.*

augmentative communication system   Any of a number of ways, such as communication boards, designed to help disabled individuals to communicate.

aural rehabilitation   The provision of therapy and training to individuals with hearing impairment.

autism   Childhood disorder, probably neurological in origin, characterized by stereotypic behavior, and a broad range of social, communicative, and intellectual deficiencies.

automaticity (automated)   The potential of a process to be completed with great speed after long practice, without allocating to it conscious attention. When a cognitive process becomes automatic, it does not require extra time or processing capacity.

baby talk   One of many names for the speech register used with young children. See *CDS.* The term is sometimes used to refer to the speech of young children, as well.

basic level category   The level of abstraction that is most generally appropiate in a given situation or for the given speaker, *dog,* rather than *animal* or *collie,* for instance.

behavioral modification   Guiding one's own or another's overt behavior, which is one of the many uses of language.

behaviorist   One who believes generally that the principles of learning can be used to explain most behavior and that observable events, rather than mental activity, are the proper objects of study.

binding principles   According to government and binding theory, these are part of the rules of our grammar that dictate the relation between words such as pronouns and their referents.

biological capacity   Innate factors, which are those present in the organism by virtue of its genetic makeup.

bottom-up model (processing)   A term taken from artificial intelligence to depict the *direction* of processing. In bottom-up models, reading is conceptualized as dependent on accurate decoding of the letter strings that make up words.

bound morpheme   A morpheme that occurs only bound to other morphemes; it cannot stand alone (e.g., the *s* in *cats*).

Broca's aphasia   See *Broca's area.*

Broca's area   Area of the left hemisphere in the frontal region. Damage to this area results in aphasia characterized by difficulty in producing speech.

canonical form   A sequence of phonological features expressing the properties that a group of highly similar words have in common.

caregiver   Any nurturing communicative partner with whom an infant interacts. Although traditionally mothers' speech has been studied, we now know that fathers, older siblings, and others can affect a child's linguistic development.

categorical perception   Two sounds with the same magnitude of acoustic difference are heard as different sounds if they fall into different phonemic categories, but they are heard as the same sound if they are from the same phonemic category.

CDS   Child-directed speech. The special speech register used when talking to children, including short sentences, greater repetition and questioning, and higher and more variable intonation than that of speech addressed to adults. See *Baby talk.*

cerebral palsy   A congenital motor disability that can affect an individual's ability to produce oral language. Various subgroups of cerebral palsied individuals exist (i.e., ataxic, spastic), reflecting damage to distinct areas of the brain before or at birth.

child-directed speech   See both *CDS* and *baby talk.*

childhood aphasia   Aphasia in a child, brought on by a traumatic accident, stroke, or other event that caused brain damage.

chronic otitis media   Middle-ear infection that may be present for months or years. See *otitis media.*

circumlocution   A way of talking *about* something without naming it directly.

classical concept   A concept that can be characterized by unchanging criteria: For instance, a *bachelor* can be defined as one who is not married.

classical conditioning   A form of learning in which previously neutral stimuli (e.g., words) through repeated pairings with other stimuli come to elicit similar responses. First described by Pavlov.

cleft palate   A congenital disability (caused by defects in the bone or tissue separating the oral and nasal cavities) that impairs control of the oral air pressure necessary for the articulation of many speech sounds.

closed-class word   In language, this is one of a small group of words with a role that is basically grammatical in nature, such as articles and prepositions in English. Also called *function word,* q.v.

cochlear implant   Device that is surgically implanted in the inner ear in to stimulate the acoustic/auditory nerve of a person suffering from deafness.

code-oriented   One kind of style exhibited by children learning language. Code-oriented children emphasize reference to things in their language.

code switching   Switching from one language, or dialect, to another in the course of a conversation.

collective monologue   A type of egocentric speech described by Piaget in which children appear to take turns but the content of their messages is completely unrelated or related only by accident.

color term   Any word that refers to a color, e.g., "magenta."

comment   An early communicative function, also called a *declarative,* in which an infant calls a caregiver's attention to something in the surroundings, often by gesturing or pointing.

communication boards   Devices that allow speech-impaired individuals to gesture toward written or pictorial images to assist their communication efforts.

communicative competence   Linguistic competence plus knowledge of the social rules for language use. The speaker has phonological, morphological, syntactic, and semantic knowledge and the additional knowledge necessary to use language appropriately in social situations.

communicative temptation tasks   Tasks designed to elicit communication efforts from an infant.

communicative functions   The purposes for which language is used. For instance, even infants use language to express rejection, requests, and comments.

competence   Linguists' term for the inner knowledge one has of language and all of its linguistic rules and structures.

competition model   A model of language development based on PDP networks that assumes that various cues in the language environment compete with one another. The most available and reliable cues will be learned first. Developed by Bates & MacWhinney.

compound word   A word composed of two or more free morphemes, (e.g., *blackboard, merry-go-round*).

comprehension   The understanding of language. Comprehension typically precedes *production*, q.v., and is governed by a different set of constraints.

conduction aphasia   An aphasic syndrome characterized by inability to repeat; typically resulting from damage to the arcuate fasciculus.

confrontation naming   The ability to name items when provided with visual stimuli.

congenital   Present at birth, but not necessarily genetic in origin.

consonant   Any speech sound made by constricting the vocal tract enough to impede air flow through the mouth. Consonants include stops, affricates, fricatives, nasal stops, and liquids. Glides (semi-vowels) are sometimes grouped with consonants.

consonant clusters   Two or more consonants that occur together in a word, without intervening vowels. Permissible sequences and position within the word (initial, medial, or final) are dictated by the phonological rules of the language.

constraints   Limits or biases that children bring to the task of acquiring language. A constraint may dictate a cognitive strategy in the interpretation of words. One early constraint leads children to assume that a new word refers to a *whole object,* rather than to a part of the object.

content word   Also called *open class word.* Nouns, verbs, and modifiers within a language are considered content words; words such as articles and auxiliary verbs are considered function words or functors.

content validity   A measure of the goodness of a test, based on the relation between the contents of the test and what it purports to be testing. A language test with high content validity would test many areas representing real language use.

controlling interactional style   See *intrusive interactional style.*

convergent validity   Truth or consensus arrived at as a result of investigation by different investigators, often using divergent methods.

coordinations   Grammatical combinations that can involve two or more sentences, connected by conjunctions, or combined phrases (e.g., *Sue and Bill ate and drank*).

core group   A small subset of the vocabulary of a child, used very frequently.

cue availability   In the competition model, a measure of the frequency of appearance of any particular cue in the language environment.

cued speech A manual system used by some deaf children and their teachers/parents, that uses handshapes near the mouth to help make lipreading easier.

d-structure In linguistic theory *d-structure* refers to the level of a grammar that captures the relationship between subject and object in a sentence.

decibel (dB) A measure of the loudness of a sound.

declarative communicative function See *comment*.

decontextualized language Language that makes reference to people, events, and experiences that are not part of the immediate context.

deep orthography An orthography (spelling system) in which there is a relatively variable relation (e.g., more than one-to-one) between graphemes and phonemes (see *shallow orthography*).

deictic terms From the Greek *deiktikos* (able to show); words that are used as linguistic pointers, e.g., *here, there*. Also called *deixis*.

dementia Loss of mental ability, typically through neurological impairment, such as Alzheimer's disease.

dementing disease Any disease that causes a loss of mental ability.

derivational morpheme A morpheme that can be used to derive a new word. See *derived word*.

derived word A complex word made from a base morpheme to which various affixes have been added: for instance, *unhappiness* is derived from *happy* by the addition of the affixes *un-* and *-ness*.

descriptive adequacy Characteristic of a model or theory that assures that it is capable of describing and cataloguing all relevant behaviors and distinguishing them from those that are not relevant.

developmental disfluency A stage of normal child language development during which many children demonstrate stuttering-like behaviors.

developmental dysphasia Congenital language disability in the absence of obvious cognitive, perceptual or neurological deficits. A more current term is *specific language impairment*.

dialect A systematic subvariety of a language spoken by a sizable group of speakers sharing characteristics such as geographical origin or social class.

diphthongized Said of vowels that change as they are produced, usually finishing with a glide.

disfluencies Breaks in the ongoing rhythm of speech, such as those caused by hesitations, repetitions, or the use of fillers like "um," "well," etc.

Down syndrome A congenital condition, usually caused by trisomy of the 21st chromosome, often characterized by short stature, typical epicanthic eyefolds, and mental retardation of varying degrees.

dramatist One kind of individual style displayed by children learning language, who prefer to represent human interaction in their symbolic play.

dummy syllable A place holder, or empty phonological form. Some children learning language use a dummy syllable in place of all unstressed initial syllables.

dyslexia (developmental dyslexia) Any one of a number of conditions that lead to a specific impairment in learning to read; dyslexias are typically linguistic processing problems, rather than difficulties with perception.

early communicative function   The prelinguistic child's early expression of intentionality (e.g., requesting or commenting), often accomplished through gaze or gesture.

early language delay (ELD)   Difficulty with language production and failure to combine words by the age of two, in the presence of good comprehension.

echolalia   Repetition of all or part of another's utterance as one's turn in a conversation; common in children with autism, but also seen in normally developing young children.

egocentrism; egocentric speech   Piaget's concept meaning the inability to take another person's perspective. Speech not adapted to listener needs, e.g., using color terms to direct the action of a blindfolded listener.

emergent literacy   Children's understanding about reading and writing before they actually acquire these skills; this understanding is enhanced in households that engage in many reading and writing activities.

empiricism   A theoretical approach emphasizing observable, environmental explanations of behavior.

environmental print   Writing found on traffic signs, food and household goods packaging, etc. Often the first words a child recognizes.

etiology   The cause of a particular problem, such as hearing loss, that may arise from a large number of genetic and environmental conditions.

expansion   A parent's repetition of a child's utterance that supplies necessary forms that the child has omotted.

expository writing   Writing that depends upon logic, rather than chronology, as its organizational principle. Hierarchically organized language that is associated with the paradigmatic mode of thinking.

expressive style   A speech style observed in toddlers that is characterized by the use of many personal-social terms.

expressive writing   Informal, personal writing, such as letters to friends.

Extended Optional Infinitive account of SLI   The hypothesis that children with specific language impairment have failed to progress beyond the early stage of typical development during which children learning English appear to believe that marking of tense in main clauses is optional.

facilitated communication (FC)   A method, largely discredited, of aiding communication efforts of people with autism by holding and guiding their arms as they write.

fast mapping   Children's ability to form an initial hypothesis about a word's meaning very quickly, after hearing it only once or twice; in-depth learning requires multiple exposures to the word in many different contexts, however.

feature-blind dysphasia   A grammatical deficit characterized by difficulty in using grammatical morphemes, such as the forms of the past tense. Some researchers have claimed that this disability is genetically determined.

focal colors   Among colors, those that are the most typical, the reddest reds and bluest blues.

folk etymology   An explanation of a word's origin that is not based on the actual historical record, but rather on common sense or custom: "It's called *Friday* because that's the day you eat fried fish."

format/scaffold   In Vygotskyian theory, adults are thought to provide intellectual interaction that serves as a scaffold, or format, that makes it possible for children to develop at a much faster rate than they could without this helpful intervention.

Fragile X sayndrome A genetic disorder, most often seen in males. The X chromosome is defective, and the affected individual may have communication problems.

free morpheme A morpheme that can stand alone (e.g., *cat*), as opposed to a bound morpheme.

free-word association A word association in which the subject responds freely with the first word that comes to mind.

free variation Allophones that can appear in the same environment without changes in meaning are said to be in *free variation.* For instance, /t/ can be released, unreleased, aspirated, unaspirated when one says "hat."

fricative A speech sound produced partly or wholly by airstream friction, such as /s/ or /v/.

functional articulation disorders Disturbances in articulation with no known etiology or cause.

functional category A grammatical category within the d-structure of a sentence, containing inflectional, complementizer, and other similar elements.

functionalism A theoretical approach emphasizing the functions or uses of any behavior (e.g., the function of requesting) rather than the structure of the behavior itself.

gaze aversion Failure to make appropriate eye contact. Parents of autistic infants often will notice gaze aversion as the very first sign of abnormality

gaze coupling A type of mutual eye contact that is very important to caregivers in establishing the original affective bond with the infant.

generalization A learning principle, whereby what is learned in specific context is extended to new instances.

Generalized Slowing Hypothesis An explanation of SLI that is based on the observation that children with SLI need about one-third more time to execute a range of perceptual and motor functions than typically developing children. SLI is believed to be related to the children's limited processing capacity.

glide A speech sound made with slightly more vocal tract constriction than a vowel and having shorter duration than a vowel. The sounds /j/ and /w/ are glides. They are also referred to as semi-vowels.

global aphasia Aphasia resulting from extensive brain damage; the patient has poor comprehension and little voluntary language. See *aphasia.*

glottal Pertaining to the glottis.

glottis The opening at the upper part of the larynx, between the vocal folds.

government and binding theory (GB) A model of grammar descended from earlier Transformational Generative models. It proposes only one type of transformation (movement of elements), the specification of possible grammatical frames for lexical items and their mapping onto the syntax of sentences, and universal constraints on possible syntactic rules, among many other notions.

grammar Finite set of rules shared by all speakers of a language that allows generation of all possible sentences.

grapheme The written symbol of a particular writing system; e.g., a letter in the alphabet.

grapheme–phoneme correspondence rules Rules that define the relationship between a letter or group of letters and the sound they represent.

hearing impairment   Loss or inability to hear sounds; children who cannot hear sounds below 60 decibels do not usually develop typical oral language.

high amplitude sucking (HAS)   A technique used to study infant perceptual abilities. Typically involves recording an infant's sucking rate as a measure of her attention to various stimuli.

hyperlexia   Unusually advanced lexical ability.

illocutionary act/intent   The goal or intentions of a speaker, which may be to persuade, inform, or make a request, for instance. Austin's label in speech act theory, for the speaker's purpose in producing an utterance.

imitation   A kind of learning, in which the learner observes a model and performs the same actions that the model has performed. Imitation can be immediate or delayed.

immersion   Settings in which a group of learners are all taught a new language through the medium of the new language

imperative trap   An attempt to increase one's power by addressing an unusually direct request to a listener

imperative communicative function   An early communicative function, in which an infant indicates that she wants the caregiver to perform some action.

Index of Productive Syntax (IPsyn)   A method of evaluating children's spontaneous language that relies upon scoring a sample for the presence of various grammatical forms.

indirect request   A form of request whose surface structure does not indicate that the utterance is a request (e.g., a hint)

infant-directed speech   Speech directed at infants that contains special modifications (e.g., high fundamental frequency, variable intonation). See *baby talk, CDS.*

inhibition   In the sense used by cognitive psychologists, the ability to ignore irrelevant stimuli. This seems to become more difficult with advancing age.

innate   Present at birth, part of an organism's essential nature.

intentional communication   Any communicative act that an individual engages in purposefully.

interdental   Speech sound made by placing the tongue between the teeth: The initial sounds of "this" or "thing" in English.

internalized representation   The mental, or inner cognitive image or map of external reality.

intonation contour   The pattern of rhythmic stress and pitch across an utterance. In English, a falling pitch at the end of an utterance typically indicates a statement, whereas a final rising pitch usually marks an interrogative.

intrusive interactional style   A way of interacting with an infant in which the caregiver is constantly controlling and redirecting the child's attention.

invented spelling   Systematic, rule-governed spelling that is created (invented) by developing writers.

IPsyn   See *Index of Productive Syntax.*

irony   Using words to convey the opposite of their literal meaning, e.g., "It's so clean in here," said of a messy dorm room.

joint attention   Situation in which two individuals are paying attention to the same thing at the same time, as in reading a book together.

kinship term   Word that refers to familial relationships (e.g., *aunt, cousin*).

labial   Any speech sound made by bringing the lips close together or making them touch one another. The English labials are /p/, /b/, and /m/.

labiodental   Any speech sound made by bringing the lower lip close to or in contact with the upper teeth. The English labiodentals are the fricatives /f/ and /v/.

LAD   Language Acquisition Device. The innate mental mechanism that, according to linguistic theorists, makes language acquisition possible.

language acquisition device   See *LAD.*

language age (LA)   A measure of a child's language development, based on her mean length of utterance.

lateralization   The process whereby one side of the brain becomes specialized for particular functions; for instance, the left side becomes *lateralized* for language.

learnability theories   Various models of language acquisition based on several assumptions concerning the nature of children, known learning mechanisms, and the structure of language and the logical inferences that may be drawn from these assumptions. Developed by Pinker, Wexler, and others.

letter recognition   Detection of the features of a letter.

lexical category   One of the categories of the d-structure that includes content words and their meanings, according to GB theory.

limited scope formulae   Simple combinatorial rules followed by children at the two-word stage of language development.

linguistic competence   See *competence.*

lipreading (speechreading)   Decoding the language of a speaker by close attention to the face and mouth, without being able to hear the speaker's voice.

liquid   A consonantal speech sound made with less oral constriction than a fricative but more constriction than a glide. The English *liquids* are /l/ and /r/.

locutionary act   Austin's label, in speech act theory, for the act of saying a sentence that makes sense and refers to something.

logical form   The component of the s-structure in government and binding theory that captures the meaning of the sentence and connects it to other parts of cognition.

long-term memory abilities   The capacities to retrieve and manipulate information that has been permanently stored in memory.

low-structured observation   A method of studying young children that often relies upon free play with a standard set of toys.

MacArthur Communicative Development Inventories (CDI)   Norms that are available for various aspects of language development, based on a large study that collected mothers' reports on their children's communicative behaviors. There are two scales, one infants and one for toddlers.

manual approach to deaf education   Any of a number of sign systems using the hands that have been developed to further the linguistic development of deaf children.

manually coded English   A sign system meant to represent English (rather than ASL).

matched guise model   An experimental paradigm in which listeners make judgments about the characteristics of speakers of different languages or dialects, without knowing that the supposed speakers are actually just one person who is multilingual. This makes it possible to show attitudes toward the language, since the speaker is constant.

mean length of utterance.   See *MLU.*

means-ends concept   Children at Stage 4 of the Piaget's sensorimotor stage of cognitive development begin to understand *causality* (have a concept of *means-ends*), and learn to communicate intentionally, lending support to the notion that certain cognitive developments might be prerequisites to language acquisition.

mental age (MA)   A measure of a child's intelligence, based on answers to age-graded questions (typical of standard IQ tests.) For instance, a six-year-old who can answer questions that are most typically answered only by eight-year-olds, will be said to have a mental age of eight.

mental retardation (MR)   A cognitive deficit of varying etiology. Individuals with *mental retardation* score two or more standard deviations below the mean on IQ tests, with measurable IQS of 70 or less.

message-oriented   An individual style of language acquisition that emphasizes the social situation, rather than reference to things.

metalinguistic knowledge (awareness) Knowledge about language, for instance an understanding of what a word is and a consciousness of the sounds of language. The ability to think about language.

metaphor   Figure of speech in which one thing is called by the name of another to indicate the similarities between them: "This room is a pig pen."

minimal pair   A pair of words that differ in meaning and whose sounds are the same except for one phonetic segment. For example "ram/ran" form a *minimal pair* differing only in the final consonant; "ram/rim" form a minimal pair differing only with respect to the vowel.

MLU   Mean length of utterance. A measure applied to children's language to gauge syntactic development; the average length of the child's utterances is calculated in morphemes.

model   An attempt to explain any currently unexplained phenomenon by reference to a possibly similar, but understood phenomenon.

modeling   A therapeutic technique in which the therapist enacts the desired behavior as a model for the client.

model adequacy   Characteristic of a theory or model that includes principles that can account for the relevant behaviors.

modulated babble   Babble with intonation contours resembling those of adult speech. Because intonation carries some aspects of meaning, modulated babble can be used (especially in conjunction with gesture) for communicative purposes even though the sound sequences themselves are meaningless.

monophthongs   Vowel sounds that do not change into glides as they are pronounced. In English, the vowel in "hot" is a *monophthong,* whereas the vowel in "hate" is *diphthongized,* q.v.

morpheme   A minimal meaningful unit of language. A *free morpheme* (e.g., "cat") can stand alone. A bound morpheme (e.g., the plural **s** on "cats") must always be connected to another morpheme.

morphology   The rules that govern the use of morphemes in a language; for instance the *morphology* of English requires that plural endings vary according to the last sound of the word stem.

morphophonology   The rules governing sound changes that accompany the combination of morphemes in a language.

mutual exclusivity   A cognitive bias shown by children, who typically avoid labeling anything at more than one level of generality:

hence they may refer to their pet as a "dog," but not also as an "animal."

narrative mode Thinking that reflects human intentions and is organized around chronology.

narratives Stories, usually about the past. A minimum narrative consists of two sequential clauses, temporally ordered, about a single past event.

narrative writing Writing that uses the natural flow of time as its organizational principle.

nasal, nasal stop A speech sound made with the velum lowered so that air can escape through the nose. English nasals include /m/, /n/, and /ŋ/ (the sound at the end of *sing*).

nativism A theoretical approach emphasizing the innate, possibly genetic contributions to any behavior.

nativist One who believes that language (or other development) is basically preprogrammed in the individual, not the product of learning.

natural processes The errors patterns and the rules describing them that result from children's early attempts to produce words, while they are still learning to control their articulatory apparatus.

negation The process of making a sentences negative, usually by adding "no" or "not" and auxiliary articles, when appropriate.

negative evidence Evidence concerning language errors or unacceptable combinations of sounds or words.

neglected children Children whose caregivers have not given them sufficient physical, emotional, or intellectual support to ensure healthy development.

neologism A new, made up word, often not a word in the language, as when a Wernicke's aphasic patient refers to an ashtray as a "fremser."

nominalist fallacy The belief that simply naming a phenomenon also sufficiently explains that phenomenon.

nominal strategy Choice of words by young children who prefer to use nouns in their early two-word sentences, rather than pronouns.

nonreflexive vocalizations Describing a process that has some voluntary component. Reflexive crying in infants, soon develops into *nonreflexive crying*.

novel name-nameless category principle A strategy followed by young language learners, who assume that if they hear a new word in the presence of an object whose name they do not know, the word refers to that object.

null-subject parameter See *parameter*.

object permanence The understanding that an infant gains during the latter part of the first year that objects continue to exist even though they may no longer be visible.

observer effect Changes in behavior that occur because a subject is being observed.

obstruent Any speech sound that constricts the vocal tract enough to cause airstream friction or that closes it off entirely. The *obstruents* of a language consist of the stops, affricates, and fricatives.

ontological categories Concepts about how the world is organized that young children have before they begin to learn language.

open-class word See *content word*.

operant conditioning A type of learning in which the learner emits a behavior in order to receive a reward. The learner thus *operates* on the environment.

oralist approach to deaf education An approach to deaf education that emphasizes auditory training, articulation ability, and lip-reading.

ostension　Pointing to referent; a technique used by mothers in teaching basic level categories. ("That's a taxi over there.")

otitis media　Infections of the middle ear that may, if chronic, affect a child's speech and language development.

overextension　Used here to refer to a child's use of a word in a broader context than is permissible in the adult language; for instance, an infant may call all men "daddy." Parents who call tigers "kitty" are also producing overextensions.

overlaid function　Said of most speech functions, because the organ systems on which they depend have a different primary function; thus, articulation of phonemes is *overlaid* on the tongue, an organ with a primary function involving eating.

overregularization errors　A common tendency among children and second language learners, *overregularization* involves applying regular and productive grammatical rules to words that are exceptions: "hurted" and "mouses," for example.

overregularized　An irregular form that has been (incorrectly) made regular (*foots, holded*).

palatal　A speech sound made on the hard palate. In English, the initial sound of "shirt" is a *palatal*.

paradigmatic　In word association tests, said of a word that is the same part of speech as a stimulus word (thus in the same paradigm).

paradigmatic mode　Thinking that is logical and scientific

parallel distributed processing (PDP)　Information theory term that refers to activity taking place at many levels at once, rather than sequentially, as in *serial processing*. PDP models explain grammatical development by analogy with the kinds associative links that computers can forge.

parameter　According to current theory, a parameter is a kind of linguistic switch that the young learner "sets" after exposure to the language; one of a finite number of values along which languages are free to vary. For example, the so-called pro-drop (null subject) parameter distinguishes languages such as English and German, which do not permit omission of lexical subjects, from languages such as Spanish or Italian, which do. See *null subject parameter*.

Parkinson's disease　A progressive disease, subcortical in nature, with primary effects in speech, rather than language.

passive　Sentence in which the object of action is highlighted: *The girl was kissed by the chimpanzee.*

patterner　A child who displays a style of early language acquisition that emphasizes physical characteristics and patterns in the world of objects.

PCF　See *phonetically consistent form*.

performance　Linguist's term for the production of speech. Contrasts with *competence*, which is almost always greater than *performance*.

perlocutionary act/effect　Austin's term in speech act theory for the effect that any particular utterance has on a listener. See *locutionary act, illocutionary intent*.

pervasive developmental disorder (PDD)　One of a number of generalized developmental syndromes, related to autism, but typically not as severe.

phone　An individual speech sound, the realization of a *phoneme* in a particular context.

phoneme   A speech sound that can signal a difference of meaning; two similar speech sounds *p* and *b* represent different phonemes in English because there are pairs of words with different meanings that have the same phonetic form except that one contains *b* where the other contains *p*, e.g., "pet" and "bet." See *minimal pair.*

phonetic form   A major component of the s-structure, according to government and binding theory. The *phonetic form* is the actual sound structure of the sentence.

phonetically consistent form (PCF)   A consistent sound pattern used in a consistent situation, not derived from the adult language. See *protoword.*

phonological working memory   Processing capacity for the sounds of language. One theory holds that SLI may be at least partially due to deficits in *phonological working memory.*

phonology   Study of the sound system of language. The sounds the language uses, as well as the rules for their combination.

phonotactics   The study of the permissible sequences of sounds in a language.

phrase structure rules   A major part of the *d-structure* (q.v.), according to GB theory, that captures the relation between subjects and predicates.

Piagetian Stage 4   A substage of the sensorimotor period of cognitive development that occurs between eight and twelve months, when infants begin to understand the relation between actions and outcomes.

place of articulation   The point or points in the vocal tract where the upper and lower articulators come closest together in the production of a particular phone.

poverty of imagination   In linguistic theory, the notion that just because one cannot imagine how language might be learned this does not prove that it was not learned (is innate).

pragmatics   The rules for the use of language in social context, and in conversation, or the study of these rules.

preferential looking paradigm   An experimental design used with prelinguistic infants that tracks their eye movements when they are presented with verbal stimuli.

prelingual hearing impairment   Hearing impairment that occurs before the infant has learned to speak. Such impairments are typically more devastating than a loss that occurs after language is established.

prelinguistic/preverbal   Occurring before the infant can speak.

prime/priming   Presentation of a stimulus (verbal or pictorial) meant to facilitate the retrieval of a target response. A subject who has seen the words *hospital, doctor* will recognize the word *nurse* more quickly than a subject who has not been similarly primed.

principles   Rules or maxims. Basic tenets of a theory.

principle of contrast   Children's assumption that no two words have the same meaning. Hence, they assume that a new word will not refer to something for which they already have a name.

principle of mutual exclusivity   See *mutual exclusivity.*

principle of relevance   A conversational maxim that holds that what a speaker says is supposed to be relevant to the conversation.

probabilistic concept   A concept that is characterized by a variable set of criteria, unlike a *classical concept.* For instance "bird" is a probabilistic concept, because no criterion defines it exclusively; a creature need not fly, have a beak or feathers to qualify as a bird.

production   The process of speaking.

productive, productivity   Referring to the regular forms of a language that are used in the formation of new words, regular plural endings, for instance.

progressive phonological idiom   A word in a child's vocabulary that is pronounced more accurately than most other words of the same general adult target form. Idioms are an exception to the child's current set of rules and are progressive in the sense that they anticipate the ability the child will soon have.

pronominal strategy   A preference for pronouns, rather than nouns, exhibited by some young children in their early speech. See *nominal strategy.*

prosodic features   Aspects of the speech stream, such as stress and intonation, that convey differences in the meaning of words or sentences.

prototype   An instance of a category that best exemplifies it; for instance, a robin is a *prototypical* member of the category "bird," because it has all of the important defining features.

protoword   A sequence of sounds (used by a child) that has a relatively consistent meaning but is not necessarily based on any adult word. The terms *phonetically consistent form* and *vocable* are also used for this general notion.

reading as decoding   An approach to reading instruction that emphasizes the teaching of decoding skills, such as grapheme–phoneme correspondence rules.

reading for meaning   An approach to reading instruction that emphasizes inferential skills and treating texts as sources of meaning.

recast   A form of parental utterance that restates the child's immature utterance in acceptable adult form.

reduplicated babble   Babbling in which consonant-vowel combinations are repeated, such as "bababa." Also called *repetitive babbling.*

referent   The actual thing to which a particular word alludes—an actual cat, for instance, as opposed to the meaning of the word, which is a mental construct.

referential   Said of speech that makes reference to the outside world, for instance speech that names objects, as contrasted with speech that is *expressive* or more social in nature.

referential communication   The manner in which one talks about a particular referent among an array of possible referents.

referential style   A speech style observed in toddlers that is characterized by the use of nouns, and few personal social terms. See *expressive style.*

reflexive vocalization   A sound made involuntarily, such as a vegetative sound, a burp, cough, newborn cry, and so on.

register   A form of language that varies according to participants, settings, and topics, such as CDS.

regression   A change backward from behavior that is more adult-like to behavior that is a poorer approximation of the adult model and representative of earlier stages of development.

regression hypothesis   The theory (not currently upheld) that in aphasia speech is lost in mirror image fashion to the order of acquisition.

rejection   One of the communicative functions seen in infants; the purposeful termination of an interaction, for instance pushing a toy away while vocalizing.

relative clause   A dependent clause that begins with a relative pronoun (*that, where, who,* and so on).

request Another communication function in infancy. Consistent gestures or vocalizations are used to get the partner to do something or to help the child achieve a goal.

responsive interactional style Manner of interacting with an infant that allows the infant to set the pace and determine the topics engaged in.

restricted-word association A type of word association in which the subject has been asked to limit responses according to some criterion (to words that rhyme with the stimulus, for instance).

riddles Word games, usually in the form of questions, that play on linguistic ambiguity.

ritualistic behavior Repetitive or constrained behavior often engaged in by children with autism.

rote/holistic style A style of early language acquisition characterized by the child's learning a number of phrases, or unanalyzed expressions. Contrasts with *analytic style.*

routine A speech form that occurs as part of a routinized event (e.g., greetings, or "trick or treat" on Hallowe'en).

s-structure One of the major levels of a grammar, according to government and binding theory. The s-structure contains the linear arrangement of words in the sentence.

sarcasm A use of language meant to wound others or convey contempt, often accomplished by the use of exaggerated intonation patterns and ironic devices (saying "Thank you SO MUCH!" to the person who sat on your hat and crushed it). See *irony.*

scaffold A supportive linguistic/communicative context supplied by mothers and other adults to young children. See *format.*

script Abstract knowledge about familiar, everyday events.

secondary intersubjectivity An attainment of infants at around ten months, in which they are now able to manage a three-term interaction consisting of the speaker, the listener, and an outside object or referent.

segmentation Separation of the stream of speech into its constituents, for instance breaking words into syllables and phonemes.

self-organizing system A model of children's early phonological development that relies on the child's own cognitive system and the presence of internal feedback mechanisms.

semantic aggravator Word or phrase that intensifies a request (e.g., "or else," "right now").

semantic development The acquisition of words and their many meanings and the development of that knowledge into a complex hierarchical network of associated meanings.

semantic feature One of the criteria by which a concept is defined and distinguished from other concepts. For instance, + male and + relative are two features of the concept *brother.*

semantic knowledge See *semantic development.*

semantic mitigator Word or phrase that softens a request (e.g., "please," reasons.)

semantic network A word and all of the words that are related to it through various hierarchies of meaning. See *semantic development.*

semantics The study of the meaning system of language.

semantic relations Characterizing the limited set of meanings conveyed by children's early utterances.

semantic transparency Obvious meaning. One of the principles children use in making new words, "plant man" for "gardener," for instance.

semivowel   See *glide.*

sensorimotor stage   In Piagetian theory, the first eighteen months, approximately, of a child's life, when the major mode of cognition is through the senses and the action of the body.

sentence modalities   The basic forms sentences may take, including declaratives, questions, and imperatives.

serial processing   An information processing term that refers to linear cognitive activity (e.g., first seeing a letter, then the next one, then reading the word, then understanding it). Contrasts with *parallel processing,* in which cognitive activity takes place on many levels at once.

set test   A word association or production test in which the subject is asked to respond with only a particular category of words, such as words begining with a certain letter.

shallow orthography   An orthography in which there exists a close relationship (one-to-one) between graphemes and the phonemes they represent (see *deep orthography*).

shape bias   A constraint on early word learning that leads the child to assume that a new word refers to the shape of an object rather than to its color, texture, or other properties.

shaping   A method of bringing about a desired behavior in an organism by rewarding (reinforcing) successive approximations of the target behavior. According to learning theorists, parents shape children's babbling into words and sentences.

short-term memory abilities   Capacities involved in processing information that has not been stored in long-term memory.

sign system   An educational communication system that translates an oral language into a manual code. In general, the syntax of a *sign system* is borrowed from the oral language upon which it is based.

signifying   A type of sarcastic or witty language play used by some African Americans to make indirect comments upon socially significant topics.

simple monologue   A type of egocentric speech described by Piaget in which a child talks to him- or herself.

simplicity   One of the principles children follow in creating new words. They extend forms they already know to cover new situations, creating words like *bicycler* for one who rides a bicycle.

SLI (specific language impairment)   Delayed or deviant language development in a child who exhibits no cognitive, neurological, or social impairment.

social cognition   Knowledge about other people that makes interpersonal interaction possible.

social routine   Routinized speech used in social settings, such as "bye bye."

sociolinguistics   An approach to the study of language variation and adaptation that considers the ways social constructs (class, gender, role, status, etc.) impact upon language, and that makes use of observation of natural conversations.

sound play   See *reduplicated babble; modulated babble.*

species specific   Refers to the fact that language as we know it is specific to our species, and not to others.

species uniform   Refers to the observation that the major milestones of language occur in the same way and at the same general time in all members of the species.

specific language impairment   See *SLI.*

speech acts   Utterances used by speakers in order to accomplish things in the world (such as requesting or apologizing).

speech-language pathologist   A professional who had been trained to assess, diagnose, and treat speech and language problems.

speechreading   See *lipreading.*

speed of processing   The rate at which an individual manages information. One of the hallmarks of aging is a decrement in speed of processing.

stem allomorphy   A change in the sound (regardless of the spelling) of the stem of a word when an affix is added. For example, the /d/ at the end of "allude" becomes /ž/ when *-ion* is added.

stress   Greater prominence on one or more syllables in a word; this may be due either to greater actual loudness, a marked change (usually a rise) in pitch, or greater length of the syllable.

structuralism   A theoretical approach emphasizing the organization or structure of a behavior as opposed to its use or function.

structured observation   A research design that imposes some consistency on observation by keeping some things constant; for instance, by bringing children into a laboratory playroom and giving each the same toys.

stuttering   Lack of fluency in speech, characterized by prolonged or repeated segments, often produced with extreme tension.

submersion   Language learning setting in which one second language learner is surrounded by native speakers.

subtractive bilingualism   Bilingualism characterized by the loss of one's original language while learning a second language.

surface hypothesis model of SLI   The hypothesis that children with SLI have difficulty processing grammatical forms that are unstressed, or have little salience.

syntagmatic   Reflecting a linearly ordered relationship between sentential constituents; in word association, a word that typically follows the stimulus word in sentence.

syntax   The rules by which sentences are made, such forms as passives, declaratives, interrogatives, imperatives.

synthetic   Characteristic of languages that combine several grammatical inflections (e.g., third person, plural, past) into one form. Contrasts with *agglutinated,* q.v.

taxonomic principle   The assumption that a new word can be extended to members of the same category.

telegraphic speech   Speech that consists of content words, without functors, much like a telegram.

text presentation   According to GB theory, the type of language that children learning language are exposed to. It contains no *negative evidence* (q.v.).

thematic roles (semantic roles)   The components of GB grammar that connect the lexicon to the logical form component of the s-structure, assigning noun phrases to roles such as *agent* or *location.*

theoretical adequacy   Characteristic of a theory or model that contains principles that not only account for observed behaviors, but are the actual principles individuals use to attain those behaviors.

theory of mind   Assumptions individuals hold about the state of knowledge of others. Children must develop a theory of mind in order to speak to others at an appropriate level.

top-down (model)   A term taken from artificial intelligence research to depict the direction of processing. *Top-down* (or concept-driven) indicates that processing moves from the level of concepts downward to basic level data. Top-down reading models conceptualize reading as involving the generation and testing of hypotheses.

topic-associating narrative   Narrative that links several episodes thematically.

topic-focused narrative   A narrative about a single person or event, that has a clear beginning, middle, and end. Contrasts with *topic-associating* style.

total communication   A method of interacting with individuals with language impairments using a combination of spoken language and signs.

transformational syntax   A part of Transformational Generative Grammar, developed by Noam Chomsky, a grammar in which surface structure is derived from deep structure by the application of transformational rules.

transformational rule   In Chomsky's latest grammar, *transformational rules,* such as [move a], meaning move any part of the sentence to a new position, applied to the d-structure produce various syntactic surface forms while retaining the meaning or intent of the original.

underextension   Use or understanding of a word that does not include its full range; assuming, for instance, that "dog" refers only to collies.

universal grammar (UG)   Hypothetical set of restrictions governing the possible forms all human languages may take.

universality   Property assumed to characterize all human languages.

variegated babble   Babbling that includes a variety of sounds, such as "babideeboo." See *reduplicated babble; modulated babble.*

velar   Any speech sound produced by having the back of the tongue touch or come near the underside of the velum, or soft palate (see *velum*). The English velars are the consonants /k/, /g/, and /ŋ/.

velum   Also called the soft plate; the soft extension of the hard palate. The velum plays two major roles as an articulator: First, it can be raised to close off the passage from the pharynx into the nasal cavity and lowered to open this passage; second, the back of the tongue rises to touch the velum in the production of the velar stops.

verbal aggression   Aggression achieved through language.

verbal humor   Humor achieved through language.

verbal transformation effect   Phenomenon that occurs after a given word has been listened to repeatedly. The listener begins to hear new words.

vernacular   The common, everyday language of a community.

vocable   A consistent sound pattern used in a consistent situation, not derived from the adult language (also called *protoword* or *phonetically consistent form*).

vocal motor scheme   A scheme or program of motor activity that underlies a canonical form. The scheme is a tightly linked sequence of articulatory gestures (including timing of jaw and tongue movements, velum position changes, and vocal cord vibration). The gestures of a vocal motor scheme are not completely specified; instead, certain details—for example, one position or manner of articulation—can be varied as the child tries to make the output resemble a particular adult target word. See *canonical form.*

voicing   Said of a speech sound (stop, fricative, etc.) produced with vocal cord vibration, for example, /a/, /z/. In the case of English, this term is usually also extended to the stops /b,d,g/.

voice onset time (VOT)   A measure that describes the point during the production of a speech sound at which vocal cord vibration, or voicing, begins.

vowel A speech sound made with a relatively unobstructed flow of air. Semivowels have some restriction but the air is not stopped and there are no friction sounds—/w/ or /y/.

Wernicke's aphasia Aphasia characterized by fluent but relatively empty speech, poor comprehension, and neologisms in severe cases. See *aphasia*.

Wernicke's area Speech area in the posterior region of the left hemisphere. Damage to *Wernicke's area* results in *Wernicke's aphasia*.

wh- question A question preceded by a *wh-* word, such as *who, what, why, where, when,* (or *how*) that requires specification of the missing element in the answer.

whole language (language experience) A reading for meaning approach that stresses involvement with "whole," or meaningful, texts.

Williams syndrome (WS) An inherited atypicality that includes elfin appearance, poor spatial ability, and hyperlexia.

word and stress patterns Part of the phonological system of the language, these patterns dictate intonation and loudness/intensity of the prosodic envelope of a word or sentence.

word associations Words that come to mind as a result of hearing other words. See *free-word association*.

word recognition The recognition that letter strings represent conventional words.

word retrieval The act of accessing a word that one knows.

working memory The ability to keep information in mind while processing; working memory declines with age, and this decline has been linked to comprehension problems.

yes/no question A question that may be responded to by saying "yes" or "no."

zone of proximal development In Vygotskyian theory, the range of behaviors available to a child in the helpful presence of a guiding adult.

Index

512

Sabbadini, L., 377
Sabo, H., 359
Sabo-Abramson, H., 478
Sabsay, S., 361
Sachs, J., 53, 135, 141, 180, 221, 257, 269, 274, 293
Sadker, D., 416
Sadker, M., 416
Saffran, E., 477
Saffran, J. R., 80
Sagart, L., 84
Sailor, W., 262, 361
Salehi, M., 225
Salerno, R., 141
Salmelin, R., 385
Salzberg, C., 361
Sampson, G., 285, 286
Samuelson, L., 130
Sander, L., 264
Sanders, P., 234
Sankoff, G., 461
Sarachan-Deily, A., 352
Sarcasm, 150, 414
Sarno, M. T., 473
Satake, E., 473
Satterly, D., 294
Savage-Rumbaugh, E. S., 10, 14, 15
Savin, H., 269
Saxton, M., 273
Scaffold, 59
Scarborough, H. S., 173, 370, 387, 428, 435
Scarcella, R., 440
Scardamalia, M., 438
Scarpa, E., 333
Schatschneider, C., 434
Scheetz, N., 349, 352
Scher, D., 427
Scherer, N., 367
Scherr, P., 475
Schick, B., 355
Schiefelbusch, R., 382
Schieffelin, B. B., 52, 59, 230, 237, 337
Schildroth, A., 350
Schlesinger, H., 356
Schlisselberg, G., 199
Schlundt, D., 240
Schmitz, F., 385
Schneiderman, M., 263
Schnitzler, A., 385
Schocken, I., 240
School years
    language and literacy in, 7–9, 409–454
        bilingualism, 439–441
        decontextualized language, 418–426
            metalinguistic development, 423
            metapragmatic awareness, 425–426
            metasemantic and metasyntactic awareness, 424–425
        narratives, 419–421
            narratives across cultures, 421–422
            other forms, 422–423
        literacy experiences at home, 426–428
        peers and media, interactions with, 410–418
            gender differences, 416–418
            language play, verbal humor, irony, 412–414
            media, influence of, 415–416
            on their own, 410–412
            verbal aggression, 414–415
        reading, 428–435

writing, 435–439
Schopler, E., 362, 365
Schreiner, C., 375
Schultz, N., 466
Schultz, T., 150
Schwaneveldt, R., 284
Schwartz, E., 370
Schwartz, J., 266
Schwartz, M., 477
Schwartz, R. G., 100, 134, 327
Scovel, T., 460
Scoville, R., 45
Scribner, S., 425
Scripts, 237
Seaman, D., 378
Sebeok, T., 271
Secondary intersubjectivity, 51
Secord, W., 385
Sedey, A., 358
Segal, E., 256
Segmentation, 148–150, 430
Sehgal, S., 358
Seibert, J., 46
Self-organizing system, 89
Seltzer, M., 142
Semantic aggravators, 220
Semantic development, 3–4, 125–161
    adult speech, influence of, 139–143
    early words, 133–139
        description of, 134–136
        differences between comprehension and production, 138–139
        invented words, 138
        unconventional word/meaning mappings, 136–138
        vocabulary, study of, 133
    later semantic development, 143–146
        complex concepts, 143–145
        semantic networks, 145–146
    metalinguistic development, 147–152
        humor, metaphor, irony, 150–151
        segmentation, 148–150
        word definitions, 151
    relations between words and referents, 126–129
        concepts, 127–129
        mental images, 127
    theoretical perspectives, 129–133
        developmental theories, 130–131
        learning theory, 129–130
        principles and strategies, 131–133
Semantic feature view, 128
Semantic knowledge, 430
Semantic mitigators, 220
Semantic networks, 145
Semantic relations, 176–177
Semantic transparency, 138
Semantics, 23
Senechal, M., 427
Sensorimotor stage, 50
Sentence modality, 187–188
Serial processing, 281
Serpell, R., 427
Set tests, 146
Sevcik, R., 362
Seymour, H., 224
Shady, M. E., 169, 180
Shand, N., 58
Shane, H., 362
Shanker, S. G., 15
Shankweiler, D., 435
Shape bias, 132

Shaping, 260–261
Shapiro, J., 238, 239
Shatz, M., 45, 139, 141, 219, 220, 221, 235, 275, 295, 334
Shaywitz, B. A., 16, 418, 435
Shaywitz, S. E., 16, 418, 435
Sheehan, C., 368
Sheldon, A., 225
Shenkman, K., 374
Sherzer, J., 414
Shi, R., 169
Shinnar, S., 367
Shipley, E., 257
Shore, C., 330
Shriberg, E., 424
Shriberg, L. D., 98, 374, 384
Shuff-Bailey, M., 140
Shultz, J., 215
Shuy, R., 459
Shwe, H. I., 45
Sigman, M., 362, 365
Sign systems, 354
Signifying, 222–223
Silliman, E., 239
Silva, P., 348, 370
Silveri, M., 473
Simmons, J., 362, 365, 366
Simon, E., 372
Simonsen, H. G., 333
Simplicity, 138
Sinclair, H., 4, 148, 424
Sinclair-deZwart, H., 277, 279
Singer, D. G., 415
Singer, D. L., 415
Singleton, J. L., 271
Siqueland, E. R., 79, 273
Sithole, N. M., 80
Ska, B., 464
Skinner, B. F., 27, 259, 470
Slobin, D. I., 4, 32, 150, 187, 196, 267, 269, 270, 278, 285, 317, 318, 366, 419
Sluckin, A., 414
Smit, A. B., 104
Smith, A., 16
Smith, B., 468
Smith, C., 135
Smith, C. B., 57
Smith, E., 129, 262, 284
Smith, F., 432
Smith, H., 146
Smith, J., 48, 359
Smith, K. E., 58
Smith, L., 130, 132, 139
Smith, N., 322, 351, 360
Smith, N. V., 91, 94, 101, 102
Smoczynska, M., 333, 421
Smyth, P., 148
Snow, C. E., 2, 4, 5, 8, 55, 56, 151, 227, 228, 231, 235, 236, 239, 273, 287, 288, 289, 291, 295, 297, 318, 409, 418, 422, 424, 426, 427, 428, 432, 433, 434, 439, 440, 441, 460, 461
Snyder, F. H., 337
Snyder, L., 49, 269, 276, 278, 279, 319, 321, 325, 352
Snyder-McLean, L., 361
Sobel, E., 476
Social interactionist approach, 286–297
    social interactive language learning, 289–292